ECONOMICS OF HEALTH AND MEDICAL CARE

SIXTH EDITION

LANIS L. HICKS, PHD

Professor and Associate Chair
Department of Health Management & Informatics
School of Medicine
University of Missouri, Columbia

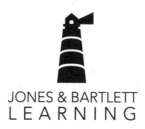

JONES & BARTLETT
L E A R N I N G

World Headquarters
Jones & Bartlett Learning
5 Wall Street
Burlington, MA 01803
978-443-5000
info@jblearning.com
www.jblearning.com

Jones & Bartlett Learning books and products are available through most bookstores and online booksellers. To contact Jones & Bartlett Learning directly, call 800-832-0034, fax 978-443-8000, or visit our website, www.jblearning.com.

Production Credits:
Publisher: Michael Brown
Managing Editor: Maro Gartside
Editorial Assistant: Kayla Dos Santos
Editorial Assistant: Chloe Falivene
Production Assistant: Alyssa Lawrence
Senior Marketing Manager: Sophie Fleck Teague
Manufacturing and Inventory Control Supervisor: Amy Bacus
Project Management Services: Lapiz Online
Cover Design: Kristin E. Parker
Cover Image: © John Foxx/Stockbyte/Thinkstock
Printing and Binding: Edwards Brothers Malloy
Cover Printing: Edwards Brothers Malloy

To order this product, use ISBN: 978-1-4496-6539-5

Library of Congress Cataloging-in-Publication Data
Hicks, Lanis L.
  Economics of health and medical care.—6th ed. / Lanis Hicks.
    p. ; cm.
  Rev. ed. of: Economics of health and medical care / Philip Jacobs, John Rapoport. 5th ed. Aspen Publishers. c2002.
  Includes bibliographical references and index.
  ISBN 978-1-4496-2986-1 (pbk.)—ISBN 1-4496-2986-5 (pbk.)
  I. Jacobs, Philip, 1943- Economics of health and medical care. II. Title.
  [DNLM: 1. Economics, Medical—United States. W 74 AA1]

  338.4'736210973—dc23
                                    2012019556

  6048

Printed in the United States of America
18   10 9 8 7 6 5 4

Contents

New to This Edition

Throughout the 6th edition, data have been updated to reflect changes that have occurred in the economy and in the healthcare system. Also, the bibliographies at the end of each chapter have been updated and expanded, providing additional resources for the users. The glossary at the end of the book has also been updated and expanded to incorporate new and additional terminology in health care, as well as provide additional definitions of basic economic terminology.

The Medicare program has been expanded, and so additional information on the new Part C and Part D components of Medicare have been included, as has discussion of the conversion of the original Diagnosis-Related Group (DRG) classification system to the new Medicare Severity Diagnosis Related Groups (MS-DRG) system. The information on Medicaid has been updated to incorporate the implications of healthcare reform on the programs and on the states. High-risk pools have been incorporated into the discussion of insurance, and the discussion of employer-based insurance has been expanded. A section on the theory, conditions, and role of insurance markets has also been included, along with an expanded discussion of moral hazard, including Nyman's model.

On the topic of demand, additional information has been included on normal and inferior goods, expectations, and on substitution effects. In addition, the implications of being uninsured have been included and additional discussion of rationing was added. On the topic of supply, the type of ownership relative to its performance is now included. The terms *not-for-profit* and *for-profit* have been replaced with the terms *tax-exempt* and *investor-owned*, respectively, to transition to current use in the field.

With respect to provider payment, a discussion of critical access hospitals is included, as is an analysis of the shift to nonpatient revenues and the factors impacting the shift. The type of ownership relative to performance is also discussed. The impact of the Patient Protection and Affordable Care Act of 2010 on bundled payments is included, and the discussions on capitation and salaried physicians were expanded. Discussion of the DRG payment system for hospitals, including an example of calculations, Resource-Based Relative Value Scale (RBRVS) payment system for physicians, and Resource Utilization Groups IV (RUGs-IV) system for long-term care are included. A discussion of Medicare's pay-for-performance program has also been included.

The previous chapter on economic evaluation of health services has been moved up in the text to introduce the concepts and methods of economic evaluation earlier to the student. The chapter now includes a section on the steps in performing any economic analysis, and the Incremental Cost-Effectiveness Ratio (ICER) method of evaluation is included. There is also expanded discussion on the net–benefit approach and the benefit–cost ratio approach, as well as a discussion of life tables.

A new chapter has been added at the end, examining the evolving issues in health care. A number of current issues are introduced and their implications for efficiency in the production and consumption of healthcare services are mentioned in more detail. The impact of focusing on value-added services in health care is described, as is the potential implications of the healthcare system incorporating consumer engagement in the delivery of care.

Acknowledgments

I would like to thank the authors of the previous editions, Philip Jacobs and John Rapoport, for allowing me to revise and update their book. The organization and structure of the earlier edition provided a strong base for this edition.

I would also like to thank two staff members who converted my writing and additions into a polished manuscript for submission. Thank you Veronica Kramer and Margaret Rossano for your assistance on this undertaking, especially during the changes occurring in our department.

About the Author

Lanis L. Hicks, PhD, Professor and Associate Chair in the Department of Health Management and Informatics, University of Missouri, School of Medicine, is a health economist. Her research interests are rural health, workforce requirements, and economic evaluations. She has focused on evaluating the cost-effectiveness of technologies in the delivery of health care, evaluating the economic impact of healthcare policies, and has been involved with a multidisciplinary team identifying and evaluating measures of quality in nursing homes and the relationship between cost and quality. Currently, she is Principle Investigator and Director of the Missouri Health Information Technology Assistance Center, which provides assistance to healthcare professionals and hospitals to enable them to adopt, implement, and achieve meaningful use of electronic health records. She has been on faculty at the University of Missouri since 1978. In recognition of her contributions, Dr. Hicks was the recipient of the 1999 National Rural Health Association's Distinguished Researcher award.

Introduction

This book is an introduction to the economic approach to understanding healthcare issues and problems. The approach is based on the identification of scarcity as a major cause of many of today's healthcare problems. Scarcity can be defined as a deficiency in the quantity and/or quality of available goods and services compared with the amounts that people desire. Perhaps the most glaring deficiency in the United States today is the lack of health insurance coverage on the part of roughly 50 million people, many of whom consequently have difficulty obtaining adequate care, especially primary care. Although there are others as well who have inadequate access to care, the size of the uninsured population has become a bellwether of the access problems in the U.S. healthcare system.

Yet the fundamental difficulty is not merely that there is "not enough" to go around. Side by side with problems of scarcity are problems of "too much." In 2010, total expenditures on health care in the United States reached over $2.6 trillion, over 7.5% of the gross national product (GNP), the dollar sum of all final goods and services produced. In 1965, healthcare expenditures were only 5.6% of the GNP. Included in these expenditures are high-cost services whose impact on health has been questioned, including large-volume "little ticket" items, such as radiographs and lab tests, which make up about a quarter of all hospital costs (Angell, 1985); high-cost procedures, such as coronary artery bypass grafting and transplants, costly intensive care services, and new drugs, whose effectiveness is often still undocumented; and some hospital services for the terminally ill, which consume a disproportionate share of the healthcare dollar (Zook and Moore, 1980; Long, et al., 1984). A number of commentators have asserted that a considerable amount of "flat of the curve" medicine, that is, medical care that produces little or no improvement in health, is being practiced (Enthoven, 1980). Accusations of "too much," when uttered side by side with cries of "not enough," point to the importance of studying the entire resource allocation process in health care.

Economics is the science that deals with making choices and the consequences of resource scarcity; health economics addresses the consequences of resource scarcity in the healthcare industry. Because of its broad scope, economics does not provide a body of rigid doctrines about scarce resources. Rather, economics offers an overall viewpoint intended to help in understanding the many problems related to various types of scarcity.

This book focuses on how to *do* economics; that is, how to think about economic problems in a systematic way. It divides the discipline into three separate areas, which can be regarded as the three main tasks of economics: description, explanation, and evaluation. The exposition of these tasks in a health context is the objective of this book; the performance of these tasks should be regarded as the objective of the reader.

Accomplishing these tasks involves asking specific questions and searching for answers to them. It should be stressed that searching for relevant questions is as critical a part of the process of analyzing economic problems as searching for answers. By formulating a problem in the context of scarcity, a deeper understanding of it can be obtained, and discovery of a solution or a means of accommodation might be the end result.

THREE MAJOR TASKS OF ECONOMICS

The three major tasks of economics covered in this book—description, explanation, and evaluation—will usually not be performed in isolation from one another. Rather, descriptive economics will be used to complement explanations and evaluations of events. But even though these tasks may be intermingled in economic analysis, the specific task being performed should be kept clearly in mind.

Descriptive Economics

Description involves the identification, definition, and measurement of phenomena. By performing this task, we obtain some notion of existing facts. It should be pointed out that this task basically amounts to fact-finding. There is, at this stage, no explanation of why the facts are what they are and no evaluative pronouncement or judgment. Of course, the selection of which phenomena to describe is usually motivated by an ultimate explanatory or evaluative purpose.

For example, the statement that, in 2008 Americans 65 years and older visited physicians' offices 6.9 times per year on average, while those in the 18- to 44-year-old age group paid 2.2 visits per year (National Center for Health Statistics, 2011), falls within the realm of description.

Explanatory Economics

The second task of economics is explaining and predicting certain phenomena. This task involves conducting a cause-and-effect analysis. In undertaking such a task, we are moving one step beyond description; we are now identifying the causes of certain events that have occurred. This task is performed with the aid of models that classify various causal factors (assuming there is more than one) in a systematic framework. Based on this framework, hypotheses are developed about the net effect of each causal factor on the phenomena we want to explain. We do not do any further analysis at this stage. That is, we do not pass judgment on whether the phenomena we have observed are present in the desired amounts.

As an example of an explanation, suppose we want to determine why those in the 65-year-old and above age group utilized more medical care than those in the 18- to 44-year-old age group. First, we would develop a framework that incorporates the major causal factors relevant to this phenomenon. Let us say that our framework contains two essential causal factors: (1) the health status of each group and (2) the price paid by the members of each group for their medical care. Using these causal factors, we might then hypothesize that quantity of medical care demanded will increase when health status is lowered and when consumers pay less for their medical care. These causal factors relate to our example because (1) the health status of the older group is lower and (2) government-sponsored health insurance for the elderly reduces the amount the older group pays for medical care. Assuming these facts to be true, our hypothesis would predict that the older group will demand medical care in greater quantities. Should these increased quantities also be available, then the older group will utilize more medical care.

Evaluative Economics

The third task of economics is evaluation. This task involves judging or ranking alternative phenomena according to some standard or relative position of alternatives. An acceptable standard is chosen, then used to rank alternative ways of distributing scarce resources. In choosing the standard, one major criterion is acceptability. Standards are easy to come by; however, many are controversial, and the standard chosen should have some degree of acceptability.

Alternative quantities of economic variables can be evaluated using a standard; that is, alternative uses of scarce resources. For example, if we choose a standard that says that the more medical care one has the better off one is, then, according to this standard, the older group in our example is better off than the younger group. Furthermore, any measure that raises the utilization of the younger group (by lowering the price paid by this group and by increasing the resources available for use by this group) would, according to our standard, improve the well-being of the younger group (Hemenway, 1982). Evaluative economics is also used to compare alternative uses of resources in order to achieve an identified goal or to allocate resources more efficiently in the achievement of alternative goals.

TOOLS USED IN ECONOMIC ANALYSIS

Several tools are used in economic analysis. One general tool is graphic analysis. The purpose of graphic analysis is to illustrate relationships among economic variables. Also helpful are models that allow us to draw inferences about the relationships we might expect to occur when specific underlying conditions are present. Such tools help us to be explicit about the underlying factors that are present in the workings of the resource allocation process.

Economic Variables

An economic variable is an economically relevant phenomenon whose value or magnitude may vary. Examples of economic variables include prices, costs, incomes, and quantities of commodities. An economic variable can be measured along a scale, once appropriate units of measurement have been chosen. For example, price can be measured in cents or dollars per unit, and quantities can be expressed in terms of number of visits, number of hospital days, number of hospital beds, and so on. Two examples of units of measurement are shown in **Figure I-1**. Along the vertical axis, values of the price of medical care are shown. The price per visit to a physician, which is the economic variable being examined, is expressed in terms of dollars. Along this axis, the price can be 0, 100, 200, 300, and so on.

Along the horizontal axis are alternative values of the quantity of visits to a physician's office. These are measured in terms of number of visits.

Relationship Between Economic Variables

The next step, after the identification and measurement of economic variables, is to determine the relationship between these variables. The relationship shows how one variable changes with respect to another variable.

These relationships can be causal or noncausal. For example, we can state that one variable (total healthcare costs) has increased, while another

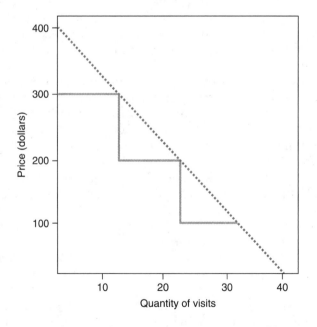

Figure I-1 Relationship Between Price and Quantity of Visits. The dashed line shows continuous values, and the solid line shows discrete values.

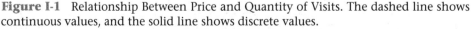

variable (time) has also increased. This is an example of a noncausal relationship, because it is not time itself that has caused the costs to increase. As time has passed, other influencing variables have changed, and these have caused the healthcare costs to increase.

In a causal relationship, when the value of one economic variable changes, the value of a second economic variable also changes as a result. For example, if the price falls for a visit to the doctor, the lower price causes more visits to be demanded. Causal relationships are usually expressed in the form of hypothetical statements (e.g., "If price falls, then the quantity demanded will increase").

Graphic Representation of Relationships

Let us start with a simple relationship between price and quantity of visits: When the price is $400, the quantity of visits is 0; when the price is $300, the quantity of visits is 10; when the price is $200, the quantity of visits is 20; and when the price is $100, the quantity of visits is 30. Associated with each price is a specific quantity: 0 visits with $400, 10 visits with $300, and so on. Each of the associations can be represented by a point, as shown in Figure I-1. All these points together form the relationship. If we knew only these values, we could draw this relationship diagrammatically as the solid line in Figure I-1. This solid line is known as a step function and relates only to the values specified. However, we could go further and generalize about the nature of our function by saying that the values between $0 and $100 (or $100 and $200) and between 0 and 10 visits (or 10 and 20 visits) could also be specified as part of the relationship. We could draw a continuous curve joining all the points specified in the relationship in order to represent the values not explicitly expressed, such as $155, 5 visits, and so on (consider the dashed line in Figure I-1). Once we have drawn a continuous curve, we have a more complete specification of the relationship between price and quantity. Any value of price, within our specified ranges, has an associated quantity of visits.

The Direction of Relationships

We can now be more specific about the nature of the relationship between the two variables. The first characteristic to be examined is the direction of the relationship. A relationship can have four possible directions, as shown in **Figure I-2**. First, the relationship may be positive, as shown by curve B. Here higher values of price are associated with higher values of quantity of visits. If there was a causal relationship between them, and if the direction of causation ran from price to quantity, we would hypothesize that as price increases, so does quantity. The opposite type of relationship is shown by curve D. The relation is a negative—the greater the price, the smaller the quantity. Thus, higher values of price are associated with lower values of quantity of visits. The remaining cases show where variables are unrelated. For curve C, whatever the quantity of visits, the price stays the same (i.e., $200). Curve A shows that the quantity of visits will remain the same (i.e., 30 visits) no matter the price.

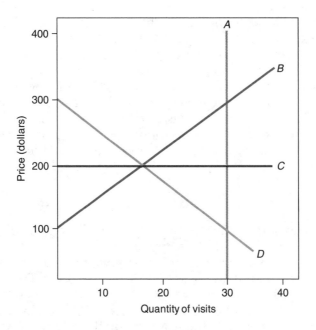

Figure I-2 Direction of Relationships: Curve *A*, constant quantity of visits for all prices; Curve *B*, price and quantity positively related; Curve *C*, constant price; and Curve *D*, price and quantity negatively related.

The Slope of Relationships

The slope of a geometric relationship shows how much of a change in one variable is associated with a given change in a related variable. In causal terms, slope can be expressed as the magnitude of response. Several examples are shown in **Figure I-3**.

Curve *F* touches the price axis where the price equals $200. This price is associated with a quantity of visits of 0. If we raise the price by $50 to a level of $250, the associated new quantity of visits is 10, as shown by *F*. A $50 increase in the price is associated with a 10 visit increase in quantity. The slope of *F* is thus 50/10 with regard to the quantity axis (or 10/50 with regard to the price axis). Because *F* is a straight line, the slope remains constant at every point on the line. (Some nonlinear relationships are presented later.)

Line *E* also has a positive slope. As can be seen in Figure I-3, *E* shows a greater change in price associated with a given change in quantity than does *F*. From the initial price of $200 and 0 visits, a quantity change of 10 visits is associated with a price change from $200 to $300. The slope is thus 100/10 with regard to the quantity axis (or 10/100 with regard to the price axis). Comparing *E* and *F*, we can say that for the same quantity change, the price change in *E* must be double that in *F*.

Lines *G* and *H* can be regarded in a similar manner, but now the direction of these relationships is such that a higher price is associated with a lower

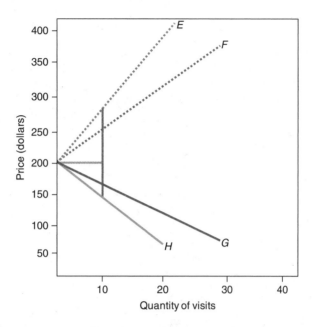

Figure I-3 Slope of Relationships. In relationship *E*, the price increases more than in relationship *F* for a given increase in quantity. In relationship *H*, the price decreases more than in relationship *G* for a given increase in quantity.

quantity. In the relationship represented by line *G*, a fall in price of $50 is associated with an increase in quantity of 10 visits. The slope is, thus, the same as the slope of *F*, but in the opposite direction. Line *H* shows a change in price of $100 associated with a quantity change of 10—the same as line *E*, except the slope is in the opposite direction. Where the two variables change in the same direction (as occurs in curves *E* and *F*), the slope is considered to be positive; where the change is in the opposite direction (as occurs in lines *G* and *H*), the slope is considered to be negative.

The Position of Relations

The next characteristic of a relationship is its position. In **Figure I-4**, two lines, *J* and *K*, are shown with similar slopes but different positions. Each line exhibits a $100 change in price associated with a change of 10 visits. Line *J* shows no visits at a price of $300, 10 visits at a price of $200, and so on. By comparison, *K* shows 10 visits at a price of $300, 20 visits at a price of $200, and so on. The essential point of this figure is to show how the two lines are positioned with respect to each other. Line *K* is higher than *J* in the sense that, at any specific price, the related quantity of visits for *K* is greater than the related quantity for *J*.

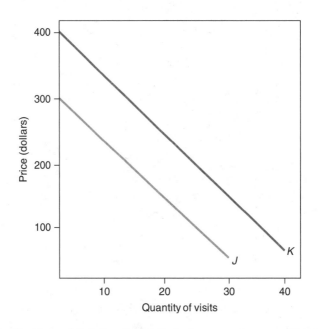

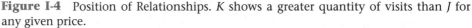

Figure I-4 Position of Relationships. *K* shows a greater quantity of visits than *J* for any given price.

The Shape of Relationships

The examples so far have involved only linear relationships, in which the change in one variable with regard to a given change in another variable is fixed. This is not the only type of relationship, however. Sometimes we also encounter nonlinear relationships. For this type of relationship, the magnitude of the response will vary along the curve. Lines *L* and *M* in **Figure I-5** are both nonlinear relationships.

M indicates the correspondence between the total cost of production of lab tests and the number of tests produced. At a quantity of 0, the total cost is $10; at a quantity of 1, it is $11; at a quantity of 2, it is $14; and at a quantity of 3, it is $19. The slope of the relationship changes as more lab tests are produced. For the first test, the slope is such that a $1 change in cost is associated with a change of one lab test. The next change of one lab test is associated with a $3 change in cost, and the next with a $5 change in cost. The slope with reference to the lab test axis increases as the number of lab tests increases. *M* is a smoothed-out version of this relationship.

Line *L* shows declining slopes with increasing production. A total cost of $0 is associated with a 0 level of output. An output level of 1 is associated with a cost of $5, an output level of 2 is associated with a cost of $8, and an output level of 3 is associated with a cost of $9. The slope of the relationship between 0 and 1 units of production, with regard to the production axis, is 5/1; for the next unit of production, it is 3/1; and for the next it is 1/1.

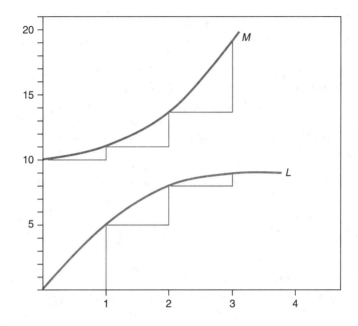

Figure I-5 Shape of Relationships. *M* shows higher additional costs at successively higher levels of lab tests produced. *L* shows lower additional costs at successively higher levels of tests.

The Nature of Economic Propositions

Many statements in this book regarding the resource allocation process in the healthcare field are basically attempts to spell out the consequences of certain conditions. The propositions are hypothetical statements of the form "if . . . then . . . ."

For example, we might claim that if certain conditions *x*, *y*, and *z* hold, then, as a consequence, phenomenon *q* will occur. In making this statement, we essentially make a prediction of what will cause the phenomenon we want to explain. The "if" portions of these statements are called *conditions* or *assumptions*; the "then" portions are *conclusions*, *implications*, or *predictions*.

As an example, let us form a model to explain how much medical care an individual will demand. Our model contains initial assumptions. The first, A1, is that the price of medical care charged to an individual is $5 per visit; this $5 includes all services provided by the doctor, including transfusions, intravenous feedings (should they be needed), and so on. The second assumption, A2, states that the individual has a weekly income of $100 that can be spent on any of a number of goods and services. This assumption brings the example within the realm of economics, since scarcity is now introduced. The third assumption, A3, is about the behavior of the individual; the individual has as an objective the consumption of medical care only; he does not want to consume any other good or service. We also assume that this is entirely feasible.

If the individual does not consume food, for example, he would begin to starve and have to visit a physician, where, for a fee of $5, he could receive nutrition intravenously.

What are the implications of these assumptions? The main implication is that the individual will consume 20 physician's office visits. Given his economic situation, this is all he can afford to consume, and given that he wants only medical care and can survive by consuming this service, then he will not consume less than 20 visits. This implication is a prediction of our model; the prediction is based on the initial conditions or assumptions of the model. Predictions are derivatives of the assumptions and can be regarded as the consequences that would result if the assumptions were to hold.

Let us now replace one of our initial assumptions, A1, with the assumption that the price of medical care is $1 per visit. Now our model implies that the quantity of visits will be 100. With a fall in price, the quantity demanded will increase. This is a prediction of our model when we consider all the assumptions and do a comparative analysis.

We can also predict the consequences that would result if the individual's income increases. Suppose we replace assumption A2 with the assumption that the individual's weekly income is $110. This new assumption, coupled with the original assumptions A1 and A3, yields the conclusion that the quantity of visits demanded will increase. By performing a comparative analysis of the original conditions and the new conditions, we can conclude that an increase in income will lead to an increase in the quantity of medical care demanded.

The mere predicting or deriving conclusions about the resource allocation process is not the end of our task, however. Our conclusions are implications about what would result if the assumptions we have posited in the model are adequate approximations of the conditions that exist in reality. In explanatory economics, implications are tested against actual data to see if what we predicted actually does occur. The true test of an explanatory model is how well it explains or predicts actual phenomena. In evaluative economics, our task is somewhat different—we compare the actual against the ideal set of events. Nevertheless, whether we are deriving explanatory or evaluative principles, we put our propositions into a logical form that allows us to incorporate a number of variables into our analysis simultaneously.

OUTLINE OF CONTENTS

This book introduces the analysis of healthcare economics in the context of the three tasks mentioned above: description, explanation, and evaluation. Part I, which consists of Chapters 1 and 2, describes the economic dimensions of the healthcare field. Part II, consisting of Chapters 3–11, presents explanatory analyses of a number of health-related issues. Part III, which consists of Chapters 12–18, develops evaluative analyses of several important aspects of healthcare resource use. The analyses in the book focus on three distinct markets: the medical care market, the health insurance market, and the labor market. Throughout the book, tools are developed to analyze the economic behavior of all three markets.

Chapter 1 contains a discussion of the output of the healthcare sector. Three types of output are identified: (1) health care, which consists of activities designed to improve health; (2) health itself; and (3) health insurance coverage. Types of input, such as the hiring of healthcare personnel, are also discussed. Measurements of each type of output are presented. In Chapter 2, economic dimensions of the healthcare sector are identified and some measures of these dimensions are presented. In particular, economic flows of the various components of the healthcare system are described, and the concept of cost is analyzed.

Chapter 3, the first explanatory chapter, develops a model to explain the demand for medical care by consumers. A number of separate factors are identified as influences on the demand for medical care. These are incorporated into a single model that allows us to predict the effects of each factor when all other relevant factors are held constant. In this chapter, the demand for medical care is presented as if medical care were an ordinary commodity in the consumer's budget.

However, medical care has several characteristics that, when combined, warrant special treatment. These include the importance of medical care in influencing health status, uncertainty when illness occurs, people's concern about others' health status and healthcare consumption, and the asymmetry in the medical knowledge possessed by providers and consumers. In Chapter 4, a number of these characteristics are introduced and analyzed in light of the standard model developed in Chapter 3.

Chapters 5–7 focus on the behavior of healthcare providers, such as physicians, hospitals, and laboratories. Chapter 5 discusses the relationships between resource use and output, quality of care and output, and cost of care and output. All these relationships are examined with regard to each individual provider. Chapter 6 presents an analysis of the supply behavior of individual providers and of groups of providers (i.e., market supply). The behavior of investor-owned providers and the behavior of tax-exempt providers are treated separately because tax-exempt and government providers play such an important role in the healthcare field. The chapter also considers a model of the supply behavior of health insurers as well as a model of the demand for labor (which is based on the supply model). Chapter 7 deals with one important aspect of supply analysis—provider payment. In health care, there are many examples of providers being paid by a third party (an insurer or the government). The important economic concept of the principal–agent relationship is introduced and is used to analyze alternative payment schemes for physicians, hospitals, long-term care providers, and health maintenance organizations.

Chapter 8 examines a standard textbook explanation of how the market resource allocation process works. This is the competitive market model, which has drawn a good deal of attention recently. Included in this chapter is an exposition of a phenomenon that has received considerable attention in health economics: supplier-induced demand. Not all market behavior is competitive. Chapter 9 looks at the concept of market power, how it is acquired by suppliers and demanders, and how its acquisition affects market phenomena (e.g., prices, quantity, and quality of output).

Chapters 10 and 11 consider two types of markets whose functioning is closely tied to health care. Chapter 10 describes the market for health insurance, and Chapter 11 presents an analysis of the labor market and of several variants of this market that are associated with health care.

The third part of the book focuses on evaluation and health policy issues. There is a great deal of controversy over whether healthcare markets can ensure that health care is delivered efficiently to consumers. One way to study this issue is to gauge whether specific interventions improve health status in an efficient way. Benefit-cost and cost-effectiveness analyses are two techniques by which we can judge the economic impact of various interventions and policies on health status. Chapter 12 offers an introduction to these tools.

Chapter 13 introduces the topic of evaluation by identifying several alternative standards that have been used in evaluating resource use in the healthcare field. These standards include efficiency and equity. Two frameworks used to evaluate efficiency are presented: the narrower efficiency framework and the broader "extra-welfarist" framework. A set of specific goals for the healthcare system is derived from these welfare analyses.

Chapter 14 discusses alternative types of healthcare finance, such as out-of-pocket payment, health insurance, and taxation. It uses economic models to identify the burden of each type of financing.

Chapter 15 discusses two major public insurance programs, Medicare and Medicaid. It presents specific policy problems and, using the explanatory economic models developed in Chapters 3–11, evaluates the effects of policy measures in light of specific policy goals.

Chapter 16 focuses on methods to reform health insurance and healthcare markets. It discusses various proposals for restructuring the health insurance market so that the preferred risk selection of the health insurers might discriminate less against high-risk individuals, thereby increasing the equity of these markets. Chapter 16 also introduces the emerging concept of "consumerism."

The role of government policy in influencing the performance of the healthcare market is the topic of Chapter 17. Two views of regulation are presented there. According to the first, the public-interest approach, the government establishes regulations to ensure that providers act in the public interest. Evidence of the effectiveness of this approach has not been very convincing. The second view of regulation is based on a wider picture of the market. According to this view, the government is a participant in a marketplace that encompasses both the suppliers and demanders of the exchanged product as well as politicians and regulators. In this marketplace, various regulations and laws that have an impact on the supply–demand situation are "traded." The market outcome is thus influenced by regulation. Faced with discontent over the results of traditional market regulation, some observers have proposed that the medical market should be reshaped in the competitive mold. Also included in Chapter 17 is an analysis of antitrust regulation, a topic of considerable policy interest in recent years.

Chapter 18 includes a brief overview of some of the most important issues facing the healthcare industry in today's environment and the implications of these issues for the efficient functioning of the healthcare system.

HOW TO USE THIS BOOK

There is a considerable amount of material in this book, much more than might be included in a typical introductory course in healthcare economics. As a rough guide, a typical student without any prior economics background should be able to cover a chapter a week. In a 14-week course, perhaps 13 chapters could be covered comfortably. Although more advanced students could handle more, instructors will probably want to be selective in covering the subjects.

This book could be used as the main text for a basic healthcare economics course for public health students as well as for a similar course in which the emphasis is more on health policy, management, and finance. Our suggestions for coverage in each kind of course are listed below.

At the end of each chapter, we have provided a set of questions and problems. The student is encouraged to work through these problems, as it is easier to learn and retain the material by doing actual problems and testing yourself. At the end of the book, we provide the answers to odd-numbered problems. The answers to the other problems are contained in the instructor's manual.

Orientation	**Chapters**
Public health	1–6, 8–9, 11–14, 17
Health finance, management, and policy	1–10, 12–13, 15–16

BIBLIOGRAPHY

Aaron, H. J. and Schwartz, W. B. (1984). *The painful prescription*. Washington, DC: Brookings Institution.

Aaron, H. J. and Schwartz, W. B. (1990). Rationing health care: the choice before us. *Science, 247*:418–422.

Angell, M. (1985). Cost containment and the physician. *JAMA, 253*:1203–1207.

Arrow, K. H. (1972). Problems of resource allocation in United States medical care. In Kunz, R. M. and Fehr, H. (Eds.). *The challenge of life*. Basel, Switzerland: Birkhauser-Verlag.

Brook, R. H. (2010). What if physicians actually had to control medical costs? *JAMA, 304*(13):1489–1490.

Core, J. E. and Donaldson, T. (2010). An economic and ethical approach to charity and to charity endowments. *Review of Social Economy, 68*(3):261–284.

Culyer, A. J. and Newhouse, J. P. (2000). *Handbook of health economics*. Vol. 1A and 1B. Amsterdam, Netherlands: Elsevier Publishers.

Debrand, T. and Dourgnon, P. (2010). Building bridges between health economics research and public policy evaluation. *Expert Review of Pharmacoeconomics & Outcomes Research, 10*(6): 637–640.

Dranove E. (2000). *The Economic Evolution of American Health Care*. Princeton, NJ: Princeton University Press.

Earl-Slater, A. (1999). *Dictionary of health economics*. Abingdon, England: Radcliffe Medical Press.

Enthoven, A. C. (1980). *Health plan*. Reading, MA: Addison-Wesley.

Evans, R. G. (1984). *Strained mercy*. Toronto, Canada: Butterworths.

Fein, R. (2010). Values in health policy and health services research. *Health Services Research, 45*(3):851–870.

Feldstein, P. J. (2005). *Health economics*. (6th ed.). Clifton Park, NY: Thomson Delmar Learning.

Folland, S., Goodman, A. C., and Stano, M. (2009). *Economics of health and health care*. (6th ed.). Upper Saddle River, NJ: Prentice Hall.

Fuchs, V. (1998). *Who shall live? Health, economics, and social choice.* Singapore: World Scientific Publishing Company, Ltd. E. Sons.

Getzen, T. E. and Allen, B. H. (2007). *Health economics.* New York: John Wiley.

Greenberg, M. and Lowrie, K. (2010). Kenneth J. Arrow: understanding uncertainty and its role in the world economy. *Risk Analysis, 30*(6): 877-880.

Hemenway, D. (1982). The optimal location of doctors. *New England Journal of Medicine, 306*:397–401.

Hicks, L. (2011). Making Hard Choices: Rationing Health Care Services. *The Journal of Legal Medicine, 32*:27–50.

Jack, W. P. (2000). *Principles of health economics for developing countries.* New York, NY: Oxford University Press

Littenberg, B. and Newhauser, D. (1981). To hell with economics? *American Journal of Public Health, 71*:363–365.

Long, S. H., Gibbs, J. O., Crozier, D. I., et al. (1984). Medical expenditures of terminal cancer patients during the last year of life. *Inquiry, 21*:315–327.

McPake, B. and Normand, C. (2008). *Health Economics: An International Perspective.* (2nd ed.). New York: Taylor and Francis.

Mooney, G. H., et al. (1986). *Choices for care.* (2nd ed.). London, England: MacMillan Press.

Mooney, G. H. (1994). *Key issues in health economics.* New York, NY: Harvester Wheatsheaf.

National Center for Health Statistics. (2011). Health, United States, 2010: With Special Features on Death and Dying. Hyattsville, MD: U.S. Department of Health and Human Services.

Reinhardt, U. (1985). Future trends in the economics of medical practice and care. *American Journal of Cardiology, 56*:50C–58C.

Reinhardt, U. (1987). Resource allocation in health care. *Milbank Quarterly, 65*:153–176.

Rice T. and Unruh, L. *The Economics of Health Reconsidered.* (3rd ed.). Chicago, IL: Health Administration Press.

Sacristan, J. A., Costi, M., Valladares, A., and Dilla, T. (2010). Health economics: the start of clinical freedom. *BMC Health Services Research, 10*:183.

Senterre, R. E. and Neun, S. P. (2007). *Health economics.* (5th ed.). Mason, OH: South-Western Cengage.

Weisbrod, B. (1975). Research in health economics: A survey. *International Journal of Health Services, 5*:643–661.

Weisbrod, B. A. (1991). The health care quadrilemma: An essay on technological change, insurance, quality of care, and cost containment. *Journal of Economic Literature, 29*:523–552.

Wilensky, G. R. (2010). Health economics. *Studies in Health Technology & Informatics, 153*:179–193.

Zook, C. and Moore, F. D. (1980). High cost users of medical care. *New England Journal of Medicine, 302*:996–1002.

PART I: Descriptive Economics

Chapter 1

Output of the Healthcare Sector

OBJECTIVES

1. Describe the product *medical care* and its components.

2. Define the concepts of *risk* and *risk shifting* and show why they are relevant to medical care.

3. Describe health care and its components.

4. Describe the concept of *health outcome*.

5. Explain the theoretical relationship between health and medical care, and demonstrate the meaning of the term *flat-of-the-curve medicine*.

1.1 INTRODUCTION

In this chapter, we introduce the descriptive elements in the study of the healthcare system. This involves identifying the phenomena with which we are concerned, defining them so we can know their nature precisely, and measuring them so we can obtain an understanding of their magnitude. At this stage, we wish only to discover what phenomena exist, not what causes them (explanation) or in what quantities they should exist (evaluation).

The processes generated within the healthcare system can be looked at in two ways. The first approach is to directly examine factors that influence health. These health-influencing factors can be classified as lifestyle elements, such as diet, sleep, and other individual behaviors; environmental factors, such as air and water purification; genetic factors; and medical care, such as examinations and treatments. Section 1.2 focuses on the definition and measurement of medical care. It identifies and defines the phenomena associated with medical care and discusses measures that indicate how much medical care is provided. Section 1.3 describes another aspect of the healthcare system: risk shifting. Because most medical expenditures do not occur with certainty, individuals will place a value on buying insurance to cover possible losses. Risk shifting provides benefits to consumers and is an important output of the healthcare sector.

The second approach stems from the assertion that the true end of the healthcare sector is not the care itself, but rather the health that results from this care. When measuring the output of health care, according to this approach, the measure should be how much health is being produced. If it is believed that the volume of medical care provided is not necessarily a good indicator of the benefits provided, a more fundamental approach would be to measure what medical care is ideally supposed to produce, that is, health. Section 1.4 examines issues of definition and measurement associated with health.

Section 1.5 focuses on the output of the healthcare system derived from the education of healthcare personnel. The healthcare system includes the training of the professionals who work within the system, and these individuals will produce output (health care) during their training and after it is completed. In economic terms, the output of the education and training production process is called "human capital."

1.2 MEDICAL CARE

Medical care is a process during which certain inputs, or factors of production (e.g., healthcare provider services, medical instrument and equipment services, and pharmaceuticals), are combined in varying quantities, usually under a physician's supervision, to yield an output. An individual visiting a physician's office receives an examination involving the services of the physician or a nurse practitioner, nurse, or medical technician, and the use of some equipment. The inputs vary from one visit to another. One patient may receive more friendly treatment than another, and healthcare providers vary in their thoroughness, knowledge, and technique. Thus, the quality of one visit may differ considerably from the quality of another.

Much of the difficulty in measuring the medical care process stems from the issue of quality. If physician care is measured by the number of patient visits to a physician's office, two cursory examinations count as two visits. But one cursory examination followed by a thorough examination involving a battery of tests also counts as two visits, even though more medical care was provided.

It should be stressed that *quality* is a very broad term, and its meaning is elusive (Donabedian, 1988). For example, organizations providing medical care can have substantially different characteristics. To begin with, they can differ in terms of structure, that is, the amount and type of training of the care providers and the type of medical equipment used. Further, differences in structure are associated with the use of different techniques in the provision of care. For example, a computerized axial tomography (CAT) scan machine that takes cross-sectional radiographs is generally considered to provide a higher quality product than a standard radiology machine (Sisk, Dougherty, Ehrenhaft, Ruby, & Mitchner, 1990). A second aspect of the quality of care involves the process of providing care, in particular, the amount of personal attention providers devote to consumers, and incorporates what is actually done in the provision and receipt of care. Examples of quality-of-care measures that reflect the degree of personal attention given to consumers include the volume of services performed per individual and patient evaluations of physician performance.

Another set of characteristics is associated with outcomes, or the effects of care on the health status of the individual or the populations. In this instance, the measure of outcomes deals with the accuracy of diagnoses and the effectiveness of treatments in producing health. Examples of measures reflecting this set of characteristics include hospital mortality rates adjusted for patient condition, the rates of other adverse events in hospitals, such as postsurgical infections, or the reduction in influenza because of immunizations.

All of these characteristics, as well as others, have been identified as aspects of quality. The challenge of measuring quality, then, derives from the fact that there are many ways of viewing quality and many different ideas as to what constitutes quality. For this reason, the raw measure "visits" should be only guardedly used as a measure of physician care.

The measurement of hospital care requires the same caution. Hospital output has frequently been measured by bed days or by the number of cases admitted to the hospital. Over time, however, the typical admitted patient receives a greater intensity of services as a result of advances in technology. To count an admission in 1965 as having the same output as an admission in 2011 (given the type of case) would be to neglect the greater intensity of services likely to be provided at the later date.

Despite these objections, physician visits as a measure of the output of medical care and hospital admissions or bed days as a measure of the output of hospital care have frequently been used because of their immediate availability. Recently, efforts have been made to develop additional measures that incorporate the changing quality of inputs per admission or per bed day.

Output measurements are usually conducted to make comparisons, either against other output measures or against some standard. There are two types of output comparisons: time series and cross-sectional comparisons. A time series comparison measures the output of the same good or service at different times. A cross-sectional comparison measures the output of the good or service among different groups at the same time (e.g., the medical care provided to consumers in different age groups, ethnic groups, or geographic areas, or with different diagnoses).

Medical care output can be measured at three sources:

1. The providers can be surveyed to determine how much medical care they have produced.
2. The payers for medical care can be surveyed to determine for how much medical care they have paid.
3. The consumers can be surveyed to determine the quantity of consumption or utilization.

With perfect measurement, all three sources will yield the same results; however, because of measurement difficulties, considerable differences will arise. A continuing source of data on medical care received by consumers is the National Health Interview Survey, an annual nationwide sample survey of households on health-related matters compiled for the U.S. Public Health Service. Much of the information from this survey is summarized in the Public Health Service's annual compendium of health-related data, *Health United States* (www.cdc.gov/nchs/hus.htm).

The National Health Interview Survey (www.cdc.gov/nchs/nhis.htm) is also the major source of data on medical care administered by physicians outside the hospital. This care is measured by the number of visits to physicians (the numbers of visits are often adjusted for the size of the relevant populations to yield utilization rates), with utilization defined as the amount of services consumed. As an illustration of the use of time series data, comparisons were made of physician's office visits per year for individuals in the 65 and over age group. For this group, visits per person were 4.5 in 1975, also 4.5 in 1985, 5.3 in 1995, and 6.9 in 2008. These numbers indicate that there was no increase in the output of physician office care for this group between 1975 and 1985, but that a marked increase did occur in the following decades (see U.S. Department of Health and Human Services, 1994, 1999, 2011). Also, one visit in 1975 was counted as the equivalent of one visit in 2008 because quality-difference adjustments were not made. It is very likely that quality did increase in this period because of new technology, better equipment, and better training. Unfortunately, this aspect of output is usually neglected in data collection efforts (Freiman, 1985).

An alternative way of measuring physician output is to focus on procedures or services. Procedures (e.g., an appendectomy) can be measured in a number of dimensions (e.g., average time of performance, complexity, overhead expenses), and based on these dimensions, comparable weights can be developed for each procedure (Hsiao & Stason 1979; Hsiao et al., 1992). This approach better captures the differences among various physician tasks.

There are several different measures of hospital output. One way of measuring output is to examine the number of admissions on a per-population basis. In 1964, there were 190 admissions per 1,000 population, while in 2007 there were 114 admissions. However, the length of stay per admission has changed radically in this time period, from 12 days per admission to 4.8 days. As a result, total days in hospital per 1,000 population fell from 2,292 to 540. The number of days is a better measure of resources used than admissions, but even days does not tell the whole story, as it leaves out the consideration of quality (U.S. Department of Health and Human Services, 1999, 2011).

Because of the vast differences in types of illnesses, in disease severity, and in medical treatment patterns (including quality of care), hospital output is difficult to characterize from an economic viewpoint. One method of doing so that captures a mixture of illness types and severities, as well as treatment patterns, is the diagnosis-related group (DRG) classification system. The DRG system has many variants, but all of them are simply patient classification systems. In the 1998 version of the DRG system, which was used by the Health Care Financing Administration to reimburse hospitals, hospital inpatient output was divided into 511 different groups based on the major reason for hospitalization, whether the case was medical or surgical, patient age, and the presence of significant complications and comorbidities (conditions in addition to the primary). In 2007, the Centers for Medicare and Medicaid introduced the Medicare Severity Diagnosis-Related Groups (MS-DRG), expanding the number of groups to 745. While the MS-DRGs do not measure quality, they do incorporate more data on the severity of illness of the patients within the diagnosis.

In a nationwide study of hospital costs conducted at the Agency for Health Care Policy and Research (AHCPR), average annual charges for specific DRGs were as follows: normal delivery, $3,094; craniotomy without complications, $32,594; liver transplant, $204,000 (Agency for Healthcare Research and Quality, 1997). Despite the fact that the DRG system develops average costs among groups, the range of costs within, as well as between, DRGs was considerable; this variation is reduced, but not eliminated, with the MS-DRG system.

DRGs do not measure "quality of care." To gather a picture of hospital product quality, we must look at data collected from hospitals. Hospital output data are available from *Vital and Health Statistics* (Series 13), published by the Public Health Service; *Hospital Statistics,* the annual compendium of the American Hospital Association (AHA), and various issues of *Hospitals: Journal of the American Hospital Association.* The Hospital Compare website (http://www.hospitalcompare.hhs.gov) provides another source of quality measures in hospitals, including patients' perceptions regarding their hospital stays.

The AHA formerly published a series of indexes that extensively covered the concept of measuring quality changes in hospital care over time (Phillip, 1977). This index attempted to measure the quality change of a day of care by changes in service intensity, which was defined as the quantity of real services that go into one typical day of hospitalization. The AHA's Hospital Intensity Index (HII) incorporated 46 services, including the number of dialysis treatments, obstetric unit worker hours, and pharmacy worker hours. A weighted average of these 46 services was calculated annually on data from a sample of hospitals to derive an average number of services per patient day offered during the year. With the calculation for 1969 as a baseline (the value for that year equals 100), the annual averages formed an index that measured changes in the service intensity component of output over time. Although these data are no longer published, they did provide an excellent illustration of how important service intensity is as a component of medical care output. While intensity of service has been associated with quality of hospital services, there is no evidence that increased intensity always results in increased quality of care. There are a number of other factors impacting actual quality of care delivered.

In Table 1-1, national data are shown for three components of hospital utilization between 1980 and 2007. The three general measures are hospital patient days per 10,000 population, hospital discharges per 10,000 population, and average lengths of stay (ALOS) in days. These three categories are then presented as crude rates and as age-adjusted rates. The crude rates are simply numbers of events that occurred. The age-adjusted rates are statistical calculations to adjust the population to a "standard" distribution. Age-adjusted rates enable better comparisons among populations with different age distributions, which is particularly important in health care, because there are substantial differences in health simply because of the aging process. For example, if there is interest in comparing hospital utilization across different areas, and one area has a high rate of younger individuals (possibly because of a college town within its borders), compared to another area with an older population, the age-adjusted rate can be used to reduce the confounding impact of age differentials.

Table 1-1   Output in Short-term, Acute Care Hospitals in the United States

Year	Days of Care per 10,000		Discharges per 10,000		Average Length of Stay	
	Crude	Age Adjusted	Crude	Age Adjusted	Crude	Age Adjusted
1980	12,166.8	15,027.0	1,676.8	1,746.5	7.3	7.5
1985	9,576.6	10,017.9	1,484.1	1,522.3	6.5	6.6
1990	7,840.5	8,188.3	1,222.7	1,252.4	6.4	6.5
1995	6,201.7	6,386.2	1,157.4	1,180.2	5.4	5.4
2000	5,546.5	5,576.8	1,128.3	1,132.8	4.9	4.9
2005	5,620.9	5,541.7	1,174.4	1,162.4	4.8	4.8
2007	5,538.4	5,404.1	1,143.9	1,124.0	4.8	4.8

Data Source: Adapted from Table 99. NCHS (2011). Health, United States, 2010: With Special Feature on Death and Dying. Hyattsville MD. NCHS. CDC/NCHS: National Hospital Discharge Survey.

As can be seen in Table 1-1, the utilization of hospitals has been declining since 1980. The decline was large in the 1980s and early 1990s, and has leveled off somewhat in recent years, especially in terms of the length of stay of individuals admitted to hospitals. The age-adjusted number of days of care per 10,000 population in 2007 was only about 40% of what it was in 1980. The decline in days of care reflect both a decrease in the number of times individuals were admitted/discharged from the hospitals and the average length of time they stayed in the hospital once admitted.

1.3 RISK SHIFTING AND HEALTH INSURANCE

Another type of healthcare sector output is risk shifting through the purchase of health insurance. Illnesses are often unexpected and accompanied by monetary losses. These losses can be in the form of medical expenses, lost earnings from work, and other expenses. Individuals can be said to face a *risk* of losing some of their wealth, which means that the existence of the loss and its amount are uncertain. This risk creates concern on the part of the consumers, and they are usually willing to pay something to avoid the risk.

One way of dealing with the risk is to shift it to someone else. Insurers are organizations that specialize in accepting risk. When an insurer accepts a large amount of risk, the average loss to the insurer becomes predictable. Of course, there are costs of operating such a risk-sharing organization. These include the administrative expenses associated with determining probabilities, setting prices, selling policies, and adjudicating claims. The owners also expect a return on their investment (profits). These expenses and profits are included in the fee (called a *premium*) that each individual must pay to obtain insurance. The essential point here is that, in its own right, risk shifting is an additional output that is distinct from the output called *medical care*. Someone can obtain medical care without risk shifting (by paying for it when the product is received). Such an individual is still faced with the risk of incurring losses, but has done nothing to shift the risk. It is the *additional* activity of shifting the risk in advance—taking action to reduce the loss should illness occur—that is the output.

There are a variety of ways in which risk can be shifted. It can be done privately, by the purchase of insurance. Insurance organizations, such as Blue Cross Blue Shield, Prudential, and Aetna, sell health insurance policies, either directly to individuals (individual policies) or through groups, such as employers and professional associations (group policies). In addition, health maintenance organizations (HMOs) act as both insurers and providers of care. The government also acts as a payer of healthcare bills for large numbers of individuals, although, strictly speaking, it is not an insurer; most of its revenues are in the form of taxes, not premiums, and often the covered individuals are not the ones who pay these taxes. Thus, the government does not manage its healthcare related expenditures on an insurance (risk assessment) basis. Government-style risk sharing is referred to as *risk pooling*.

Health insurance can cover all an individual's expenses. Full insurance has become quite costly, and so insurers have come to resort to "cost-sharing" provisions, in which insured persons pay a portion of their healthcare bills and the insurer covers the rest. These provisions allow the insurers to limit expected payouts and charge the insured persons lower premium rates. In cost-sharing arrangements, the risk shifting is not complete.

Cost sharing can be done in several ways. The insurance policy can require the individual to cover the first dollars of expenses—a deductible—and the insurer then pays all, or a portion, of the rest. For example, the individual might be required to pay a deductible of $100 before the insurer begins to kick in. The insurer can also specify a limit above which payments will cease. For example, it might cover expenses up to a lifetime limit of $1,000,000. Beyond that, the individual would again bear the risk. So-called catastrophic insurance can be obtained to cover very large losses.

The amount and type of insurance coverage is inextricably tied to the workings of the medical care market. Thus, although insurance and medical care should be thought of as separate products, they do affect one another. In the case of insurance coverage, distribution issues have arisen as a cause for concern. In the United States in 2010, some 18.5% or roughly 49.1 million people under age 65 were uninsured (CDC, 2011). Among those lacking insurance were a number of children (8.2% of those under 10), a fact that has generated a considerable amount of concern.

This number of uninsured children is much lower than previously, mainly the result of the implementations of the SCHIP (State Children's Health Insurance Program). Additionally, many employed individuals have no insurance. Because employment is the traditional source of health insurance in the United States, the lack of insurance among workers is viewed as a worrisome development (Monheit & Short, 1989).

The mere possession of some sort of coverage does not guarantee adequate risk protection. Medicare is a government plan that covers hospital expenses and (optionally) medical and drug expenses for individuals age 65 and older. Because of the cost-sharing arrangements incorporated into the program, many of those who are covered under Medicare still face a substantial financial risk should they become ill. Indeed, 70% of those who are age 65 and older now purchase private supplemental insurance plans, also called "Medigap" policies, to cover the risk resulting from the cost-sharing elements (Health Care Financing Administration, 1998).

At the same time, it also should be pointed out that a complete absence of risk on the part of insured individuals (the shifting of the entire risk onto insurers) has its problems as well. A totally riskless policy may be very expensive, because individuals are more prone to demand care when it has a zero price (as under full insurance coverage). The costs of such care must still be covered by the insurer, and so premiums must increase to cover these costs.

1.4 HEALTH STATUS

1.4.1 Concepts

The concept of health seems so familiar to us that we can almost reach out and touch it. It seems easy to distinguish the 97-pound weakling from the bodybuilder who kicks sand in his face at the beach or to recognize a radiant complexion when we see one in a facial soap commercial on television. More precise measures, however, are hard to obtain. The categories "healthy" and "unhealthy" are not exact. The main reason for this is that we have not defined health precisely. Lacking such a definition, two observers can have different opinions as to whether one person is healthier than another. An essential task of the scientific method is to obtain widespread agreement about the nature of a phenomenon. If we lack an operational definition, we can hardly expect two independent observers to reach agreement about the status of the phenomenon. A definition is useful if it helps pinpoint the characteristics of the phenomenon we are trying to describe and eventually measure.

Health is not an easy concept to define with any degree of precision. As the English epidemiologist Sir Richard Doll remarked concerning the concept of health, "Positive health seems to be as elusive to measure as love, beauty, and happiness" (Doll, 1974). Yet, in an effort to give some hold on the concept, the World Health Organization (2000) has defined health as "a complete state of physical, mental and social well-being, and not merely the absence of illness or disease." This is a very broad definition, and the characteristics of health suggested by it are not easy to pinpoint and measure. The definition stresses that there are three components of health, and even if a person is physically healthy, he or she can still be lacking in the other categories.

1.4.2 Measures of Individual Health

For many years, health was identified by the presence of disease (morbidity) or by death (mortality). Individual measures, such as the diagnosis rates for certain conditions or rates of hospitalization, were used as indicators for morbidity. Mortality was usually adjusted for such population factors as age and gender. More recently, mortality has been addressed in terms of premature mortality, with the difference between expected age of death and the actual age of death being forwarded as a measure of life-years lost prematurely. Thus, if the expected age of death for a male aged 20 is 75, then a 20-year-old man who dies in a car accident is considered to have lost 55 years of life.

Researchers have been looking for other measures of health with a more positive focus. Attempts at identifying and measuring health have focused on certain characteristics we would expect in a healthy person. These characteristics include the physical functioning of the individual's body in relation to some norm, the physical capability of the individual to perform certain acts (e.g., getting up or dressing), the social capabilities of the individual (i.e., how well he or she interacts with others), and how the individual feels. These characteristics are, by no means, distinct from one another, a fact that has led to much disagreement among researchers who have tried to invent a unique measurement of health status. Different research efforts have focused on clinical characteristics; on individual capabilities (Boyle & Torrance, 1984; Culyer, 1976); on the physical functioning of people's bodies in relation to some norm (Kass, 1975; Williamson, 1971); and on a mixture of physical, mental, and social characteristics (Breslow, 1972).

Despite the considerable difficulties in arriving at widely accepted indexes of health status, the importance of the topic ensures that researchers will keep trying. One widely used measure is the 15-D (for 15 health dimensions), which categorizes health status into 15 groups, as shown in Table 1-2. These groups include breathing, hearing, moving, and so on. Subjects rate each dimension on a 5-point scale. For the breathing dimension, for example, a "1" would indicate normal breathing, and a "5" would indicate that the individual experiences breathing difficulties almost always. Within each dimension, each point on the scale is assigned a value, which scores the functioning level. For example, normal breathing is scored as 1.0000, and level 5 breathing is scored as 0.0930. The 15-D investigators have assigned a second set of weights to each of the 15 dimensions. These weights were obtained from community surveys and reflect the importance of each dimension. Example weights are shown in Table 1-2. For example, breathing has an importance weight of 0.0805. The 15 importance weights sum to 1.0000.

Investigators can use instruments such as the 15-D to provide measures of an individual's quality of life. Further, a time dimension can be added to provide a measure of quality-adjusted life years, or QALYs. Investigators often standardize these measures, with a score of 1.0000 being the highest level of health and 0.0000 being the lowest (or perhaps even death). Thus, for example, a group of patients with asthma had an average overall 15-D score of 0.89 (out of a maximum possible score of 1.00) (Kaupinnen et al., 1998). If the condition persisted for 1 year, then the average patient's quality of life index would be 0.89 QALYs for the period. The individual would have lost 0.11 QALYs due to his asthmatic condition. The figure 0.11 represents the loss of full health over the year. If the condition persisted over 2 years, then the individual would have experienced 1.78 QALYs during that period.

The translation of health-related quality of life (HRQOL) measures into QALYs has one very convenient benefit. By evaluating death as 0.0000, one can compare interventions, some of which result in death. For example, if one

Table 1-2   Health Dimensions in the 15-D Health-related Quality of Life Index

Dimension	Importance Weight
Breathing	0.075
Mental functioning	0.044
Speech	0.065
Vision	0.075
Mobility	0.046
Usual activities	0.057
Vitality	0.074
Hearing	0.104
Eating	0.040
Eliminating	0.033
Sleeping	0.090
Distress	0.079
Discomfort/symptoms	0.072
Sexual activity	0.084
Depression	0.062
Total	1.000

Source: Adapted from H. Sintonen. The 15D Instrument of Health-related Quality of Life: Properties and Applications, *Annals of Medicine 33*: 328–335, ©2001.

person lived for 5 years at a QALY value of 0.5 rather than being dead (QALY value of 0.0000), then the difference in QALYs would be 2.5000–0.0000, or 2.5 QALYs. Of course, there are conceptual problems with placing a 0.0000 value on death; death is beyond the conscious experience of people, and so they may have great difficulty comparing different levels of health with death.

The 15-D weights can be used both to assess the HRQOL of an individual over time or to compare different individuals or groups. For example, women with breast cancer can take different forms of chemotherapy. The 15-D can measure differences in health-related quality of life among the interventions. There are several general HRQOL measures in use (Bowling, 1995); those used mostly by economists include the Euroquol 5D (Kind, 1996) and the Health Utilities Index (Feeny et al., 1996). In addition, there are a large number of HRQOL measures for specific diseases (Bowling, 1995).

1.4.3 Population Health Measures

The most commonly used population health measures have been mortality rates and morbidity (usually hospitalization) rates. Mortality, or death rates, are standardized by age and sometimes gender and can be expressed for the entire

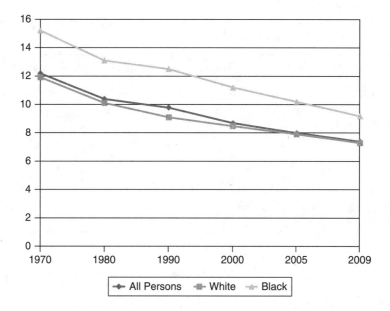

Figure 1-1   Age-adjusted Death Rates by Group, United States, 1970–2009 (Deaths per 100,000 Residents).

Source: 1970–2005 data from U.S. Census (2010). Statistical Abstract of the United States, 2010, Table 107; Table A: National Center for Health Statistics, National Vital Statistics Reports, Deaths: Preliminary data for 2009.

population or for subgroups, such as Whites and Blacks. In Figure 1-1, we show the trends in death rates for the total population and for Whites and Blacks from 1970 to 2009 in the United States. All rates have been falling, but the death rate for Blacks is substantially above that for Whites. Death rates are also used for subgroups; for example, the neonatal mortality rate, which expresses deaths up to the first 28 days of life as a percentage of total live births, was 4.5 in 2006. For the White and Black populations, the respective rates were 3.7 and 9.1 (U.S. Department of Health and Human Services, 2011).

Increasingly, analysts have been focusing on survival time as an indicator of health status. They choose survival-time indicators because these place emphasis on the duration component of health status; a person's well-being is a function of the time spent in each health state, not merely the health state at a given moment in time. Measures that look at survival time adopt this important dimension of health. One such measure is that of potential years of life lost (PYLL) before a target age. The analyst selects a target age below which most individuals are expected to live. Deaths that occur at an age earlier than the target age are considered to be premature. The measure of premature deaths is considered to be one of the best population-level indicators of health. This indicator for Whites and Blacks in the United States is shown in Table 1-3. The PYLL for males, expressed in terms of 100,000 persons, is almost 14,000 life years, while for females it is only about half that, at 7,400. The number for Blacks, on the other hand, is almost 18,000 compared to Whites at less than 10,000.

Table 1-3   Years of Potential Life Lost before Age 75, per 100,000 Population under 75 Years of Age, United States, Selected Years (Age Adjusted)

Year	Total	Males	Females	White	Black
1980	10,448.4	13,777.2	7,350.3	9,554.1	17,873.4
1990	9,085.5	11,973.5	6,333.1	8,159.5	16,593.0
2000	7,578.1	9,572.2	5,644.6	6,949.5	12,897.1
2005	7,299.8	9,206.1	5,425.7	6,775.6	11,890.7
2007	7,083.5	8,919.9	5,274.2	6,614.2	11,259.8

Source: Adapted from National Center for Health Statistics, *Health, United States, 2010, Table 25.* Department of Health and Human Services, 2011.

Of course, mortality rates do not take quality of life into account. In an effort to incorporate both mortality and quality of life into a single index, analysts at the World Health Organization have developed an index called *healthy adjusted life expectancy* (HALE) (WHO, 2010), which reflects the average number of years an individual can expect to live in "good health." To estimate HALE, the investigators determine the prevalence of both fatal and non-fatal conditions in each country and adjust life years in light of disability rates due to diseases and injuries. The results for selected countries are displayed in Table 1-4. This table shows the life expectancy for males and females in seven countries, including the United States, both adjusted (2007) and unadjusted

Table 1-4   Life Expectancy at Birth and Healthy Life Expectancy (HALE) at Birth, Selected Countries

Country	Life Expectancy at birth, 2008			Healthy Life Expectancy (HALE) at birth, 2007		
	Total	Males	Females	Total	Males	Females
Argentina	76	72	79	67	64	69
Australia	82	79	84	74	72	75
Japan	83	79	86	76	73	78
New Zealand	81	78	83	73	72	74
Switzerland	82	80	84	75	73	76
United Kingdom	80	78	82	72	71	73
United States	78	76	81	70	72	68

Source: Reprinted with permission from: World Health Organization. World Health Statistics, 2010. Geneva Switzerland. Accessed April 19, 2012 from http://www.who.int/whosis/whostat/EN_WHS10_Full.pdf and http://www.who.int/whosis/whostat/EN_WHS2011_Full.pdf.

(2008) for disability. For the United States, the life expectancy at birth was 78 years before adjusting for disability. After making disability adjustments, this figure was reduced to 70 years. The difference (8 disability-adjusted years) is the reduction in quality of life of those who survived. The greater the gap between the two figures, the poorer the measure of health of the surviving population. For those countries shown in the table, the gap is between 7 and 9 disability years.

1.4.4 Outcome

The final output of the healthcare sector is health. If there is a close relationship between health and medical care, then indicators of *medical care* output can be used as indicators of the true output of the healthcare sector. It has been contended that there is not necessarily such a correspondence, and that the quantity of medical care utilized is, therefore, not a good indicator of output.

The true output of the healthcare sector is measured by the net change in health produced by the medical care provided. That is, output is measured not by the level of the health index (e.g., by the infant mortality rate) but rather by the *change* in the index due to the medical care, in other words, the effects of the care. For example, if the infant mortality rate fell from 12 to 10 deaths per 1,000 births subsequent to a program to introduce a new drug, the output of the program would be that proportion of the reduction in infant mortality that was due to the program. It may be that other factors, such as the mothers' diets, also contributed to the change in infant mortality. The presence of such confounding factors creates difficulties in finding an accurate measure of output; medical care is seldom the only factor contributing to changes in health status. Other factors may be difficult to identify (e.g., changes in personal behaviors) and equally difficult to measure.

In addition to the identification of confounding factors, there is the problem of measuring changes in health status. The previous discussion illustrates how many difficulties are posed in trying to measure levels of health status. The measurement of changes in health status merely adds to these problems. For example, assume that an individual with a gastrointestinal disorder will have a quality-of-life index of 0.5 for a seven-week period in the absence of any treatment. She can be treated using one of two different drugs. With the less effective drug, Treatment A, the individual will have a quality-of-life index of 0.7 for two weeks, of 0.8 for an four additional weeks, and 1.0 for the seventh week (see Figure 1-2). With Treatment B, the individual will have a quality of life of 0.8 for two weeks and will be completely cured after that. Over the entire seven week period, the individual would have a total quality-of-life measure of 3.5 quality-adjusted weeks with no treatment, 5.6 quality-adjusted weeks ([2 · 0.7] + [4 · 0.8] + 1.1.0) with Treatment A, and 6.6 weeks with Treatment B.

The outcome measure will depend on what the alternative is. If the alternative is no care, then the outcome for Treatment A is 2.1 quality-adjusted weeks, and for Treatment B, it is 3.1 quality-adjusted weeks. That is, the outcome is the difference in the value of the index between the two treatments (Williams, 1985).

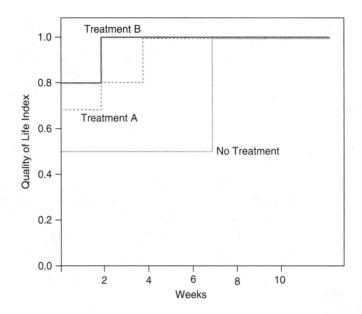

Figure 1-2 Quality of Life Indexes Under Three Alternative Treatment Options. With no treatment (see thin solid line), the individual has a quality of life index of 0.5 over 7 weeks and then recovers fully (quality of life level 1.0). Under Treatment A (broken line), the quality of life index is 0.7 for 2 weeks, 0.8 for the next two weeks, and 1.0 thereafter. Under Treatment B (darker solid blue line), the quality of life index is 0.8 for 2 weeks and full recovery (1.0) thereafter.

It has been contended that, in general, there is a limit to how much good medical care can do; as more medical care is provided (to the same individuals), the additional output becomes less. This is illustrated in Figure 1-3, in which health is shown on the vertical axis and the quantity of medical care on the horizontal axis. The medical care "outcome" curve, showing the relation between health and medical care, is drawn to indicate that there would be some level of health without any medical care (H_0) and that additional levels of medical care make some contribution to health. However, the additional (marginal) contribution declines as the quantity of medical care increases. Such an output curve assumes all other factors (environmental, genetic, personal) are held constant and only medical care varies. The additional output is expressed as $\Delta H/\Delta M$, where ΔM is the additional medical care and ΔH is the additional health. Note that, because of the way the curve is drawn, $\Delta H/\Delta M$ declines in value as more medical care (M) is provided. This eventual flattening of the output curve has given rise to the expression "flat-of-the-curve medicine" (Enthoven, 1980). Drawing the curve in this way geometrically illustrates that, as medical care provision is increased, the additional effectiveness of medical care declines.

Researchers have attempted to establish the relationship between medical care and health in different ways. Several early studies attempted to identify a statistical relationship between mortality rates and various measures of medical input per capita using state data (Auster et al., 1969) and national data (Stewart, 1971). Both studies found a small relationship or none at all. One explanation

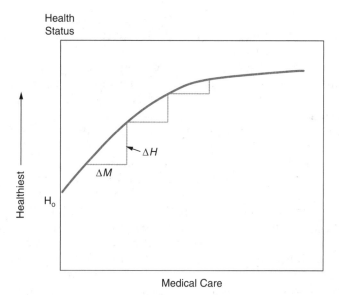

Figure 1-3 Hypothesized Relationship Between Health and Medical Care. In this figure, additional units of medical care have a diminishing impact on health; eventually, a situation of low medical productivity, termed "flat-of-the-curve medicine," is reached.

given was that we may have reached the leveling-out point on the curve. Furthermore, it was estimated that the self-care components of health care (e.g., quitting smoking, eating right, getting exercise) may, indeed, be more important than the medical care components (Newhouse & Freidlander, 1979). However, subsequent statistical research that examined specific groups, such as infants, did find significant evidence of the impact of medical care (Hadley, 1982).

Because such studies are so broadly focused, their results are often difficult to interpret, and it may be that health output is more reasonably measured only by experimental means. Setting up clinical trials, in which one group receives a certain treatment and another group with similar characteristics (a control group) does not, is an experimental method of establishing output. The difference in cure rates, if any, between the two groups could be taken as a measure of the output produced by the resources (Cochrane, 1972). In a number of instances, less aggregated studies have sometimes failed to turn up evidence that certain medical practices impact health (e.g., no relationship was found between appendicitis death rates and appendectomies performed) (see Enthoven, 1980, chap. 2). However, such findings should not automatically be generalized (Angell, 1985). Although it may have some analytic appeal, a broad-brush approach may pass over many situations in which we are not on the "flat of the curve."

1.5 CONSUMPTION AND INVESTMENT OUTPUT

The production of any output requires the use of inputs, including services and supplies. These inputs themselves have to be produced. Many of them are capital inputs, which means that they are durable and last for fairly long periods of time. The totality of resources at any point in time is called a *stock*. In contrast, the amount of activity that occurs during a given time period is called a *flow*.

An output is measured over a given period of time, such as a year. Outputs fall into two classes: those that serve current wants, such as the treatment of patients; and those that serve future wants, such as the production of capital inputs. The use of output for current wants is called *consumption* activity. In health care, much of the output is used up as soon as it is produced. Curing a common cold using drugs is a consumption activity, because the treatment is brief. The production of capital resources is called *investment* activity; the effects themselves are designed to last for several years or more.

Capital inputs can be of the physical variety (radiological equipment) or the human variety (trained radiologists and radiology technicians). Physical capital is the stock of physical means of production. Examples include equipment and buildings. Human capital is the stock of talents, skills, and knowledge embodied in individuals. An example of investment in physical capital is the production of radiology machines. Undergraduate and postgraduate medical education is an example of investment in human capital.

One feature of the healthcare sector is that much of the human capital investment activity is a by-product of medical care consumption activity. Much undergraduate medical education and most postgraduate medical education occur in hospitals and clinics. In many cases, education and patient care activities are inseparable, physically and financially. For many years, teaching hospitals have relied on labor from medical interns and residents for patient care. Because the supply of physicians, including the ratio of specialists to primary care physicians, has become such an important issue in the United States, much attention is being paid to the process by which physicians and specialists are produced.

There is a distinct relationship between capital and production activities. Imagine a given stock of capital at the beginning of 2010 (e.g., magnetic resonance imaging [MRI] machines). Net new investment is the additional stock added during the year (new machines produced minus any machines retired). The stock at the beginning of 2011 is the original capital stock plus the net new investment in MRIs. Important related concepts include the capacity of the capital equipment, actual production, and the percent utilization (or occupancy) rate. If there are 1,000 MRIs in existence, and it takes one hour to produce one image, then the daily capacity is 24,000 images and the yearly capacity is 8.76 million images. If, in any year, 2 million images were produced, the utilization rate would be 23%.

Measures of capacity have a particular importance in the healthcare field. Some analysts believe that the supply of resources directly influences the demand. Commonly used terms and sayings such as "supplier-induced demand" and "an available bed is a filled bed" reflect this view. One of its implications is that, in order to control consumption activity, the investment of capital inputs must be controlled.

EXERCISES

1. Distinguish among three different views of the quality of medical care and provide examples of types of care that would be considered indicators of quality by each view.
2. What is risk and how can people reduce it? Is it costless to do so?
3. What is the difference between morbidity and utilization? Identify an indicator that has been used to measure both, and state a reason why it is not an ideal measure of morbidity.
4. What is the World Health Organization's definition of health? How does this differ from the concept of utilization? Why is it important to distinguish between these two concepts?
5. What is a health-related quality-of-life index? What is the difference between "social importance" weights and "level values" in constructing such indexes?
6. What is a quality-adjusted life year? How can it be used to compare differences in health status between someone who is healthy and someone who is not? Can it be used to compare health outcomes of someone who is ill with someone who has died?
7. What is the weakness of using an unadjusted mortality rate as an indicator of population health status?
8. Which issues in the measurement of population health do potential years of life lost (PYLL) and disability-adjusted life expectancy (DALE) address?
9. Specify a hypothesized relationship between medical care and health. How does flat-of-the-curve medicine fit in with this concept?
10. Indicate at which point flat-of-the-curve medicine is experienced in the following example (imagine that antibiotics have been prescribed for a given population of 1,000 elderly persons).

Number of Prescriptions	Hospitalizations for Community Acquired Pneumonia
0	60
100	50
200	40
300	32
400	28
500	28

BIBLIOGRAPHY

Measurement of Medical Care

Agency for Healthcare Research and Quality. (1997, September). *Statistics from the Nationwide Inpatient Sample for 1994 Hospital Inpatient Stays.* AHCPR pub. no. 97-0056. Retrieved April 7, 2001, from http://www.ahcpr.gov/ data/hcup/1991

Bailey, R. (1970). Philosophy, faith, fact and fiction in the production of medical services. *Inquiry, 7,* 37–53.

Berry, R. E. (1973). On grouping hospitals for economic analysis. *Inquiry, 10,* 5–12.

Centers for Disease Control. (1986). Premature mortality in the United States: Public health issues in the use of years of potential life lost. *MMWR Supplements, 35*(2S), 1s–11s.

Centers for Disease Control. (2011). *Lack of health insurance and type of coverage. Health insurance coverage. Early release of selected estimates. Based on date from the January–September 2010 National Health Interview Survey.* Retrieved from http://www.cdc.gov/nchs/data/nhis/earlyrelease/insur201103.htm

Fasolo, B., Reutskaja, E., Dixon, A., & Boyce, T. (2010). Helping patients choose: How to improve the design of comparative scorecards of hospital quality. *Patient Education & Counseling, 78*(3), 344–349.

Freiman, M. P. (1985). The rate of adoption of new procedures among physicians. *Medical Care, 23,* 939–945.

Hornbrook, M. (1982). Hospital case mix: Its definition, measurement, and use. Parts 1, 2. *Medical Care Review, 39,* 1–43, 73–123.

Horowitz, M. D. (2010). Health care report cards and baseball statistics: Is there a linkage? *American Journal of Medical Quality, 25*(6), 488–489.

Hsiao, W. C., & Stason, W. B. (1979). Toward developing a relative value scale for medical and surgical services. *Health Care Financing Review, 1,* 23–39.

Hsiao, W. C., Braun, P., Dunn, D. L., Becker, E. R., Yntema, D., Verilli, D. K. . . . Chen, S.-P. (1992). An overview of the development and refinement of the resource-based relative value scale. *Medical Care, 30* (Suppl.), NS1.

Lave, J. R., & Lave, L. B. (1971). The extent of role differentiation among hospitals. *Health Services Research, 5,* 15–38.

May, E. L. (2011). The efficient healthcare organization: Creating a new standard in healthcare. *Healthcare Executive, 26*(2), 14–16, 18.

Phillip, P. J. (1977, April 20–26). HCI/HII: Two new AHA indexes measure cost, intensity. *Hospital Financial Management.*

Reder, M. W. (1967). Some problems in the measurement of productivity in the medical care industry. In V. R. Fuchs (Ed.), *Production and productivity in the service industries.* New York, NY: Columbia University Press.

Russell, L. B. (1976). The diffusion of new hospital technologies in the United States. *International Journal of Health Services, 6,* 557–580.

Sisk, J. E., Dougherty, D. M., Ehrenhaft, P. M., Ruby, G., & Mitchner, B. A. (1990). Assessing information for consumers on the quality of medical care. *Inquiry, 27,* 263–272.

U.S. Department of Health and Human Services. (1994). *Health, United States, 1993.* Hyattsville MD: National Center for Health Statistics.

U.S. Department of Health and Human Services. (1999). *Health, United States, 1998.* Hyattsville MD: National Center for Health Statistics.

U.S. Department of Health and Human Services. (2011). *Health, United States, 2010.* Hyattsville, MD: National Center for Health Statistics.

Measurement of Health

Ahlburg, D. (1997). *Measuring health* (2nd ed.). Buckingham, England: Open University Press.

Beckles, G. L., & Truman, B. I. (2011). Morbidity & mortality weekly report. Education and income—United States, 2005 and 2009. *Surveillance Summaries, 60*(Suppl.), 13–17.

Beckles, G. L., Zhu, J., & Moonesinghe, R. (2011). Diabetes—United States, 2004 and 2008. *Morbidity & Mortality Weekly Report. Surveillance Summaries, 60*(Suppl.) 90–93.

Bowling, A. (1995). *Measuring disease.* Buckingham, England: Open University Press.

Boyle, M. H., & Torrance, G. W. (1984). Developing multiattribute health indexes. *Medical Care, 22*, 1045–1057.

Breslow, L. (1972). A quantitative approach to the World Health Organization definition of health: Physical, mental, and social well-being. *International Journal of Epidemiology, 1*, 347– 355.

Casarett, D., Shreve, S., Luhrs, C., Lorenz, K., Smith, D., De Sousa, M., & Richardson, D. (2010). Measuring families' perceptions of care across a health care system: Preliminary experience with the family assessment of treatment at end of life short form (FATE-S). *Journal of Pain & Symptom Management, 40*(6), 801–809.

Culyer, A. J. (1972). Appraising government expenditure on health services: The problems of "need" and "output." *Public Finance, 27*, 205–211.

Culyer, A. J. (1976). *Need and the national health service.* London, England: Martin Robertson.

Cutler, D. M., & Richardson, E. (1998). The value of health, 1970–1990. *American Economic Review, 88*, 97–100.

Donaldson, C., Atkinson, A., Bond, J., & Wright, K. (1988). Should QALYs be programme-specific? *Journal of Health Economics, 7*, 239–257.

Eddy, D. M., Pawlson, L. G., Schaaf, D., Peskin, B., Shcheprov, A., Dziuba, J., Bowman, J., & Eng, B. (2008). The potential effects of HEDIS performance measures on the quality of care. *Health Affairs, 27*(5), 1429–1441.

Feeny, D., Furlong, W., Boyle, M., & Torrance, G.W. (1996). Health utilities index. In B. Spilker (Ed.), *Quality of life and pharmacoeconomics in clinical trials*. Philadelphia, PA: Lippincott-Raven.

Freedman, D. S., C. Centers for Disease, et al. (2011). Obesity—United States, 1988–2008. *Morbidity & Mortality Weekly Report. Surveillance Summaries, 60*(Suppl.), 73–77.

Garrett, B. E., Dube, S. R., Trosclair, A., Caraballo, R. S., & Pechacek, T. F. (2011). Cigarette smok-ing–United States, 1965–2008. *Morbidity & Mortality Weekly Report. Surveillance Summaries, 60*(Suppl.) 109–113.

Goldsmith, S. B. (1973). A re-evaluation of health status indicators. *Health Services Reports, 88*, 937–941.

Gonnella, J. S., Hornbrook, M. C., and Louis, D. Z. (1984). Staging of disease. *JAMA, 251*, 637–644.

Hall, H. I., Hughes, D., Dean, H.D., Mermin, J.H., & Fenton, K.A. (2011). HIV Infection—United States, 2005 and 2008. *Morbidity & Mortality Weekly Report. Surveillance Summaries, 60*(Suppl.) 87–89.

Hellinger, F. J. (1989). Expected utility theory and risky choices with health outcomes. *Medical Care, 27*, 273–279.

Hornbrook, M. C. (1983). Allocative medicine. *Annals: American Association of Political and Social Science, 468*, 12–29.

Israel, S., & Teeling-Smith, G. (1967). The submerged iceberg of sickness in society. *Social Policy and Administration, 1*, 43–57.

Kass, L. R. (1975). The pursuit of health. *Public Interest, 40*, 11–42.

Kanny, D., Liu, Y., & Brewer R.D. (2011). Binge drinking—United States, 2009. *Morbidity & Mortality Weekly Report. Surveillance Summaries, 60*(Suppl.) 101–104.

Kauppinen, R., Sintonen, H., & Tukiainen, H. (1998). One-year economic evaluation of intensive versus conventional patient education and supervision for self-management of new asthmatic patients. *Respiratory Medicine, 92*, 300–307.

Keenan, N. L. & Shaw, K. M. (2011). Coronary heart disease and stroke deaths—United States, 2006. *Morbidity & Mortality Weekly Report. Surveillance Summaries, 60*(Suppl.), 62–66.

Kind, P. (1996). The EUROQUOL instrument: An index of health related quality of life. In B. Spilker (Ed.), *Quality of life and pharmacoeconomics in clinical trials*. Philadelphia, PA: Lippincott-Raven.

MacDorman, M. F., & Mathews, T. J. (2011). Infant deaths—United States, 2000–2007. *Morbidity & Mortality Weekly Report. Surveillance Summaries, 60*(Suppl), 49–51.

Martin, J. A. (2011). Preterm births—United States, 2007. *Morbidity & Mortality Weekly Report. Surveillance Summaries, 60*(Suppl), 78–79.

Mathers, S. D., Sadana, R., Salomon, J.A., Murray, C.J.L., & Lopez, A.D. (2000). *Estimates of DALE for 191 countries: Methods and results*. Global Programme on Evidence for Health Policy Work Paper No. 16. Geneva, Switzerland: World Health Organization.

Sintonen, H. (1981). An approach to measuring and valuing health states. *Social Science and Medicine, 15C*, 55–65.

Sintonen, H. (1995). *The 15D-measure of health-related quality of life. II. Feasibility, reliability, and validity of its valuation system*. West Heidelberg, Australia: National Centre for Health Program Evaluation.

Sintonen, H., & Pekurinen, M. 1992. A fifteen-dimensional measure of health-related quality of life and its applications. In S. R. Walker & R. M. Rosser (Eds.), *Quality of life assessment*. Dordrecht, The Netherlands: Kluwer Academic.

Smith, G. T. (1988). *Measuring health: A practical approach*. Chichester, England: Wiley.

Sullivan, D. F. (1966). Conceptual problems in developing an index of health. *Vital and Health Statistics*, series 2, no. 17, pub. no. HRA 74-1017. Washington, DC: U.S. Department of Health, Education and Welfare.

U.S. Congress, Office of Technology Assessment. (1988). *The quality of medical care*. Pub. no. OTA-H-386. Washington, DC: U.S. Government Printing Office.

Williams, A. (1985). The nature, meaning, and measurement of health and illness. *Social Science and Medicine, 20*, 1023–1027.

Williamson, J. W. (1971). Evaluating quality of patient care. *JAMA, 218*, 564–569.

World Bank. (1993). *World development report: Investing in health*. Washington, DC: World Bank.

World Bank. (2000). *World development indicators*. Washington, DC: World Bank.

World Health Organization. (2000). *The world health report 2000*. Geneva, Switzerland: World Health Organization.

World Health Organization. (2010). *The world health report 2010*. Geneva, Switzerland: World Health Organization.

The Health–Medical Care Relationship

Anderson, B. O., & Azavedo, E. (2010). Balancing resource constraints against quality of care. *World Journal of Surgery, 34*(11), 2537–2538.

Anderson, E. F., Frith, K. H., & Caspers, B. (2011). Linking economics and quality: Developing an evidence-based nurse staffing tool. *Nursing Administration Quarterly, 35*(1), 53–60.

Angell, M. (1985). Cost containment and the physician. *JAMA, 254*, 1203–1207.

Auster, R., et al. (1969). The production of health. *Journal of Human Resources, 4*, 412–436.

Bauer, D. T., & Ameringer, C. F. (2010). A framework for identifying similarities among countries to improve cross-national comparisons of health systems. *Health & Place, 16*(6), 1129–1135.

Cochrane, A. (1972). *Effectiveness and efficiency*. New York, NY: Oxford University Press.

de Brantes, F., D'Andrea, G., & Rosenthal, M. (2009). Should health care come with a warranty? *Health Affairs, 28*(4), w678–w687.

Doessel, D. P., & Marshall, J. V. (1985). A rehabilitation of health outcome in quality assessment. *Social Science and Medicine, 21*, 1319–1328.

Doll, R. (1974). Surveillance and monitoring. *International Journal of Epidemiology, 3,* 305–314.

Donabedian, A. (1988). The quality of care. *JAMA, 260,* 1743–1748.

Enthoven, A. C. (1980). *Health plan.* Reading, MA: Addison-Wesley.

Erickson, P., Kendall, E.A., & Anderson, J.P. (1989). Using composite health status measures to assess the nation's health. *Medical Care, 27,* S66–S76.

Gage, T. B., Fang, F., O'Neill, E.K., & DiRienzo, A.G. (2010). Racial disparities in infant mortality: What has birth weight got to do with it and how large is it? *BMC Pregnancy & Childbirth, 10,* 86.

Hadley, J. (1982). *More medical care, better health?* Washington, DC: Urban Institute.

Jankovic, S., Raznatovic, M., Marinkovic, J., Jankovic, J., Kocev, N., Tomic-Spiric V., & Vasiljevic, N. (2011). Health-related quality of life in patients with psoriasis. *Journal of Cutaneous Medicine & Surgery, 15*(1), 29–36.

Jardim, R., Barreto, S. M., & Giatti, L. (2010). Self-reporting and secondary informant reporting in health assessments among elderly people. *Revista de Saude Publica, 44*(6), 1120–1129.

Kripalani, S., Jacobson, T. A., Mugalla I.C., Cawthon, C.R., Niesner, K.J., & Vaccarino, V. (2010). Health literacy and the quality of physician-patient communication during hospitalization. *Journal of Hospital Medicine (Online), 5*(5), 269–275. http://aspiruslibrary.org/literacy/Kripalani.pdf

Newhouse, J. P., & Friedlander, L. J. (1979). The relationship between medical resources and measures of health. *Journal of Human Resources, 15,* 200–218.

Newson, R. S., Witteman, J. C. M., Franco, O.H., Stricker, B.H., Breteter, M. M., Hofman, A., & Tiemeier, H. (2010). Predicting survival and morbidity-free survival to very old age. *Age, 32*(4), 521–534.

Russell, L. B. (1986). *Is prevention better than cure?* Washington, DC: Brookings Institution.

Scheffler, R. M., Knaus, W. A., Wagner, D. P., & Zimmerman, J. E. (1982). Severity of illness and the relationship between intensive care and survival. *American Journal of Public Health, 72,* 449–454.

Stewart, C. T. (1971). Allocation of resources to health. *Journal of Human Resources, 6,* 103–122.

Truman, B. I., Smith, K. C., Roy, K., Chen, Z., Moonesinghe, R., Zhu, J., Crawford, C.G., & Zaza, S. (2011). Rationale for regular reporting on health disparities and inequalities—United States. *Morbidity & Mortality Weekly Report. Surveillance Summaries, 60*(Suppl.), 3–10.

Williams, A. (1974). Measuring the effectiveness of the health care system. *British Journal of the Preventive Medicine Society, 28,* 196–202.

Health Insurance

Cafferata, G. C. (1984, September 18). *Private health insurance coverage of the Medicare population.* National Health Care Expenditures Study, data preview. Rockville, MD: National Center for Health Services Research.

Choudhry, N. K., Rosenthal, M. B., & Milstein, A. (2010). Assessing the evidence for value-based insurance design. *Health Affairs, 29*(11), 1988–1994.

Claxton, G., DiJulio, B., Whitmore, H., Pickreign, J., McHugh, M., Finder, B., & Osei-Anto, A. (2009). Job-based health insurance: Costs climb at a moderate pace. *Health Affairs, 28*(6), w1002–w1012.

Dave, D. M., Decker, S. L., Kaestner, R., & Simon, K.I. (2010). The effect of Medicaid expansions on the health insurance coverage of pregnant women: An analysis using deliveries. *Inquiry, 47*(4), 315–330.

Dror, D. M., Radermacher, R., Khadilkar, R., Schout, P., Hay, F., Singh, A., & Koren, R. (2009). Microinsurance: Innovations in low-cost health insurance. *Health Affairs, 28*(6), 1788–1798.

Health Care Financing Administration. (1998). *A profile of Medicare chartbook.* Baltimore, MD: Health Care Financing Administration.

Kirby, J. B., & T. Kaneda (2010). Unhealthy and uninsured: Exploring racial differences in health and health insurance coverage using a life table approach. *Demography, 47*(4), 1035–1051.

Monheit, A. C., & Short, P. F. (1989). Mandating health coverage for working Americans. *Health Affairs, 8*(Winter), 22–38.

Moonesinghe, R., Zhu, J., & Truman, B. I. (2011). Health insurance coverage—United States, 2004 and 2008. Morbidity & Mortality Weekly Report. *Surveillance Summaries, 60*(Suppl.), 35–37.

Price, J. H., Khubchandani, J., Dake, J.A., Thompson, A., Schmatzried, H., Adeyanju, M., Pringle, D., Zullig, K. J., ... Esprit, L. G. (2010). College students' perceptions and experiences with health insurance. *Journal of the National Medical Association, 102*(12), 1222–1230.

Short, P. F., & Farley, P. (1988). *Uninsured Americans: A 1987 profile.* Rockville, MD: National Center for Health Services Research.

U.S. Census Bureau. (1999). *Health insurance coverage 1998.* Washington, DC: U.S. Census Bureau.

Vesely, R. (2011). Thinking smaller in 2011. Insurers expect lower profits as they cope with higher costs, new regulations. *Modern Healthcare, 41*(6), 14.

Data Sources

American Community Survey (The American Community Survey is a nationwide survey designed to provide communities a fresh look at how they are changing) http://factfinder.census.gov/servlet/DatasetMainPageServlet?_program=ACS&_submenuId=datasets_2&_lang=en

American Hospital Association. *Hospital statistics.* Chicago, IL: American Hospital Association. Various years.

FedStats (Celebrating over 10 years of making statistics from more than 100 agencies available to citizens everywhere) http://www.fedstats.gov/

U.S. Census Bureau (To serve as the leading source of quality data about the nation's people and economy.) http://www.census.gov/

U.S. Department of Health and Human Services. *Health, United States.* Rockville, MD: National Center for Health Statistics.

U.S. Department of Health and Human Services. *Morbidity and Mortality Weekly Report.* Atlanta, GA: Centers for Disease Control and Prevention.

U.S. Department of Health and Human Services. *NCHS Monthly Vital Statistics Report.*

U.S. Department of Health and Human Services. *Vital and Health Statistics.* Rockville, MD: National Center for Health Statistics.

Chapter 2

Economic Dimensions of the Healthcare System

OBJECTIVES

1. Identify the key economic units in the healthcare market.
2. Describe the flows of money and services in an uninsured and an insured healthcare market.
3. Describe the flows of money in the Medicare and Medicaid programs.
4. Describe the flows of money and services in a health maintenance organization and a preferred provider organization.
5. Describe the meaning of managed care and how it may affect the flow of services in a healthcare market.
6. Define the concept of cost.
7. Identify the key components in the cost of healthcare services.
8. Understand the growth of costs in the American healthcare system over time.
9. Compare the magnitude of healthcare costs in the United States to other developed countries.
10. Understand the concept of "cost of illness" or "economic burden of illness," and describe how cost-of-illness studies have helped us to understand the overall impact of various illnesses in the United States.

2.1 INTRODUCTION

The purpose of this chapter is twofold: to introduce readers to some basic concepts used in describing healthcare activity and to provide a description of some of the key elements of health care in the United States. To achieve its purpose, it focuses on three aspects of economic activity. First, it will examine the basic economic units that participate in the healthcare economy. Second, it explains how simple flow analysis can be used to describe the economic relationships among the various units. Finally, it presents the concept of economic cost, which is used in measuring the amount of economic activity performed to produce economic output, as well as the potential impact of illness.

It should be pointed out that this chapter describes what happens over time as a result of activity in the healthcare economy. It identifies the economic units and their characteristics and describes the flows of money and services that occur.

Section 2.2 identifies the main "actors" in our analysis—the economic units of the healthcare sector—and describes some of their central characteristics. It also identifies the concepts economists use to study how these units are organized. Finally, using flow diagrams, it shows how transactions among the various economic units can be understood.

Of considerable importance is the measurement of the magnitude of economic activity. Section 2.3 elucidates the concept of "economic cost," which is a measure of economic activity in terms of money. This concept is used to measure various aspects of healthcare activity, including the total expenditures on healthcare services, the total economic costs of illness, and the burden of economic costs on various groups.

2.2 ECONOMIC UNITS AND ECONOMIC FLOWS

2.2.1 Economic Units

Units observed for economic analysis include individuals and organizations. In examining the activity of consuming health care, one can take the economic unit to be an individual or a household. Both alternatives are commonly employed by economists in describing and explaining economic activity. One reason the household is so frequently used is that more consistent data can be collected at this level. For example, if one examined housewives' consumption of health care in relation to their *personal* incomes, a biased picture of the relationship might emerge, because their consumption of health care is more closely related to the income of their households. The roles of individuals include those of demanders of health care and health insurance, employees, and taxpayers. Employers are also economic units in the healthcare system, primarily in their role as demanders of healthcare insurance for their employees.

Insurers are firms that have the function of taking on the healthcare expenditure risk of their customers. They collect premiums from their customers and reimburse the providers for the care they provide for their customers. Providers of health care can include physicians, nurse practitioners, nurses, hospitals, long-term care facilities, and providers of various forms of ambulatory care.

There has been a trend in recent years toward the integration of units. "Horizontal integration" is a term that refers to the joining together of providers (and sometimes consumers) of the same type. Physicians have joined group practices. Hospitals and long-term care facilities have joined chains. And there have been some instances of small businesses joining together to form group purchasing cooperatives for health insurance. There has also been a considerable movement toward "vertical integration," which is the amalgamation of purchasers and sellers. Insurers and providers have joined together to create health maintenance organizations (HMOs).

2.2.2 Flows Between Units

Economic flows can involve both money and services. Generally, a flow will summarize a transaction in which a service or good is exchanged for money. Such transactions occur in simple markets, with the degree of concentration influencing the terms of the exchange. The market for lettuce is a simple market in which vendors provide lettuce to consumers in exchange for money. The exchange is at a price that is determined, in part, by how concentrated the vendor market is. In this section, we are concerned with describing which flows take place, not with the terms of the transactions. Further, as we shall see presently, the flows in typical healthcare markets are much more complex than those in markets for lettuce because they often contain two sets of flows—one for insurance and one for healthcare services.

2.2.2.1 Flows in a "Generic" Healthcare Market

The flows in a simple, or "generic," healthcare market are shown in Figure 2-1. In this market, consumers purchase health insurance from insurers. The cash payments by the consumers and employers are called *premiums*. When a consumer uses services that are covered by the insurer, the insurer *reimburses* the provider for the services.

The contract between the insurer and the consumer can have another very important dimension. The consumer can purchase varying degrees of insurance coverage. If the consumer is partially covered, the insurer reimburses the provider for only a portion of the bill; the consumer must pay the remainder. The consumer's portion is called a *copayment* (or an *out-of-pocket payment*). If the consumer is fully insured, there is no

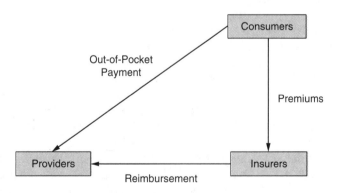

Figure 2-1 Flow of Funds in a Typical Healthcare Market. Consumers purchase insurance from third-party insurers, who pay providers for services. Providers include physicians, hospitals, nursing homes, and other healthcare organizations, and professionals.

out-of-pocket payment. The reimbursement provided by the insurer is payment in full for the services.

The economic importance of out-of-pocket payments is that they are borne by the consumer. It is this cost that governs the consumer's decision as to how much of the service he or she demands. Among the types of direct consumer payments are deductibles, which are fixed upfront payments; and coinsurance, which are payments related to quantity used. For example, an insurance policy might have a deductible of $200 and a coinsurance rate of 10%. This means that the consumer pays the first $200 for services rendered before insurance coverage begins. After the deductible is used up, the consumer pays 10% of the bill and the insurer reimburses the other 90%. Typically, hospital care has the highest coverage, with over 95% of expenses being covered; physician care has a lower degree of coverage (91% on average), and nursing home care has less still (71%).

With regard to insurer payments, there are numerous bases on which providers can be reimbursed. Hospitals can be reimbursed on the basis of a given budget or on a unit basis—per patient day, per case, or per service. Over the decades, there has been a movement on the part of insurers toward reimbursing hospitals on a per-case basis, recognizing differences in resource use among different case types. In this instance, hospital cases are categorized into *diagnosis-related groups* (DRGs), and a separate reimbursement rate is set for each DRG. Each time a patient is admitted to the hospital, the hospital is paid a rate corresponding to the patient's particular DRG. Physicians are largely reimbursed on a fee-for-service basis, and long-term care facilities on a per diem (per day) basis.

2.2.2.2 Introducing the Employer

In 2011, only about 58% of all private health insurance was provided through employers (Kaiser Family Foundation, 2011). A basic set of flow relationships for employer-provided health insurance is shown in Figure 2-2. In these circumstances, both the employer and the employee pay a share of the premiums. Typically, the employer pays about three-fourths of the premium, although the percentage will vary depending on the plan and upon the size of the firm. In 2011, the number of employers offering insurance to employees was still only about 60%, down from the 69% in 2010, but similar to the 2009 figure. (Kaiser Family Foundation, 2011).

Note that the employer's share of the premiums is not a "free" benefit given to the employee; it is, rather, a form of compensation received by the employee. Total compensation takes the form of money benefits (wages) and nonmonetary benefits, such as health insurance coverage. From a financial standpoint, the employer is affected the same by either form of compensation: a dollar in wages costs the same to the employer as a dollar in noncash benefits. But the employee will have a preference because of income tax regulations. In 2011, average family premiums for health insurance exceeded $15,000, and premiums for an individual were over $5,400 (Kaiser Family Foundation, 2011).

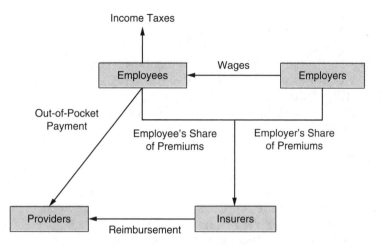

Figure 2-2 Healthcare Services and Insurance Markets with Employer Provided Health Insurance. Employers and employees typically share premiums. Health insurance premiums are a tax-free benefit to the employee.

Unlike wages, many noncash benefits are not subject to income tax. Thus, noncash benefits, such as health insurance, are cheaper to obtain if they are "purchased" through an employer rather than paid for out of after-tax income. As an example, assume that a family's tax rate is 20% and that the family wants to buy $100 of health insurance. If the employee takes compensation in the form of wages, the employee must earn $125 in order to have $100 after paying the 20% tax (20% of $125 is $25). The employee need earn only $100 if compensation is taken in the form of benefits. Or put another way, $100 of compensation in the form of nontaxable benefits will buy more health insurance than the employee could with $100 in wages. The economic importance of this is that present taxation arrangements make health insurance cheaper and encourage more of it to be bought.

It was mentioned earlier that when economic units are bigger or have a larger share of the market, they may be able to obtain better terms when selling or purchasing services. One type of arrangement that has been increasing in importance is the employer coalition, which is formed by businesses in local markets. Coalition members share information on provider prices, utilization trends, and so on, and they also cooperate with each other in developing benefit designs (e.g., common copayment arrangements). The original purpose of forming coalitions was to develop a sort of countervailing power in the market so that the buyers—the employers—would be able to exert some degree of market influence over price (McLauchlin, Zellers, & Brown, 1989). Another type of arrangement is the health insurance purchasing coalition (HIPC), which is a coalition of purchasers of insurance designed to garner the benefits associated with group purchasing (Reinhardt, 1993). HIPCs have been set up in some states to improve the access of smaller purchasers to health insurance.

The Patient Protection and Affordable Care Act, passed in 2010, provided funds to states to establish high-risk insurance pools to provide access to uninsured individuals with preexisting medical conditions who had been unable to obtain private health insurance coverage in the past because of these conditions. The intent of these temporary high-risk insurance pools (officially called the Preexisting Condition Insurance Plan) is to fill the gap until 2014, when insurance companies will no longer be able to deny coverage or charge excessive premiums to individuals because of their preexisting medical conditions. Beginning in 2014, consumers with preexisting conditions will be able to access affordable care through health insurance exchanges, which are also being established by the Affordable Care Act. Under the reform law, the premiums are set to not exceed 100% of the standard nongroup rate in the state and cannot vary by age by more than 4 to 1. While many states had offered different forms of high-risk pool insurance plans in the past, the premiums charged by these plans (usually 125 to 200% of prevailing individual market premiums) were still often prohibitive for individuals, effectively shutting them out of the insurance market.

2.2.2.3 Medicare

Many individuals are insured by government programs. Medicare is a program of the federal government that covers individuals 65 years old and over, certain disabled groups, and individuals with certain kidney diseases. Medicare is a form of limited national health insurance. The essential flows in Medicare are shown in Figure 2-3.

Medicare currently has four parts. Part A, Hospital Insurance (HI), helps cover inpatient care in hospitals, skilled nursing facilities (for limited services, not long-term care or custodial care), hospice, and home health care.

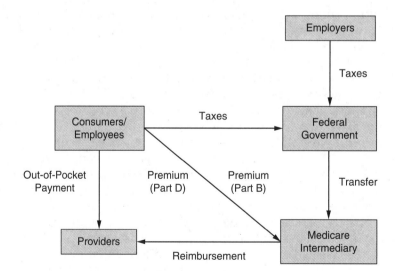

Figure 2-3   Medicare Part A, B, and D Flows. Consumer and employer taxes include the payroll tax, which is paid into the Hospital Insurance Trust Fund (part of the federal government). Medicare enrollee premiums are only for Parts B and D.

If an individual has paid Medicare taxes while working, there is no premium associated with enrollment in Part A (see Figure 2-3 for essential flows in Medicare). Eligible individuals are automatically enrolled in Part A upon obtaining eligible status. Part A is largely financed by a federal payroll tax paid by both employers and employees. In 2011, this tax was 2.9% of every dollar of salary and wages (taxable earnings); the employee's rate was 1.45%, as was the employer's rate. These taxes are placed in the Hospital Insurance Trust Fund, forming the bulk of the revenues for funding hospital and other institutional expenditures.

Because of the way the Trust Fund was established, it cannot be supplemented, to any great extent, by other forms of receipt, such as general taxes, without major changes in the legislation. Because expenditures from the fund have been greater than tax revenues, there are concerns that the Trust Fund will be bankrupt soon. The projections made in the 1980s regarding potential deficits by the end of the century led to major changes in the 1990s in the method by which Medicare reimbursed hospitals, converting from a cost-based reimbursement system to the prospective payment system based on DRGs. In addition, beginning in 2013, the healthcare reform law increases the Medicare HI payroll tax for higher-income taxpayers by 0.9 percentage points, in which higher-income taxpayers are defined as earnings of more than $200,000 per individual and $250,000 per couple.

Although Part A Medicare has no premiums, the level of copayments is high. In 2010, there was a deductible of $1,100, which covered the first 60 days of care for each spell of illness, and for anyone needing 61 to 90 days of hospitalization, there was a copayment of $275 for each day. If someone exceeded 90 days of care during a year, they could draw upon a lifetime reserve totaling 90 days. For many enrollees, the out-of-pocket payments have been considerable, and many individuals have purchased a private form of insurance called *Medigap*, which covers Medicare direct expenses. For individuals needing long-term facility service, there was a payment required in 2010 of $137.50 per day for days 21 through 100; home health requires no copayment.

Medicare Part B is the Supplementary Medical Insurance (SMI) program, and it helps pay for physician, outpatient, home health, and preventive services. It also pays for ambulance services, clinical laboratory services, durable medical equipment, outpatient mental health care, kidney supplies and services, and diagnostic tests. Enrollment in Part B is voluntary, and does require a monthly premium; the premium was $110.50/month in 2010, although 73% of beneficiaries were not required to pay the increase from the 2009 amount of $96.40 because there was no cost-of-living increase in Social Security benefits. The Affordable Care Act also added a free annual comprehensive wellness visit and personalized prevention plan to the benefits. The Act also added an income-related monthly Part B premium for individuals with annual incomes greater than $85,000 and for couples with incomes of $170,000 in 2010; this premium ranged from $154.70 to $353.60 in 2010. The reform law freezes these thresholds at 2010 levels through 2019. In addition, Part B benefits include an annual deductible ($155 in 2010), and most Part B services are subject to a coinsurance of 20%, although, beginning in 2011, no coinsurance and deductibles will be charged for preventive services rated as A or B by the U.S. Preventive Services Task Force (USPSTF). Revenues for Part B come from premiums, copayments, and general taxation.

Part C, Medicare Advantage (MA) plans, are private health plans that pay for Medicare benefits under Part A, Part B, and Part D. Medicare Advantage enrollees typically pay the monthly Part B premium plus an additional premium directly to their plan. While health maintenance organizations were originally an option, other private plans are now covered. In 2010, areas in which the plans were available offered, on average, 33 different plans from which beneficiaries could choose. These plans provide all benefits covered under traditional Medicare, plus many offer additional coverage, including prescription drugs. Plans must use any extra payment they receive (rebates) to provide additional benefits, such as lower premiums, lower cost sharing, or vision, hearing, preventive dental care, podiatry, chiropractic, and gym memberships. In 2010, the weighted monthly premium was $48.

The Medicare Prescription Drug, Improvement, and Modernization Act (MMA) was enacted in 2003, creating Medicare Part D, a voluntary outpatient prescription drug benefit plan that began in 2006. Enrollees in Part D generally pay a monthly premium; the plan is also funded through general revenues. Part D is very complex in terms of coverage and implementation. The law requires a standard benefit that must be covered or an alternative equal in value (actuarially equivalent); enhanced benefits can also be offered, and most Part D plans have a coverage gap, called the "doughnut hole." In 2010, there was a $310 deductible and 25% coinsurance up to an initial coverage limit of $2,830 in total drug costs under the standard benefit. Enrollees then paid 100% of their drug costs until they spent $4,550 out of pocket, not including premiums. Then the individual pays 5% of drug costs or a copayment of $2.50 per generic prescription or $6.30 per brand prescription for the rest of the year. The standard benefit amounts increase annually by the rate of per capita Part D spending growth. The health reform law provides enrollees with any spending in the doughnut hole in 2010 with a $250 rebate and gradually phases in coverage in the gap between 2011 and 2020.

2.2.2.4 Medicaid

Medicaid (Figure 2-4) is a joint cooperative federal-state program introduced in 1966 to cover certain low-income and categorically defined individuals. Federal guidelines set basic minimum criteria for eligibility, but each state's program is unique and operates differently. Medicaid is the largest health insurance program in the country. States set their own eligibility requirements within the federal parameters; select the services that will be offered and specify the amount, duration, and scope of services; design delivery systems; determine payments for services; and administer the program. To secure Medicaid eligibility, the person must be in one of the statutorily recognized categories or eligibility groups. There are six broad coverage categorical groups: children, pregnant women, adults in families with dependent children, adults and children with disabilities or are blind, and older persons. In addition, Medicaid is a means-tested entitlement program, and so individuals who meet the categorical criteria must also have incomes below the

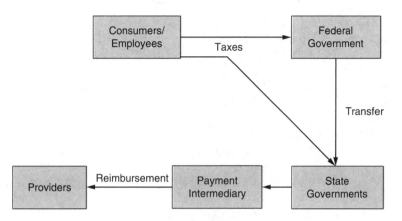

Figure 2-4 Flow of Funds for Medicaid Program. Federal government transfers to state governments are for federal share of the combined state-federal program. Beneficiaries pay no premiums, and direct consumer payments are minimal to providers.

income standard for the category. Because of the complicated combinations of categorical and financial factors, the mixture of mandates and options, and discretion afforded each state, eligibility varies considerably state-to-state. Federal policy, however, generally prevents Medicaid eligibility being extended to childless, nondisabled, nonelderly adults, and individuals who have primary addictive disorders, regardless of income. Currently, Medicaid covers more than two-thirds of all nursing home residents.

The Balanced Budget Act of 1997 created the State Children's Health Insurance Program (S-CHIP) to assist states in providing insurance coverage to low-income children who were not eligible for Medicaid but couldn't afford private insurance. In 2009, the Children's Health Insurance Program (CHIP) Reauthorization Act was passed and prohibits states from implementing eligibility standards, methodologies, or procedures that are more restrictive than those in place as of March 23, 2010, with the exception of waiting lists for enrolling children in CHIP. Under health reform, CHIP is maintained through 2019.

The Affordable Care Act contains provisions for dramatic expansion of the Medicaid program. Almost half of the expected gains in health insurance coverage under health reform are expected to be achieved through expansions in the Medicaid program. Historically, nonelderly adults without dependent children were not eligible for Medicaid. Under the health reform law, the categorical exclusion of these adults ends in 2014, expanding Medicaid eligibility to reach adults under 65, and provides states the option of beginning the coverage in 2010 instead of waiting until 2014.

2.2.2.5 Health Maintenance Organizations

Managed care refers to forms of insurance coverage in which enrollee utilization patterns and provider service patterns are monitored by the insurer, or an intermediary, with the aim of containing costs. An HMO is one type of managed care organization.

Payment of most HMO premiums are on a "capitation" basis. That is, there is a set fee for each enrollee, and the HMO receives a single annual amount for each enrollee, whether it provides much or little care. This form of payment puts the HMO at risk for all expenses incurred when serving enrollees, which incidentally means that the HMO serves as an insurer as well as a provider. Enrollees in HMOs may also be expected to pay a small copayment amount (e.g., $10) each time they visit a provider.

Traditionally, an HMO had one of two forms: either it was a self-contained unit that functioned as insurer and provider, or it was an amalgamation of private practice physicians (called an independent practice association) who were separately reimbursed by the HMO on a discounted fee-for-service basis. Recently, several new forms of HMOs have sprung up, many owned by traditional insurance companies, such as Blue Cross or commercial companies. These new types receive the capitation fee and contract out for services with providers that the HMO enrollees use.

One of the salient features of any HMO is the restriction of access to providers. Whereas under traditional coverage individuals can go to any provider, enrollees in an HMO must use a group of designated providers in order for the services to be covered. This closed-panel arrangement allows the HMO to monitor the providers and possibly have some impact on provider behavior. The providers on the panel may be employees of the HMO or contractors; in either case, monitoring providers is more likely to be feasible than if the enrollees have an unrestricted choice of providers. Such monitoring can potentially encourage providers to practice in a more conservative, less costly manner.

Beginning in the 1980s, HMO enrollment expanded rapidly, reaching a peak in 1999. In 2010, an estimated 66 million individuals had HMO-type coverage. HMO coverage is offered to enrollees of Medicare and Medicaid, as well as those who are traditionally covered. A simple flow diagram for HMO coverage is presented in Figure 2-5. Typically, HMO receipts would include employer contributions as well. It should be noted that, unlike in the case of traditional insurance coverage, there is typically no pass-through from insurer

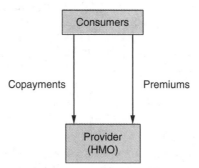

Figure 2-5 Flow of Funds for an HMO. Consumers pay premium to the HMO, which is also the provider. Copayment levels vary among plans, and some plans do not require any copayment.

to provider; the insurer is, in essence, the provider. However, there are some types of HMOs that do contract with independent providers.

2.2.2.6 Preferred Provider Organizations

A major drawback of HMO coverage is that enrollees can only choose from a limited panel of providers to have services covered. In many cases, an enrollee may be attached to or prefer a specific physician. If the physician is not on the provider panel, the enrollee must pay the provider's full price. Preferred provider organizations (PPOs) were designed to expand consumer choice while maintaining many of the monitoring benefits of managed care.

A PPO will contract with certain providers ("preferred providers") who agree to charge lower prices and submit to utilization monitoring in exchange for being designated as a preferred provider (see Figure 2-6). The PPO will then contract on behalf of these providers with insurance companies to gain their business. The insurers offer their enrollees a dual pricing system—one price for those who use the preferred providers and a higher price for those who use nonpreferred providers. This price differential might take the form of varying copayment rates; for example, a low (or zero) copayment rate for those who use the preferred group and a higher direct payment for those who use nonpreferred providers. This creates an economic incentive for the consumers to use the preferred group, but it allows partial coverage when a consumer chooses a nonpreferred provider.

Preferred providers gain from the fact that they will likely get a greater volume of business from the enrollees. Their agreeing to submit to some form of utilization monitoring will, if the monitoring is successful, translate into lower utilization patterns and lower premiums, which, in turn, translates into savings for the employer and employees.

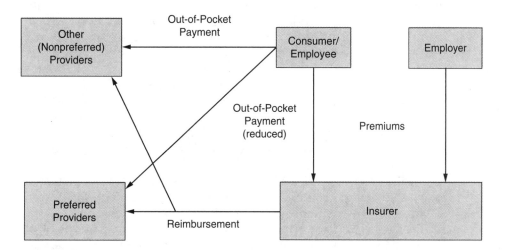

Figure 2-6 Outline of Flows in a Preferred Provider Arrangement. The preferred provider organization (PPO), not shown, arranges the preferred reimbursement rate from the preferred providers and conducts reviews of utilization. The PPO could be the preferred provider, the insurer, or an independent organization.

A PPO can be a separate contractor that receives a fee from the insurer. It can be part of the insurance company itself, or it can be owned by provider groups and used as a marketing mechanism. In fact, there are many types of PPOs. What distinguishes them from HMOs is their allowance of greater choice of provider. Recently, however, HMOs have been relaxing their closed panel restrictions in favor of coverage that is more similar to PPO coverage. An HMO that allows members to seek care from nonpanel providers for a differential fee is called a point-of-service (POS) plan.

PPOs have been growing in popularity in recent years. Between 1993 and 2011, the proportion of all insured persons who were enrolled in PPOs increased from 26% to 55% (Kaiser Family Foundation, 2011). In fact, their popularity has earned them a place in a popular health insurance package now offered by many employers: the "triple option" package. With such a package, the employer offers each employee a choice among types of coverage: traditional coverage, HMO coverage, and PPO coverage. In order to make the three types roughly comparable, the employer can alter the out-of-pocket payments and employee premiums. For example, for traditional care (the least restrictive in terms of consumer choice) the employer might set higher copayments and premiums, and enrollees who choose the more restrictive managed care options might be offered lower copayments and premiums.

2.2.2.7 The Meaning of Managed Care

Managed care is most frequently associated with HMOs and PPOs, because these types of organizations were the first to try to control the utilization of care. In a traditional HMO, providers are typically employed by the HMO or are contractually tied to it and subject to some degree of regulation. More recently, indemnity insurers have also introduced regulatory controls over providers, such as second-opinion requirements for surgery, length-of-stay reviews, and drug formularies. Providers transact with indemnity insurers at arm's length, and so indemnity insurers have had to develop such mechanisms to restrain utilization. Also, HMOs have been changing in form. In many cases, providers are more loosely tied to the HMO than has been true historically. In this type of arrangement, controlling utilization requires the establishment of contractual mechanisms. For example, providers who serve HMO members often have to obtain permission from the HMO before initiating expensive therapies in order for the services to be covered.

The regulatory function of indemnity and contractual HMOs is shown in Figure 2-7. In this diagram, the financial flows are shown as before. The flow of services from the providers to the consumers is also shown. A dotted line from the insurer to the service flow line indicates the care-management function established by the insurer. Under managed care, the service flow is regulated.

In order to set standards for providers, HMOs engage in profiling, which involves collecting comparative data on the treatment patterns of providers. Using this information, the insurers can set benchmarks that can be used to regulate the utilization of care. In addition to specific controls on services, managed care organizations can also affect utilization through choosing providers to employ or with whom to contract. A cost-efficient practice style may be one characteristic such an organization is seeking when recruiting new providers.

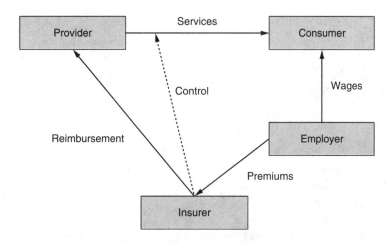

Figure 2-7   Flow of Money and Services that Are Consistent with any Insurance Arrangement. What is added is a control function by which the insurer establishes some form of control over the provider, thus regulating the flow of services from the provider to the consumer.

2.3 COST OF ACTIVITIES

Having identified productive activities as efforts involving resource inputs whose aim is to create goods or services we now need to find some common measure. The concept of cost is often used. In the context of a flow, cost is taken to be the magnitude of the resources devoted to an activity during a given period of time. Several different meanings can be attached to this concept. One definition of cost is the money outlay, or expenditure, that has been paid to the providers for their services. For example, if an optometrist performs an eye pressure test, the money cost is simply what is paid for the optometrist's services. Money cost is a convenient way to measure the magnitude of an activity, but it is not always a complete measure. The same optometrist may do the same test for free; in this case, the money cost would be zero. Yet some activity has taken place, and this activity has used scarce resources.

In the healthcare sector, there are many examples of free (i.e., zero money cost) services. Clinical teachers in medical schools frequently donate their efforts. Volunteer collectors for such organizations as the American Heart Association, United Way, and March of Dimes donate their time. The notion of *opportunity cost*, defined as the value of the most valuable alternative course of action given up for the chosen course of action, is used as a measure that does not depend on whether providers are paid in money for their services. Opportunity cost is relevant when a resource has several alternative uses. If the resource is used in activity A, the opportunity cost is what that resource would have earned if it had been used in alternative activity B, in which B is the highest valued alternative employment for that resource. For example, if an optometrist who performs a refraction for free in a clinic could have obtained a fee of $100 had he or she performed it in the office, by valuing this service at $100,

Table 2-1   National Health Expenditures by Type of Service, United States, 2010

Expenditure Category	Amount (billions of dollars)	Percent of Total
National Health Expenditures	2,593,644	100.0%
Health Consumption Expenditures	2,444,600	94.3%
Personal Health Care	2,186,013	84.3%
Hospital Care	814,045	31.4%
Professional Services	688,625	26.6%
Physician and Clinical Services	515,483	19.9%
Other Professional Services	68,357	2.6%
Dental services	104,785	4.0%
Other Health, Residential, and Personal Care	128,533	5.0%
Home Health Care	70,172	2.7%
Nursing Care Facilities & Continuing Care Communities	143,078	5.5%
Retail Outlet Sales of Medical Products	341,559	13.2%
Prescription Drugs	259,061	10.0%
Durable Medical Equipment	37,736	1.5%
Other Non-Durable Medical Products	44,762	1.7%
Government Administration	30,069	1.2%
Net Cost of Health Insurance	146,029	5.6%
Government Public Health Activities	82,489	3.2%
Investment	149,045	5.7%
Research	49,267	1.9%
Structures and Equipment	99,778	3.8%

Source: Derived from Centers for Medicare & Medicaid Services, NHE60-10_Final.csv. Accessed on April 4, 2012 from https://www.cms.gov/Research-Statistics-Data-and-Systems/Statistics-Trends-and-Reports/NationalHealthExpendData/NationalHealthAccountsHistorical.html.

we make it comparable to services performed for a fee. Whenever a service is provided at a price below its alternative value, the money cost will not take into account the portion of cost that is, in effect, subsidized; opportunity cost is a better measure of the true size of the total resources committed to an activity.

Costs can be categorized, among other ways, as direct or indirect. *Direct costs* are money expenditures, while *indirect costs* (also called *lost-productivity costs*) are unpaid resource commitments. Although these are unpaid, they may still have significant opportunity costs.

Table 2-1 shows the value of all direct national health expenditures for one year (2010) in the United States (Centers for Medicare and Medicaid, 2010). These expenditures amount to $2,593.6 billion. The largest portion of funds went to hospital care (31.4%), followed by physician care (19.9%). The prescription drug portion has been growing considerably, and in 2010, it equaled 10.0% of the total. In 1980, it had been only 4.7% of the total.

The growth in health expenditures, on a per capita basis, is shown in Figure 2-8. Since 1970, the growth has been steady. In 1990, health expenditures equaled $2,853 per person. By 2010, they had reached $8,402 per person.

A frequently used benchmark for health spending is total health spending expressed as a ratio of the total of all final goods and services produced in the economy during a year (the gross domestic product [GDP]). In 2010, the ratio for the United States was 17.9%. That is, of all final goods and services, 17.9% were healthcare services. The ratio of national health expenditures to the GDP is generally considered a critical indicator of resource use in the healthcare

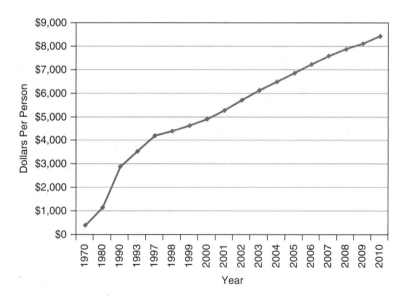

Figure 2-8 Per Capita Health Expenditures, United States, 1970–2010.

Source: National Health Expenditures Tables, Table 1, Centers for Medicare and Medicaid Services. Accessed April 4, 2012 from http://www.cms.gov/Research-Statistics-Data-and-Systems/Statistics-Trends-and-Reports/NationalHealthExpendData/Downloads/tables.pdf.

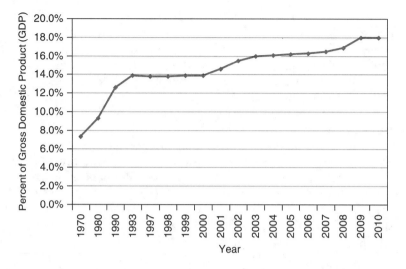

Figure 2-9 National Health Expenditures as a Percent of Gross Domestic Product (GDP), United States, 1970–2010.

Source: National Health Expenditures Tables, Table 1, Centers for Medicare and Medicaid Services. Accessed April 4, 2012 from http://www.cms.gov/ResearchStatistics-Data-and-Systems/Statistics-Trends-and-Reports/NationalHealthExpendData/Downloads/tables.pdf.

sector. In fact, as seen in Figure 2-9, this ratio had been growing steadily and significantly over the past several decades (Centers for Medicare and Medicaid, 2010). While there was a relatively stable period in the mid to late 1990s, when government spending was reduced, there has been a rapid increase the past couple of years, reflecting the depressed economy. As seen in Figure 2-8, per-capita spending on health care was unabated after 1993. In fact, the national economy experienced tremendous growth during the 1990s, and this increase (which is the denominator in the ratio of health spending to GDP) helped reduce the ratio. In recent years, the ratio has increased again. When compared with other developed countries, the United States has a very costly healthcare system. As can be seen in Figure 2-10, the health spending to GDP ratio is much lower for other countries (World Health Organization, 2011). In Germany, in 2008, for example, the ratio was 10.5%, in Japan it was 8.3%, and in the United Kingdom it was 8.7%. Investigators have focused on this statistic as an important indicator of the economic performance of the healthcare system (Anderson, 1997).

The data provide us with some idea of the direct costs of services provided. They do not, however, provide an indication of the total "burden" of costs—direct and indirect—that falls on all members of society as a result of illness. This total measure composes what are called the *social costs*.

Ideally, a cost-of-illness study will include all of the relevant resources that are influenced by the illness. The economic effects of illness can be experienced for years, and they can have a very broad impact in terms of the types of resources that are affected.

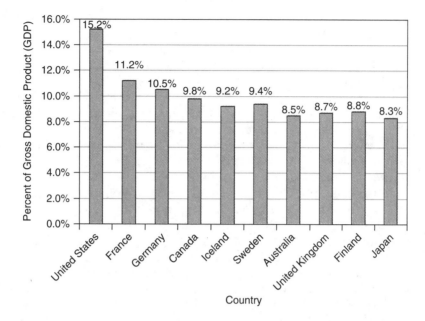

Figure 2-10   Health Expenditures as a Percentage of GDP, Selected Countries, 2008.

Source: Reprinted with permission from: World Health Organization. World Health Statistics, 2011. Geneva Switzerland. Accessed April 19, 2012 from http://www.who. int/whosis/whostat/EN_WHS10_Full.pdf and http://www.who.int/whosis/whostat/ EN_WHS2011_Full.pdf.

An illness can be diagnosed years after it was acquired. For example, a person can be affected with the hepatitis C virus for many years before finally being diagnosed. It is only when he or she has been diagnosed that one can measure the economic impact of the illness. Furthermore, the illness can generate economic costs for years after it has been diagnosed, even after the person has died. Chronic diseases last for years, and resources can be used as long as an illness lasts. If the person with the disease dies prematurely because of the disease, earnings that would have been experienced, but were not, are an indirect cost and part of the economic picture. The following resource components might be affected by the illness: healthcare resources used in diagnosis and treatment (also called *direct care costs*); direct nonhealth resources, such as transportation, special diets, and household goods; patient loss of work time due to illness and injury (also called *indirect care costs*); and other related indirect costs, such as work time lost by unpaid caregivers. The collection of all of these data is expensive, and so most studies will not include all the components.

Cost-of-illness studies can be conducted on a prevalence or incidence basis. With a prevalence basis, the annual costs of all existing cases during a year (including newly and previously diagnosed) are included. The future mortality-related costs for all persons with the disease who died during the year are also included (Rice, 1990). In contrast, an incidence-based analysis includes all present and future costs *only for cases newly diagnosed during the year.* In theory, one can also conduct an incidence-based analysis for cases that were contracted during the year, although this is seldom done for chronic diseases because of a lack of data. The cost of a premature death would include the lost work time from future deaths.

The prevalence approach is useful for budgeting purposes. For many purposes, the incidence approach is preferred, although it is much easier to obtain prevalence data than incidence data. If we are conducting a study on the economic effects of preventing or detecting illness, we should obtain data on the costs of all downstream events of the illness. The incidence approach would provide that information. If we used the prevalence approach, we would be obtaining the cost of many of the cases in midstream.

Data on the cost of several of the more economically important illnesses are shown in Figure 2-11. The costliest condition is injuries, with direct costs of $145.1 billion and indirect costs of $556.8 billion. The disease with the highest direct medical costs is heart disease, with annual costs of $257.6 billion. However, persons who suffer from injuries are generally younger than those who suffer from heart disease, and so their indirect costs are higher. Diabetes and cancer have roughly the same total cost of illness, but diabetes generally occurs in older persons, and so the ratio of direct to

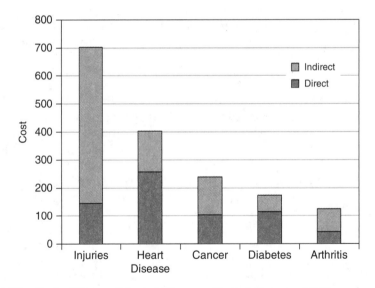

Figure 2-11   Cost of Illness, Selected Diseases, United States, c. 2006.

Source: DeNavas-Walt, C., et al. US Census Bureau, Current Population Reports, P60-238, Income, Poverty, and Health Insurance Coverage in the United States: 2009, US Government Printing Office, Washington DC, 2010. Department of Health and Human Services. Fact sheet–Temporary High Risk Pool Program. http://www.hhs.gov/ociio/initiative/hi_risk_pool_facts.html. Dunlop D., et al. Change. The costs of arthritis. Arthritis and Rheumatism (Arthritis Care Research), 2003. 49(1): 101–113. George A. Mensah, David W. Brown. An Overview of Cardiovascular Disease Burden in the United States. Posted 01/16/2007; Health Affairs, 2007: 26(1): 38–48. Kaiser Family Foundation. www.Statehealthfacts.org

indirect costs is greater for diabetes. Arthritis has low direct costs because the cost of treatment is much lower than for the other illnesses shown in the graph.

Cost-of-illness studies can provide valuable information that can be used in budgeting decisions and in cost-effectiveness studies. Cost-of-illness studies focus on the economic component of trends in disease and consequently are useful for policymakers. It is important for policymakers to have a notion of the impact of disease changes on expenditures. Much debate and misunderstanding has surrounded this topic. It should be understood that cost-of-illness studies are descriptive studies. One should not use the results of these studies by themselves to make policy recommendations. For these studies to be useful for evaluation purposes, the investigator must add additional information. Put another way, cost-of-illness studies describe what has happened. This can be most useful. But decision making requires more information—we must know why costs are what they are and what our objectives are.

EXERCISES

1. What is the difference between an insurance premium and a deductible?

2. Through what mechanism do most people in the United States purchase private health insurance?

3. What population does the Medicare program cover? What is Part A Medicare? Is there a premium, deductible, or coinsurance for Part A Medicare?

4. What is Part B Medicare insurance? Is there a premium, deductible, or coinsurance for Part B?

5. What is Part C Medicare insurance? Is there a premium, deductible, or coinsurance for Part C?

6. What is Part D Medicare insurance? Is there a premium, deductible, or coinsurance for Part D?

7. What populations does Medicaid cover? In general, is there a deductible or coinsurance for Medicaid? Why is there no premium?

8. On what basis is an HMO reimbursed? What is the relationship between the insurer and the provider in the HMO?

9. What distinguishes a preferred provider organization from a traditional health maintenance organization?

10. What is "managed" in managed care?

11. When would it be preferable to use opportunity costs rather than money costs?

12. What are direct and indirect costs?

13. What is a cost-of-illness study? What is the difference between measuring the cost of illness using the prevalence and incidence approaches?

BIBLIOGRAPHY

Overall Dimensions

Angell, M. (1985). Cost containment and the physician. *JAMA, 253*, 1203–1207.

Bauerschmidt, A. D. (1969). Sources and uses of healthcare funds in South Carolina. *Business and Economics Review of the University of South Carolina, 3*, 2–7.

Feldman, E., Hall, P. H., Smith, J., Monheit, A. C., Martin, S., & Kaiser, L. (2010). The promise and pitfalls of the federal health care reform law for nonprofit health care organizations and the people they serve. *Inquiry, 47*(4), 278–284.

Hall, M. A. (2011). The sausage-making of insurance reform. *Hastings Center Report, 41*(1), 9–10.

Hoffman, C., & Schwartz, K. (2008). Eroding access among nonelderly U.S. adults with chronic conditions: Ten years of change. *Health Affairs, 27*(5), w340–w348.

Holman, K. H., & Hayward, R. A. (2011). How to make market competition work in healthcare. *Medical Care, 49*(3), 240–247.

Letsch, S.W., Levit, K. R., & Waldo, D. R. (1988). National health expenditures, 1987. *Health Care Financing Review, 10*(winter), 109–122.

Levit, K. R., Freeland, M. S., & Waldo, D. R. (1989). Health spending and the ability to pay. *Health Care Financing Review, 10*(Spring), 1–12.

Monheit, A. C. (2010). The free lunch society. *Inquiry, 47*(4), 272–277.

Mullner, R., & Hadley, J. (1984). Interstate variations on the growth of chain-owned proprietary hospitals. *Inquiry, 21*, 144–151.

Rice, D. P., & Feldman, J. J. (1983). Living longer in the United States. *Milbank Quarterly, 61*, 362–396.

Sutcliffe, E. M. (1972). The social accounting of health. In M. M. Hauser (Ed.), *The economics of medical care*. London, England: George Allen and Unwin.

Costs, Prices, and Expenditures

Anderson, G., & Knickman, J. R. (1984). Patterns of expenditure among high utilizers of medical services. *Medical Care, 22*, 143–149.

Burner, S. T., & Waldo, D. R. (1995). National health expenditure projections, 1994–2005. *Health Care Financing Review, 16*, 221–242.

Centers for Medicare and Medicaid Services (2010). NHE60-10_Final.csv.

http://www.cms.gov/Research-Statistics-Data-and-Systems/Statistics-Trends-and-Reports/National-HealthExpendData/Downloads/tables.pdf

Chernew, M. (2010). Health care spending growth: Can we avoid fiscal Armageddon? *Inquiry, 47*(4), 285–295.

Cromwell, J., & Pushkin, D. (1989). Hospital productivity and intensity trends. *Inquiry, 26*, 366–380.

Freeland, M. S., Anderson, G., & Schendler, C. E. (1979). National hospital input price index. *Health Care Financing Review, 1*(Summer), 37–61.

Fuchs, V. R. (1990). The health sector's share of the gross national product. *Science, 247*, 534–538.

Ginsburg, D. H. (1978). Medical care services in the consumer price index. *Monthly Labor Review, 101*, 35–40.

Hellinger, F. J. (1990). Updated forecasts of the costs of medical care for persons with AIDS. *Public Health Reports, 105*(January), 1–12.

Hellinger, F. J. (1993). The lifetime cost of treating a person with AIDS. *JAMA, 270*, 474–478.

Kaiser Family Foundation (2011). *Employer Health Benefits, 2011 Annual Survey*. Menlo Park CA: Author.

Kelly, J. V., Ball, J. K., & Turner, B. J. (1989). Duration and cost of AIDS hospitalizations in New York. *Medical Care, 27*, 1085–1098.

Klarman, H. E. (1972). Increases in the cost of physician and hospital services. *Inquiry, 7*, 22–36.

Long, S. H., Gibbs, J. O., Crozier, J. P., Cooper, D. I., Jr., Newman, J. F., Jr. & Larsen, A. M. (1984). Medical expenditures for terminal cancer patients during the last year of life. *Inquiry, 22*, 315–327.

Malakoff, D. (2011). Can treatment costs be tamed? *Science, 331*(6024), 1545–1547.

McCall, N. (1984). Utilization and costs of Medicare services by beneficiaries in their last year of life. *Medical Care, 22*, 329–342.

Moonesinghe, R., Zhu, J., & Truman, B. I. (2011). Health insurance coverage—United States, 2004 and 2008. *Morbidity & Mortality Weekly Report. Surveillance Summaries, 60*(Suppl.), 35–37.

Moscone, F., & Tosetti, E. (2010). Health expenditure and income in the United States. *Health Economics, 19*(12), 1385–1403.

Pope, G. (1990). Physician inputs, outputs, and productivity; 1976–1986. *Inquiry, 27*, 151–160.

Rice, D. P., Hodgson, T. A., & Kopstein, A. N. (1985). The economic cost of illness. *Health Care Financing Review, 7*(Fall), 61–80.

Scitovsky, A. A. (1984). The high cost of dying. *Milbank Quarterly, 62*, 591–608.

Scitovksy, A. A., & McCall, N. (1977). *Changes in the cost of treatment of selected illness*. Publication no. HRA 77-3161. Hyattsville, MD: National Center for Health Services Research.

Scitovsky, A. A., & Rice, D. P. (1987). Estimating the direct and indirect costs of acquired immuno-deficiency syndrome in the United States, 1985, 1986, and 1991. *Public Health Reports, 102*, 5–17.

Sisk, J. E. (1987). The cost of AIDS: A review of the estimates. *Health Affairs, 6*(2), 5–21.

Sloan, F. A., Perrin, J. M., & Valvona, J. (1985). The teaching hospital's growing surgical caseload. *JAMA, 254*, 376–382.

Thygeson, M., Van Vorst, K. A., Maclosek, M. V., & Solberg, L. (2008). Use and costs of care in retail clinics versus traditional care sites. *Health Affairs, 27*(5), 1283–1292.

Vesely, R. (2011). Thinking smaller in 2011. Insurers expect lower profits as they cope with higher costs, new regulations. *Modern Healthcare, 41*(6), 14.

World Health Organization (2011). *World Health Statistics, 2011*. Geneva, Switzerland: Author.

Zook, C. J., & Moore, E. D. (1980). High cost users of medical care. *New England Journal of Medicine, 302*, 996–1002.

New Institutions

Chernew, M. (2010). Bundled payment systems: Can they be more successful this time. *Health Services Research, 45*(5, Pt. 1), 1141–1147.

Choudhry, N. K., Rosenthal, M. B., & Milstein, A. (2010). Assessing the evidence for value-based insurance design. *Health Affairs, 29*(11), 1988–1994.

Christianson, J. B., Ginsburg, P. B., & Draper, D. A. (2008). The transition from managed care to consumerism: A community-level status report. *Health Affairs, 27*(5), 1362–1370.

Cox, T. (2010). Legal and ethical implications of health care provider insurance risk assumption. *JONA's Healthcare Law, Ethics, & Regulation, 12*(4), 106–116.

de Lissovoy, G., Rice, T., Gabel, J., & Gelzer, H. J. (1987). Preferred provider organizations one year later. *Inquiry, 24*, 127–135.

Dobson, A., DaVanzo, J. E., El-Gamil, A. M., & Berger, G. (2009). How a new "public plan" could affect hospitals' finances and private insurance premiums. *Health Affairs, 28*(6), w1013–w1024.

Dror, D. M., Radermacher, R., Khadilkar, S., Schout, P., Hay, F., Singh, A., & Koren, R. (2009). Microinsurance: Innovations in low-cost health insurance. *Health Affairs, 28*(6), 1788–1798.

Gabel, J., Ermann, D., Rice, T., & de Lissovoy, G. (1986). The emergence and future of preferred provider organizations. *Journal of Health Politics, Policy, and Law, 11*, 305–321.

Gruber, L. R., Shadle, M., & Polich, C. L. (1988). From movement to industry: The growth of HMOs. *Health Affairs, 7*(3), 197–208.

Havighurst, C. C. (2008). Disruptive innovation: The demand side. *Health Affairs, 27*(5), 1341–1344.

Hudson, C. G., & Chafets, J. (2010). A comparison of acute psychiatric care under Medicaid carve-outs, HMOs, and fee-for-service. *Social Work in Public Health, 25*(6), 527–549.

Lee, M., Jr. (2011). Trends in the law: The Patient Protection and Affordable Care Act. *Yale Journal of Health Policy, Law, & Ethics, 11*(1), 1–7.

McLaughlin, C. G. Zellers, W. K., & Brown L. D.(1989). Health care coalitions: characteristics, activities, and prospects. *Inquiry, 26*, 72–83.

Robinson, J. C. (2010). Applying value-based insurance design to high-cost health services. *Health Affairs, 29*(11), 2009–2016.

Sengupta, A. (2011). Medical tourism: Reverse subsidy for the elite. *Signs, 36*(2), 312–319.

Health Insurance

Berry, M. D. (2011a). Medicaid copayments. Issue brief. *Issue Brief-Health Policy Tracking Service*, 1–4.

Berry, M. D. (2011b). Medicaid eligibility. Issue brief. *Issue Brief-Health Policy Tracking Service*, 1–14.

Berry, M. D. (2011c). Medicaid provider tax. Issue brief. *Issue Brief-Health Policy Tracking Service*, 1–7.

Berry, M. D. (2011d). Medicaid reimbursement. Issue brief. *Issue Brief-Health Policy Tracking Service*, 1–24.

Berry, M. D. (2011e). Medicaid waivers. Issue brief. *Issue Brief-Health Policy Tracking Service*, 1–19.

DiCarlo, S., & Gabel, J. (1989). Conventional health insurance: A decade later. *Health Care Financing Review*, 10(Spring), 77–89.

Gabel, J. Liston, D., Jensen, G., & Marsteller, J. (1994). The health insurance picture in 1993. *Health Affairs, 13*, 325–336.

Gilmer, T. P., & Kronick, R. G. (2009). Hard times and health insurance: How many Americans will be uninsured by 2010? *Health Affairs*, 28(4), w573–w577.

Health Policy Tracking Service, A. S. o. T. R. W. (2011a). Benefits and services. Issue brief. *Issue Brief-Health Policy Tracking Service*, 1–26.

Health Policy Tracking Service, A. s. o. T. R. W. (2011b). Mandated benefits. Issue brief. *Issue Brief-Health Policy Tracking Service*, 1–27.

Health Policy Tracking Service, A. S. o. T. R. W. (2011c). Medicaid restructuring. Issue brief. *Issue Brief-Health Policy Tracking Service*, 1–33.

Qian, X., Russell, L. B., Valiyeva, E., & Miller, J. E. (2011). "Quicker and sicker" under Medicare's prospective payment system for hospitals: New evidence on an old issue from a national longitudinal survey. *Bulletin of Economic Research, 63*(1), 1–27.

Reinhardt, U. E. (1993). Reorganizing the financial flows in American health care. *Health Affairs, 12*, 172–193.

Rotwein, S. Boulmetis, M., Boben, P. J., Fingold, H. I., Hadley, J. P., Rama, K. L., & Van Hoven, D. (1995). Medicaid and state health care reform: process, programs, and policy options. *Health Care Financing Review, 16*(Spring), 105–120.

Rubin, R. M. Wiener, J. M., & Meiners, M. R. (1989). Private long-term care insurance: simulations of a potential market. *Medical Care, 27*, 182–193.

Short, P. F. (1988). Trends in employee health insurance benefits. *Health Affairs, 7*(3), 186–196.

Smeeding, T. M., & Straub, L. (1987). Health care financing among the elderly. *Journal of Health Politics, Policy, and Law, 12*, 35–52.

Data

Anderson, G. F. (1997). In search of value: An international comparison of cost, access, and outcomes. *Health Affairs, 16*(6), 163–171.

Blackwell, D. L. (2010). Family structure and children's health in the United States: Findings from the National Health Interview Survey, 2001–2007. *Vital & Health Statistics-Series 10: Data From the National Health Survey*, (246), 1–166.

Eastwood, G. M., Peck, L. & Young, H. (2011). A call for a pragmatic approach to data collection. *Critical Care & Resuscitation, 13*(1), 59.

Health Insurance Association of America. (1999). *Sourcebook of health insurance data 1999–2000.* Washington, DC: Health Insurance Association of America.

Huang, H., Sim, H. G., Chong, T. W. Yuen, J. S., Cheng, C. W., & Lau, W. K. (2010). Evaluation of data completeness of the prostate cancer registry after robotic radical prostatectomy. *Annals of the Academy of Medicine, Singapore, 39*(11), 848–853.

Klerman, J. A., Davern, M., Call, K. T., Lynch, V., & Ringel, J. D. (2009). Understanding the current population survey's insurance estimates and the Medicaid "undercount." *Health Affairs, 28*(6), w991–w1001.

Levit, K., Cowan, C., Lazenby, H., Sensenig, A., McDonnell, P., Stiller, J., & Martin, A. (2000). Health spending in 1998: Signals of change. *Health Affairs, 19*(1), 124–132.

Organization for Economic Cooperation and Development. (2000). *OECD health data 2000.* Paris, France: Organization for Economic Cooperation and Development.

U.S. Department of Health and Human Services. (1999). *Health United States, 1999.* Hyattsville, MD: U.S. Department of Health and Human Services.

World Health Organization. (2000). *World health report 2000.* Geneva, Switzerland: World Health Organization.

Cost of Illness

Allen, J. M. (2010). Economic/societal burden of metastatic breast cancer: A US perspective. *American Journal of Managed Care, 16*(9), 697–704.

Barnett, S. B. L., & Nurmagambetov, T. A. (2011). Costs of asthma in the United States: 2002–2007. *Journal of Allergy & Clinical Immunology, 127*(1), 145–152.

Blaiss, M. S. (2010). Allergic rhinitis: Direct and indirect costs. *Allergy & Asthma Proceedings, 31*(5), 375–380.

Byford, S., Torgerson, D. J., & Raftery, J. (2000). Economic note: cost of illness studies. *BMJ, 320*, 1335.

Cholbi, M. (2010). The duty to die and the burdensomeness of living. *Bioethics, 24*(8), 412–420.

Cipriano, L. E., Romanus, D., Earle, C. C., Neville, B. A., Halpern, E. F., Gazelle, G. S., & McMahon, P. M. (2011). Lung cancer treatment costs, including patient responsibility, by disease stage and treatment modality, 1992 to 2003. *Value in Health, 14*(1), 41–52.

Cutler, D. M., McClellan, M., Newhouse, J. P., & Remler, D. (1998). Are medical prices declining? Evidence from heart attack treatments. *Quarterly Journal of Economics, 63*, 991–1024.

Frank, R. G., Busch, S. H., & Berndt, E. R. (1998). Measuring prices and quantities of treatment for depression. *American Economic Review, 88*, 106–111.

Gergen, P. J. (2011). Surveillance of the cost of asthma in the 21st century. *Journal of Allergy & Clinical Immunology, 127*(2), 370–371.

Gilden, D. M., Kubisiak, J., & Zbrozek, A. S. (2011). The economic burden of Medicare-eligible patients by multiple sclerosis type. *Value in Health, 14*(1), 61–69.

Gustavsson, A., Jonsson, L., McShane, R., Boada, M., Wimo, A., & Zbrozek, A. S. (2010). Willingness-to-pay for reductions in care need: Estimating the value of informal care in Alzheimer's disease. *International Journal of Geriatric Psychiatry, 25*(6), 622–632.

Heinrich, S., Rapp, K., Rissmann, U., Becker, C., & Konig, H. H. (2010). Cost of falls in old age: A systematic review. *Osteoporosis International, 21*(6), 891–902.

Hodgson, T. A. (1999). Medical expenditures for major disease. *Health Care Financing Review, 21*(Winter), 119–164.

Hodgson, T. A., & Cohen, A. J. (1999). Medical care expenditures for selected circulatory diseases. *Medical Care, 37*, 994–1012.

Hodgson, T. A., & Meiners, M. R. (1982). Cost of illness methodology: A guide to current practices and procedures. *Milbank Quarterly, 60*, 429–462.

Keeler, E. B., Manning, W. G., Newhouse, J. P., Sloss, E. M., & Wasserman, J. (1989). The external costs of a sedentary lifestyle. *American Journal of Public Health, 79*, 975–981.

Kelley, A. S., Ettner, S. L., Morrison, R. S., Du, Q., Wenger, N. S., & Sarkisian, C. A. (2011). Determinants of medical expenditures in the last 6 months of life. *Annals of Internal Medicine, 154*(4), 235–242.

Lang, H. C. (2010). Willingness to pay for lung cancer treatment. *Value in Health, 13*(6), 743–749.

Leger, D., & Bayon, V. (2010). Societal costs of insomnia. *Sleep Medicine Reviews, 14*(6), 379–389.

Mariotto, A. B., Yabroff, K. R., Shao, Y, Feuer, E. J., & Brown, M. L. (2011). Projections of the cost of cancer care in the United States: 2010–2020. *Journal of the National Cancer Institute, 103*(2), 117–128.

McClellan, M., & H. Noguchi. (1998). Technological change in heart-disease treatment. *American Economic Review, 88*(2), 90–96.

Moore, R., Mao, Y, Zhang, J, & Clarke, K. (1997). *Economic burden of illness in Canada, 1993.* Ottawa: Health Canada.

Naci, H., Fleurence, R., Birt, J., & Duhig, A. (2010). Economic burden of multiple sclerosis: A systematic review of the literature. *Pharmacoeconomics, 28*(5), 363–379.

Pike, C., Birnbaum, H. G., Schiller, M., Sharma, H., Burge, R., & Edgell, E. T. (2010). Direct and indirect costs of non-vertebral fracture patients with osteoporosis in the US. *Pharmacoeconomics, 28*(5), 395–409.

Rice, D. P. (1990). Cost-of-illness studies: Fact or fiction? *Lancet, 344*, 1519–1520.

Rice, D. P., Hodgson, T. A., & Kopstein, A. N. (1985). The economic cost of illness: A replication and update. *Health Care Financing Review, 7*(Fall), 61–80.

Rice, D. P., Kelman, S., & Miller, L. S. (1990). *The economic costs of alcohol and drug abuse and mental illness: 1985.* San Francisco: University of California, Institute for Health and Aging.

Sheill, A., Gerard, K., & Donaldson, C. (1987). Cost of illness studies: An aid to decision-making? *Health Policy, 8*, 317– 323.

Strombeck, B., Englund, M., Bremander, A., Jacobsson, L. T., Kedza, L., Kobelt, G., & Petersson, I. F. (2010). Cost of illness from the public payers' perspective in patients with ankylosing spondylitis in rheumatological care. *Journal of Rheumatology, 37*(11), 2348–2355.

Sullivan, P. W., Ghushchyan, V. H., Slejko, J. F., Belozeroff, V., Globe, D. R., & Lin, S. L. (2011). The burden of adult asthma in the United States: Evidence from the Medical Expenditure Panel Survey. *Journal of Allergy & Clinical Immunology, 127*(2), 363–369, e361–e363.

Ungar, W., & Coyte, P. (2000). Measuring productivity loss days in asthma patients. *Health Economics, 9*, 37–46.

Withrow, D., & Alter, D. A. (2011). The economic burden of obesity worldwide: A systematic review of the direct costs of obesity. *Obesity Reviews, 12*(2), 131–141.

Zook, C. J., Savickis, S. F., & Moore, F. D. (1980). Repeated hospitalization for the same disease. *Milbank Quarterly, 58*, 454– 471.

PART II: Explanatory Economics

Chapter 3

Demand for Medical Care: A Simple Model

OBJECTIVES

1. Identify two hypotheses used to predict the behavior of quantity demanded for a healthcare service.

2. Explain the demand hypothesis and distinguish between the concepts of *demand* and *quantity demanded.*

3. Know the individual factors that influence demand and explain how each affects the demand curve.

4. Explain how we can derive an individual's demand curve for medical services from basic assumptions about the economic behavior of consumers.

5. Explain how to derive a market demand curve from data on individual demand curves.

6. Define the concept of elasticity of demand and explain how to measure the concept using data on prices and utilization.

7. Know the various types of health insurance arrangements and explain how each affects the out-of-pocket or direct price and the demand curve for medical services.

3.1 THE CONCEPT OF DEMAND

The purpose of explanatory economics is to predict economic behavior. When analyzing demand behavior, our attention focuses on the quantity demanded by consumers of a specific good or service. To perform the analysis, we use a demand model that serves two purposes: It provides a categorization of the separate factors that might cause demand or quantity demanded to increase or decrease, and it provides a specific hypothesis about how economic factors (e.g., price and income) influence demand or quantity demanded.

Models are devices we use to obtain our results. A model is a representation of reality, not a complete description of it. The purpose of a model, however specified, is to present us with an "If . . . then . . ." type of explanation. In the case of the demand model, the reasoning is of this form: "If factor x increases, then demand or quantity demanded will increase (or decrease, depending on what factor x is)." A good model screens essential causal factors and incorporates them into a logical, coherent system. Models enable simpler explanations of complex situations to be undertaken. Using these simpler models enables exploration of the actions and consequences of complex situations to be studied and understood. Using diagrams and equations, economic models attempt to explain events occurring in the world.

Even though every model is conjectural, it should tell us something about movements in real phenomena (e.g., the quantity of medical care demanded). In assessing a model, it is therefore sufficient to examine whether its predictions concerning movements in selected phenomena are realized by comparing the predictions with actual movements in the phenomena as measured by data. In other words, accuracy of prediction is the test of an explanatory model.

This chapter introduces a simple model of the demand for a good or service. Section 3.2 sets forth the model, using an individual's demand for medical care as an example. Section 3.3 takes us behind the scenes and shows how the model of demand can be derived. Several key shortcomings of the simple model, when applied to the medical care context, are emphasized; these shortcomings are central to the extended analyses of the chapter on additional topics in the demand for health and medical care. Section 3.4 examines the factors influencing the market demand for the good or service. Section 3.5 develops the concept of *elasticity*, a tool used to measure the magnitude of the hypothesized movements, and Section 3.6 presents the demand analysis when insurance is present. Finally, Section 3.7 presents some actual estimates of the demand relationship.

3.2 INDIVIDUAL DEMAND: THE PRICE-QUANTITY RELATIONSHIP

3.2.1 Demand and Quantity Demanded

We begin our exposition of the price-quantity relation with a specification of the terms of reference and definitions of the variables used. The unit of analysis is the individual consumer. In the present context, we examine the economic behavior of a typical, or representative, consumer. This behavior involves attaining or attempting to attain goods and services. Because our focus is on health care, the service *physician care* is used as the major example. Physician care is defined as examinations and treatments administered by physicians to their patients. Physician care is only one of many goods and services in the healthcare sector. Thus, when following the analysis, keep in mind that the relationships specified in this chapter can be applied to other health-related goods and services as well, including hospital services, pharmaceuticals, dental care, home care, preventive measures, nutritional services, nursing care, and the services of other health professionals.

As the model of physician care is developed, certain assumptions are made in order to simplify the complex healthcare market, making it easier to understand. In making assumptions, attention can be focused on the major issues associated with a problem. Once the simpler model is understood, then the more complex world can be more easily understood. The assumptions made will vary with different situations or different questions to be studied. Assumptions will also vary with the length of time in which the situation occurs; assumptions involving short-run situations may be very different from those involving long-run situations.

Having identified the service in our analysis, we must next find an appropriate unit of measurement. Here we encounter a problem that is pervasive in medical care organization analysis: defining and measuring quality differences among units of medical care. Examinations and treatments can vary in thoroughness, such as in the physician's technical competence or in the physician's bedside manner, among other factors. Quality differences constitute differences in these characteristics. When analyzing physician care as a service, all these variations should be kept in mind. In this chapter, we will abstain from quality differences to avoid complicating our initial entrance into explanatory economics.

Our service, physician care, is measured by the number of visits to a physician by the typical consumer. Each visit is assumed to be identical with all others. Finally, we specify the time span as being one year. Given this time frame, our service measure becomes the number of physician visits per year.

With this background, the demand hypothesis used to predict the effect of a change in direct per-unit price on the quantity demanded of a good or service can be presented. The hypothesis is that the lower the out-of-pocket price (the endogenous variable) offered to consumers (all other factors held constant), the greater the number of units of that good or service they will demand. A number of conventions, or interpretations, are related to this hypothesis. By "quantity demanded," we mean the quantity demanded at any specific price, all other causal factors held constant. Quantity demanded is the amount that the consumer is willing and able to buy at the specified price. By "demand," we mean the set of quantities demanded at various prices, all other causal factors held constant. By "out-of-pocket price," we mean the price paid directly by consumers for a particular unit of the good or service. By "all other factors," we mean those variables other than price that influence consumer demand behavior. The economic approach to consumer behavior is to specify an initial relation between out-of-pocket price and quantity demanded and then to introduce other causal factors to see how they affect the basic demand relation.

One such demand relation, assuming all other factors remain unchanged, is illustrated diagrammatically as line d_1 in Figure 3-1. The specific relation shown by this line, or curve, entails that at a price of $7 per visit, the consumer would be willing to visit the physician twice a year; at a price of $6 per visit, the consumer would be willing to make three visits; and so on. Assuming that the quantities demanded at all other prices trace out a straight-line relation, d_1 represents a particular demand curve at one specific level of

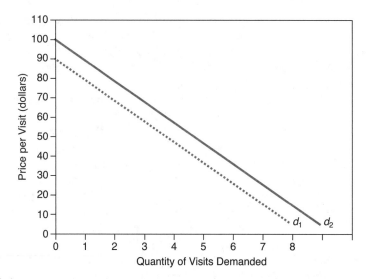

Figure 3-1   The Demand Relationship, the Famous Downward Sloping Demand Curve. Curves d_1 and d_2 show the quantity demanded increasing as the direct price decreases. Each curve represents a separate level of demand. With reference to curve d_1, curve d_2 represents an increase in demand, not just an increase in quantity demanded.

demand. The lowercase letter d is used to indicate that we are representing the behavior of a single individual.

The downward slope of the demand curve is explained by the possibility of substitution. Substitution occurs when goods and services can be used in place of each other to satisfy a desire or need to a similar level. This economic approach implies that very few, if any, goods or services are absolute musts. Substitutes exist for most goods or services; some are almost identical and others are less similar. The longer the time span during which the consumer adapts his or her behavior to any substitutes, the more relevant they become. A sore throat, for example, can be treated by a physician or by resorting to drugs or home remedies. Furthermore, even if the malady is treated by a physician, alternative types of broad-spectrum antibiotics can be used. In recent years, use of outpatient treatment instead of hospitalization has been suggested for many types of ailments. In the long term, health foods and other preventive services are substitutes for medical care in maintaining desired health levels. In these, as well as other instances, the hypothesized relation applies: the lower the price of any specific alternative, the more it will be demanded.

Other hypotheses than this demand relation might be put forward to explain consumer demand behavior. One alternative hypothesis that has received much attention in medical care literature is that at higher prices, individuals will still demand and pay for the same quantity of medical care. This alternative hypothesis would be represented by a vertical demand curve representing a perfectly inelastic demand curve. Similar vertical demand curves have also been hypothesized for other items considered necessities, such as housing, basic foods, and even alcohol.

Having two alternative hypotheses, we are faced with the problem of determining which is the more useful for explaining actual behavior. Debating the issue by itself cannot resolve the controversy, however. The hypothesis chosen should be the one that most closely fits the actual data. The empirical testing of hypotheses is discussed in Section 3.7.

Before proceeding with qualifications to our hypothesis, we should emphasize that we are focusing solely on consumer behavior. Our hypothesis relates only to how much the consumer is willing to buy at any price. At this stage, we are not inquiring about whether the amount demanded will be supplied or even available.

3.2.2 Changes in Demand

The effects of factors other than the out-of-pocket price on the economic behavior of consumers are introduced by way of their influence on the basic price-quantity relationship. These other exogenous factors can be placed into four broad categories: (1) income, (2) prices of other (related) goods and services (3) tastes, and (4) expectations. Each category is considered in turn.

3.2.2.1 Income

The income of the consumer is generally assumed to be positively related to demand. That is, if income increases, the quantity demanded at each price will be greater if the good or service is a normal good. If the good or service is inferior, then the increase in income will result in a decrease in demand, other factors being equal. The basic relation between income and demand can be illustrated with the use of demand curves. In Figure 3-1, curve d_1 can now be interpreted as representing a level of demand at some initial level of income. Let us suppose that, from this initial level, income increases. The hypothesized effect on demand is such that at a price of \$7, there will be three visits demanded instead of two; at a price of \$6, there will be four visits demanded instead of three, and so on. The new demand level, corresponding to the higher income level, can be represented by the curve d_2. In the diagram, the relative position of the two curves summarizes the net influence of income on consumer behavior. A shift in demand from curve d_1 to curve d_2 is called an *increase* in demand, as opposed to a change in quantity demanded with a change in price, represented by movement along a static demand curve.

The same reasoning can be applied in reverse to a fall in income. This decline causes the consumer to demand less of the good or service at each price. The change in the level of demand might, for example, be represented by a shift from d_2 to d_1. This is called a *decrease* in demand, reflecting a reduction in quantity demanded at every price.

Income is frequently defined as an individual's earnings in a specific time period. It is a variable used to measure the ability of the individual to afford medical care, but it is only an approximate measure. Another measure of an individual's ability to purchase medical care is the individual's level of wealth, including bonds, bank deposits, real estate, and other assets, minus any debt, such as bank loans and mortgages. A third measure is after-tax income.

This measure is particularly important to take into account when considering changes in tax rates and their effects on purchasing power. Whatever measure is used should be a good approximation of the individual's ability to pay for medical care.

3.2.2.2 Prices of Related Good and Services

The demand for a particular good or service is also influenced by the quantities of related goods and services consumed. The quantities of these related goods and services are, in turn, influenced by their prices. Two classes of good and service relationships are of concern to us: complements and substitutes. A complementary good or service is one whose use is generally accompanied by the use of the good or service in question. Examples might include penicillin and syringes, the services of a surgeon and the hospital's surgical services, and the services of a radiologist and radiographic film. The hypothesis relating the demands of complementary goods and services is as follows: a fall in the price of a good or service increases the quantity demanded of that good or service, and it also leads to an increase in the demand for goods and services that are complements. Similar reasoning, in reverse, applies to an increase in the price of one good or service in a complementary set. As an example of this relationship, we can hypothesize that a fall in the out-of-pocket price of the surgical services involved in tonsillectomies will lead to an increase in the quantity of services demanded; it will also increase the demand for hospital room services.

Complements play an important role in medical care demand. The close relationship between radiology machines and radiologist services has frequently led to the assertion that much hospital demand is really determined by the quantity of physician services consumed.

The second type of good or service relationship is that of substitution. A substitute is a good or service that can replace the original good or service. The hypothesis is that a fall in the price of a good or service increases the quantity demanded and leads to a reduced demand for substitute goods and services. This relationship can be illustrated using an example of two substitute services, such as postoperative recuperation time in the hospital versus home care. A rise in the price the patient pays for an additional day of hospital care decreases the quantity of hospital days demanded. At the same time, it increases the demand for home care.

Substitution was also the reason given for the downward slope of the demand curve for any good or service. For example, quantity of inpatient care demanded is negatively related to patient price, because inpatient care can be substituted for home care when the price of inpatient care falls and vice versa. This assumes, of course, that the price of home care remains constant. A rise in the price of home care leads to additional substitution, which is accounted for, in our model, by an outward shift in the inpatient care demand curve. The slope of the demand curve of any good or service, as well as how much it shifts when substitute prices change, depends on how similar the patient perceives the substitutes to be. Services, such as inpatient and outpatient surgery (e.g., for hernia repair and tonsillectomies), are highly substitutable, as are nursing home care and home care, in many instances.

3.2.2.3 Tastes

Consumer taste is a catchall category covering a large number of other factors that might influence demand. Tastes have sometimes been called *wants*, a term connoting the intensity of desire for particular goods and services. The elements that influence the intensity of an individual's desire for medical care include health status, educational background, gender, age, race, and upbringing. Any of these can explain differences among individuals in the intensity of desire for medical care. That is, with other factors (incomes, prices of other goods and services, and so on) held constant, these differences can be used to explain why one individual's demand curve is d_1 (Figure 3-1) whereas another's is d_2. (The explanation might simply be that the health status of the first individual is lower than that of the second individual.)

Tastes are usually considered to be fixed from the standpoint of economic analysis, although some economic models recognize that advertising by firms can influence consumer tastes. Although tastes differ among individuals, they are hypothesized, for most goods and services, to be stable over fairly short periods of time. If they are stable, once the factors that underlie tastes are accounted for, differences in demand can be attributed to differences in incomes, prices of other goods and services, and factors influencing tastes. However, controversy exists over the stability of individual tastes for medical care. In addition to the dependence of tastes on health, which is itself transitory, physicians potentially can exert considerable influence over tastes for medical care. Changing tastes have played a large role in health economics. Because of this, it is necessary to go behind the scenes to discover the role of tastes in medical care demand.

3.2.2.4. Expectations

Consumers' expectations about the future may impact current demand for a good or service. For example, if consumers expect their incomes to be higher in the near future, then they may purchase more goods and services currently and save less. Another example of the impact of expectations is if consumers expect prices to increase, then they may purchase additional services at the current price.

3.3 DERIVING THE DEMAND RELATIONSHIP

In Section 3.2, the demand for medical care was analyzed as if medical care were an ordinary good or service, like carrots or shoes. However, certain characteristics of medical care make it unlike many ordinary goods and services. We must pay closer attention to these characteristics to determine if and when standard demand analysis is appropriate for medical care. To do this, we present a theoretical model focusing on the conditions that are required for the demand relationship to hold; special attention is paid to whether these conditions are likely to be met in the case of medical care.

The factors influencing a consumer's behavior with regard to the demand for a good or service can be placed under the categories of tastes, incomes, prices, and expectations. Let us assume that a typical individual has a choice of purchasing only two goods and services. These two goods and services are carrots and physician care (as measured by physician's office visits). In what follows, we will specify the assumptions underlying our model for the demand for these two products.

3.3.1 Tastes

Tastes are essentially desires for products. These desires, or wants, are quantified using an index that we call *utility*. Although it is a hypothetical construct, the concept of utility is very valuable as an instructive device. It is often equated with the notion of satisfaction. The utility of carrots for a hypothetical individual is shown in Table 3-1. The numbers in this table were devised to show an increasing total amount of utility (total utility) as more carrots are consumed, but more importantly, they were devised so that the increases gradually diminish.

The concept used to represent the increases in utility from successive quantities of a good or service is called *marginal utility*, which is the change in total utility resulting from a unit change in the consumption of the good or service. Thus, the marginal utility for the first carrot is 6; it is 5 for the second, and so on. This decrease in the size of the utility of successive quantities of a good or service is called *diminishing marginal utility*. Note that, in general, total satisfaction will still increase. This is a key assumption of demand analysis. The same assumption can be applied to medical care as well, but the circumstances in which the relationship of diminishing marginal utility will hold needs to be explored in greater detail. We therefore list the conditions that must occur.

3.3.1.1 Health Status

The initial health status of the individual (H) is given and known by the individual. That is, the individual knows what medical condition she has.

Table 3-1 Relationship Between Quantity Consumed of Two Goods and Services and Utility of (Satisfaction Derived from) the Goods and Services

Quantity	Medical Care		Carrots	
	Total Utility	Marginal Utility	Total Utility	Marginal Utility
1	22	22	6	6
2	42	20	11	5
3	60	18	15	4
4	76	16	18	3
5	90	14	20	2
6	102	12	21	1

3.3.1.2 Consumer Information

The relationship between medical care (*MC*) and health status (*H*) is also known by the individual. That is, the individual knows how "productive" medical care will be influencing his/her health. Part of this reflects the fact that the individual has a good understanding of his/her health problems.

3.3.1.3 Productivity of Medical Care

In general, we assume that the marginal productivity of medical care in influencing health is constant. As more units of medical care (visits) are consumed, equal additions to health status will result. Obviously, there must be a limit to how healthy an individual can become, and we will show what happens when this assumption is altered. For the moment, we will hold with the assumption of constant productivity.

3.3.1.4 Quality

The quality of medical care is also assumed to be constant. All visits provided by the physicians are of the same quality.

3.3.1.5 Other Taste-Influencing Variables

It should be noted that the utility function is dependent on a host of other variables, each of which may influence the individual's intensity of desire for medical care. These variables include the individual's education, upbringing or culture, marital status, and age, among others. For example, it is believed that higher levels of education increases an individual's desire for good health. Thus, we should be aware that in the back of any taste function lies a series of formative factors that cause the utility-quantity relation to be what it is. In this example, we will assume that there are no other sources of utility except for medical care and carrots.

Given these assumptions, we can hypothesize the type of relationships between utility and medical care shown in Table 3-1, in which each added visit results in a smaller increment of additional utility, unless the individual is a competitive bodybuilder, the hypothesis is a plausible one.

3.3.2 Income

The second variable in our demand model is the individual's income. We will assume that the individual's income is $10 for the time period and that the individual lacks any accumulated wealth usable for purchasing care.

3.3.3 Prices of Other Goods and Services

Other variables include the prices charged for medical care and carrots. We will initially set these at $1 per carrot and $4 per physician's office visit. The purpose of our analysis is to predict what happens when the price of medical care changes and, in the process, to make explicit what variables are initially being held constant in the analysis.

3.3.4 Behavioral Assumption: Utility Maximization

Finally, we come to our behavioral assumption, which is what sets the model in motion. Our assumption is that the individual is a utility maximizer (i.e., the individual desires to gain the most satisfaction, or benefit, from his or her income).

3.3.5 Predictions

The model's conclusion stems from these assumptions together with assumptions about price changes. Let us first determine what quantities of medical care and carrots are demanded at the initial prices. In doing this, we need to focus on the marginal utility (MU) per dollar of expenditure, or the ratio of marginal utility to price (P), which is expressed as MU / P. It is this variable that expresses the satisfaction per dollar of expense for each alternative use. At a price of $1 per carrot, buying a carrot will be the best bet for the first $1 of expenditure, because the first carrot yields 6 units of utility. The next item purchased will not be another carrot, because an additional expenditure here would yield 5 units of utility per $1, whereas a visit to the doctor would yield 5.5 units (22 units / $4). Therefore, the individual makes a visit to the doctor. The individual has now spent a total of $5 and has $5 left. The next items of expenditure will be a carrot and another visit to the doctor (indeed, both have an MU / P ratio of 5). At this point, the individual will have used up all income and will have achieved an equal marginal utility per dollar for the last purchases of each good or service. The total utility (53) is the highest that can be attained with $10. This equality of MU / P in each use indicates that the individual's income cannot be reallocated to a different mix of carrots and visits to obtain more utility.

To show that the individual is maximizing utility, let us assume that, after the second carrot, the individual allocates the remaining $4 to the purchase of carrots instead of medical care. The marginal utility of the third, fourth, fifth, and sixth carrot would be 4, 3, 2, and 1, respectively. The individual would now be getting 1 unit of utility per $1 of expenditure instead of the 5 units obtainable by purchasing medical care. The total utility would be 43. That is, the individual would have been better off with two carrots and two visits than with this alternative set of purchases.

Having shown that there is a utility-maximizing "equilibrium" quantity for each good or service, let us now change the assumption about prices of other goods and services and lower the price of medical care to $3. A carrot will still cost $1. This fall in the price of medical care results in an increase in the utility per dollar of medical care for all visits and makes medical care more valuable in dollar terms. Under this altered assumption, the individual will maximize utility by "consuming" three physician visits and consuming only one carrot.

The essential implication of this analysis is that when the price of medical care falls, the quantity demanded increases (assuming all other variables, including other prices as well as incomes and tastes, remain the same, ceteris paribus). This is therefore a derivation of the demand relationship. It should be noted that the model holds only when other variables are held constant. Changing them will shift the demand relationship in one direction or the other, depending on the variable and the degree of change. For example, a more educated person may perceive health as having a greater utility relative to carrots, thus causing a shift in tastes. This will shift the demand for medical care as well.

With regard to one particular loose end, our assumption about the productivity of medical care, let us consider the probable effect of a more realistic assumption. In particular, let us assume that medical care has diminishing marginal productivity with respect to health. If additional units of health diminished in size with successive visits, this would make the marginal utility of medical care fall more quickly and would reduce the relative desirability of additional units of medical care. There would still be a downward-sloping demand curve, but it would be shifted inward, in comparison to the situation in which the productivity of medical care was constant.

3.4 MARKET DEMAND

The model developed previously provided a means of analyzing an individual's demand for medical care. To generalize the model to explain market demand, we must make an additional assumption. (By "market" we mean the network of buyers and sellers of a good or service.) The assumption is that the more individuals there are who seek the product, the greater will be the market demand and the quantity demanded in the market at any price.

This is illustrated in Figure 3-2, which shows the demand curves of three individuals: d_b is Mr. B's demand curve, d_k is Ms. K's demand curve, and d_j is Mrs. J's demand curve. At a price of $20 per visit, Mr. B will demand 3 visits, Ms. K will demand 2, and Mrs. J will demand none. At $15 per visit, Mr. B., Ms. K., and Mrs. J will demand 5 visits, 4 visits, and 1 visit, respectively. At $10, the number of visits will be 7, 6, and 4, respectively. Using information on individual demand curves, and on the number of individuals, we can derive a market demand curve.

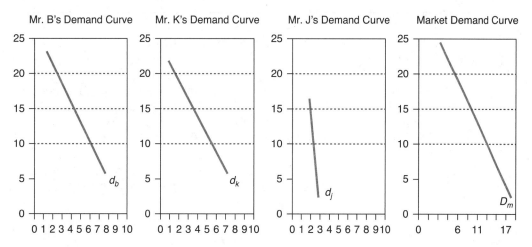

Figure 3-2 Derivation of the Market Demand Curve from Individual Demand Curves. The quantity demanded at each price by all consumers in the market is the sum of the individual quantity demand. The market demand curve is the horizontal sum of all individual demand curves.

Given the three individual demand curves, the market quantity demanded at a given price will be the sum of the quantities demanded by all three individuals at that price. At a price of $20, the quantity demanded in the market will be 5 visits; at $15, the quantity will be 10; and at $10, it will be 17. The market demand curve is shown in Figure 3-2 as D_m and is the horizontal sum of the demands of the three individuals demanding visits.

We can now divide the factors influencing market demand into two categories: (1) factors influencing individual demand only and (2) factors influencing market demand. The former includes prices, incomes, and tastes. If any of these change, individual demand, or the quantities demanded, will also change. If individual demand curves shift out, market curves, being based on individual curves, will shift out as well. In addition to responding to changes in individual curves, market demand is influenced by changes in the number of participants in the market. For example, an influx of people into an area will cause market demand to increase. It is also possible that people in the area who did not demand any medical care at higher prices will become consumers of care as the price falls. As this indicates, demand does not have to remain constant over time.

3.5 MEASURING QUANTITY RESPONSIVENESS TO PRICE CHANGES

In the preceding sections, we developed a model that enabled us to predict how a particular factor will affect quantity demanded or demand. Thus, we can predict that, when the out-of-pocket price falls, the quantity demanded will rise; that is, there is an inverse relationship between price and quantity demanded. We can now ask, by how much will the quantity demanded rise? The answer to this question is likely to play an important role in setting policy.

The concept used to measure quantity responsiveness to out-of-pocket price changes is the concept of *price elasticity of demand*. Price elasticity is designed to measure the responsiveness of demand to a price change at a given point or between two given points on a single demand curve. That is, it attempts to measure responsiveness when the only factor undergoing change, and thereby influencing the quantity demanded, is price.

The elasticity of demand is designed to measure changes independent of the units of measurement. That is, the measure of elasticity is a measure of relative magnitudes and will not change if cents rather than dollars are used to measure price or units rather than thousands are used to measure quantity. Elasticity is, thus, a pure measure of the magnitude of change. The formula used for small changes in price is the percentage change in quantity demanded divided by the percentage change in price. In symbolic terms, this is written

$$E_p = \frac{\Delta Q / Q}{\Delta P / P}$$

in which E_p is price elasticity, Q is the original quantity, P is the original price, and ΔQ and ΔP are changes in Q and P. This formula is known as a *point elasticity formula*. The point elasticity formula is appropriate for very small changes along the demand curve. If the change in price is at all appreciable, an average elasticity measure over the range of the demand curve covered by the change is more appropriate. This measure, known as the *arc elasticity of demand*, is written as

$$E_p = \frac{(Q_2 - Q_1) \, / \, (Q_2 + Q_1)}{(P_2 - P_1) \, / \, (P_2 + P_1)}$$

in which Q_1 and P_1 refer to one price and quantity set and Q_2 and P_2 refer to a second set at another point on the same demand curve. In fact, both the price and quantity changes are expressed as ratios to average price and quantity levels, that is, as $(P_1 + P_2) \, / \, 2$ and $(Q_1 + Q_2) \, / \, 2$. The 2s would cancel out, leaving us with the formula as presented.

An example will help to illustrate the use of this formula. Assume that the Richland County Health Department charges \$3.00 per syphilis test, and that, in May, it performed 1,200 tests. In June, the County Council decided to raise the charges to \$3.25 per test. Only 1,150 people requested tests in June. What is the price elasticity of demand?

The elasticity measure of a price change is supposed to be a measure of responsiveness along a demand curve, that is, when all factors other than price remain constant. If other factors have, indeed, remained constant, we can use the elasticity formula as an approximation of the responsiveness of quantity demanded to price changes. If other factors have changed, we must make some adjustment to take into account the extent to which these other factors influenced the quantity demanded. In our example, assume that these other factors remained constant and that only price influenced quantity. In this case, we can use the price elasticity formula directly:

$$E_p = \frac{(1,150 - 1,200) \, / \, (1,150 + 1,200)}{(3.25 - 3) \, / \, (3.25 + 3)} = -0.53$$

The elasticity of demand at that point is -0.53. (The minus sign is frequently dropped from discussions, so one will often see the price elasticity quoted as the absolute value, for example, 0.53. The reader should remember that, in the case of price elasticity, the negative sign, if dropped, is taken for granted.) We thus have a figure indicating the responsiveness of quantity to price.

Price elasticity is related to how total consumer expenditures respond to a change in the out-of-pocket price. For any elasticity measure whose absolute value is less than 1, total out-of-pocket expenditures will increase with a decrease in price; at such points on the demand curve, demand is said to be inelastic. When demand is relatively inelastic, the demand curve is steeper. In our example, total expenditures ($P \times Q$) were \$3,600.00 before the price change and \$3,737.50 after. Receipts from this source rose by \$137.50 because of the nature of the responsiveness at that point on the demand curve. An elasticity measure of -0.53 is thought of as relatively unresponsive, that is, a small relative price rise or fall will generate a smaller relative quantity change. If price increases by 1%, the quantity will decrease by only about 0.5%, and the total amount spent on syphilis tests will increase. With an elasticity of -0.53, a reduction in price will lower total expenditures (i.e., total consumer expenditures in terms of dollars), because the relative increase in quantity purchased will not be sufficient to overcome the relatively greater price decrease. Thus, if the Richland County Health Department wants more revenue, and does not care about how many tests are performed, it should raise its price to $3.25.

Demand curves can also have unitary elastic and elastic portions. When the elasticity measures –1, demand responsiveness is said to be *unitary elastic*. In the case of a small change in price, total expenditures will remain constant. When the demand responsiveness is elastic (i.e., greater than 1 in absolute value), it means that the relative change in quantity consumed exceeds the relative change in price. If there is a small increase in price, the decrease in quantity will be relatively greater, and total expenditures will fall. If there is a small decrease in price, total expenditures will rise. When demand is relatively elastic, the demand curve has a flatter slope.

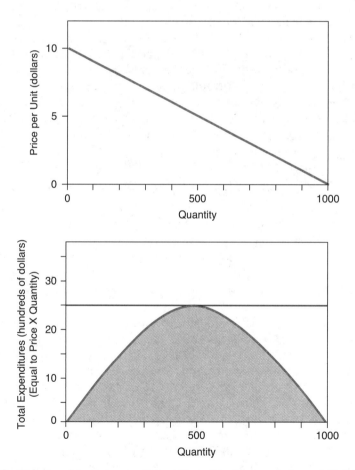

Figure 3-3 Relationship Between Price, Quantity Demanded, and Total Revenue. Graph A shows the basic relationship between quantity demanded and price. Graph B shows the relationship between total expenditures (which equal price times quantity) and quantity. Graph B is derived from Graph A.

These relationships are shown in Figure 3-3. A straight-line demand curve for vaccinations is shown in Graph A. At a price of $10, no vaccinations are demanded, but as the price falls in $1 increments, vaccination demand increases by 100. Thus, at a price of $9, there will be 100 vaccinations demanded; at a price of $8, there will be 200 demanded; and so on. Graph B shows the total expenditures generated at each level of sales. Thus, if 100 vaccinations are sold, $900 in expenditures is generated, and so on (see Table 3-2 for the actual values). Over a range, total expenditures increase, but eventually the increase levels off to a maximum, and beyond that point total expenditures begin to decline.

There is a connection between the elasticity along a specific segment of the demand curve and the total expenditures specific to relevant points on the curve. At relatively high prices and low quantities on a straight-line demand curve, only a relatively small change in price (in terms of percentage) is needed to induce a relatively large change in the quantity demanded. The lower expenditures resulting from the fall in unit prices is therefore more than offset by the large increase in quantity demanded, and so total expenditures will increase. For example, in Table 3-2, for a reduction in price from $9 to $8, the arc elasticity of demand along that segment of the curve is –4.76. Demand is therefore said to be elastic, and if that reduction in price is instituted, total expenditures will increase (in this case, from $900 to $1,600). As we move down the demand curve, the relative price change becomes smaller in relation to the associated quantity change. Thus, the absolute value of elasticity falls. But as long as this value in absolute terms is greater than 1 (i.e., we are on the elastic portion of the curve), total expenditures will increase, although not by as much as in higher priced segments. Eventually, the elasticity takes on a value of –1. At this point, price and quantity changes offset each other exactly, and total expenditures stay constant (we are at the top of the total

Table 3-2 Price for Vaccinations, Quantity Demanded, and Total Expenditures

Price	Quantity Demanded	Total Expenditures
$10	0	$0
9	100	900
8	200	1,600
7	300	2,100
6	400	2,400
5	500	2,500
4	600	2,400
3	700	2,100
2	800	1,600
1	900	900

expenditures curve). As prices fall further, we move on to the inelastic portion of the demand curve. Price reductions offset quantity increases, and total expenditures fall.

Thus, along any single straight-line demand curve, the elasticity of demand will decrease with successive reductions in price. While elasticity is related to slope, it is not identical with the slope of the curve. For example, the slope of a linear curve is constant, but the elasticity varies along the linear demand curve. Slope is defined as "rise over run," in which rise reflects the change in price and run reflects the change in quantity. As indicated, slope is the ratio of changes in two variables, and elasticity is the ratio of percentage changes in two variables.

Further insight into the concept of elasticity can be gained by examining elasticity for two different demand curves at a single price. Assume that two demand curves in two different markets for physician visits cross at a price of $3, as in Figure 3-4. The consumers in Market 2 are more responsive to price reductions than are those in Market 1.

Let *AD* be the demand curve in Market 1 and *BC* be the demand curve in Market 2. Now let the price fall by 10 cents. Consumers in Market 1 demand 10,300 visits, whereas those in Market 2 demand 10,500. The arc elasticity in Market 1 is

$$E = \frac{300 / 20{,}300}{-0.10 / 5.90} = -0.87$$

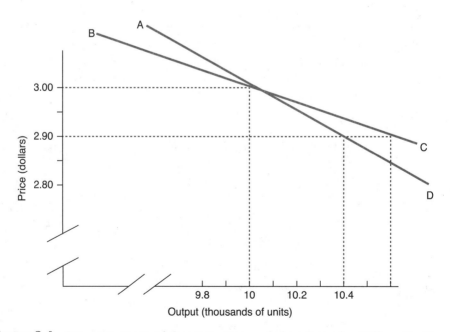

Figure 3-4 Responsiveness of Quantity Demanded to Price for Differently Sloped Demand Curves. Curve BC shows a greater responsiveness of quantity demanded to price than curve AD.

The arc elasticity in Market 2 is

$$E = \frac{500 \,/\, 20{,}500}{-0.10 \,/\, 5.90} = -1.44$$

As can be seen, demand curve *BC* is for a more responsive group of consumers, and the elasticity for a given quantity will be greater in absolute value than that of a less responsive group.

3.6 INSURANCE, OUT-OF-POCKET PRICE, AND QUANTITY DEMANDED

A major factor in considering the demand for medical care is the role that insurance plays in influencing the out-of-pocket price of medical care. There are a number of different types of insurance arrangements that consumers can obtain, and these will affect the out-of-pocket price and hence, the quantity demanded in different ways. We will examine the important alternatives.

In analyzing the effect of alternative insurance arrangements, we initially specify a demand curve in which the consumers have no insurance and hence, pay the full price charged by the provider (e.g., a physician). This curve, in which full price equals the out-of-pocket price, is labeled D_n in Figure 3-5.

Now let us introduce the first type of insurance arrangement: a coinsurance arrangement. A coinsurance is a payment by the patient of a proportion of the charged price; the insurance company pays the remainder of the charged price. For example, with a 20% coinsurance rate and a charged price of $20 per visit, the patient pays the provider 20% of the charged price, $4, and the insurance

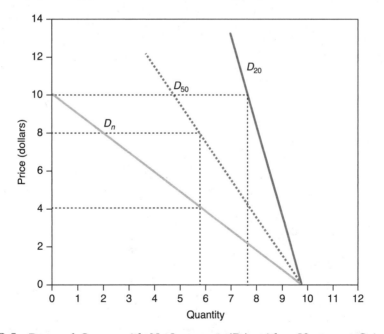

Figure 3-5   Demand Curves with No Insurance (D_n), with a 50-percent Coinsurance (D_{50}), and with a 20-percent Coinsurance (D_{20}). When there is a coinsurance rate, D_n also represents the relation between the quantity demanded and the out-of-pocket price.

company pays the remaining $16. In analyzing the impact of a coinsurance contract on demand, we assume that, even though the consumer has purchased an insurance contract, demand behavior is still governed by the demand curve D_n. What changes is that the out-of-pocket price and charged price now differ from one another. At any given charged price, the consumer faces a lower out-of-pocket price and hence, will move down the demand curve D_n.

If the coinsurance rate is 50%, the demand curve facing the provider is D_{50} (Figure 3-5). Here, at any charged price, the out-of-pocket price is one-half the charged price, and the consumer demands a quantity determined by the out-of-pocket price and the demand curve D_n. In fact, D_n becomes the demand curve relating quantity to out-of-pocket price. Thus, if the provider's charge were $8 per visit (in Figure 3-5), the consumer with a 50% coinsurance contract would pay a $4 out-of-pocket price and the quantity demanded would be six visits. If the coinsurance rate was 20%, the market demand curve facing the providers would be D_{20}. A charged price of $10 would mean an out-of-pocket price of $2 and a quantity demanded of eight. As the coinsurance rate falls, the market demand curve facing the providers shifts out, but the curve D_n continues to represent the relation between quantity demanded and out-of-pocket price.

Next, we examine the impact of an indemnity contract, which sets a fixed per-unit amount up to which the insurer will pay in the event of a service being used. For example, if an individual has pediatric coverage, an indemnity contract might specify that the insurer will pay up to $4 per visit. If the price is greater than $4, the consumer is responsible for the balance. In Figure 3-6, D_n is again the demand curve with no insurance coverage. Now, let the individual purchase an indemnity contract that requires the insurer to reimburse the provider up to $4 per visit. The demand curve facing the provider becomes D_{n+i}, which is the D_n curve raised by $4 at all points. The

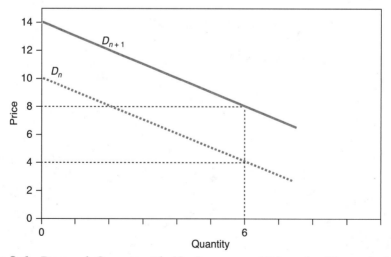

Figure 3-6 Demand Curves with No Insurance (D_n) and with an Indemnity (Copayment) Amount of $4 ($D_{n+1}$). When there is a copayment, D_n also represents the relationship between the quantity demanded and the out-of-pocket price.

position of D_{n+i} is such that, at each price charged, the out-of-pocket price will be $4 less than this, and the quantity demanded will reflect this lower out-of-pocket price. In Figure 3-6, a charged price of $8 means an out-of-pocket price of $4 and a quantity demanded of six. An increase in the amount by which the insurer indemnifies the consumer would shift D_{n+i} upward. The curve D_n would remain the same.

Finally, we examine the impact of a deductible, which is a fixed total amount that the insurer deducts from the bill; the consumer must spend up to this amount before coverage begins. Until the consumer spends this amount, he or she pays the full price for each additional unit consumed (the price paid for the next additional unit is called the *marginal out-of-pocket price*). The marginal out-of-pocket price before the deductible is reached is the charged price. If there is no coinsurance in addition to the deductible, the marginal out-of-pocket price, after the deductible is met, is zero.

To analyze the impact of a deductible on demand, we will slightly reinterpret the demand curve. Assume that the curve shows the value to the consumer of each additional visit (the marginal value). If the patient consumes one visit, the value of the visit is $9. The second visit has a smaller marginal value, in this case $8. The two visits together would have a value of $17. These numbers, and the value of additional visits, are contained in Table 3-3. The table shows a declining marginal value for successive visits, which is consistent with what we assumed in deriving the demand hypothesis.

Let us now assume a market price of $8 and a deductible of $32. At this market price, the out-of-pocket marginal price to the consumer will be $8 per visit until (and if) the deductible is met. Thereafter, it will be zero (if there is no coinsurance as well). In answering the question of how many visits will be demanded, we must look at the consumer's valuation of visits in

Table 3-3 Schedule of Value of Additional Medical Visits to Patient and Total (Summed) Value of All Units of Care

Quantity	Value of Additional Unit of Care to Consumer	Total Value of All Care Received up to Given Quantity
1	$9	$9
2	8	17
3	7	24
4	6	30
5	5	35
6	4	39
7	3	42
8	2	44
9	1	45
10	0	45

Table 3-3 and compare these with the marginal out-of-pocket price and the deductible level. At first we might be tempted to say that only the first two visits are worth at least the marginal out-of-pocket price and so only two will be demanded. One would then conclude that, having spent $16 in total, the consumer did not meet the deductible, and so the visits will end at two.

But our consumer is truly a logical "economic person" and will look more carefully at all the options. The consumer realizes that he or she could buy the third and fourth units and, in doing so, use up the deductible of $32. Once the deductible is used up, the rest of the visits demanded would be free! Indeed, if the individual consumed nine units, the value to him or her of all of them would be $45, well in excess of the outlay of $32 for the first four units. In general, we can say that, with a deductible, the amount demanded will be determined by the consumer's comparison of the additional value of all extra units with the additional out-of-pocket cost of all extra units. Even if the marginal value of the next visit (third, in this case) is less than its marginal out-of-pocket price, overall it will pay the individual to spend more in order to receive the benefits of the post deductible units. If, however, the deductible was $100 and the charged price $8, the individual would stop consuming at two units because there would be no other quantity of consumption at which the total value to the individual exceeded what the individual had to pay.

Frequently, a deductible and a coinsurance are found together in the same policy. In our example, a $32 deductible is combined with a 20% coinsurance (on units of care after the deductible has been reached). With a charged price of $8, the individual would then pay a marginal out-of-pocket price of $1.60 for each unit consumed after four. The individual would overspend the deductible in this case, but would demand only eight visits, because the ninth, costing $1.60, would have a marginal value of only $1.

3.7 ELASTICITY OF DEMAND ESTIMATES

Demand responsiveness can be measured by natural experiments and controlled trials. A natural experiment (in the demand context) occurs, for example, when a change in insurance coverage is implemented by an insurer. We can use the results of such a policy action to determine demand responsiveness by conducting before-and-after comparisons of the data. Assuming all else has remained the same (e.g., that an increase in a deductible has not driven the sicker insureds to buy more complete insurance elsewhere), we can use the data to measure the degree of responsiveness. Natural experiments, unfortunately, often do not provide sufficient information. The investigators have no control over insurer policy decisions and are therefore restricted to researching the changes in price and coverage introduced by the insurers.

A more flexible, but also more expensive, approach is to do a controlled experiment. In this approach, study groups are selected randomly (to avoid any bias due to self-selection, such as sicker individuals choosing more complete insurance coverage) and assigned to specific categories (e.g., 20% coinsurance, 40% coinsurance, etc.). Differences in utilization (which are assumed to be caused by differences in demand) can be measured, and thus, a measure of demand responsiveness can be obtained.

An example of a natural experiment in the demand field occurred in 1977, when the United Mine Workers introduced a $250 deductible for inpatient services and a 40% coinsurance for physician and outpatient visits up to a maximum family liability of $500. Prior to this, the insureds had no out-of-pocket expenses.

Scheffler (1984) conducted a study of the impact of this cost sharing on hospital admissions, average length of hospital stay, the probability that an insured would have at least one physician visit, and the number of times an insured visited a physician. According to the analysis, in the five months prior to introduction of the hospital deductible (the comparison period), the hospital admission rate was 6.8 per 1,000 enrollees, and the average length of stay per hospitalization was 5.42 days. The corresponding figures for the five months after introduction (the study period) were 4.8 per 1,000 for admissions and 6.45 days per hospitalization. The longer average length of stay in the study period may have been due to the fact that only sicker cases were hospitalized, with individuals with typical short lengths of stay now not being admitted to the hospital at all. With regard to physician visits, the study's results indicated that the proportion of the population seeing a physician at least once fell from 44% in the comparison period to 28% in the study period, and the average number of visits of those who did see a physician at least once fell from 2.3 to 1.6.

The results of this experiment, like the results of other such studies, convincingly demonstrate the immediate impact of cost-sharing policies on utilization. But do the reductions in utilization last? Are there bad consequences farther down the line? One study (Scitovsky & McCall, 1977) verified that reductions in physician visits did last several years, but several others have raised doubts as to whether longer-term impacts occur.

By far, the best-known controlled experiment in this area is the six-site Health Insurance Experiment conducted by the Rand Corporation (Newhouse et al., 1981). In this study, 2,756 families agreed to participate in an experiment in which each family was assigned to one of five groups with different coinsurance rates. The rates included free care (0 coinsurance), 25, 50, and 95% coinsurance, and a deductible with 95% coinsurance (all services, such as physician visits and hospitalization, were covered under the single rate). Those families with greater potential out-of-pocket expenses than their preexperiment coverage were compensated accordingly. Upper limits were placed on each family's out-of-pocket expenses. The families participated for three to five years.

The results dramatically indicated the differential impact of higher out-of-pocket expenses. For example, those with free care incurred average expenses for all services of $401, whereas those with 25, 50, and 95% coinsurance incurred expenses of $346, $328, and $254, respectively. Furthermore, these differentials held up over several years. Because the experiment was designed to control for all other intervening factors (e.g., health status, income, etc.), the results have had a considerable impact in health policy circles. The fact is that such controlled results are seldom obtained.

Several questions have been raised concerning the applicability of the study's results. First, the experiments affected only a small portion of the entire healthcare market in each of the six communities studied. If coinsurance rates were raised for the entire market, or a substantial portion of the market, would providers (physicians) react and generate additional demand, thus changing the results? Furthermore, the aged (and presumably the fragile) were omitted from the study. Would their responses be any different?

Despite the unanswered questions, such studies have moved us closer toward developing a quantitative measure of the impact of out-of-pocket price on demand. As seen previously, demand elasticity depends on the starting point on an individual's demand curve, which, in turn, is affected by the individual's level of insurance. A rough estimate of demand elasticity when consumers have 0 to 25% coinsurance is –0.2 (Newhouse, Phelps, & Marquis., 1980).

Such an estimate can be used in the following way. If the price for a physician visit is $100, the coinsurance rate is 10%, and initially there are 120 visits, what would be the expected number of visits after the coinsurance rate is raised to 20%? The answer (assuming an elasticity of –0.2) is obtained by solving for Q_2 (visits in Period 2), in which

$$E = \frac{(Q_2 - Q_1) \, / \, (Q_2 - Q_1)}{(P_2 - P_1) \, / \, (P_2 + P_1)}$$

or

$$-0.2 = \frac{(Q_2 - 120) \, / \, (Q_2 + 120)}{(20 - 10) \, / \, (20 + 10)}$$

The result gives a value for Q_2 of 104 visits (rounded to the nearest integer). In this case, the total price did not change, although the coinsurance rate and therefore the out-of-pocket price did. A similar analysis could be done if the charged price and the copayment rate had both been changed.

A number of studies have been conducted analyzing demand in the nursing home market. Nursing home care is a healthcare service whose demand has distinct characteristics that have an impact on its elasticity of demand. First, there are a significant number of self-pay (uninsured) patients in this market; in 2009, out-of-pocket payments accounted for 29% of all nursing home expenditures. For those patients who are not covered by public insurance (primarily through Medicaid), the out-of-pocket price becomes an important variable, because private insurance for long-term care is still a minor factor. Second, there are close substitutes for nursing home care. Home health care is, in many instances, a viable alternative to nursing home care. Also, some patients who are hospitalized and could be moved to a skilled nursing care facility "economize" on skilled nursing home care by remaining in the hospital longer and transferring later or not at all. The existence of close substitutes increases the elasticity of demand for nursing home care.

Lamberton and colleagues (1986) conducted a cross-county study of nursing home demand in South Dakota. In analyzing the relationship between nursing home days and such variables as price, income, and home care visits, they estimated an elasticity of demand for private patients of –0.76.

They also detected a significant negative relationship between home care visits and nursing home care, which substantiated the hypothesis that the two forms of care are substitutes. These results, which show that nursing home care has greater elasticity of demand than hospital care, were expected. Given the current interest in expanding long-term care insurance, an elasticity of this magnitude indicates that the demand for long-term care would increase substantially, if long-term care insurance were to increase (because the out-of-pocket price of long-term care would be lowered).

EXERCISES

1. Distinguish between demand and quantity demanded.
2. State two distinct hypotheses about the relationship between price and quantity demanded.
3. Indicate how each of the following factors will change the individual demand curve for aspirin tablets:
   a. an increase in income
   b. an increase in the price of Tylenol (a substitute)
   c. an increase in the price of bottled water (a complement)
   d. an increase in the number of people with headaches
   e. the discovery that aspirin, if taken regularly, reduces the severity of heart attacks
4. Determine whether and how each of the following factors would shift the demand curve for chiropractic visits:
   a. an increase in the out-of-pocket price of chiropractic visits
   b. an increase in back problems
   c. a reduction in the out-of-pocket price for chiropractic visits
   d. an aging of the population
   e. an increase in the out-of-pocket price of back surgery (a substitute for chiropractic services)
   f. a reduction in the price of radiographs (a complement of chiropractic services)
   g. an advertising campaign that makes people more aware of the benefits of chiropractic care
5. What will be the effect on the market demand for aspirin in North Dakota, if the population of North Dakota increases?
6. In a small town in Florida, a food supplement sold for $2.00 a bottle in May. In total, 2,000 bottles were sold. In June, nothing else changed but the price of the supplement, which was increased to $2.20. A total of 1,900 bottles were sold. What is the elasticity of demand?
7. Smith has insurance coverage for drugs. The insurance company will pay 50% of the price charged by the pharmacy. Smith went to the store in May. The price of aspirin was $0.50 per tablet. Smith bought 60 for the month. Next month, Smith found that the

pharmacy had raised the price to $0.60 per tablet. Smith bought only 50 tablets. What is the elasticity of demand for aspirin?

8. Estimate the elasticity of demand for physician checkups from the following market data from a small state. The population in the state has remained the same.

Month	Average Age of Population	Persons with Flu	Out of Pocket Price	Number of Check-ups
October	40	Many	$30	5,000
November	40	Few	$35	3,000
December	45	Few	$40	2,500
January	40	Many	$35	4,800

9. Determine whether and how each of the following factors would shift the demand for home care:
   a. an increase of $10 in the price per day charged by nursing homes, with the government picking up the entire price increase
   b. an increase, from $12 to $15, in the price paid out of pocket by users of home care
   c. an increase in the number of people being discharged early from hospital
   d. an increase in productivity among home care providers
   e. an increase in the percentage of low-income people in a given population

10. A social survey taken in the town of Maple Ridge yielded the following information for five consecutive years. Determine from the results of these surveys what direct effect price has on quantity demanded (i.e., elasticity) of physician visits.

Year	Average Health	Average Income	Direct Price Per Visit	Quantity Demanded (visits per person)
1	Good	$10,000	$5	3
2	Good	$10,000	$5	3
3	Poor	$6,000	$5	5
4	Poor	$6,000	$4	6
5	Poor	$4,000	$4	5

11. The elasticity of demand for physician visits was determined to be −0.2. The president of the local health insurance company wants to add a copayment of $0.50 onto each physician visit. Currently, there is no copayment. The number of insured people is 3,000,000, and currently, the population uses 2.4 visits per capita. How many visits will they use after the introduction of the copayment?

12. Currently, there is a $0.50 copayment on drugs. The HMO has decided to raise this to $1.00 per prescription. The cost of a prescription is $6.00, which means the HMO's contribution to the total cost will fall from $5.50 to $5.00. Currently, the elasticity of demand is about −0.5 for prescriptions, and the HMO members use 2.2 prescriptions per capita. How much will be demanded after the new copayment is put into effect, and how much money will this save the HMO?

BIBLIOGRAPHY

Consumer Demand: Analysis and Surveys

Frech, H. E., & Ginsburg, P. B. (1975). Imposed health insurance in monopolistic markets. *Economic Inquiry, 13*, 55–69.

Gilligan, P., Winder, S., Ramphul, N., & O'Kelly, P. (2010). The referral and complete evaluation time study. *European Journal of Emergency Medicine, 17*(6), 349–353.

Ginsburg, P. B., & Manheim, L. (1973). Insurance, copayment and health services utilization. *Journal of Economics and Business, 25*, 142–153.

Higginson, I., Whyatt, J., & Silvester, K. (2011). Demand and capacity planning in the emergency department: How to do it. *Emergency Medicine Journal, 28*(2), 128–135.

Joseph, H. (1971). Empirical research on the demand for health care. *Inquiry, 8*, 61–71.

Mukatash, G. N., Al-Rousan, M., & Al-Sakarna, B. (2010). Needs and demands of prosthetic treatment among two groups of individuals. *Indian Journal of Dental Research, 21*(4), 564–567.

Mushkin, S. J. (1974). *Consumer incentives for health care.* New York, NY: Neale Watson.

Patterson, P., Millar, B., & Visser, A. (2011). The development of an instrument to assess the unmet needs of young people who have a sibling with cancer: Piloting the sibling cancer needs instrument (SCNI). *Journal of Pediatric Oncology Nursing, 28*(1), 16–26.

Rice, T., & Morrison, K. R. (1994). Patient cost sharing for medical services. *Medical Care Review, 51*, 235–287.

Robertson, B. D., & McConnel, C. E. (2011). Town-level comparisons may be an effective alternative in comparing rural and urban differences: A look at accidental traumatic brain injuries in north Texas children. *Rural & Remote Health, 11*(1), 1521.

Tomura, H., Yamamoto-Mitani, N., Nagata, S., Murashima, S., & Suzuki, S. (2011). Creating an agreed discharge planning for clients with high care needs. *Journal of Clinical Nursing, 20*(3/4), 444–453.

Empirical Studies

Alexander, D. L., Flynn, J. E., & Linkins, L. A. (1994). Estimates of the demand for ethical pharmaceutical drugs across countries and time. *Applied Economics, 26*, 821–826.

Beck, R. G. (1974). The effect of co-payments on the poor. *Journal of Human Resources, 9*, 129–142.

Bennett, K. M., Vaslef, S., Pappas, T. N., & Scarborough, J. E. (2011). The volume-outcomes relationship for United States level I trauma centers. *Journal of Surgical Research, 167*(1), 19–23.

Burns, K. M., Evans, F., & Kaltman, J. R. (2011). Pediatric ICD utilization in the United States from 1997 to 2006. *Heart Rhythm, 8*(1), 23–28.

Chiswick, B. R. (1976). The demand for nursing home care. *Journal of Human Resources, 11,* 295–316.

Coulson, N. E., Terza, J. V., Neslusan, C. A., & Stuart, B. C. (1995). Estimating the moral-hazard effect of supplemental medical insurance in the demand for prescription drugs by the elderly. *American Economic Review, 85,* 122–126.

Davis, K., & Russell, L. B. (1972). The substitution of outpatient care for inpatient care. *Review of Economics and Statistics, 54,* 109–120.

De Angelis, G., Murthy, A., Beyersmann, J., & Harbarth, S. (2010). Estimating the impact of healthcare-associated infections on length of stay and costs. *Clinical Microbiology & Infection, 16*(12), 1729–1735.

Dent, A., Hunter, G., & Webster, A. P. (2010). The impact of frequent attenders on a UK emergency department. *European Journal of Emergency Medicine, 17*(6), 332–336.

Duan, N., Manning, W. G. Jr., Morris, C. N., & Newhouse, J. P. (1983). A comparison of alternative models for the demand for medical care. *Journal of Business and Economic Statistics, 1,* 115–126.

Duke, J., Wood, F., Semmens, J., Edgar, D. W., Spilsbury, K., Hendrie, D., & Rea, S. (2011). A study of burn hospitalization for children younger than 5 years of age: 1983–2008. *Pediatrics, 127*(4), e971–e977.

Eichner, M. J. (1998). The demand for medical care: What people pay does matter. *American Economic Review, 88,* 117–121.

Einav, L., & Finkelstein, A. (2011). Selection in insurance markets: Theory and empirics in pictures. *Journal of Economic Perspectives, 25*(1), 115–138.

Epstein, A. J., Polsky, D., Yang, F., Yang, L., & Groeneveld, P. W. (2010). Coronary revascularization trends in the United States, 2001–2008. *JAMA, 305*(17), 1769–1776.

Freiburg, L., & Scutchfield, F. D. (1976). Insurance and the demand for hospital care. *Inquiry, 13,* 54–60.

Gold, M. (1984). The demand for hospital outpatient services. *Health Services Research, 19,* 384–412.

Gourin, C. G., Forastiere, A. A., Sanguineti, G., Marur, S., Koch, W. M., & Bristow, R. E. (2011). Volume-based trends in surgical care of patients with oropharyngeal cancer. *Laryngoscope, 121*(4), 738–745.

Hall, J. P., Fox, M. H., & Fall, E. (2010). The Kansas medicaid buy-in: Factors influencing enrollment and health care utilization. *Disability & Health Journal, 3*(2), 99–106.

Hellinger, F. (1977). Substitutability among different types of care under Medicare. *Health Services Research, 12,* 11–18.

Hershey, J. C., Luft, H. S., & Gianaris, J. M. (1975). Making sense out of utilization data. *Medical Care, 13,* 838–851.

Holtmann, A. G., & Olsen, E. O. (1978). *The economics of the private demand for outpatient health care.* Publication no. NIH-78-1262. Bethesda, MD: John E. Fogarty Center of the National Institutes of Health.

Hurd, M. D., & McGarry, K. (1997). Medical insurance and the use of health care services by the elderly. *Journal of Health Economics, 16,* 129–154.

Johnston, D., Samus, Q. M., Morrison, A., Leoutsakos, J. S., Hicks, K., Handel, S. . . . Black, B. S. (2011). Identification of community-residing individuals with dementia and their unmet needs for care. *International Journal of Geriatric Psychiatry, 26*(3), 292–298.

Kazer, M. W., Bailey, D. E., Jr., Colberg, J., Kelly, W. K., & Carroll, P. (2011). The needs for men undergoing active surveillance (AS) for prostate cancer: Results of a focus group study. *Journal of Clinical Nursing, 20*(3/4), 581–586.

Keeler, E. B., & Rolph, J. (1983). How cost spending reduced medical spending of participants in the health insurance experiment. *JAMA, 249,* 2220–2222.

Lamberton, C. E., Ellingson, W. D., & Spear, K. R. (1986). Factors determining the demand for nursing home services. *Quarterly Review of Economics and Business, 26*, 74–90.

Maulik, P. K., Mendelson, T., & Tandon, S. D. (2011). Factors associated with mental health services use among disconnected African-American young adult population. *Journal of Behavioral Health Services & Research, 38*(2), 205–220.

Mosen, D. M., Schatz, M., Gold, R., Mularski, R. A., Wong, W. F., & Bellows, J. (2010). Medication use, emergency hospital care utilization, and quality-of-life outcome disparities by race/ethnicity among adults with asthma. *American Journal of Managed Care, 16*(11), 821–828.

Nelson, A. A. Jr., Reeder, C. E., & Dickson, W. M. (1984). The effect of a Medicaid drug copayment program on the utilization and cost of prescription services. *Medical Care, 22*, 724–736.

Newhouse, J. P., Phelps, C. E., & Marquis, M. S. (1980). On having your cake and eating it too. *Journal of Econometrics, 13*, 365–390.

Newhouse, J. P., Manning, W. G., Morris, C. N., Orr, L. L., Keeler, E. B., Leibowitz, A., ... Brock, R. H. (1981). Some interim results from a controlled trial of cost sharing in health insurance. *New England Journal of Medicine, 305*, 1501–1507.

O'Sullivan, A. K., Sullivan, J., Higuchi, K., & Montgomery, A. B. (2011). Health care utilization and costs for cystic fibrosis patients with pulmonary infections. *Managed Care, 20*(2), 37–44.

Pinkhasov, R. M., Wong, J., Kashanian, J., Lee, M., Samadi, D. B., Pinkhasov, M. M., & Shabsigh, R. (2010). Are men shortchanged on health? Perspective on health care utilization and health risk behavior in men and women in the United States. *International Journal of Clinical Practice, 64*(4), 475–487.

Ravn, H. B., Lindskov, C., Folkersen, L., & Hvas, A. M. (2011). Transfusion requirements in 811 patients during and after cardiac surgery: A prospective observational study. *Journal of Cardiothoracic & Vascular Anesthesia, 25*(1), 36–41.

Reeder, C. E., & Nelson, A. A. (1985). The differential impact of a copayment on drug use in a Medicaid population. *Inquiry, 22*, 396–403.

Schatz, M., Zeiger, R. S., Yang, S. J., Chen, W., Crawford, W. W., Sajjan, S. G., & Allen-Ramey, F. (2010). Persistent asthma defined using HEDIS versus survey criteria. *American Journal of Managed Care, 16*(11), e281–e288.

Scheffler, R. M. (1984). The United Mine Worker's health plan. *Medical Care, 22*, 247–254.

Scitovsky, A. A., & McCall, N. (1977). Coinsurance and the demand for physician services. *Social Security Bulletin, 40*(May), 19–27.

Stewart, K. E., Phillips, M. M., Walker, J. F., Harvey, S. A., & Porter, A. (2011). Social services utilization and need among a community sample of persons living with HIV in the rural south. *AIDS Care, 23*(3), 340–347.

Strickland, B. B., Jones, J. R., Ghandour, R. M., Kogan, M. D., & Newacheck, P. W. (2011). The medical home: Health care access and impact for children and youth in the United States. *Pediatrics, 127*(4), 604–611.

Toy, E. L., Beaulieu, N. U., McHale, J. M., Welland, T. R., Plauschinat, C. A., Swensen, A., & Duh, M. S. (2011). Treatment of COPD: Relationships between daily dosing frequency, adherence, resource use, and costs. *Respiratory Medicine, 105*(3), 435–441.

Venkatraman, G., Likosky, D. S., Morrison, D., Zhou, W., Finlayson, S. R., & Goodman, D. C. (2011). Small area variation in endoscopic sinus surgery rates among the Medicare population. *Archives of Otolaryngology—Head & Neck Surgery, 137*(3), 253–257.

Warner, J., & Hu, T.-W. (1977). Hospitalization insurance and the demand for inpatient care. In B. C. Martin (Ed.), *Socioeconomic issues of health*. Chicago, IL: American Medical Association.

Wulfman, C., Tezenas du Montcel, S., Jonas, P., Fattouh, J., & Rignon-Bret C. (2010). Aesthetic demand of French seniors: A large-scale study. *Gerodontology, 27*(4), 266–271.

Yu, J., Harman, J. S., Hall, A. G., & Duncan, R. P. (2011). Impact of Medicaid/SCHIP disenrollment on health care utilization and expenditures among children: A longitudinal analysis. *Medical Care Research & Review, 68*(1), 56–74.

Zgraj, O., Clarke Moloney, M., Motherway, C., & Grace, P. A. (2010). Provision of general paediatric surgical services in a regional hospital. *Irish Journal of Medical Science, 179*(1), 29–33.

Chapter 4

Additional Topics in the Demand for Health and Medical Care

OBJECTIVES

1. Identify the wider implications of changes in the demand for health services.

2. Identify the private, external, and social demand for health services.

3. Explain how changes in the quality of care will influence the demand for health care.

4. Explain how time costs influence the demand for health services.

5. Explain the factors that influence the demand for health.

6. Explain the roles of the principal and the agent in determining the demand for medical care when the consumer has imperfect information about his or her health status and the productivity of medical care.

7. Explain the model of the demand for preventive health services when the consumer is uncertain about his or her health status.

8. Explain the concept of discounting by which the consumer places lower valuations on future health benefits than on present benefits.

4.1 INTRODUCTION

Earlier in the text, the demand for medical care was introduced as if medical care were an ordinary everyday good or service. Some types of medical care *are* ordinary everyday goods and services. Pediatric well-child visits, the consumption of aspirin, and visits to a dentist are routine occurrences for many people. However, the circumstances surrounding many types of medical care are quite unlike the circumstances surrounding the use of everyday goods and services (Culyer, 1971). As a result, the traditional model must be modified to incorporate special factors. This chapter brings these factors into consideration by showing how they influence the demand relation as developed elsewhere in the text.

In section 4.2, we examine the economic implications of one alleged characteristic of medical care—that it is indispensable for life and health. In section 4.3, we analyze the implications for medical care demand when individuals other than direct consumers are concerned with the consumption of medical care by direct consumers. In this context, we look at the relationships among private, external, and social demand. In section 4.4, we examine the influence of quality differences on medical care demand. Section 4.5 is concerned with situations in which the money paid for medical care is not an adequate reflection of the total resource commitment made by the patient in acquiring medical care. In particular, patients devote a great deal of traveling and waiting time in obtaining medical care. This section develops a more general picture of the cost of medical care, including the role of time costs. In section 4.6, we analyze the consumer's choice behavior in terms of the demand for health rather than the demand for medical care. In this analysis, medical care and other resources are viewed as inputs in the production of a more fundamental good: health. As such, the demand for health care is a derived demand; it is derived from the demand for better health.

In Section 4.7, we discuss the role of the physician as an agent for the patient; under certain circumstances, the physician will participate in the process of determining demand, a situation that can lead to "supplier-induced demand." The demand for medical care is not always determined under conditions of certainty. Often, the patient will not know when he or she will require medical care. Under these uncertain conditions, the individual consumer may purchase care on a prepaid basis (insurance); as well, the consumer will decide whether or not to engage in certain activities that influence health, such as exercise, smoking, and eating certain foods. In Section 4.7, we present a preliminary introduction to the topic of demand under conditions of uncertainty. Finally, many health-related activities will have effects that extend into future time periods. Individuals' valuations of benefits in future time periods will be less than those in the current time period. In Section 4.7, we introduce the concept of discounting of future benefits.

4.2 IMPLICATIONS OF HEALTH CARE FOR LIFE AND HEALTH

One of the most widely cited characteristics of medical care is its ability to improve health. In some instances, if a person does not obtain timely medical care, he or she may die or become permanently disabled. Where this condition holds (e.g., after a heart attack or a serious traffic accident), the question of substitutes, or price of services, will have little importance. Presumably, the person would be willing to disburse all of his or her wealth to receive lifesaving medical care, and the demand curve would be vertical, reflecting absolute inelasticity of demand.

However, such instances amount to a very small portion of the total number of situations that cause individuals to seek medical care. In the vast majority of cases, alternative courses of action are available, and individuals have the time to consider the options. In fact, medical care should be viewed as a spectrum of services and goods rather than as a good or service only sought and consumed in an emergency. The less a situation calls for immediate action, and the greater the relevance of substitutes, the less steeply sloped the demand curve is for medical care. For example, dental checkups can be given annually, monthly, or weekly. Few would consider monthly or weekly checkups to be necessary, or even reasonable. Substitutes are important even in emergency situations: individuals and planners have a wide variety of alternatives they can choose in advance of dire circumstances. Some of these choices are reflected in living wills and advanced directives, reflecting an individual's desires in cases of medical events.

Even though most medical problems are not of emergency proportions, a reduction in medical care consumption can lead to a deterioration in health. In studying such a possibility, it may be desirable to analyze medical care demand from the longer perspective of a multiperiod analysis. The imposition of a copayment on drugs or physician visits will generally lead to a reduction in the quantity demanded in Period 1. There is nothing in the theory of demand that says which units of medical care will no longer be demanded. Some units may have been unnecessary to begin with, but some may have been highly desirable (from the point of view of their effects on health status). When medical care is desirable, a reduction in its consumption in Period 1 may lead to a decline in health status in Periods 2, 3, or 4, and to possible increases in medical care demand in these subsequent periods.

This phenomenon was first examined following the imposition of a $1 copayment for each of the first two doctor's visits and $0.50 for each of the first two prescriptions in the California Medicaid program. An original study (Roemer, Hopkins, Carr, & Gartside, 1975) stated that reductions in doctor's office visits and diagnostic tests after the copayment's introduction were accompanied by increases in hospitalization rates in subsequent periods. Although the data methods of the study were questioned, with no conclusive results (Chen, 1976a; 1976b; Dyckman, 1976; Hopkins, Gartside, & Roemer, 1976), the study raised the issue of the importance of examining the wider effects of demand-reducing measures. A subsequent study, based on the national Rand Health Insurance Experiment (Brook et al., 1983), examined the effects of reductions in use due to copayments on subsequent consumer health status and found that they were generally not adverse, except for certain groups. In particular, for poor individuals with hypertensive conditions, free care was associated with better blood pressure control and reductions in the risk of early death. There is a likelihood that, for selected groups, reductions in demand can have considerable impact on subsequent health status and medical care demand (Fein, 1981; Relman, 1983).

Research does indicate that the price of healthcare services is relevant to the demand for many healthcare services, especially when viewed in terms of the impact of insurance on the utilization of healthcare services. For example, O'Neill and O'Neill (2009) reported that, in 2005, about 80% of insured women between the ages of 40 and 64 had received a mammogram during the past two years, but only 49% of uninsured women had received one. Similarly, 84% of insured women between the ages of 20 and 64 had received Pap Smear tests during the past two years, but only 63% of uninsured women had received one. For the total population between the ages of 18 and 64, only 50% of those uninsured had received a routine physical during the past two years, compared to 78% of the insured population in that age cohort. While these are not direct measures of the impact of higher price on the demand for healthcare services, they can be used as proxies for determining the inverse relationship between price and quantity demanded in the market for selected healthcare services.

The consequences of being uninsured can be significant. A recent Urban Institute study (Dorn, 2008), estimated that applying the conservative increased risk of mortality associated with being uninsured of 15% to individuals between the ages of 25 and 64 resulted in over 101,000 excess deaths between 2000 and 2006, with 16,000 of them occurring in 2006.

For individuals with insurance, cost sharing can still have a substantial impact upon the demand for healthcare services. Zeber, Grazier, Valenstein, Blow, & Lantz (2007) found that increasing pharmacy copayments did result in a reduction in prescription utilization; however, following the reduction was a higher inpatient utilization resulting from cost-related nonadherence to treatment regimen. Similar impact findings were reported by Doshi, Zhu, Lee, Kimmel, & Volpp (2009), in which an increase in copayments for lipid-lowering medication adversely impacted medication adherence, including among those at high coronary heart disease risk.

4.3 EXTERNAL AND SOCIAL DEMAND FOR MEDICAL CARE

In the analysis in the chapter on demand for medical care, it was assumed that the sum of all individual's own demands for medical care was the same as the total societal demand for medical care. Investigators have questioned the reasonableness of this assumption. For certain social goods, such as medical care and education, it has been asserted that individuals would be willing to pay something to enable others to consume them. This is not true for all goods and services. Many individuals would be willing to pay something to help ensure that a heart attack victim could reach a hospital on time; they would not be so generous if a person's car had broken down and he or she "needed" $400 for repairs. Furthermore, people's generosity probably extends only to certain types of medical care. The need for medical care with substantial health implications for the recipients (e.g., inoculations or care for the aged) elicits great concern; someone's desire to undergo cosmetic surgery does not.

To formalize the analysis of this phenomenon, let us focus on the consumption of a single individual, called A. The service whose demand we are analyzing will now be defined as individual A's consumption of medical care. A's demand for his or her own consumption may be called *private* or *internal demand.*

Assume that the rest of society can be characterized as individual B, who may also have a demand for A's own consumption of medical care. Such a demand can be characterized in the same way as A's own demand. In particular, as the price is lowered, B's demand for A's consumption of medical care will increase. This demand is in addition to A's own demand and can be called an *external demand*, because it comes from a force external to the consumer of the service. Examples of policies to influence the social demand for medical care are Medicare and Medicaid. When society determined that the elderly and certain categories of low-income individuals weren't consuming sufficient medical care, policies were implemented to subsidize their purchase of additional services.

If we define society as the sum total of A and B, then society's demand for A's consumption of medical care will depend on the private demand of A and the external demand of B. This total demand can be called *community* or *social* demand.

The effect of the external demand is to increase the quantity demanded (of medical care for A) at any given price, assuming that the external demand is greater than zero at that price. (It may well be, as in the case of the external demand for auto repair, that this external demand is zero at a particular price or at all prices.) (See Figure 4-1.) The old phrase that "society wants everyone to have a decent level of medical care" can be recast in terms of this analysis. Society is the sum of all individuals, and the social demand for an individual's consumption of a given good or service is the sum of all private and external demands. The statement that "society wants everyone to have a decent level of medical care" can be interpreted to mean that, at the given price, there is a social demand for a "decent" level of care for each person.

There are a sufficiently large number of manifestations of external demands for medical care to impress on us how real this phenomenon is. The existence of philanthropic giving to such organizations as the American Heart Association, the United Way, the American Cancer Society, and the National Research Foundation provides evidence that donors are truly committed to

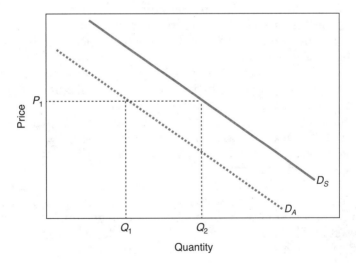

Figure 4-1 Social Demand for Medical Care. At the price of P_1, individual A would purchase Q_1 units of medical care. But because society values A's use of medical services, society determines that at price P_1 individual A should consume Q_2 units of medical care. As a result, subsidies or other actions must be provided to increase A's demand for medical services to society's level of Q_2. Society's demand for A, therefore, is the distance between Q_1 and Q_2.

enabling others to consume the services of these organizations, including health education and research. The majority of hospitals in the United States began as tax-exempt (not-for-profit) organizations with large charitable components. In recent years, these charitable components have decreased because of the growth of government health programs, such as Medicare and Medicaid. Such programs themselves may be an expression of external demands expressed through the "political marketplace." Before the introduction of Medicare and Medicaid, physicians contended that a great deal of their medical services were provided as a form of charity.

4.4 INFLUENCE OF QUALITY ON THE DEMAND FOR MEDICAL CARE

In the chapter on the demand for medical care, the analysis of medical care demand was based on the assumption that each unit of medical care was like any other unit. Of course, this is not always the case. One of the more problematic tasks in analyzing resource allocation in medical care is coming to terms with quality differences.

Quality is not a single attribute, but rather a series of attributes, any of which can make the product appear better or worse to the consumer (Congress of the United States, 1988). In this section, we will assume that the consumer is fully aware of how each of these attributes that determine the quality level of a product will affect him or her. Furthermore, we will regard quality as subjective, that is, in terms of how the consumer values these attributes of the good or service.

There are three attributes of medical care that are used to identify quality (Donabedian, 1988): (1) the *structure* of the resources provided (e.g., the qualifications of the clinicians and the type of facilities); (2) the *process* of medical care (e.g., the thoroughness with which the diagnostic services are carried out or the comfort or luxury of the particular services provided); and (3) the *outcome*, or the level of medical excellence of the services. The latter attribute is associated with the accuracy of a diagnosis, the effectiveness of a treatment in restoring health, the effectiveness of a preventive course of action, and so on. Assuming that these aspects of quality can be accurately assessed, a consumer can make a personal evaluation of the overall quality levels associated with alternative units of medical care and can rank these alternative units according to their quality levels.

How might consumers behave when faced with different overall medical care quality levels? A reasonable hypothesis is that a higher quality level will increase the importance of medical care in relation to other goods and services at all levels of medical care consumption. This will result in an outward shift of the demand curve for medical care.

One qualification must be mentioned. If the quality of care is low, the demand may be less. But if low-quality care results in subsequent illness (e.g., if rheumatic fever develops from a failure to check for strep throat or if a patient with chicken pox contracts Reye's syndrome because he or she was prescribed aspirin), it may lead to a greater demand for care, in subsequent time periods (see Figure 4-2).

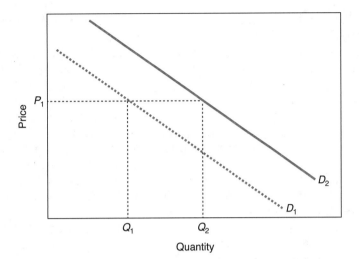

Figure 4-2 Increase in Demand for Medical Care with Improved Quality of Care. Demand curve D_1 reflects an individual's initial demand for medical care. When the quality of care is viewed as increasing, or improved, then the individual's demand for medical care will shift outward to demand curve D_2, increasing the quantity demanded at each price of medical care. Notice that a change in quality shifts the entire demand curve, and doesn't cause just a movement along the original demand curve.

4.5 TIME AND MONEY COSTS

Until now, we have measured the resource commitment necessary to obtain a unit of medical care by the per-unit out-of-pocket money price of that good or service. Thus, if a unit of medical care costs $5, then $5 was treated as an accurate measure of what a person had to give up (the opportunity cost) to obtain a unit of medical care. Yet the resources devoted to consuming a good or service include more than the money price of the good or service; when obtaining medical care, people have to travel to and from the physician's office and wait to see the physician and be examined. The effort and time expended are personal resources and are part of the totality of resources committed to obtaining medical care.

The value of the time spent by a person travelling and waiting is referred to as the time cost of obtaining medical care. The associated resource commitment is equivalent to the amount that could have been earned if the person had not visited the physician (assuming the person does forgo income in undertaking this action). If the person does not forgo income, valuable time is still given up. In this case, the opportunity cost of time would be taken to be equivalent to the value to the person of the activity given up. This latter magnitude is very difficult to measure, so for our purposes, we will assume that all time spent in obtaining health care can be measured in terms of the person's wage rate.

The total cost to, or total resource commitment made by, the person for each unit of health care can be expressed as $(w \times t) + p$, in which t is the amount of time involved in obtaining a unit of health care, w is the wage that would have been earned had the person worked during this time, and p is the money price of the health care.

We can use this expression to substitute total per-unit cost for money price in our demand analysis. If we regard the good or service as medical care and the total cost per unit of this good or service as $(w \times t) + p$, we can develop a more general hypothesis about the consumption of medical care. Our new hypothesis is this: as the total per unit cost (time cost plus money price) falls, more medical care is demanded. To give an example, if the time required for a visit to the doctor is one hour, the wage forgone is $10 per hour, and the money price of a visit is $20, the total per-unit cost is $30. If the money price is set at zero by a government program, the total cost falls to $10 per visit. Medical care may still be too costly for some people, even at a zero out-of-pocket money price. If the government wishes to encourage consumption beyond this point, it might have to take steps that would lower waiting or travel time (e.g., by relocating a clinic to a more populous area).

Framing the analysis of demand in terms of total cost provides additional insight regarding issues of distribution. Even though money costs may be the same for all consumers, total costs may vary because of variations in w and t. For example, w may vary among consumers because some may have their wages docked if they take time off from work, whereas others may not. And t may vary because of variations in distances from care providers. Our generalized demand hypothesis states that, other things being equal, the quantity demanded will vary inversely with the total per-unit cost. When medical care is offered for "free," that is, at a zero money price, variations in quantity demanded will be determined by variations in time costs. In this circumstance, individuals who incur the lowest time cost will demand the greatest quantities. Perhaps those who pay the lowest time costs and hence demand the greatest quantities are not the same as those with the most acute medical conditions. In this case, medical care would be rationed to those who are willing to wait and not to the most ill. This problem arises when a program lowers the direct money price to zero while failing to increase supply sufficiently to meet the increased quantity demanded. An excess demand results, and queues may form. This raises the time cost, which becomes the mechanism by which medical care is rationed. Rationing, in and of itself, is not negative but simply a fact of life. Rationing is simply about making choices. If resources are limited, resulting in everyone not having everything they want, then choices will have to be made about how the limited resources will be used and who will be able to receive the resources. The issue becomes what is the best mechanism by which to ration the service to achieve the best or society-desired result.

4.6 THE DEMAND FOR HEALTH

In the chapter on the output of the healthcare sector, we showed that the output of the healthcare sector can be regarded either as health care or as health. An alternative formulation of consumer behavior in this area has been presented in terms of the demand for health (Grossman, 1972b). Health care can be regarded as an end in itself, something people want for its intrinsic characteristics or as a means to an end. For example, better health, by enabling a person to earn more income and purchase other goods and services, would function as a means for attaining a higher level of consumer consumption.

In this analysis, we assume health to be an end in itself that can be created or produced by the activities individuals undertake. These activities can include receiving medical care, engaging in self-care (exercise and proper diet), and so on. Such activities are substitutes for one another, because each contributes to achieving the desired end. The cost of each alternative activity can be expressed in terms of the resources an individual would have to commit in order to produce one healthy day. Because each activity will normally require time and purchased inputs on the part of the consumer, the cost of one healthy day can be expressed as follows:

$$c = (a \times w) + (b \times p)$$

In this equation, c is the unit cost (cost per one healthy day produced) of the activity; a is the amount of time required to produce one healthy day by engaging in the activity; b is the amount of purchased inputs required in conjunction with a to produce one healthy day; w is the opportunity cost of the individual's time and thus a measurement of the size of the resource commitment of one unit of time; and p is the price of one unit of purchased input. The cost of one healthy day (c) depends on a, b, w, and p. For each health-producing activity, there will be a different c. If one activity, say self-care, is very productive (i.e., a and b are small), then the cost of producing an extra healthy day through self-care will be low. On the other hand, if self-care is not very effective in producing health, then a may be very high and c, in turn, will likely be high. Recall that, although the unit price of purchased inputs (p) may be high, the number of units required to produce a healthy day (b) may be low. Thus, purchased input–intensive activities, such as medical care, are not necessarily more costly than other health-producing activities.

One prediction of this model is that, if the value of c of one type of health-producing activity rises relative to the value of c for another type, individuals will substitute in favor of the lower cost alternative. For example, if waiting time in a doctor's office (a) becomes lengthy, the cost of medical care will rise. Self-care becomes relatively less expensive under these circumstances, and individuals will engage in more self-care activities.

It is unlikely that a and b will remain constant across all levels of an activity. Instead, it is probable that the more an activity (e.g., physician care or self-care) is engaged in, the more a and b will increase. That is, it will take successively larger doses of personal effort and purchased inputs to yield a unit of health, reflecting diminishing marginal productivity. For this reason, several health-producing activities will be demanded by an individual. For example, the individual will probably demand both medical care and self-care. However, if a factor changes (e.g., there is an increase in the amount of waiting time necessary to obtain medical care), this will cause a shift in demand (e.g., more self-care and less medical care will be demanded).

Viewing the demand for health-related resources in this way allows us to incorporate the full resource commitment of alternative ways of producing health. In such a framework, medical care becomes one of several alternatives, and a broader picture of health-related resources can be obtained. However, while the picture is broader, it is also more complex, and for many purposes, such a broad and complex picture is not required.

4.7 AGENCY THEORY AND SUPPLIER-INDUCED DEMAND

Many consumers do not know the effect of medical care on health, and physicians have been regarded as having two main roles: (1) to act in an advisory capacity and inform patients of their level of health and the activities and treatments that might improve their health; and (2) to undertake treatments upon which their patients have decided. When we introduce the physicians into the demand analysis, we widen the framework, for the patient's demand is now also dependent on the interaction with the physician.

As we saw in the chapter on the demand for medical care, a patient's perception of the level of his or her health and the probable effect of medical care on the patient's health, can influence the patient's demand for medical care. Because the physician potentially has influence over both of these factors, the physician can conceivably change the patient's demand for medical care by providing pertinent information. For example, telling a patient that he or she has a dangerous, but possibly curable, neoplasm will almost certainly increase that patient's demand for cancer treatment.

If we assume that the physician knows the patient's health level and the effectiveness of medical care in producing health, and if the physician has an awareness of the patient's tastes and other circumstances (prices and income), then, assuming the physician behaves as a "perfect agent," he or she will prescribe and/or provide a quantity of medical care such that the patient him- or herself, if fully informed, would have chosen. However, principal–agent relationships are such that the agent (physician) may not behave in the best interests of the principal (patient). A deviation of the agent from the principal's own interests is called *supplier-induced demand*.

Supplier-induced demand will arise when there is a potential divergence of interest between the principal and the agent. Despite this divergence, there must still be a basis for the two to engage in a contractual relationship. However, when the principal uses the services of the agent, he or she, in effect, has entered into an agreement that the agent will meet the principal's needs. Problems with the relationship will arise when there is uncertainty and information asymmetry that makes it difficult for the two parties to agree on a fixed price, agree on a predetermined service that the agent will provide, and develop an adequate mechanism to monitor and enforce the agreement.

As an example of a principal–agent relationship that would not be plagued by agency problems, imagine a private home care nursing agency administering intravenous drugs on a daily basis to a bedridden client. The home care nurse will agree to show up at a specified time each day and administer the drugs. The client can clearly specify the contract with the agency. Also, the client can easily monitor the performance of the nursing agency, and if the nursing agency does not perform adequately, the client can terminate the contract.

When the patient interacts with a provider, there are four types of costs which he or she incurs, in addition to the price, wait, and travel costs:

1. Search costs, or the costs of determining specifications of the services needed and the prices of these services;
2. Contract costs, or the costs of reaching an agreement with the provider as to what services are to be provided;
3. Monitoring costs, or the costs of identifying the desired outcomes, collecting data on these outcomes, and determining whether the outcomes have been achieved; and
4. Enforcement costs, or the costs of ensuring that the provider meets the agreed criteria

These costs are especially important in the present circumstances. The patient (principal), lacking relevant information, relies on the physician (agent) to provide advice on health status and alternative treatments and in many instances, to provide the recommended therapy. In some circumstances, the physician's interests may diverge from those of the patient. The physician can then engage in supplier-induced demand by providing advice and therapies that are in his or her own interests rather than the interests of the patient. Despite the divergences of interests, the patient may still contract with the physician because, given the costs of engaging in the medical care process, what is provided by the physician may be the best alternative (Dranove & White, 1987).

Thus, supplier-induced demand is a phenomenon that has been linked to agency theory. Supplier-induced demand may be encouraged by certain payment mechanisms that provide incentives to physicians to deliver more services, such as fee-for-service. Under fee-for-service, the physician is paid for each unit of service performed, and so one of the conditions needed for principal–agent problems to arise—the divergence of interests—will be present. Monitoring and enforcement costs may be very high for the patient, therefore the physician has both the incentive and the ability to engage in demand-inducing practices. In the chapter on provider payment, the effect of the basis of payment on provider supply is discussed regarding supplier-induced demand.

There are limits to such a process. For one thing, with repeated events (e.g., common colds), the patient eventually gains information that can be used to evaluate health and medical productivity. In addition, information sharing between patients, between patients and other physicians (second opinions), or on the Internet, limits the degree to which a physician can sway the patient with incomplete or misinformation. That is, the patient's monitoring abilities are improved. Deliberate misrepresentation of information would be contrary to the physician's ethical codes. Finally, the assumption that the *physician* has perfect information about the patient's health status and the productivity of medical care is not always realistic. Diagnosis and treatment are often undertaken under conditions of uncertainty. Under such conditions, a physician experiments to obtain the best treatment. Although the physician can still generate demand, it is impossible to say with certainty how much of the "experimentation" was intentional demand generation and how much was honest experimentation.

4.7.1 Demand Under Uncertainty: The Demand for Health Promotion

The simple analysis of demand for medical care in the chapter on demand for medical care was based on the assumption that the consumer knows with certainty what his or her state of health will be during the relevant time period. This underlying assumption is not plausible for many medical problems. In these cases, a consumer cannot be certain whether or not a problem will occur. The consumer does know, however, that he or she *might* be sick during a particular period and might have to visit a healthcare provider and even be hospitalized. Issues related to the uncertain appearance of illness have a bearing on a number of health-related activities (Kenkel, 1991; Russell, 1984; Scheffler & Paringer, 1980). For example, people adopt healthy or unhealthy lifestyles; these lifestyles are often resource intensive and will have an impact on the likelihood that the individuals will be sick.

The basic theory of the demand for health promotion activities presents a systematic view of how certain underlying variables—tastes, wealth, the cost of health promotion, the likelihood of an illness, and the loss resulting from the illness—can influence the decision to engage in these activities. The assumptions of the model are as follows:

1. *Time frame.* All activities and consequences occur in the current time period.

2. *Level of wealth.* Our second assumption is that our individual initially has a level of wealth of $1,000.

3. *Consumer tastes.* We assume that, when an illness occurs, it leads to medical care expenses that constitute a loss of wealth. To specify what this loss means to the individual, we must introduce a concept to characterize the individual's well-being at alternative levels of wealth—the concept of utility. Utility is a measure of consumer satisfaction and reflects the maximum amount of resources (money) an individual will exchange for a particular bundle of goods and services. One hypothetical individual's taste for wealth is presented in the form of an index of utility in Table 4-1. This index shows the level of utility that is associated with each specific level of wealth. Thus, a level of wealth of $1,000 is associated with a level of utility of 100, a level of wealth of $990 is associated with a level of utility of 99.8, and so on. The size of specific numbers in the utility index is arbitrary. What is important is that higher wealth gives higher utility (i.e., increased wealth makes the individual "better off"). We further assume that the function is characterized by diminishing marginal utility. That is, each additional $10 of wealth results in less additional utility than the previous $10. For example, at $850, an extra $10 will yield 3 extra units of utility; at $860, an extra $10 will yield 2.8 extra units; and so on.

Table 4-1   Relationship Between Wealth and Utility

Wealth	Total Utility	Marginal Utility
$800	57.0	4.2
810	61.2	4.0
820	65.2	3.8
830	69.0	3.6
840	72.6	3.4
850	76.0	3.2
860	79.0	3.0
870	81.8	2.8
880	84.4	2.6
890	86.8	2.4
900	89.0	2.2
910	91.0	2.0
920	92.8	1.8
930	94.4	1.6
940	95.8	1.4
950	97.0	1.2
960	98.0	1.0
970	98.8	0.8
980	99.4	0.6
990	99.8	0.4
1000	100.0	0.2

If an individual has a diminishing marginal utility for wealth, he or she is said to be *risk averse*. The basic idea is that, for a given wealth level, a loss of a given amount of wealth (e.g., $10) is of greater subjective importance (utility) to the person than would be a gain of an equal amount. Utility is the subjective index of the relative importance of wealth.

In this model, a utility function is unique to an individual. Thus, it does not imply that additional wealth means less to a rich person than it does to a poor person. This kind of comparison, called *interpersonal comparison*, would involve specifying different people's utilities on the same scale.

4. *Medical expenses in the event of illness.* Our fourth assumption is that, if the individual becomes sick, he or she will face medical expenses of

$150. This expenditure is assumed to restore the loss in health fully so that $150 is the full value of the loss when the individual is sick.

5. *The cost of health promotion activities.* The consumer uses up resources when engaging in health promotion, including time, professional services, and supplies. In our example, we will assume that these costs total $20.

6. *Likelihood of illness.* A sixth assumption concerns the element of uncertainty. We will assume that we can assign probabilities to the various possible health states the individual may experience. Let us say that, without any health promotion activities, there is a 0.3 probability of illness (i.e., of 10 people in similar circumstances, 3 will become ill) and a 0.7 probability the individual will remain well and will not incur any medical costs. These are the only two possibilities, so the sum of the probabilities equals 1. With health promotion activities, the probability of being healthy increases to 0.9 and the probability of being ill falls to 0.1.

7. *Behavioral assumption.* The final assumption is that the individual wants to maximize the expected value of his or her utility. Thus, the individual will choose that course of action from which he or she can expect to receive the highest level of utility.

The model's conclusions are obtained by determining how, under these assumed conditions, the individual will behave so as to maximize expected utility (i.e., which of the two options, engage in health promotion or do not engage in health promotion, will be chosen). Under the option of not engaging in health promotion, the expected utility for the individual is 92.8 [(0.7 × 100) + (0.3 × 76.0)]. This is because when the individual is healthy, he or she has a utility of 100.0 (corresponding to a wealth of $1,000), and when he or she is ill, the utility is 76.0 (corresponding to a wealth level of $850). If the individual engages in health promotion activities, the expected utility will be derived from the probabilities and utility levels when he or she is healthy or ill, but has spent $20 on health promotion activities (which occur whether the individual is healthy or not). Therefore, the expected utility is 95.3 [(0.9 × 99.4) + (0.1 × 69.0)]. The individual is better off when he or she engages in health promotion activities under these circumstances, and so we predict that he or she will choose that option.

However, this will not always be the case. If any of our basic assumptions change, so will our conclusion. The individual will be less likely to engage in health promotion when any of the following occurs: the cost of health promotion increases, health promotion has a reduced impact on illness, or the individual experiences an increase in risk aversion.

4.7.2 Limitations of the Model

The theory of the demand for health care under conditions of uncertainty has the virtue of explicitly organizing some of the variables that are central to the decision to engage in activities that promote health. As presented, however, it has an important limitation.

The reader may find it strange that the utility function, which is supposed to measure satisfaction, does not include health. This is, indeed, a shortcoming of the model, because well-being can depend on health status as well as wealth. The model looks only at financial aspects of the situation, in effect assuming that the care consumed fully and instantly restores health, with no utility implications of either the illness or the process of getting care. Clearly, this is an unrealistic assumption. Including health status creates a much more complicated model that is more difficult to apply, and while it is important to understand that we have abstracted from reality, this should not detract from the value of the model. The present model has the virtue of focusing on the benefits of risk shifting, which is an economic good that is distinct from medical care.

4.7.3 Discounting Future Values

Another factor that affects health promotion behavior is the individual's valuation of benefits in different time periods. Health promotion activities, such as the use of condoms, smoking cessation, vaccinations, and clean needles (for drug users), and unhealthy activities, such as smoking, engaging in unsafe sex, and excessive drug use, generally do not have good or bad impacts on health immediately. It takes a long time, sometimes years, for individuals to experience adverse health effects. The timing of health benefits will have an influence on the demand for health-related activities that promote these benefits.

It is generally assumed that $1,000 in current benefits will be worth more to an individual than $1,000 in benefits one year from now. The value of the preference for earlier rather than later periods can be expressed in terms of a discount rate, called r. If an individual is asked how much money he or she would accept at the end of 2012 rather than have $1,000 at the beginning of 2012, the person might take $1,100 at the end of the period. In other words, $1,000 on January 1, 2012, would be worth as much as $1,100 one year later. The discount rate is 0.1, and the discounting equation is be expressed as $1,000 \times (1 + 0.1) = $1,100, or symbolically as $1,000 \times (1 + r) = $1,100. This may be rewritten as $1,000 = $1,100/(1 + r)$. This equation says that, in the individual's eyes, $1,100 one year hence will be equivalent to $1,100/(1 + r)$, or $1,000, now. The discount rate for an individual is derived largely from introspection—from an acceptance that a given future amount and a lesser current amount provide the same satisfaction *at the present moment*.

The same principle holds for comparisons between December 31, 2012, and December 31, 2013. That is, $1,000 at the end of 2012 is equivalent to $1,100 at the end of 2013 if the individual's discount rate is 0.1. By inference, then, $1,000 at the end of 2013 would be worth $1,000/[(1 + r) \times (1 + r)]$ on January 1, 2012 (also expressible as $1,000/(1 + r)^2$). Similarly, $1,000 on December 31, 2014, would be worth $1,000/(1 + r)^3$ at the start of 2012, and so on. Generally, improved health, or added life, yields a stream of benefits. That is, a saved life on January 1, 2012 will yield benefits in 2012 (valued as of December 31, 2012), 2013 (valued as of December 31, 2013), 2014 (valued as of December 31, 2014), and so on. If the benefits are $2,000 each year, the *present* value of future benefits can be expressed as $2,000 + 2,000/(1 + r)$ + $2,000/(1 + r)^2$, and so on, for as long as benefits last. The letter usually used to symbolize the annual benefits is B, with subscripts 0, 1, 2, . . . for right now (0), one year hence (1), two years hence (2), and so on. In our current example, $B_0 = B_1 = B_2$, and the present value of benefits can be expressed symbolically as

$$B_0 + B_0 / (1 + r) + B_0 / (1 + r)^2$$

If the number of years that benefits will last is quite large, and the value of the benefits for every year is the same, the present value of the benefits can be expressed as B_0/r. If benefits of $10,000 a year will last forever, and if the discount rate is 0.1, the present value of these benefits will be 10,000/0.1, or $100,000. Benefits lasting for long periods can be approximated using this formula.

The discount factor can be quite substantial for benefits that will not be experienced for many years. For example, hepatitis C may not be recognized for 20 years. If hepatitis C imposes health-related costs of $1,000 in 20 years, and the discount rate is 10%, then the present value of these imposed costs is $148.64 [$1,000 / (1 + 0.1)^{20}]$.

Not everyone will have the same discount rate. An individual who has a very strong preference for current satisfaction rather than future benefits will have a high interest rate, perhaps 15% or 20%. On the other hand, a person who places very great importance on future satisfaction will have a very low discount rate, perhaps 2% or even 0%. In the latter case, there would be no discount rate, and present and future values would be the same.

Discounting has typically been done with a handheld calculator or with present value tables; currently, most calculators and computer software

Table 4-2 Calculation of Present Value of Benefits Under Alternative Discount Rates

Part A: Discounting Factors					
Discount Rate	$(1 + r)$	$(1 + r)^2$	$(1 + r)^3$	$(1 + r)^4$	$(1 + r)^5$
0.04	1.04	1.08	1.12	1.17	1.22
0.08	1.08	1.16	1.25	1.36	1.41
0.12	1.12	1.25	1.41	1.57	1.63
Part B: Discounted Present Value of Benefits ($10,000)					
Discount Rate	$B/(1 + r)$	$B/(1 + r)^2$	$B/(1 + r)^3$	$B/(1 + r)^4$	$B/(1 + r)^5$	Present Value (row sum)
0.04	9,615	9,233	8,896	8,554	8,196	44,494
0.08	9,259	8,620	8,000	7,353	7,092	40,324
0.12	8,928	8,000	7,029	6,275	5,602	35,834

have functions to calculate present values and discounting. In Table 4-2, we show a series of discounted values, varying according to discount rates (4, 8, and 12%) and time periods (one to five years). For example, in Part A, at a discount rate of 8% and a four-year time horizon, the value of $(1 + r)^4$ is 1.36. The present value of a benefit of $10,000 that occurred in four years, discounted at a rate of 8%, would, therefore, be $7,353.

Often, benefits will repeat themselves from year to year. For example, a $10,000 benefit may be experienced in each of the next five years. If the discount rate was 4%, then the present value of the benefits for each of the next five years would be $9,615; then $9,233; and so on for five years. The present value of $10,000 for all five years together, called the annuity value, is $44,494, as shown in Table 4-2. Annuity tables would contain present values summed over each time horizon.

EXERCISES

1. A copayment was placed on the use of physician checkups. As a result, poor people reduced their demands for checkups, and their health status was reduced. How might this affect the demand for subsequent health care?
2. Name three different ways of identifying quality. How would increased quality affect the demand for medical services?
3. Mrs. Smith earns $20 an hour. Normally, she has to drive into St. Cloud from her home (150 miles away) for a medical consultation. The drive is 2.5 hours each way. Mrs. Smith usually has a one-hour wait, and the consultation takes about an hour. Mrs. Smith estimates that the cost of the transportation is 50 cents a mile. What are Mrs. Smith's travel and waiting costs for each visit?
4. Mrs. Siegal has two alternative activities to help relieve her backache. In the first, she can visit a physiotherapist. The total time for a physiotherapist visit, including travel and waiting, is two hours. Mrs. Siegal earns a wage of $20 an hour. Physiotherapists charge $50 per visit, and Mrs. Siegal does not have any health insurance. As a second alternative, Mrs. Siegal can take pain killers. Each pill costs 50 cents, and Mrs. Siegal needs to take 30 pills per month. The two treatments are not equally effective. The physiotherapy visits yield 10 additional healthy days per month, while the pills yield 6 healthy days.
   a. If Mrs. Siegal can choose only one alternative, and if she wants to maximize the most healthy days per dollar that she gets, which option will she choose?
   b. If the price of a pill increases to $3, which option will she choose?
5. What is information asymmetry and how does it result in a principal-agent problem?

6. What are the costs that an individual or organization must incur in order to contract with another individual or organization?
7. What is supplier-induced demand? How is it related to a principal-agent problem?
8. Mrs. Backman has a utility function like that in Table 4-1. Her wealth level is $900. If she is ill, she incurs costs of $50 in medical expenses. This is a one-time expense and will leave her at a lower wealth level (in this case, $850). Without any special diet or exercise, she has a 20% chance of being sick. She can purchase vitamins for $20, in which case her chance of being sick will fall to 10%. Using expected utility as her objective, should she purchase the vitamins?
9. Mr. Manos has a discount rate of 10%. To him, it is worth $2,000 to be very well and $1,900 to be moderately well. It is the beginning of the year 2012. Mr. Manos can engage in exercise, which will make him very well during the year 2014 but will leave him only moderately well for the years 2012 and 2013. Alternatively, he can take medicine, which will make him very well in 2012, but its effects only last one year. Therefore, if Mr. Manos takes the medicine, he will only be moderately well in the years 2013 and 2014. What is each alternative worth to Mr. Manos as of the present?

BIBLIOGRAPHY

General

Culyer, A. J. (1971). The nature of the commodity "health care" and its efficient allocation. *Oxford Economic Papers, 23,* 189–211.

Donabedian, A. (1988). The quality of care. *JAMA, 260,* 1743–1748.

Kluge, E. W. (2007). Resource allocation in healthcare: Implications of models of medicine as a profession. *Medscape General Medicine, 9*(1), 57.

Pawlson, L. G., Glover, J. J., & Murphy, D. J. (1992). An overview of allocation and rationing: Implications for geriatrics *Journal of the American Geriatrics Society, 40*(6), 628–634.

Persad, G., Wertheimer, A., & Emanuel, E. J. (2009). Principles for allocation of scarce medical interventions. *The Lancet, 373,* 423–431.

Petrou, S., & Wolstenholme, J., (2000). A review of alternative approaches to healthcare resource allocation. *Pharmacoeconomics, 18*(1), 33–43.

Utilization and Subsequent Health Implications

Bhandari, A., & Wagner, T. (2006). Self-reported utilization of health care services: Improving measurement and accuracy. *Medical Care Research and Review, 63*(2), 217–235.

Brook, R. H., Ware, J. E. Jr., Rogers, W. H., Keeler, E. B., Davies, A. R., Donald, C. A., Goldberg, G. A. .... Newhouse, J. P. (1983). Does free care improve adults' health? *New England Journal of Medicine, 309,* 1426–1434.

Carlsen, F., & Grytien, J. (2000). Consumer satisfaction and supplier-induced demand. *Journal of Health Economics, 15*(5), 731–753.

Chen, M. K. (1976a). Penny-wise and pound foolish: Another look at the data. *Medical Care, 14,* 958–963.

Chen, M. K. (1976b). More about penny-wise and pound foolish: A statistical point of view. *Medical Care, 14,* 964–968.

Chernew, M., Gibson, T. B., Yu-Isenberg, K., Sokol, M. C., Rosen, A. B., & Fendrick, A. M. (2008). Effects of increased patient cost sharing on socioeconomic disparities in health care. *Journal of General Internal Medicine, 23*(8), 1131–1136.

Congress of the United States. (1988). *The quality of medical care.* Washington, DC: Congress of the United States, Office of Technology Assessment.

Cutler, D. M., McClellan, M., & Newhouse, J. P. (1998). What has increased medical-care spending bought? *American Economic Review, 88*(2), 132–136.

Domino, M. E., Martin, B. C., Wiley-Exley, E., Richards, S., Henson, A., Carey, T. S., & Sleath, B. (2011). Increasing time costs and copayments for prescription drugs: An analysis of policy changes in a complex environment. *Health Services Research, 46*(3), 900–919.

Doshi, J. A., Zhu, J., Lee, B. Y., Kimmel, S. E. & Volpp, K. G. (2009). Impact of a prescription copayment increase on lipid-lowering medication adherence in veterans. *Circulation, 119,* 390–397.

Dranove, D., & White, W. D. (1987). Agency and the organization of health care delivery. *Inquiry, 24*(4), 405–415.

D'Souza, A. O., Rahnama, R., Regan, T. S., Common, B., & Burch, S. (2010). The H-E-B value-based health management program—Impact on asthma medication adherence and healthcare cost. *American Health Drug Benefits, 3*(6), 394–402.

Dyckman, Z. Y. (1976). Comment on "copayments for ambulatory care: Penny-wise and pound foolish." *Medical Care, 14,* 274–276.

Dyckman, Z. Y., & McMenamin, P. (1976). Copayments for ambulatory care: Son of thrupence. *Medical Care, 14,* 968–969.

Fein, R. (1981). Effects of cost sharing in health insurance. *New England Journal of Medicine, 305,* 1526–1528.

Flores, G. (2005). The impact of medical interpreter services on the quality of health care: A systematic review. *Medical Care Research and Review, 62*(3), 255–299.

Gibson, T. B., McLaughlin, C. G., & Smith, D. G. (2005). The long-term and short-term effects of a copayment increase on the demand for prescription drugs. *Inquiry, 42,* 293–310.

Gilman, B. H., & Kautter, J. (2008). Impact of multitiered copayments on the use and cost of prescription drugs among Medicare beneficiaries. *Health Services Research, 43*(2), 478–495.

Giuffrida, A., & Gravelle, H. (1998). Paying patients to comply. *Health Economics, 7,* 569–580.

Gruber, J. (2006). *The role of consumer copayments for health care: Lessons from the RAND health insurance experiment and beyond.* Menlo Park CA: The Henry J. Kaiser Family Foundation.

Hadley, J. (2003). Sicker and poorer—The consequences of being uninsured: A review of the research on the relationship between health insurance, medical care use, health, work, and income. *Medical Care Research and Review, 60*(2 Suppl.), 3S–75S.

Hopkins, C. E., Gartside, F., & Roemer, M. I. (1976). Rebuttal to "Comment on 'Copayments for ambulatory care: Penny-wise and pound foolish.'" *Medical Care, 14,* 277.

Jamtvedt, G., Young, J. M., Kristoffersen, D. T., O'Brien, M. A., & Oxman, A. D. (2006). Audit and feedback: Effects on professional practice and health care outcomes. *Cochrane Database of Systematic Reviews (Online), 2006*(2):CD000259. http://ovidsp.tx.ovid.com/sp-3.5.1a/ovidweb.cgi?&S=BBAOFPLJNGDDADDANCALGCOBBLOEAA00&Link+Set=S.sh.16%7c3%7csl_10

Keeler, E. B., Brook, R. H., Goldbert, G. A., Kamberg, C. J., & Newhouse, J. P. (1985). How free care reduced hypertension in the health insurance experiment. *JAMA, 254,* 1926–1931.

Knowles, J. C. (1995). Price uncertainty and the demand for health care. *Health Policy and Planning, 10,* 301–303.

Labelle, R., Stoddart, G., & Rice, T. (1994). A re-examination of the meaning and importance of supplier-induced demand. *Journal of Health Economics, 13*(3), 347–368.

Lichtenberg, F. R. (1996). Do (more and better) drugs keep people out of hospitals? *American Economic Review, 86*(2), 384–388.

Lurk, J. T., Dejong, D. J., Woods, T. M., Knell, M. E., & Carroll, C. A. (2004). Effects of changes in patient cost sharing and drug sample policies on prescription drug costs and utilization in a safety-net-provider setting. *American Journal of Health-System Pharmacy, 61*(3), 267–272.

Meissner, B. L., Moore, W. M., Shinogle, J. A., Reeder, C. E., & Little, J. M. (2004). Effects of an increase in prescription copayment on utilization of low-sedating antihistamines and nasal steroids. *Journal of Managed Care Pharmacy, 10*(3), 226–233.

Mulley, A. G. (2009). Inconvenient truths about supplier-induced demand and unwarranted variation in medical practice. *British Medical Journal, 339*, b4073.

Ndumele, C. H., & Trivedi, A. N. (2011). Effect of copayments on use of outpatient mental health services among elderly managed care enrollees. *Medical Care, 49*(3), 281–286.

O'Neill, J. E., & O'Neill, D. M. (2009). *Who are the uninsured? An analysis of America's uninsured population, their characteristics, and their health.* Washington, DC: Employment Policies Institute.

Relman, A. (1983). The Rand health insurance study: Is cost sharing dangerous to your health? *New England Journal of Medicine, 309*, 1453.

Roemer, M. I., Hopkins, C. E., Carr, L., & Gartside, F. (1975). Copayments for ambulatory care: penny-wise and pound-foolish. *Medical Care 13*(6): 457–466.

Roemer, M. I., & Hopkins, C. E. (1976). Response to M. K. Chen. *Medical Care, 14*(11), 963–964.

Stoddart, G., & Labelle, R. J. (1985). *Privatization in the Canadian health care system.* Ottawa, Canada: Health and Welfare Canada.

Wennberg, J. E. (1985). On patient need, equity, supplier-induced demand, and the need to assess the outcome of common medical practices. *Medical Care, 23*(5), 512–520.

Wennberg, J. E., Barnes, B. A., & Zubkoff, M. (1982). Professional uncertainty and the problem of supplier-induced demand. *Social Science and Medicine, 16*(7), 811–824.

Zeber, J. E., Grazier, K. L., Valenstein, M., Blow, F. C., & Lantz, P. M. (2007). Effect of a medication copayment increase in veterans with schizophrenia. *The American Journal of Managed Care, 13*(6, Pt 2), 335–346.

Demand for Health

Boucekkine, R., Desbordes, R., & Latzer, H. (2009). How do epidemics induce behavioral change? *Journal of Economic Growth, 14*(3), 233–264.

Chaloupka, F. J. (1995). Public policies and private anti-health behavior. *American Economic Review, 85*(2), 45–49.

Dorn, S. (2008). *Uninsured and dying because of it: Updating the Institute of Medicine analysis on the impact of uninsurance on mortality.* Washington, DC: Urban Institute.

Grossman, M. (1972a). On the concept of health capital and the demand for health. *Journal of Political Economy, 80*, 223–255.

Grossman, M. (1972b). *The demand for health.* New York, NY: National Bureau of Economic Research.

Grossman, M. (1982). The demand for health after a decade. *Journal of Health Economics, 1*, 1–4.

Grossman, M. (2004). The demand for health, 30 years later: A very personal retrospective and prospective reflection. *Journal of Health Economics, 23*, 629–636.

Hay, J. W., Ballit, H., & Chiriboqa, D. A. (1982). The demand for dental health. *Social Science and Medicine, 16*, 1285–1289.

Heisler, M., Langa, K. M., Eby, E. L., Fendrick, A. M., Kabeto, M. U., & Piette, J. D. (2004). The health effects of restricting prescription medication use because of cost. *Medical Care, 42*, 626–634.

Hellerstein, J. K. (1998). The importance of the physician in the generic versus trade name prescription decision. *RAND Journal of Economics, 29*, 108–136.

Jacobson, L. (2000). The family as producer of health—An extended Grossman model. *Journal of Health Economics, 19*(5), 611–637.

Kenkel, D. S. (1991). Health behavior, health knowledge, and schooling. *Journal of Political Economy, 99*(2), 287–305.

Lairson, D., Lorimor, R., & Slater, C. (1984). Estimates of the demand for health: Males in the pre-retirement years. *Social Science and Medicine, 19*, 741–747.

Mitchell, J. M., & Hadley, J. (1997). The effect of insurance coverage on breast cancer patients' treatment and hospital choices. *American Economic Review, 87*(2), 448–453.

Pezzin, L. E., & Schone, B. S. (1997). The allocation of resources in intergenerational households: Adult children and their elderly parents. *American Economic Review, 87*(2), 460– 464.

Scott, R. (2006). Investing in health (one prescription at a time): Out-of-pocket spending for medical care. *Medical Care, 44*(3), 197–199.

Vistnes, J. P., & Hamilton, V. (1995). The time and monetary costs of outpatient care for children. *American Economic Review, 85*(2), 117–121.

Wagstaff, A. (1986). The demand for health: Theory and applications. *Journal of Epidemiology and Community Health, 40*, 1–11.

Warner, K. E., & Murt, H. A. (1984). Economic incentives for health. *Annual Review for Public Health, 5*, 107–133.

Wedig, G. J. (1988). Health status and the demand for health. *Journal of Health Economics, 7*, 151–163.

Williams, A. (1985). The nature, meaning and measurement of health and illness: An economic viewpoint. *Social Science and Medicine, 20*, 1023–1027.

Economics of Disease Prevention and Health Promotion

Ayyagari, P., Grossman, D., & Sloan, F. (2011). Education and health: Evidence on adults with diabetes. *International Journal of Health Care Finance and Economics, 11*(1), 35–54.

Finkelstein, E. A., Trogdon, J. G., Cohen, J. W., & Dietz, W. (2009). Annual medical spending attributable to obesity: Payer- and service-specific estimates. *Health Affairs, 28*(5), 822–831.

Jones, L., & Bakler, M. R. (1986). The application of health economics to health promotion. *Community Medicine, 8*, 224–229.

Kenkel, D. S. (1984). The demand for preventative medical care. *Applied Economics, 26*(4), 313–325.

Kim, D., & Leigh, J. P. (2010). Estimating the effects of wages on obesity. *Journal of Occupational & Environmental Medicine, 52*(5), 495–500.

Lleras-Muney, A. (2005). The relationship between education and adult mortality in the United States. *Review of Economic Studies, 72*(1), 189–221.

Russell, L. B. (1984). The economic of prevention. *Health Policy, 4*, 85–100.

Scheffler, R. M., & Paringer, L. (1980). A review of the economic evidence on prevention. *Medical Care, 18*, 473–484.

Shepart, R. J. (1987). The economic of prevention: A critique. *Health Policy, 7*, 49–56.

Wolf, A. M., & Colditz, G. A. (1998). Current estimates of the economic cost of obesity in the United States. *Obesity Research, 6*(2), 97–106.

Healthcare Production and Costs

5.1 INTRODUCTION

The present chapter focuses on the economic behavior of healthcare providers. Examined first is how the resource commitment made by individual providers varies with the amount of production undertaken by these providers. Then, the focus is on the individual providing unit. The measure used to weigh the magnitude of the resource commitment of each providing unit is the cost to the unit of resource services. How these costs vary as the size of operations of the providing unit varies is then examined.

Before embarking on the analysis of costs, Section 5.2 considers the relationship between inputs (resources) and outputs (the input–output or production relation). The presentation is in purely "physical" terms and is designed to provide a brief summary of the role of production in determining cost. In Section 5.3, the basic cost–output relationship is explored and three alternative ways of looking at this relationship are examined. Using the cost–output relationship as the basic reference point, in Section 5.4 the various factors that affect this relationship are examined, such as changing technology, the quality of care given, the incentives offered to providers, and the size of the production unit.

In Section 5.5, the impact of one particular organizational factor on a unit's operating costs—the relatedness of the types of services produced together in the same unit—is examined. Producing services of different types in the same unit may give rise to economies and diseconomies of scope. In Section 5.6, the impact of operating scale on a unit's costs is examined. Finally, in Section 5.7, the empirical estimation of cost curves in relation to physician practices, hospitals, nursing homes, and health insurance companies is investigated.

5.2 PRODUCTION: THE INPUT–OUTPUT RELATIONSHIP

5.2.1 Basic Relationship

The economic analysis of production involves the specification of alternative combinations of inputs that yield varying levels of outputs. Typically, inputs consist of labor, capital equipment, raw materials, intermediate goods and services, knowledge, and entrepreneurial abilities. The production process itself, its organization, and the technology used lie in the realm of administrative practice and medicine. The production process has considerable impact on economic variables and can be influenced by economic factors as well.

The production process is partially determined by the technology used. Roughly defined, technology is a way of transforming inputs into outputs. Outputs consist of finished goods or services, or intermediate goods and services used by others in the production process. The production process in medical care is determined by what things are done to the patients as well as the way they are done. In this sense, there are many "technologies," even for the same illness. To bring out the essential characteristics of the production (input–output) relationship, we focus initially on one technology and then later introduce complicating factors and determine how they affect this relationship.

The simplest production process can be illustrated by the hypothetical case of a solo private practice physician who treats patients all with the same disease—the common cold. Treatment involves an examination, diagnostic tests, and a prescription of two aspirins and a glass of water. Two simplifying assumptions should be noted. First, the patients' conditions are homogeneous (the patients have equally severe cases of a single disease). Second, the treatment provided is of the same quality (all patients receive the same examination and the same tests and listen to the same instructions from the physician).

The process involves the use of various resources. These resources can be divided into two groups: fixed and variable inputs. Fixed inputs are those whose use is restricted to their current function for the time period under consideration and cannot be varied or changed in the current production period. Given their specialized nature, the high costs of transferring them to other uses, or contractual arrangements in force, fixed factors cannot be used elsewhere in the economy during the current period of production. Furthermore, the producer cannot increase the quantity during this period, or production cycle, which is assumed to be one month. In this example, fixed factors include physician office space, test equipment, and physician time.

An assumption is that office space and equipment are rented annually, and so their use for a one-year period is fixed. As for physician time, assume that the physician has, by choice, decided to remain in his or her present position for at least the next production cycle and will work 40 hours per week. Physician time is therefore a fixed factor in this instance.

Whether or not a factor is fixed depends on the time period under consideration. If the time period involved multiple production cycles, then office space, equipment, and even physician time might vary. The variable factor of production in this example is nursing time. This input can be purchased in varying quantities by the physician during the production cycle. It will be assumed that one or more nurses perform all tasks during the cycle that the physician does not.

The production process consists of three types of tasks performed using the available nursing and physician resources. The first are the administrative tasks of setting appointments, keeping records, moving patients through the office, and billing patients. The second type are technical tasks, such as the testing of blood with the rented equipment. These two tasks are performed by the nurses in this example. Finally, there is the examination itself, which is performed by the physician. For simplicity's sake, assume no patient can be processed without the involvement of a nurse, so at least one nurse must be employed. Generally, of course, the physician is able to process some patients with no help, but assume this is not the case. Also assume that, within the current ranges of resource use considered, the physician can treat all patients who ask for an appointment; his or her time limitations do not create a "capacity" problem.

Now, inquire into the number of patients who can be treated at different levels of the variable input. The specification of this production relationship will be made under the condition that whatever the level of the variable input used in conjunction with the fixed inputs, the maximum number of patients possible are being served. This condition, discussed further at the end of this section, will hold only if the human resources (nurses) have incentives to produce as much as possible. Under this condition, a production function that expresses how output will vary when inputs are changed in quantity can be specified. In specifying this function, use L to refer to the nurses' input, which is measured by hours worked. All other factors, which in this example are fixed, will be called F. Output, called Q, is measured by patient visits (each visit is assumed to be identical in nature). The production function can be written $Q = Q(L, F)$, which means that Q depends on, or is a function of, L and F.

The production function is a summary of what goes into the process—the inputs—and what comes out—the output. With F fixed, only L can vary.

Table 5-1:   Relations Between Cost and Output

(1)	(2)	(3)	(4)	(5)	(6)	(7)	(8)	(9)	(10)
Total Nursing Hours (L)	Total Visits (Q)	Marginal Product ($\Delta Q/\Delta L$)	Total Fixed Cost (TFC)	Total Variable Cost (TVC)	Total Cost (TC = TFC + TVC)	Average Fixed Cost (AFC = TFC/Q)	Average Variable Cost (AVC = TVC/Q)	Average Total Cost (ATC = TC/Q)	Marginal Cost ($\Delta TC/\Delta Q$)
8	1	1/8	100	16	115	100.0	16.0	116.0	16
15	2	1/7	100	30	130	50.0	15.0	65.0	14
20	3	1/5	100	40	140	33.3	13.3	46.7	10
24	4	1/4	100	48	148	25.0	12.0	37.0	8
30	5	1/6	100	60	160	20.0	12.0	32.0	12
38	6	1/8	100	76	176	16.7	12.7	29.3	16
50	7	1/12	100	100	200	14.3	14.3	28.6	24
64	8	1/14	100	128	228	12.5	16.0	28.5	28
100	9	1/30	100	200	300	11.1	22.2	33.3	72
140	10	1/40	100	280	280	10.0	28.0	38.0	80

By varying L, we are in fact specifying different combinations of L and F. With few nursing hours, a single nurse will perform all the nonexamination tasks and consequently cannot afford to specialize. Few patients will thus be treated. In Table 5-1, this is presented by showing only one patient treated as a result of the first eight hours of nursing input. When more patients are treated, the single nurse can begin to perform some tasks for several patients together. This concentration of tasks allows additional output to be produced with fewer additional resources. Indeed, in this example, only seven additional nursing hours are required to process a second patient.

The additional production yielded by the use of one extra unit of variable input is called the *marginal product*. It can be expressed symbolically as $\Delta Q/\Delta L$. As can be seen in Table 5-1, at the lowest level of output (one visit), an extra nursing hour adds one-eighth of a visit to the level of output. At a level of two visits, the additional output of an extra nursing hour is one-seventh of a visit. This fraction represents the marginal product. This tendency toward an increasing marginal product, created initially by the productivity gains that the concentration of tasks allows, is reinforced by productivity gains from the specialization of tasks as output continues to grow. As more patients are processed and more nursing hours and more nurses are used, some tasks can be divided among the nurses, resulting in productivity gains from specialization.

But such gains cannot be reaped forever. Eventually, a large number of routine activities will lead to boredom. It also becomes increasingly difficult to manage the activities being performed by nurses as the size of the operation increases. In addition, the fixed amount of equipment in the office

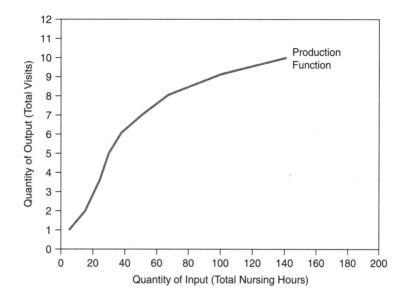

Figure 5-1 Production Function. The production function illustrates the relationship between the number of nursing hours employed in the example and the amount of total output produced in terms of the number of physician visits provided. The horizontal axis reflects the output Nursing Hours (*L*) in the first column of Table 5-1; the vertical axis reflects the output Total Visits (*Q*) in the second column of Table 5-1. Note that the production function gets flatter as the number of nursing hours increases, reflecting diminishing marginal product.

becomes heavily taxed and nurses have to wait to perform lab tests. This changes the relationship between additional inputs and additional output; to produce successively more units of output at these higher levels requires increasingly larger amounts of nursing hours. Putting the argument in terms of marginal productivity, at higher levels of output, the marginal productivity of nurses' efforts begins to decline, this property is referred to as diminishing marginal product. Thus, in our example, at a level of output of four visits, the marginal product of an additional nursing hour is one-fourth of a visit; at a level of output of five visits, the marginal product falls to one-sixth of a visit; and for six visits, the marginal product is lower still, at one-eighth of a visit. Production has reached the stage of diminishing marginal productivity. It should be noted, however, that total output is constantly rising; the assumed relationship in our production function stipulates that additional increases of output are harder and harder to come by as the size of output rises.

In viewing Figures 5-1 and 5-2, notice that these two curves reflect opposite sides of the same coin. That is, the production function gets flatter as total production (output) increases; also notice that the total cost curve gets steeper as the total production (output) increases. These two changes in the slopes of the curve occur for the same reason: diminishing marginal productivity, reflected in column 3 in Table 5-1.

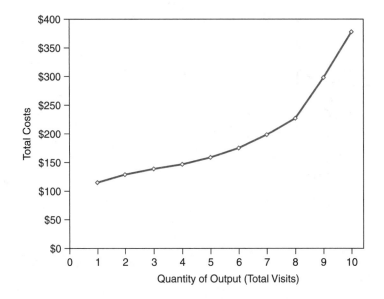

Figure 5-2   Total Cost Curve. The total cost curve illustrates the relationship between the quantity of output produced (total number of physician visits) and the total costs of production. The horizontal axis reflects the number of visits produced (*Q*) in column 2 of Table 5-1; the vertical axis reflects the total cost (*TC = TFC + TVC*) in column 6 of Table 5-1. Note that the total cost curve gets steeper as the quantity of output increases. This reflects the diminishing marginal product of the input.

The numbers used in this example were invented to illustrate the principle being hypothesized: that marginal productivity eventually diminishes. Other equally illuminating examples could have been chosen to elucidate this principle.

5.2.2 Shifts in the Relationship

We have now defined a production function and specified, in general terms, the most important property we would expect such a function to possess: the marginal product will eventually decline as more units of a variable input are added. This relationship was specified on the basis of restrictive underlying conditions. We can now examine how the productive relationship will be affected by changes in these underlying conditions. These changes will be examined using the basic production (input–output) relationship specified in Table 5-1 as a point of reference. A change in any of these underlying conditions either increases or decreases the amount of output obtained from given amounts of input. Either result will be regarded as a shift in the production relationship. An upward shift means that at each level of input, more output can be produced; a downward shift means that less output can be produced. Looking at an upward shift in marginal terms, at any level of input more additional output can be produced with an additional unit of the variable input. Expressed in output terms, at any level of output, less additional input is required to produce one extra unit of output. Stating the same thing in marginal terms, we would say that the marginal product is greater at any level of output. Thus, at a level of output of eight visits, the original production relationship was such that an extra nursing hour employed led to an increase in output of one-fourteenth of a visit. With an upward shift in the production function, an extra nursing hour might now produce one-tenth of a visit. Of course, the assumption that marginal productivity is diminishing still holds, but the entire relationship is such that now more can be obtained at any level of output.

We will now examine how changes in some of the underlying conditions affect the production relationship. The possible changes include a change in the case mix, in the severity of illness of patients, in the quality of care, in technology, in the amount of capital (*F*) that the employer uses, and in the underlying incentive structure.

First, a change in the case mix, (type and/or severity of patients seen) would occur if the physician was confronted with a number of rheumatic fever cases in addition to patients with colds. More resources would need to be expended on each of these cases, shifting the production relationship downward. The same type of downward shift would occur if the physician merely had to treat some patients with especially severe colds. These cases would require more resources and would thus shift the production relationship downward.

Second, the result of a change in the quality of care will depend on the precise meaning attached to *quality*. If greater thoroughness in performing an examination is an aspect of higher quality care, then the effect of providing higher quality care is to shift the production relationship downward, because more resources would be required for each examination. Similarly, if more extensive patient education is an aspect of higher quality care, then the production relationship will again be pushed downward.

Third, high quality is frequently associated with high technology; in other words, highly trained specialists and sophisticated equipment. Offering the benefits of advances in technology thus usually entails an increase in capital, both human and physical. More input is required to produce a single unit of output (measured as a visit), and therefore the measured relationship between input and output will shift downward. However, note that more resource-intensive visits are qualitatively different than less resource-intensive ones. We cannot say that medical resources are less productive in any of these instances. Instead, a given amount of resources will produce a lower quantity of care, but this medical care is likely to be of a higher quality.

Of course, sometimes the introduction of a new piece of equipment can increase the quantity of output without changing the quality. As an example, if a computerized blood counter replaces a manually operated counter, more tests of the same quality can be processed with the same amount of variable input (technician time). The production relationship shifts upward in this case.

A final factor influencing the production relationship is the "management" incentive system. Our production relationship was derived using the assumption that the maximum output would be obtained at any given level of resource use. Incentives enter the picture when we consider the benefits that accrue to management (the physician, in our example) as a result of the way resources are used. If management is rewarded for keeping production costs low, then management will have an incentive to use as few resources as possible per unit of output. However, incentives can be structured in such a way as to encourage use of inputs. If, for example, the management receives a fixed rate of compensation that is positively related to its costs, then it will have an incentive to use more resources to perform each task. Even though the analysis of production lies in the realm of production management and medicine, the production relationship cannot be analyzed in total isolation from the economic incentives that exist within the organization.

5.2.3 Substitution Among Inputs

The analysis of the previous section was based on the assumption that one variable input existed. In fact, there may be several variable inputs, and they may be substitutable for each other, at least to some degree. Let us suppose that there are two variable inputs, nursing time (P) and medical assistant time (N), in addition to the fixed inputs (F). The production function is now expressed as $Q = Q(P, N, F)$.

Substitutability among inputs is often analyzed by assuming the level of output (Q) is held constant and then examining, for example, how much medical assistant time must be added to the process to offset a decrease in a unit of nursing time. We will call this the marginal rate of substitution of medical assistants for nurses.

A number of areas have been identified in health care in which substitution makes sense. One study examined the use of paraprofessional surgical assistants as substitutes for physicians or surgeons in the role of assistant to the operating surgeon. The study found that trained assistants could replace physicians in this assisting role with no adverse effects on the operating surgeon's time, particularly in less complex operations (Lewit, Bentkover, Bentkover, Watkins, & Hughes., 1980). Increasingly, computer-assisted procedures are being substituted for physician-only procedures. One study (Iampreechakul, Chongchokdee, & Tirakotai, 2011) found that such substitution could decrease overall surgery time without decreasing accuracy. Another study by Patel, Youssef, Vale, and Padhya, (2011) found that the use of computer-guided endoscopic transsphenoidal surgery increased procedure time without additional personnel.

Another example of the substitutability of inputs is the use of drugs in the care of mental patients. To some extent, increased utilization of drugs reduces the amount of effort required of psychiatric hospital attendants. Also, physician assistants and nurse practitioners can perform many of the tasks that physicians traditionally perform (Kleinpell, Ely, & Grabenkort, 2008; Leski, Young, & Higham, 2010; Reinhardt, 1972), and dental technicians can perform simple tasks, such as cleaning teeth and doing easy repairs (Yee, Crawford, & Harber, 2005).

Frequently, substitution is feasible and even economical, but barriers exist to limit it. For example, licensing laws may limit the degree to which nurse practitioners can substitute for physicians. In such cases, one must separate what is feasible from what is legally or institutionally permitted.

5.2.4 Volume-Outcome Relationship

The production function has been specified as a relationship between the volume of services provided and the quantity of inputs. As noted, there is also a relationship between the quality and volume of healthcare services. This relationship has usually been specified for specific surgical procedures.

Tsao, Lee, Loong, Chen, Chiu, & Tai (2011) found that there were significantly higher quality and lower costs in high-volume kidney transplant hospitals in Taiwan than in low-volume hospitals. In a review of the literature, the authors Halm, Lee, and Chassin (2002) found that there was, in general, a positive association between higher volumes and better outcomes; however, the magnitude of the relationship varied widely among the studies, as did the methodological quality of the studies. Begg, Cramer, Hoskins, & Brennan (1998) found a significant association between volume and short-term outcomes in cancer care, which has been supported in more recent studies (Birkmeyer, Sun, Wong, & Stukel., 2007; Joudi & Konety, 2005; Ward, Jaana, Wakefield, Ohsfeldt, Schneider, Miller, & Lei, 2004).

In discussing the relationship between volume and outcome, the focus can be on the volume of services that are provided by individual providers (surgeons or surgical teams) or the service volume of a healthcare organization (Garnick, Luft, McPhee, & Mark, 1989; Roukos, 2009; Tsao et al., 2011). Surgeons individually or as part of a team, can maintain their skills better when they perform more of the same types of procedures during a specified time period. If they do only a few operations of a given type within a given time frame, they may get out of practice, their team may lose its cohesiveness and skills, and the quality of their work may deteriorate. We would therefore expect a positive relationship between the volume of a given procedure for a given practitioner or team and outcomes of the care provided.

A positive relationship between volume and outcome may also hold for an institution, but for different reasons. An institution with an especially large volume of certain procedures may hire specialized personnel and acquire specialized equipment. For example, in the area of rehabilitation, an institution with specialized personnel and equipment can return patients to normal functioning sooner. Thus, the relationship between volume and outcome can work separately for the surgical (or treatment) team and for the institution where the treatment occurs.

There is a confounding factor that can make it difficult to interpret an observed relationship between outcome and volume. If a surgical team is known to be more skilled, then the team will be sought out by patients. We would then observe a positive relationship between outcomes and volume, but the high volume may not be the cause of the team's maintenance of its skills. Thus, a policy that encourages larger volumes for surgical teams regardless of their skill levels may not be successful in improving the overall levels of outcome. A further confounding factor may be that an especially skilled surgical team may attract the most difficult cases, which would tend to worsen outcomes irrespective of provider skills. In evaluating the outcomes of the providers and/or institutions, it is important to consider the case mix and severity of the patient population. Determining the causes of the observed relationship is important for policy reasons, although it may be difficult, in practice, to uncover the real causes.

5.3 SHORT-RUN COST–OUTPUT RELATIONSHIPS

5.3.1 Production and Cost

Previously, we focused on the relationship between output and alternative combinations of inputs. In specifying the production relationship, the inputs were presented as separate entities that work together. The next step in our analysis is to present a measure of the overall commitment of resources by the provider in producing the output. One such measure, which places all inputs on a single scale measured in money terms, is cost. To a provider, cost means the value of inputs used in the production process. However, this value may not always be well approximated by money outlays.

Therefore, a broader view of cost—one that measures what the provider gives up by using all the resources committed to production, not just the ones paid for—is used in this section. Of central importance is the concept of opportunity cost, which is defined as the value that the provider gave up by not committing the resources to the next highest valued use. Another way of putting it is that the cost of resources is measured by the amount for which those resources could be sold in the market, or the market value of the resources used in the production process. This concept is particularly important when measuring the value of resources that are not paid for to others (e.g., resources that the producer owns) and hence that appear to be free. If the owner of these unpaid resources is giving up some return on them, then there is a cost associated with them, and this cost must be estimated by calculating the probable market value of the resources. These resources are often considered to be implicit costs because they don't require an outlay of money.

Because we are concerned with the functioning of an organization, the cost of resource use will be considered from the organization's point of view. Any organization can undertake a resource commitment that does not appear in its paid-out costs. Nevertheless, if the organization commits its resources to a particular use, they are part of the organization's costs and should be counted as such. On the other hand, an economic unit outside the organization may make a resource commitment that allows the organization to function. For example, a person may give blood to a blood donor clinic, a benefactor may endow a hospital with an operating room, or a physician may volunteer teaching time at a medical school. In these instances, resources are used to undertake activities, but they are not part of the resource commitment of the institution. Rather, they are part of the total resource commitment required to undertake the activity. In this chapter, we are concerned with the operations of healthcare organizations and so focus on the resource commitment made by these organizations in their activities. This leaves out the question of the total (or social) resource commitment made to perform any activity, including the commitment of donors, volunteers, benefactors, and government agencies.

In the analysis that follows, the definitions presented are placed in a time frame of one month, or a single production cycle. Given this time frame, we can divide production costs into fixed costs and variable costs. Fixed costs are defined as those that do not change, or vary, with output within the relevant time frame. Variable costs, on the other hand, increase as output increases; they vary with output in the production cycle. In the physician's practice example, the fixed costs are those that do not vary during the month; they are the costs of the fixed factors, including space and equipment rental costs and the cost of physician time. We will assume the rental values to be $50 during the period. We will also assume that the physician could have earned $50 working in a clinic rather than in a private practice; this amount measures the opportunity cost the physician faced when making the decision whether to continue to practice privately. Given that the decision to practice privately has been made, the forgoing of other ways of using work time becomes a "sunk" cost, relevant more to the past than to the present. A sunk cost is one that has already been committed and cannot be recovered. Nevertheless, it is still a cost, and is classified as a fixed cost. The total fixed costs thus, in this example, equal $100. (The cost curve of a company incorporates the return that the owners could normally get on their assets, including their time, the buildings they own, and so on. This normal return is called *normal profit*, which is associated with the risk taken, not a specific percentage. Any return above normal profit is called *economic profit* and is typically viewed as excessive and not sustainable in the long run.)

Variable costs are costs of inputs that change as the firm alters the quantity of output produced during the production cycle. In our example, the only variable input is nursing hours. Assume that the price of nursing services is $2 per hour. Thus, eight hours of services cost $16. We can now specify the relationship between the cost to the provider and the level of output. This relationship depends on the quantities of resources used (determined by the production relationship) and the money paid for, or the opportunity cost imputed to, these resource services. The relationship can be viewed in three different ways. First, we can examine costs from the point of view of the total resource commitment required to maintain production at any specific level of output. In this case, we determine how total costs vary with output. Second, we can look at the average value of resource commitment, that is, the total cost of the resource commitment required to produce the total output or total costs divided by total output. The value of this average resource commitment is called *average cost*. The third way of viewing costs is to examine the value of additional resources that must be committed to the production process to produce an additional unit of output. This value is called the *marginal cost*. We will now discuss how each of these alternative measures varies as the level of output changes.

5.3.2 Total Cost

Total cost (*TC*) is the sum of all costs incurred in producing a given level of output; total variable cost (*TVC*) is the total cost of variable inputs for any level of output; total fixed cost (*TFC*) is the total cost of all fixed factors. Total cost is the sum of the total variable cost and the total fixed cost. We now look at these types of cost with regard to the data contained in Table 5-1. The total fixed cost is $100 whatever the level of output. Therefore, this cost, plotted on the graph in Figure 5-3, is represented by a straight horizontal line (*TFC*) at the $100 level.

The behavior of the total variable cost depends on two factors: the relationship between output and variable inputs, specified in Section 5.2; and the unit cost of these variable resources. Figure 5-3 contains a total variable cost curve that reflects the data in our example.

The total cost curve (*TC*) is the vertical sum of the two curves *TVC* and *TFC* at each output level (see Table 5-1, column 6). The level of the *TC* curve is determined, in part, by the fixed cost; its shape is determined by the production function and the variation of output with variable inputs. Given the fixed per-unit price of the variable input ($2 an hour), the production function relation, translated into a cost–output relationship, entails that the addition to total costs of the extra resource commitment levels off as output increases. Thus, the total variable cost is $16 at a scale of one visit, $30 at a scale of two visits, $40 at a scale of three visits, and $48 at a scale of four visits. This leveling off of cost is shown diagrammatically by the flattening of the section between 0 and 4 of curve *TVC* in Figure 5-3. If additional

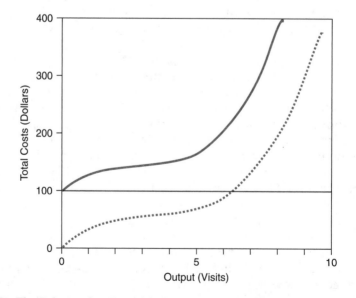

Figure 5-3 The Relationship Between the Total Fixed Cost, Total Variable Cost, Total Cost, and Level of Output. At each production level, total cost can be divided between the fixed and variable costs. The fixed cost does not vary with output. This graph is based on data from Table 5-1.

resources had been increasingly more productive beyond this scale of input, the *TVC* curve would have continued leveling off. But beyond four units of output, diminishing marginal productivity begins to set in; and in terms of costs, this means that successively greater resource commitments are needed to attain successively higher levels of output. In Table 5-1, the total variable cost rises to 60, 76, 100, 128, 200, and so on, and the total cost also rises rapidly. As seen on the curve, beyond a scale of 4, *TVC* is curving upward; at the extreme, it would become almost vertical. Thus, a considerable commitment in resources is required to move to a higher output level. The shape of *TC* is similar to that of *TVC*, except that *TC* is higher by $100.

5.3.3 Marginal Cost

Implicit in the total variable cost–output relationship is the marginal cost–output relationship. The marginal cost at any level of output is the additional cost required to move one unit higher on the output scale. It is thus defined as $\Delta TC/\Delta Q$. Because *TFC* is constant over all levels of output, the marginal fixed cost would be zero at any value, because the additional fixed resource commitment is zero at all levels of output. Thus, the marginal cost is simply the addition to total variable cost needed to produce one extra unit of output. In Table 5-1, the marginal cost (*MC*) is shown in column 10. As can be seen, the extra cost of moving to one unit of output from zero is $16, to two units from one is $14, and so on. Until we reach four units of output, *MC* is falling. However, because of the diminishing marginal productivity of variable inputs, coupled with the fact that the additional variable inputs used are all paid the same wage, producing additional units of output eventually requires successively greater resource commitment. This is reflected in rising marginal cost after the fourth visit; the fifth visit costs $12 extra; the sixth, $16 extra; and so on. The marginal cost curve is shown in Figure 5-4. Note that beyond an output of 4, marginal costs cease falling and begin to rise.

The concept of marginal cost is central to the analysis of most economic decisions. For the most part, the types of decisions that concern economists involve determining the consequences of employing additional (or fewer) resources for a particular purpose. For example, we might be concerned with the implications of placing additional surgeon-training facilities in either Boston or Boise, we might analyze the consequences of adding one or more paramedics to an existing medical practice, or we might be interested in the consequences of decreasing the number of obstetrics beds in a particular region of the country or a particular hospital. In these instances, as in most other cases of resource allocation, the allocation decision concerns whether to expand a particular facility or service or increase the available quantity of trained personnel. The concept used to measure the added resource commitment is the marginal cost.

5.3.4 Average Cost

The third way of looking at costs is to average the costs required to obtain a given level of output. The average total cost (*ATC*) is the total cost per unit of output and is defined for any level of output. It equals *TC/Q*. It measures

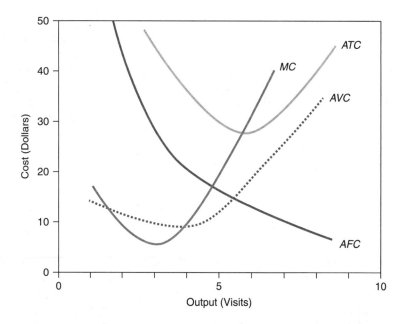

Figure 5-4 Relationship Between Cost and Output. The average cost is shown in total (*ATC*) and as separated into the two components of the total: fixed cost (*AFC*) and variable cost (*AVC*). Marginal costs (*MC*) is the addition to total cost of the next unit produced. There is a unique relationship between *MC* and both *AVC* and *ATC*: when *MC* is below *ATC* (or *AVC*), the average cost is falling; when *MC* is greater than *ATC* (or *AVC*), the average cost is increasing; and when *MC* equals *ATC* (or *AVC*), the average cost is constant; that is, it has reached a minimum point.

---

the value of the average resource commitment required to sustain a given scale of output. However, because it is useful in making comparisons, this variable has been frequently used in empirical studies.

The behavior of the average total cost depends on the behavior of the average fixed cost (*TFC/Q*) and the average variable cost (*TVC/Q*). The average fixed cost is lower at successively higher levels of output because the $100 in fixed cost is spread out over more and more output. Thus, at one visit, the average fixed cost is $100; at two visits, it is $50; and so on. The average variable cost initially falls at successively greater levels of output. At one unit of output, it is $16; at two, it is $15; at three, it is $13.30; and so on. The fall in average variable cost is made possible by the increasing productivity of additional variable inputs at low output levels. Another way of viewing this relationship is to consider that the marginal cost is initially below the average cost, which brings down the average cost as output increases. The marginal cost for the first visit is $16, and the average variable cost is $16. For the second visit, the marginal cost is $14. This brings down the average variable cost of the two visits to $15 (i.e., $30/2). The falling average variable and the average fixed cost, together, ensure that the average total cost (which is the sum of the two) will also fall as output expands. Eventually, after four visits, the marginal cost increases as output expands. Expanding output from four to five visits costs an extra $12, expanding to six visits costs another $16, and the marginal cost at seven is $24. However, as long as the marginal cost is lower than the average total cost, a further expansion of output will continue to reduce the average total cost.

For example, in Table 5-1 we can see that at five units of output, the total cost is $160 and the average total cost is $32. An expansion of output by one unit to a level of output of six would cost an additional $16. The *ATC* at six units of output decreases to $29.33 because the *MC* of the sixth unit of output is lower than the *ATC*, and so expanding output brings down the average. With a rising *MC*, this situation will not continue indefinitely. At some level of output, the *MC* will just equal the *ATC*, and at a still higher level, it will exceed it. The *ATC* must then begin to rise. In our example, the level at which the *MC* equals the *ATC* is eight visits. As seen in Table 5-1, an expansion from seven to eight visits will cost an extra $28. With an *ATC* of $28.57 at the level of seven visits, expansion to eight visits leaves the *ATC* at about the same level. An expansion to nine visits has an *MC* of $72. This is above the *ATC* at eight visits. The *ATC* increases to $33.33 at nine visits.

The average cost curves are shown in Figure 5-4 in juxtaposition to the *MC* curve. These curves are based on the data presented in Table 5-1, but have been smoothed out. The average fixed cost (*AFC*) curve declines over all levels of output. The average variable cost (*AVC*) curve declines until four visits. At five visits, the *MC* just equals the *AVC*, and so the *AVC* curve bottoms out. For output levels higher than five, the *MC* is above the *AVC*, and so the *AVC* increases with expansion of output. The *AVC* curve is thus U-shaped, indicating that at lower levels of output the *AVC* falls as output expands. The *AVC* curve then bottoms (where *MC* = *AVC*) and begins to rise. The *ATC* curve (remember, *ATC* = *AVC* + *AFC*) is also U-shaped. It is located above and slightly to the right of the *AVC* curve and also bottoms out where the rising *MC* cuts it.

The *ATC*, as already noted, has a fixed and a variable component. The relative sizes of these two components will determine at which level of output the *ATC* curve will begin to slope upward. The fixed cost component (*AFC*) always falls as output increases, because the same costs are spread over a greater output. The variable cost component (*AVC*) follows the rules of productivity and begins to rise, because eventually higher marginal costs will raise the average. The larger the fixed cost component, the greater the range over which the average total cost will fall. Hospitals have been identified as having large fixed cost components. If this is indeed true, then hospitals should experience a diminishing average total cost over a wide range of potential output levels.

The fixed cost component is related to the use of capital equipment. A heavy investment in capital equipment will create a large fixed cost. However, such equipment may permit additional procedures to be undertaken with a small additional commitment of resources up to high levels of output. In such a situation, although the fixed cost would be high, the marginal cost would be low, and the average total cost would fall over a wide range of output levels. In a related phenomenon, called *indivisibility*, expensive equipment, available in a large dose, cannot be divided into smaller units. It is operated at low levels of output at a high *ATC* and operated at high levels at a low *ATC*.

This section has identified three related cost–output measures: total cost, average cost, and marginal cost. Their shapes are dependent largely on the production relationship. As shown in Section 5.2, the production relationship is subject to shifts caused by a variety of conditions. These same conditions can cause a cost curve to change its positions, as discussed next.

5.4 COST CURVE POSITION

The position of a cost curve is determined by the same factors that influence the production relationship. These factors include the case mix and the severity of cases treated, the quality of care provided, the technology used, the amount of fixed factors employed in the production process, and the incentive system under which the provider is operating. In addition, change in input prices can affect the position of the cost curve. Each factor will be considered separately.

Given fixed inputs and fixed costs, a change in the case mix toward more complicated cases and an increase in the average severity level will increase the variable resources required per unit of output and will thus increase marginal and average costs at all output levels. The positions of both the ATC and MC curves will now be higher. The shifts in position are shown in Figure 5-5. Here, ATC_1 and MC_1 are the average total cost and marginal cost relationships before the change to a more complex case mix. This change results in a shift to ATC_2 and MC_2.

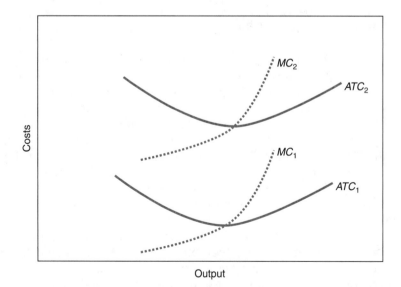

Figure 5-5 A Shift in Average and Marginal Cost Curves. Curves ATC_1 and MC_1 indicate the initial relationship between costs and output. Curves ATC_2 and MC_2 represent an upward shift in costs at every level of output.

An increase in quality, if this entails more thorough examinations or treatments, will similarly shift the cost curves upward. The adoption of a technology that uses more resources per case will have a similar effect. Many recent technological innovations have been associated with a large capital investment for equipment as well as a larger flow of variable expenditures for the services of the highly trained personnel needed to operate this equipment. Examples of such technological innovations include open-heart surgery, a procedure that intrigued economists in the 1960s; coronary care units (CCUs) or intensive care units (ICUs), which are high-cost monitoring and life support units; computed tomography (CT) scanning; magnetic resonance imaging (MRI), a revolutionary and somewhat costly advance in radiology; and laparoscopic surgery, which allows a surgeon to perform an operation through a small incision. All these examples require a heavy investment in equipment, and the effect of introducing any of them would be to shift both the fixed and variable components of the *ATC* upward, thus increasing the *ATC* for all levels of output. However, it should be remembered that an increase in the quality of services provided may accompany the introduction of new technology. One physician visit or one hospital stay is not always the same as another.

All technological innovations in medical care are not of this resource-using type, however. Innovations in pharmaceuticals have reduced the length of hospitalization required for some illnesses. Two notable examples are tuberculosis treatment and mental illness treatment. Furthermore, new laboratory equipment has allowed many tasks to be automated. This has led to falling average costs over broad ranges of output because of the low variable costs associated with the use of this equipment. Surgical interventions have also changed, with many surgical procedures becoming less invasive thereby requiring fewer days in the hospital to recuperate therefore leading to decreasing average costs.

The effect of incentives that encourage resource use is to raise the level of average cost associated with any single level of output. Assuming that a single least-cost position is associated with each output level, we can identify a least-cost average cost curve. Incentives to use resources will encourage the provider to choose a position above this curve. It has been questioned whether a cost curve that measures the cost–output relationship when given resources are not used to maximize output (i.e., a more-than-least-cost curve) is a meaningful concept. This is because more than one such average cost point may exist at any output level. There can be only one least-cost point, however, and in the least-cost case, a cost curve that supposedly represents a unique relationship between cost and output can be uniquely determined. Once a provider chooses to use more than the least amount of resources to achieve a given output level (with no change in quality), he or she can use these excessive resources to varying degrees. There is no longer a unique cost curve (Zuckerman, Hadley, & Iezzoni, 1994).

Another factor that might cause cost curves to shift is the price the provider pays for hired resources. In our example, if the physician had to pay $3 per nursing hour instead of $2, both the marginal and the average cost curves would shift upward. Conversely, if the price fell to $1, the curves would shift downward. A final factor that can influence the position of the average cost curves appears when two or more types of variable input exist. When these inputs can be substituted for each other, at least to some degree, then a substitution of a less costly for a more costly input can lower the cost curves, although other factors may push them the other way. For example, if a paramedic is substituted for a physician but takes much longer to do the same task, the total or average cost may not shift downward as a result of the substitution. Also, keep in mind that the quality of the product may become lower as a result of the substitution, and even though the output may cost less to produce, it might not be exactly comparable.

5.5 ECONOMIES OF SCOPE

We have proceeded with the discussion of costs as if a healthcare institution had a single type of output. Although this assumption helps to clarify certain relationships between costs and output, it is generally false in the case of larger institutions, notably hospitals. Hospitals are multiproduct firms that offer a large number of separate product lines, such as clinical laboratory services, emergency department services, physical therapy, and intensive care (Berry, 1973; Goldfarb, Hornbrook, & Rafferty, 1980).

The product line dimension of output should be distinguished from the case-mix dimension. Case mix refers to the complexity of the types of diseases being treated. A hospital that treats a large number of different diseases has a different case mix than one that specializes in a few. If, as is sometimes done, severity is included as a dimension of case mix, then case-mix indexes can be developed (Hornbrook & Monheit, 1985). Each hospital also has a number of services or product lines. In fact, two hospitals can have very similar case-mix measures but very different service scopes. As a consequence, the relationship between cost and scope offers itself as a possibly fruitful topic of investigation.

Economies of scope are savings derived from producing different products jointly/simultaneously in the same production unit rather than producing them individually in separate production units. Let X_1 stand for one output (e.g., family planning services) and X_2 stand for a second output (e.g., pediatric services). Let $C(X_1)$ stand for the total cost of producing X_1, let $C(X_2)$ stand for the total cost of producing X_2 in a separate setting, and $C(X_1, X_2)$ stand for the cost of jointly producing X_1 and X_2 in the same production unit. Economies of scope arise when the cost of jointly producing specific quantities of the two services [$C(X_1, X_2)$] is less than the sum of the costs of producing each service separately [$C(X_1) + C(X_2)$]. In our example, economies of scope would exist if a clinic could jointly produce given quantities of family planning services and pediatric services more cheaply than the same quantities produced in sharply separated units or departments.

Economies of scope might arise when some of the tasks involved in providing two distinct services are complementary. For example, if family planning and pediatric services require a common core of testing capabilities, then providing the two types of services in separate units would cause duplication. Savings could be achieved by combining the two services into a single unit that caters to both groups of patients. Of course, it is also possible to have diseconomies of scope. This would occur when two types of output are best produced in separate units. For example, if psychiatric patients are treated with one regimen and home health service patients with a different one, combining the psychiatric and home health services in a single unit may be more costly than keeping them separate.

In one study of the economies of scope in health care, Cowing and Holtmann (1983) estimated economies of scale and scope for 138 short-term hospitals in New York State. They divided hospital output into five diagnostic categories (actually representing different case mixes rather than service scopes): medical-surgical, maternity, pediatric, other inpatient care, and emergency department care. For four of the services (pediatric care being the exception), marginal cost fell over low ranges of output and then became constant. These results indicate substantial economies of scale in these services and suggest that merging services produced on a small scale into larger units could yield considerable savings. However, with regard to the existence of economies of scope, the findings were generally negative. These findings, if they hold up in repeated trials, indicate that, on cost grounds alone, hospitals should specialize rather than become multiproduct organizations. One must be careful not to overgeneralize, because, even though economies of scope may not be widespread, specific services may have production conditions that, when combined, yield economies of scope.

Gonzales (1997) applied the economies of scope theory to the home health industry in Connecticut. In the study, costs initially decrease as the scope of services provided increase. However, as the scope of services continued to rise, the costs of providing the services increase even more, demonstrating diseconomies of scope. The provision of services under diseconomies of scope reflects the services being provided beyond the point at which they could be produced cost effectively. Dunn, Sacher, Cohen, & Hsiao (1995), found that there were significant economies of scope in the provision of multiple surgery.

5.6 LONG-RUN COST CURVES

In deriving the cost curves in Section 5.4, the assumption was made that some of the inputs were fixed. Suppose we take a longer perspective and allow enough time for the providing unit to change its "fixed" factors—to expand or contract its physical plant, to buy and sell equipment, and to hire and fire physicians. For planning periods of sufficient length, such changes are certainly possible. An analysis of relevant issues is called a *long-run analysis*.

Indeed, the factors that are considered fixed from the perspective of the short term are no longer fixed; they too can vary. From the longer planning perspective, all resources are variable. Suppose a hospital board is planning to build a new facility from scratch. The board can choose either a 60-, 120-, or 250-bed facility, entailing a capital outlay of $2 million, $3 million, or $3.5 million, respectively. Associated with each size is the given annual capital cost of depreciation and the interest on the financing capital. During the planning period—up until the size decision is made—these capital costs can be varied (in three different levels) and thus are variable. That is, if the time horizon is sufficiently long, all costs in the production process become variable.

Associated with each facility under consideration is an average cost curve (either ATC_1, ATC_2, or ATC_3 in Figure 5-6), which includes capital costs (remember that, in the long run, there are no fixed costs). Now assume that each facility is least costly for a given range of output. For fewer than 1,000 annual admissions, ATC_1 is the least costly; for over 3,000 admissions, ATC_3 is the least costly. Depending on which level of output is chosen, one plant size will be the least costly. The dashed curve in Figure 5-6 represents the least cost that can be used to produce at any given output level (assuming we can choose the size of the facility). This is called the *long-run average cost (LRAC)* curve. It is made up of the minimum cost points at each output level. The *LRAC* is usually hypothesized, if it were represented in a smooth fashion, to be U-shaped. Such a shape would be generated by falling long-run average costs (economies of scale) at low levels of output, followed by constant and finally increasing costs (diseconomies of scale).

Before discussing such costs, it is necessary to specify whether the entity in question is a single operating unit (e.g., an individual hospital, nursing home, or ambulatory care clinic) or an entire system (e.g., a corporate chain). A single operating entity may be subject to eventual diseconomies, because the gains from specialization in certain tasks eventually run out. Also, a single hospital unit may be able to expand only by the addition of diverse units

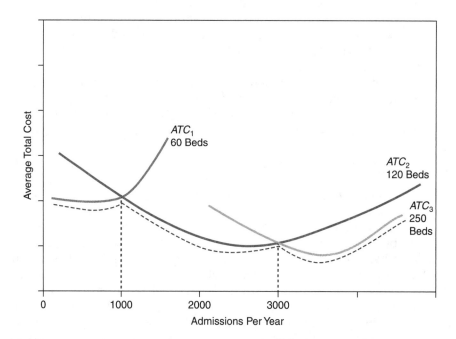

Figure 5-6 Relationship Between Short- and Long-run Average Cost Curves. Short-run curves (ATC_1, ATC_2, and ATC_3) are shown for three plant sizes (expressed in terms of bed size). The long-run average cost curve (*LRAC*) is derived from these curves (shown as the dashed line). The *LRAC* is the minimum cost point at each level of output). At 1,000 and 3,000 admissions, the LRAC curve becomes associated with the different cost curves (different plant sizes), because it becomes more economical to produce successively greater outputs with larger-sized plants.

(e.g., a CAT scanning unit or a physiotherapy department), and such units may be costly to manage in a single unit. For these reasons, the long-run cost curve of the single operating unit may exhibit diseconomies of scale.

A multiplant system, such as a multihospital corporation, may exhibit economies of scale as it expands by acquiring additional distinct operating units. Certain functions, such as purchasing, may be run more efficiently on a scale that exceeds that of an individual operating unit. Furthermore, a multi-unit system can develop standardized procedures in patient records, accounting, and the like, and can make comparisons among units. For these reasons, as a system expands, it may exhibit economies of scale, at least up to a point.

5.7 EMPIRICAL ESTIMATION OF COST CURVES

5.7.1 Background

Average, or per-unit, cost is a convenient and accessible summary of a producer's performance. To obtain the average cost at any level of output, divide total cost by total quantity. Given the convenience of this measure of performance, it is natural that analysts would use it to compare producers who produce roughly the same product, but at different levels of output. Our simple, unqualified, short-run hypothesis would lead us to expect a U-shaped relation between average cost and output. However, interproducer comparisons are fraught with complications.

Quality, case mix, and technology differences among producing units may make comparisons difficult. For this reason, as well as others cited in Section 5.4, producers may be operating on different cost curves, as shown in Figure 5-7, in which ATC_1, ATC_2, and ATC_3 are average short-run cost curves of three producers. As compared with Producer 1, Producer 2 is producing a higher quality product or serving patients with a more severe case mix, but is using the same amounts of fixed inputs. Therefore, Producer 2's cost curve (ATC_2) is above ATC_1 at all levels of output. To identify the shape of the short-run cost curve, one must control for factors that shift the curve. Assume, for example, that Producer 1's cost–output point is at x and Producer 2's is at v. Without knowing how the quality of services and other factors differed, one would not know if points x and v are on the same curve or on different curves.

In estimating long-run cost curves, one encounters even greater difficulties. Let us say that Producer 3 has a more capital-intensive operation than Producers 1 or 2 because Producer 3 has invested more heavily in capital equipment to gain economies from automation. Let us also assume that the quality and case mix of Producer 3 are similar to those of Producer 1. The true long-run cost curve for the industry (assuming that these are the only two scales of operations available) is ATC_1 up to point t in Figure 5-7 and ATC_3 for scales of output above and beyond point t. But when we start to estimate this curve, we do not know this. Among the data that are usually available for making such comparisons, we have only one observation for each producer. These observations tell us, for example, that Producer 1 is producing at 1,000 units of output with an ATC of $50, Producer 2 is producing at 1,200 units with an ATC of $80, and so on. (We may, of course, also have

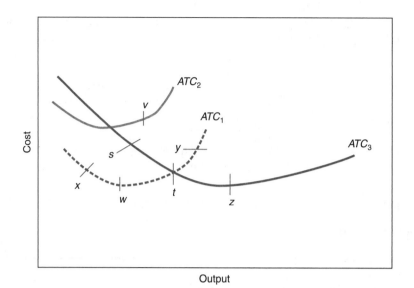

Figure 5-7   Identifying Points on the *ATC* Curve. When data are gathered from producers on their average total costs at various output levels, care must be taken in interpreting these points. Data points collected from different producers may be on similar ATC curves (such as *x*, *w*, *y*, and *t*) or on different *ATC* curves (such as *v* and *y*). The key to determining which is more likely is to identify extraneous circumstances (other than output) that might have caused producers to operate on different curves. These circumstances, if identified, would lead to the conclusion whether pairs such as *x* and *z* are on different or similar curves. The circumstances that shift the cost curve (or lead to different cost curves) include differences in input prices, quality of output, and capital equipment.

some information on some of the operating characteristics of each producer.) With this information, we have only one point on each producer's cost curve, which is not enough to tell us where on its cost curve each producer is operating.

If, for example, Producer 1 is producing at point *x* and Producer 3 at point *z*, then both are on the long-run cost curve, and an estimation of a long-run cost curve with points such as these will give us a reasonably accurate picture of what the long-run cost curve looks like. But there is no reason why we should be so lucky. Producer 1 could well be producing at a high-capacity level, such as point *y*, and Producer 3 could be at a low-capacity level, such as point *s*. Although both are on their short-run curves, neither is on its long-run curve. We would have no way of knowing this, and if we assumed that we were estimating a long-run curve, we would end up with biased results.

In fact, where on its cost curve each producer is producing depends on supply. It also depends on the producer's goals or objectives as well as the conditions underlying costs and revenues, which is the topic of the chapter on the behavior of supply. Following are brief summaries of empirical evidence on producer cost curves for several health-related activities. When reviewing this material, keep in mind the difficulties in identifying actual cost–output relations.

5.7.2 Group Practices

Group medical practices have occasionally been held up as institutions that should yield considerable economies of scale and thus help raise output while moderating increases in total costs. Because a fairly large number of group practices are in operation, it might seem that the proposition that average costs are falling would be easy to test. However, because of the considerable variation in the types of group practices, difficulties in output measurements, and problems associated with gathering appropriate data, only tentative answers have been obtained. The first statistical analysis was done using data collected on solo and group practices in the field of internal medicine (Bailey, 1968). Because the study compared practices in the same field, it circumvented problems associated with the inclusion of different production techniques used by different types of practices. The data collected showed that the average volume of services provided per physician, adjusted for the type of visit (e.g., routine visit, annual examination, or complete examination), was greater for solo practices than for group practices. Although the sample size was small, it cast some doubt on the existence of economies of scale.

There are several reasons why this finding may not be so surprising. First, the technology generally used in internal medicine is such that the gains from task specialization and the use of capital-intensive techniques may be achieved at a low level of output. For the tasks involved in operating an internal medicine practice, the *ATC* curve may reach a lower point at a scale of output supportable by one practitioner. Second, an incentive factor may be at work when several practitioners combine forces. This factor, which has a tendency to shift the *ATC* curve upward when the group is formed, is operative in situations in which members of the practice share revenues and costs. When this sharing occurs, the revenues that any single member of the group generates are shared, and the costs that he or she incurs are borne by all the members. Because of reduced burden, the individual physician can make a heavier use of nurses' time and of equipment while feeling less impact than in a solo practice. It is hypothesized that, under cost-sharing arrangements, each physician in the group will generate more costs than in a solo practice, pushing up the cost curve for the group. Furthermore, the larger the group, the higher will be the cost curve (assuming that offsetting factors do not exist; see Scheffler, 1975).

Another study analyzed interpractice variations in the relationship between staff salary costs and scale of output (measured by office visits) for a sample of single-specialty practices, although they were not all of the same specialty (Newhouse, 1973). The presence of cost sharing was found to shift the cost curve upward for group practices. Furthermore, after adjusting for this incentive factor, the cost curve was found to exhibit economies of scale, indicating that such economies do exist among practices with no cost sharing and also among practices with some cost sharing. Because of the small sample, the inattention paid to case mix, and technology differences among practices due to specialty differences, the results are not conclusive.

Pauly (1996) investigated multispecialty group practices and found that the evidence does not suggest that such group practices will obtain economies of scope because of their diversity, but that they may be able to coordinate the process of care better. Engberg, Wholley, Feldman, & Christianson (2004) concluded that mergers among health maintenance organizations that produce Medicare and other products are likely to create diseconomies of scope that increase costs.

5.7.3 Hospital Marginal Costs

The importance of the topic of hospital marginal cost is related to the objective of reimbursing hospitals for the extra resource costs they incur when their volumes change. If a hospital is being reimbursed at the level of costs in 1995, and its admissions have increased by 5%, its additional costs may be greater than, equal to, or less than 5%. If the hospital is reimbursed an additional 5% (ignoring inflation) to cover the volume differential, and actual costs had gone up by 3%, the hospital would incur a windfall gain. On the other hand, the hospital would lose out if its costs had increased by 10%.

Marginal cost variation is often measured using the ratio of marginal to average costs (M/A). Recall that if M is greater than A (or $M/A > 1$), then the average cost will increase (Section 5.3). For example, beginning from an initial output level of 1,000 admissions and an average cost of $200 per case, if output expands by 5% (50 admissions) and M is $220, then M/A is 1.1. Expansion has raised the average cost, and if the hospital was reimbursed for the additional cases at $200 per case, it would incur a loss. If the hospital was reimbursed on the basis of its prior year's costs plus the marginal cost of its additional cases, it would be fully reimbursed.

This problem has arisen in a number of instances. During the early 1970s, when price controls were set on hospital revenues, allowable revenues were set at the previous year's revenue levels, plus an inflation factor, plus a volume adjustment based on estimates of M/A (Lipscomb et al., 1978). In the Finger Lakes region of New York State, a regional reimbursement experiment was set up: hospitals were reimbursed based on a base-year cost, plus an inflation factor, plus a volume adjustment that assumed that the value of M/A was 0.4 for inpatient care and 0.6 for outpatient care (Farnand, Jacobs, & Dickson, 1986). And currently under Medicare regulations, hospitals are given extra reimbursement for cases in a particular diagnostic group whose length of stay or costs are outside diagnostic limits (outliers). The additional reimbursement is based on an M/A value of 0.6 for the extra days.

One way of estimating hospital marginal cost is to take short-term (e.g., monthly) values of operating costs and volume for a given hospital over a period (two to three years) and find the average variation in costs with a given variation in output. Another way is to relate variation in costs and outputs across hospitals. The former method will probably give a more accurate estimate than the latter of short-run marginal cost, but there are difficulties even with it. Among these are that the cost levels of inputs must be adjusted for (assuming they have changed) and that capital equipment and operating techniques must remain the same throughout the study period (otherwise the hospital will have moved from one short-run cost curve to another).

In addition, the marginal cost will depend on the measure of output (e.g., whether it is length of stay or admissions). It will vary with the amount of the volume adjustment (e.g., 2 or 5%) and the relative permanence of the adjustment as estimated by the hospital administrator. For a volume increase that is small or short-lived, the administrator may decide to tax existing resources for a time rather than immediately expand and thereby raise marginal cost. The estimate of M under these circumstances would appear to be lower than if the administrator responded more automatically.

For the preceding reasons, there is no accepted measure of the true short-run value of M/A (Lave & Lave, 1984). Estimates range from 0.2 to 0.6, but remember that the value will vary depending on a number of factors (Friedman & Pauly, 1983).

5.7.4 Hospital Economies of Scale

A large number of studies have investigated the possible existence of economies of scale in hospitals, with very mixed results (Berki, 1972; Frech & Mobley, 1995). Early studies identified economies of scale, but subsequent studies have uncovered no evidence (Lave & Lave, 1984) or conflicting evidence (Frech & Mobley, 1995). There is an explanation for the differences in findings.

As discussed earlier, the typical hospital is an organization with a complex case mix and a large number of different services. Each service has its own cost–output relation, which may exhibit economies of scale. The scope of services is greater for larger hospitals (Berry, 1973), but these hospitals may have more varied case types, so some services (e.g., cobalt therapy) that are devoted to specific case types may be operated at low capacity and high cost. A multiproduct hospital can be quite large, yet have a number of services with considerable excess capacity (Finkler, 1979b). As a result, it might exhibit a higher average cost than many smaller hospitals.

One study (Hornbrook & Monheit, 1985) that incorporated both case-mix and service scope variables to investigate economies of scale found no such economies at the hospital level. But a number of studies of individual services, such as open-heart surgery facilities, CT scanner units, therapeutic radiology facilities, and hospital laundries, have found evidence of economies of scale (Finkler, 1979a; Gregory, 1976–1977; McGregor & Pelletier, 1978; Okunade, 1993; Schwartz & Joskow, 1980). This suggests that the economies of scale that do occur in some hospital departments are offset by diseconomies of scale in others.

Yatchak (2000) found that economies of scale had recently evolved for nonteaching and teaching hospitals, reflecting the pressure of market forces associated with decreased revenues. Valdmaris (2010) found that hospitals would benefit from decreasing costs by exploiting economies of scale. Burns and Lee (2006) found that hospital purchasing alliances represented an important source of economies of scale for hospitals.

5.7.5 Nursing Home Costs

A number of studies have been undertaken in the nursing home area with a view to determining the effect on costs of operating variables, such as volume of operations, product quality, case mix, and organizational characteristics (e.g., for-profit or nonprofit status and membership in a chain) (Bishop, 1980). The relevant variable for such studies is average cost, which is the most appropriate variable for a comparison of costs in different facilities. There is no agreement as to whether total costs (which include fixed costs, such as administrative costs, interest, and depreciation) or only variable costs should be used. Using just variable costs would be appropriate when focusing on short-term operations, whereas including capital and other fixed costs would be appropriate when dealing with long-term issues. For example, one might want to find out whether a large-scale plant is more efficient than a small-scale plant. Asking which is the most efficient implies that time would be allowed to develop a plant of the appropriate size.

Studies that have examined the relationship between average cost and various causal variables have uncovered some interesting relationships. There is disagreement as to the relationship between average cost and scale of operations (Bishop, 1980; McKay, 1988). The fact that a nursing home is a member of a chain does not appear to influence its costs (Ullman, 1986). On the other hand, for-profit nursing homes have been identified as having a lower average cost that nonprofit nursing homes (Ullman, 1984).

As with all cost studies in the healthcare area, such studies have had to deal with difficulties in measuring and netting out the impact of patient case mix and the level of quality, two factors that influence the level of care and hence nursing home costs. For example, it has proven extremely hard to identify patient characteristics associated with specific levels of care. Patients differ considerably with regard to health status, and their different needs should translate into differences in the level of care or resource intensity. Several case-mix classifications (for long-term care patients) that try to take into account resource-use differences have been developed. These measures are far from perfect, but even allowing for their shortcomings, their inclusion in the cost analysis may not be sufficient to account for differences in average cost that are related to level-of-care differences. A nursing home that offers "high-quality" care as measured by resource-intensive processes (rehabilitation, nursing care) may provide more care to all patients regardless of their health status. Similarly, in a low-quality nursing home, all patients may receive fewer services than in the high-quality home, adjusting for health status. One must therefore find a quality measure that is independent of case mix or case severity in order to control for the influence of each factor on cost of care. Most measures of case mix do not adequately distinguish between case mix and severity, and so it has been very difficult to identify each factor's specific impact on cost.

Average cost is not the only relevant cost measure in nursing home analysis. Marginal cost is also important when forecasting resource use or when assessing nursing home profitability. A New York study analyzed the marginal cost of nursing homes, adjusting for variables, such as SNF/ICF days, average level of service in the institution, patient characteristics, input prices, and for-profit or nonprofit status. The marginal cost for the healthiest patients was $51 per patient day. For the least healthy patients, the marginal cost was $60. These rates can be compared with the reimbursement rate of $72, indicating a profit for patients at all levels.

5.7.6 Health Insurance Costs

Theoretically, health insurance administrative costs are potentially influenced by the scale of a firm's operations. Additionally, a very important factor affecting these costs is the ratio of group policies to all policies that an insurance company sells. Per policy, individual policies are more expensive to sell. Also, employers perform many of the functions for group policies that insurers perform for individual policies. This fact may influence public policy, because if individual and group policies have significantly different costs, the government may act to encourage holders of individual policies to obtain group policies.

One study examined health insurance administrative costs for a cross section of insurance companies that offer health insurance. The study found that both factors have a significant impact on these costs (Blair, Jackson, & Vogel,, 1975b). An unexpected finding of their study was that mutual (nonprofit) companies had lower administrative costs than stock (for-profit) companies, however, one might have expected the opposite to be true.

EXERCISES

1. The Green City Hospital treated 100 patients in May with 20 nursing hour inputs, and it treated 120 patients in June with 22 nursing hour inputs. What is the total product for each month? What is the marginal product?
2. Sweetgrass Radiology Labs has a fixed amount of radiology equipment. The laboratory can hire any number of radiology technicians per hour to produce radiographs, which are displayed on a screen. The relationship between the number of technicians hired per hour and the number of radiographs produced per hour is shown in the following table. Show the total and marginal products and indicate at each level of production whether the production function exhibits increasing, constant, or diminishing marginal productivity.

Radiograph Technician Per Hour	Radiograph Produced Per Hour
1	10
2	26
3	50
4	74
5	94
6	100

3. Given the production function between nurse hours and patient visits per day to a community clinic, how will each of the following shift this function:
   a. A change in nurse remuneration from salary to fee for service
   b. A change in the case mix of patients, with more having leukemia and fewer having common colds
   c. A change in policy to provide more thorough examinations
   d. Higher nurse wages
   e. A requirement that each patient now be told all his or her legal rights before an examination
   f. An increase in the total number of nurses who are hired
   g. An increase in the clinic's budget.
4. St. Mary's Hospital owns a prime piece of real estate in the center of town. There is a small shopping center on this piece of land. Rents for each store are $4,000 per month. The benefactor of this real estate, in her endowment to St. Mary's, stated that one of the stores should be operated as a clinic for the poor and be kept open 24 hours a day. St. Mary's has agreed to these conditions. It hires three nurses monthly at $3,000 each. Furnishings are included in the estimate of the $4,000 rent. Supplies are $10 per patient; there are 800 patients a month, each of whom come in for one visit. What are the costs of operating the clinic?
5. Given the following data for a community health center, calculate the average and marginal costs for each output level and (in the case of marginal costs) between successive output levels.

Number of Visits	Total Cost
1	$100
2	160
3	200
4	260
5	360

6. If the total fixed cost is $1,000 at 100 visits for a clinic, what will the marginal fixed cost be for 101 visits?
7. City Home Care hires a furnished office at $2,000 per month, telephones at $200 a month, and a secretary at $2,000 per month. These resources do not change, no matter how many clients are visited. Currently, CHC sees 400 patients a month, each three times (1,200 visits in total). CHC uses 30 full-time nurses with their own cars, and they are paid $4,000 per month each. There is a plentiful supply of additional nurses in town. These nurses can be hired almost on notice. Supplies are $20 per patient per month. What are the money costs of operating CHC at its current level? Approxi-

mately how much would it cost to operate CHC at a level of 1,300 visits per month?

8. The Jonesville Clinic is an inner city clinic that provides primary care for indigent persons. Three physicians volunteer five hours a week each. Normally, physicians earn $150 per hour, but the clinic is lucky to get their services for free. The clinic hires two nurses annually at $18,000 each. Overhead, including secretarial time, is $15,000 a year. Ace Pharmaceuticals donates $2,000 worth of drugs annually, and the First Street Mall donates a small office. The mall's owners could get $400 monthly in rent for the office. What is the economic cost annually of operating the clinic.

9. For each volume of output, calculate the total fixed costs.

Clinic Visits	Total Costs	Total Variable Costs
10	$1,200	$1,000
11	1,300	1,100
12	1,500	1,300
13	2,000	1,800

10. The following is an estimate by the manager of the Centerville Nursing Home for total monthly costs at alternative operating levels, measured by patient days. Calculate the total fixed cost for the Centerville Nursing Home.

Patient Days	Total Cost
0	$120,000
1	150,000
2	180,000
3	210,000
4	240,000

11. The May Clinic rents a small office in Dubuque. May pays the building owner a rent of $2,000 a month, which includes all utilities. It has signed a three-year lease. May hires a general practice physician at $50 an hour, a nurse at $15 an hour, and a secretary at $10 an hour. May assumes that each patient uses $10 in supplies. In September, the clinic was open for 200 hours, during which all personnel were available at all times to staff the clinic. During that time, 1,000 patients were seen. What were May's fixed and variable costs for the month?

12. Given the following monthly data for alternative operating levels at the St. Christopher's Ambulance, calculate the total fixed cost, average fixed cost, average variable cost, average total cost, and marginal cost for successive output levels. If St. Christopher's is

operating at a level of three trips and it wants to determine the resources needed to make another trip, which statistic will it use?

Ambulance Trips	Total Variable Cost	Total Cost
0	$0	$1,200
1	1,300	2,500
2	1,400	2,600
3	1,500	2,700
4	1,800	3,000
5	2,400	3,600
6	3,400	4,600

13. The Grinch Clinic pays its nurses $20 an hour. It also pays $100 a week rent and has other weekly overhead costs of $50. Supply costs are $1 per patient. The short-run production function, relating patient visits and nursing hours, is shown here. Given this relationship and the other specified data, calculate the total variable, total fixed, and total costs; average costs (variable, fixed, and total); and marginal costs at each output level.

Patient Visits	Nursing Hours
1	2
2	4
3	8
4	14
5	22
6	32

14. The Rushmore Clinic pays nurses an hourly wage of $10. The clinic's fixed costs in 1992 were $1,000. The schedule relating visits to nursing hours is given here.

Visits	Nurse Hours
1	10
2	25
3	50
4	100
5	200
6	400

a. Determine the average, marginal, and total costs at each operating level when the nursing wage is $10.

b. Determine the average, marginal, and total costs at each operating level when the nursing wage is $20.

c. If the clinic manager wants to compare her clinic to that of another in order to determine which was more efficient, what statistic would she use?

15. Given the following data, calculate the total fixed, total variable, and marginal costs.

Quantity	Total Cost
0	$100
1	120
2	150
3	200
4	300

BIBLIOGRAPHY

Production of Medical Care

Cromwell, J. (1974). Hospital productivity trends in short-term general non-teaching hospitals. *Inquiry, 11*, 181–187.

Deb, P., & Holmes, A. M. (1998). Substitution of physicians and other providers in outpatient mental health care. *Health Economics, 7*, 347–362.

Defelice, L. C., & Bradford, W. D. (1997). Relative inefficiencies in production between solo and group practice physicians. *Health Economics, 6*, 455–466

Djellal, F., & Gallouj, F. (2007). Innovation in hospitals: A survey of the literature. *European Journal of Health Economics, 8*(3), 181–193.

Freda, C. E. (2000). Nurse practitioner versus physician assistant. *Nephrology Nursing Journal, 27*(2), 26.

Goldfarb, M., Hornbrook, M., & Rafferty, J. (1980). Behavior of the multi-product firm. *Medical Care, 18*, 185–201.

Hart, J. T. (2004). Health care or health trade? A historic moment of choice. *International Journal of Health Services, 34*(2), 245–254.

Iampreechakul, P., Chongchokdee, C., & Tirakotai, W. (2011). The accuracy of computer-assisted pedicle screw placement in degenerative lumbrosacral spine using single-time, paired point registration along technique combined with the surgeon's experience. *Journal of the Medical Association of Thailand, 94*(3), 337–345.

Kleinpell, R. M., Ely, E. W., & Grabenkort, R. (2008). Nurse practitioners and physician assistants in the intensive care unit: An evidence-based review. *Critical Care Medicine, 36*(10), 2888–2897.

Leibowitz, A. A. (2004). The demand for health and health concerns after 30 years. *Journal of Health Economics, 23*(4), 663–671.

Leski, M., Young, M., & Higham, R., (2010). Managing inflammatory arthritides: Role of the nurse practitioner and physician assistant. *Journal of the American Academy of Nurse Practitioners, 22*(7), 382–392.

Lewit, E. M., Bentkover, J. D., Bentkover, S. H., Watkins, R. N., & Hughes, E. F. (1980). A comparison of surgical assisting in a prepaid group practice. *Medical Care, 18*, 916–929.

Lu, M. (1999). The productivity of mental health care: An instrumental variable approach. *Journal of Mental Health Policy and Economics, 2,* 59–71.

Nicholson, S., Pauly, M. V., Wu, A. Y., Murray, J. F., Teutsch, S. M., & Berger, M. L. (2008). Getting real performance out of pay-for-performance. *Milbank Quarterly, 86*(3), 435–457.

Nyman, J. A., & Bricker, D. L. (1989). Profit incentives and technical efficiency in the production of nursing home care. *Review of Economics and Statistics, 71,* 586–593.

Okunade, A., & Suraratdecha, C. (1998). Factor interchange and technical progress in U.S. specialized hospital pharmacies. *Health Economics, 7,* 363–372.

Patel, S. N., Youssef, A. S., Vale, F. L., & Padhya, T. A. (2011). Re-evaluation of the role of image guidance in minimally invasive pituitary surgery: Benefits and outcomes. *Computer Aided Surgery, 16*(2), 45–53.

Pauly, M. V. (2004). Competition in medical services and the quality of care: Concepts and history. *International Journal of Health Care Finance & Economics, 4*(2), 113–130.

Picone, G., Uribe, M., & Wilson, R. M. (1998). The effect of uncertainty on the demand for medical care, health capital and wealth. *Journal of Health Economics, 17*(2), 171–185.

Reinhardt, U. (1972). A production function for physicians' services. *Review of Economics and Statistics, 54,* 55–66.

Reinhardt, U. (1973a). Manpower substitution and productivity in medical practice. *Health Services Research, 7,* 200–277.

Reinhardt, U. (1973b). Proposed changes in the organization of health care delivery. *Milbank Memorial Fund Quarterly, 51,* 169–222.

Rosenman, R., Siddharthan, K., & Ahern, M. (1997). Output efficiency of health maintenance organizations in Florida. *Health Economics, 6,* 295–303.

Ruchlin, H. S., & Leveson, I. (1974). Measuring hospital productivity. *Health Services Research, 9,* 308–323.

Scheffler, R. M. (1975). Further consideration of the economics of group practice. *Journal of Human Resources, 10,* 258–263.

Schumacher, E. J., & Whitehead, J. C. (2000). The production of health and the valuation of medical inputs in wage-amenity models. *Social Science & Medicine, 50*(4), 507–515.

Wagner, T. H., & Jimison, H. B. (2003). Computerized health information and the demand for medical care. *Value in Health, 6*(1), 29–39.

Yee, T., Crawford, L., & Harber, P. (2005). Work environment of dental hygienists. *Journal of Occupational & Environmental Medicine, 46*(6), 633–639.

Outcome-Volume Relation

Begg, C. B., Cramer, L. D., Hoskins, W. J., & Brennan, M. F. (1998). Impact of hospital volume on operative mortality for major cancer surgery. *JAMA, 280*(15), 1747–1751.

Birkmeyer, J. D., Sun, Y., Wong, S. L., & Stukel, T. A. (2007). Hospital volume and late survival after cancer surgery. *Annals of Surgery, 245*(5), 777–783.

Bolling, S. F., Li, S., O'Brien, S. M., Brennan, J. M., Prager, R. L., & Gammie, J. S. (2010). Predictors of mitral valve repair: Clinical and surgeon factors. *Annals of Thoracic Surgery, 90*(6), 1904–1911.

Bunker, J. P., Luft, H. S., & Enthoven, A. (1982). Should surgery be regionalized? *Surgical Clinics of North America, 62,* 657–668.

Campos, G. M., Rabl, C., Roll, G. R., Peeva, S., Prado, K., Smith, J., & Vittinghoff, E. (2011). Better weight loss, resolution of diabetes, and quality of life for laparoscopic gastric bypass vs banding: Results of a 2-cohort pair-matched study. *Archives of Surgery, 146*(2), 149–155.

Fieldston, E. S., Ragavan, M., Jayaraman, B., Allebach, K., Pati, S., & Metlay, J. P. (2011). Scheduled admissions and high occupancy at a children's hospital. *Journal of Hospital Medicine (Online), 6*(2), 81–87. http://onlinelibrary.wiley.com/doi/10.1002/jhm.819/pdf

Garnick, D. W., Luft, H. S., McPhee, S. J., & Mark, D. H. (1989). Surgeon volume vs. hospital volume: Which matters more? *JAMA, 262,* 547–548.

Gourin, C. G., Forastiere, A. A., Sanguineti, G., Marur, S., Koch, W. M., & Bristow, R. E. (2011). Impact of surgeon and hospital volume on short-term outcomes and cost of oropharyngeal cancer surgical care. *Laryngoscope, 121*(4), 746–752.

Halm, E. A., Lee, C., & Chassin, M. R. (2002). Is volume related to outcome in health care?: A systematic review and methodologic critique of the literature. *Annals of Internal Medicine, 137,* 511–520.

Hamilton, B. H., & Hamilton, V. H. (1997). Estimating surgical volume-outcome relationships applying survival models: Accounting for frailty and hospital fixed effects. *Health Economics, 6,* 383–396.

Joudi, F. N., & Konety, B. R. (2005). The impact of provider volume on outcomes from urological cancer therapy. *Journal of Urology, 174*(2), 432–438.

Larochelle, M., Hyman, N., Gruppi, L., & Osler, T. (2011). Diminishing surgical site infections after colorectal surgery with surgical care improvement project: Is it time to move on? *Diseases of the Colon & Rectum, 54*(4), 394–400.

Li, Y., Cai, X., Mukamel, D. B., & Glance, L. G. (2010). The volume-outcome relationship in nursing home care: An examination of functional decline among long-term care residents. *Medical Care, 48*(1), 52–57.

Luft, H. S. (1980). The relationship between surgical volume and mortality: An exploration of causal factors and alternative models. *Medical Care, 18,* 940–959.

Luft, H. S., & Hunt, S. S. (1986). Evaluating individual hospital quality through outcome statistics. *JAMA, 255,* 2780–2784.

Luft, H. S., Hunt, S. S., & Maerki, S. C. (1987). The volume-outcome relationship: Practice makes perfect or selective referral patterns? *Health Services Research, 22,* 157–182.

Luft, H. S., Garnick, D. W., Mark, D. H., & McPhee, S. J. (1990). *Hospital volume, physician volume, and patient outcomes.* Ann Arbor, MI: Health Administration Press Perspectives.

Porter, M. P., Gore, J. L., & Wright, J. L. (2011). Hospital volume and 90-day mortality risk after radical cystectomy: A population-based cohort study. *World Journal of Urology, 29*(1), 73–77.

Ptok, H., Marusch, F., Schmidt, U., Gastinger, I., Wenisch, H. J., & Lippert, H. (2011). Risk adjustment as basis for rational benchmarking: The example of colon carcinoma. *World Journal of Surgery, 35*(1), 196–205.

Rossi, A., Rossi, D., Rossi, M., & Rossi, P. (2011). Continuity of care in a rural critical access hospital: Surgeons as primary care providers. *American Journal of Surgery, 301*(3), 359–362.

Roukos, D. H. (2009). Laparoscopic gastrectomy and personal genomics: High-volume surgeons and predictive biomedicine may govern the future for resectable gastric cancer. *Annals of surgery, 250*(4), 650–651.

Spector, W. D., Seiden, T. M., & Cohen, J. W. (1998). The impact of ownership type on nursing home outcomes. *Health Economics, 7,* 639–654.

Tilford, J. M., Roberson, P. K., Lensing, S., & Fiser, D. H. (1998). Differences in pediatric ICU mortality risk over time. *Critical Care Medicine, 26,* 1737–1743.

Tilford, J. M., Simpson, P. M., Green, J. W., Lensing, S., & Fiser, D. H. (2000). Volume-outcome relationships in pediatric intensive care units. *Pediatrics, 106,* 289–294.

Tsao, S. Y., Lee, W. C., Loong, C. C., Chen, T. J., Chiu, J. H., & Tai, L. C. . (2011). High-surgical-volume hospitals associated with better quality and lower cost of kidney transplantation in Taiwan. *Journal of the Chinese Medical Association, 74*(1), 22–27.

Varghese, T. K., Jr., Wood, D. E., Farjay, F., Oelschlager, B. K., Symons, R. G. MacLeod, K.E., Flum, D. R., & Pellegrini, C. A. (2011). Variation in esophagectomy outcomes in hospitals meeting leapfrog volume outcome standards. *Annals of Thoracic Surgery, 91*(4), 1003–1009.

Ward, M. M., Jaana, M., Wakefield, D. S., Ohsfeldt, R. L., Schneider, J. E., Miller, T., & Lei, Y. (2004). What would be the effect of referral to high-volume hospitals in a largely rural state? *Journal of Rural Health, 20*(4), 344–354.

Costs: Hospitals

Barer, M. (1982). Case mix adjustment in hospital cost analysis. *Journal of Health Economics, 1,* 53–80.

Bays, C. (1980). Specification error in the estimation of hospital cost functions. *Review of Economics and Statistics, 62,* 302–305.

Beenen, E., Brown, L., & Connor, S. (2011). A comparison of the hospital costs of open vs. minimally invasive surgical management of necrotizing pancreatitis. *HPB, 13*(3), 178–184.

Berki, S. (1972). *Hospital economics.* Lexington, MA: D.C. Heath.

Berry, R. E. (1973). On grouping hospitals for economic analysis. *Inquiry, 10,* 5–12.

Burns, L. R., & Lee, J. A. (2006). Hospital purchasing alliances: Utilization, services, and performance. *Health Care Management Review, 33*(3), 203–215.

Caldwell, C., Butler, G., & Poston, N. (2010). Cost reduction in health systems: Lessons from an analysis of $200 million saved by top-performing organizations. *Frontiers of Health Services Management, 27*(2), 3–17.

Carey, K. (1997). A panel design for estimation of hospital cost functions. *Review of Economics and Statistics, 77,* 443–453.

Cary, K., & Burgess, J. F. (1999). On measuring the hospital cost/quality trade-off. *Health Economics, 8,* 509–520.

Cassel, J. B., Webb-Wright, J., Holmes, J., Lyckholm L., & Smith, T. J.. (2010). Clinical and financial impact of a palliative care program at a small rural hospital. *Journal of Palliative Medicine, 13*(11), 1339–1343.

Cleverley, W. O., & Cleverley, J. O. (2011). A better way to measure volume—and benchmark costs. *Healthcare Financial Management, 65*(3), 78–86.

Cowing, T. G., & Holtmann, A. G. (1983). Multiproduct short-run hospital cost functions. *Southern Economic Journal, 49,* 637–653.

Craver, C., Gayle, J., Balu, S., & Buchner, D. (2011). Clinical and economic burden of chemotherapy-induced nausea and vomiting among patients with cancer in a hospital outpatient setting in the United States. *Journal of Medical Economics, 14*(1), 87–98.

Cremonesi, P., DiBella, E., & Montefiori, M. (2010). Cost analysis of emergency department. *Journal of Preventive Medicine & Hygiene, 51*(4), 157–163.

David, G., Helmchen, D. G., & Henderson, R. A. (2009). Does advanced medical technology encourage hospitalist use and their direct employment by hospitals? *Health Economics, 18*(2), 237–247.

Dranove, D. (1998). Economies of scale in non-revenue producing cost centers: Implications for hospital mergers. *Journal of Health Economics, 17,* 69–83.

Evans, R. G. (1981). Behavioural cost functions for hospitals. *Canadian Journal of Economics, 4,* 198–215.

Etzioni, R. D., Feuer, E. J., Sullivan, S. D., Lin, D., Hu, C., & Ramsey, S. D. (1999). On the use of survival analysis techniques to estimate medical care costs. *Journal of Health Economics, 18,* 365–380.

Farnand, L. J., Jacobs, P. & Dickson, W.M. (1986). An evaluation of the Finger Lakes Experimental Payment Program. *Inquiry, 23*(2), 200–208.

Feldstein, P. (1961). *An empirical investigation of the marginal cost of hospital services.* Chicago, IL: University of Chicago Graduate Program in Hospital Administration.

Finkler, S. A. (1979a). Cost effectiveness of regionalization: The heart surgery example. *Inquiry, 16,* 264–270.

Finkler, S. A. (1979b). On the shape of the hospital industry long run average cost function. *Health Services Research, 14,* 281–289.

Fournier, G. M., & Mitchell, J. M. (1997). New evidence on the performance advantages of multi-hospital systems. *Review of Industrial Organization, 12,* 703–718.

Frakt, A. B. (2011). How much do hospitals cost shift? A review of the evidence. *Milbank Quarterly, 89*(1), 90–130.

Fraser, R. D. (1971). *Canadian hospital costs and efficiency*. Ottawa, Ontario: Economic Council of Canada.

Frech, H. E., & Mobley, L. E. (1995). Resolving the impasse on hospital scale economies. *Applied Economics, 27*, 286–296.

Friedman, B., & Pauly, M. V. (1983). A new approach to hospital cost functions and some issues in revenue regulation. *Health Care Financing Review, 4*, 105–114.

Gregory, D. D. (1976–1977). Some evidence on the economic aspects of hospital cooperative ventures. *Journal of Economics and Business, 29*, 59–64.

Hadley, J., & Zuckerman, S. (1994). The role of efficiency measurement in hospital rate setting. *Journal of Health Economics, 13*, 335–340.

Hansen, K. K.,& Zwanzinger, J. (1996). Marginal costs in general acute care hospitals. *Health Economics, 5*, 195–216.

Horn, S. D., Sharkey, P. D., Chambers, A. F., & Horn, R. A. (1985). Severity of illness within DRGs: Impact on prospective payment. *American Journal of Public Health, 75*, 1195–1199.

Hornbrook, M. C., & Monheit, A. C. (1985). The contribution of case mix severity to the hospital cost–output relation. *Inquiry, 22*, 259–271.

Hsieh, H. M., Clement, D. G., & Bazzoli, G. J. (2010). Impacts of market and organizational characteristics on hospital efficiency and uncompensated care. *Health Care Management Review, 35*(1), 77–87.

Kralewski, J. E., Dowd, B., Pitt, L., & Biggs, E. L. (1984). Effects of contract management on hospital performance. *Health Services Research, 19*, 479–498.

Lave, J., & Lave, L. B. (1984). Hospital cost functions. *Annual Review of Public Health, 5*, 193–213.

Lee, M. L., & Wallace, R. L. (1972). Problems in estimating multi-product hospital cost functions. *Western Economic Journal, 11*, 350–363.

Linna, M. (1998). Measuring hospital cost efficiency with panel data models. *Health Economics, 7*, 415–429.

Linna, M., Hakkinen, U., & Linnakko, E.. (1998). An econometric study of costs of teaching and research in Finnish hospitals. *Health Economics, 7*, 291–306.

Lipscomb, J. et al. (1978). The use of marginal cost estimates in hospital cost-containment policy. In Zubkoff, M., Raskin, I., & Hanft, R. S. (Eds.), *Hospital cost containment*. New York: Watson Publishing International.

Litvak, E., & Bisognano, M. (2011). More patients, less payment: Increasing hospital efficiency in the aftermath of health reform. *Health Affairs, 30*(1), 76–80.

McCue, M. J. (2011). Capital expenditure trends in California hospitals: 2002–2007. *Hospital Topics, 89*(1), 9–15.

McGregor, M., & Pelletier, G. (1978). Planning of specialized health facilities: Size vs. cost and effectiveness in heart surgery. *New England Journal of Medicine, 299*, 179–181.

Newhouse, J. P. (1994). Frontier estimation: How useful a tool for health economics? *Journal of Health Economics, 13*, 335–340.

Schwartz, W., & Joskow, P. (1980). Duplicated hospital facilities. *New England Journal of Medicine, 303*, 1449–1457.

Sloan, F. A. Perrin, J. M., & Valvona, J. (1985). The teaching hospital's growing surgical caseload. *JAMA, 254*, 376–382.

Valdmanis, V. G. (2010). Measuring economies of scale at the city market level. *Journal of Health Care Finance, 37*(1), 78–90.

Wier, L. M., & Andrews, R. M. (2011, March). The national hospital bill: The most expensive conditions by payer, 2008. *Healthcare Cost and Utilization Project*. Retrieved from http://www.hcup-us.ahrq.gov/reports/statbriefs/sb107.pdf

Yatchak, R. (2000). A longitudinal study of economies of scale in the hospital industry. *Journal of Health Care Finance, 27*(1), 67–89.

Zuckerman, S., Hadley, J., & Iezzoni, L. (1994). Measuring hospital efficiency with frontier cost functions. *Journal of Health Economics, 13*, 335–340.

Costs: Medical Practice

Bailey, R. M. (1968). A comparison of internists in solo and fee-for-service group practice. *Bulletin of the New York Academy of Medicine, 44*(2nd series), 1293–1303.

Bailey, R. M. (1970). Economies of scale in medical practice. In H. Klarman (Ed.), *Empirical studies in health economics*. Baltimore, MD: Johns Hopkins University Press.

Cammisa, C., Partridge, G., Ardans, C. Buehrer, K., Chapman, B., & Beckman, H. (2011). Engaging physicians in change: Results of a safety net quality improvement program to reduce overuse. *American Journal of Medical Quality, 26*(1), 26–33.

Chernew, M. E., Sabi, K. L., Chandra, A., & Newhouse, J. P. (2009). Would having more primary care doctors cut health spending growth? *Health Affairs, 28*(5), 1327–1335.

Dunn, D. L., Sacher, S. J., Cohen, W. S., & Hsiao, W. C. (1995). Economies of scope in physicians' work: The performance of multiple surgery. *Inquiry, 32,* 87–101.

Engberg, J., Wholey, D., Feldman, R., & Christianson, J. B. (2004). The effect of mergers on firms' costs: Evidence from the HMO industry. *The Quarterly Review of Economics and Finance, 44*(4), 574–600.

Escarce, J. J., & Pauly, M. V. (1998). Physician opportunity costs in physician practice cost functions. *Journal of Health Economics, 17,* 129–151.

Frech, H. E., & Ginsburg, P. B. (1974). Optimal scale in medical practice. *Journal of Business, 47,* 23–36.

Hillson, S. D. Feldman, R., & Wingert, T. D. (1992). Economies of scope and payment for physician services. *Medical Care, 30,* 822–831.

Miller, T. P., Brennan, T. A., & Milstein, A. (2009). How can we make more progress in measuring physicians' performance to improve the value of care? *Health Affairs, 28*(5), 1429–1437.

Murphy, R. K., McHugh, S., O'Farrell, N., Dougherty B., Sheikh, A., Corrigan, M., & Hill, A. D. (2011). The financial imperative of physicians to control demand of laboratory testing. *Irish Medical Journal, 104*(1), 15–17.

Newhouse, J. P. (1973). The economics of group practice. *Journal of Human Resources, 8,* 37–56.

Pauly, M. V. (1996). Economics of multispecialty group practice. *Journal of Ambulatory Care Management, 19*(3), 26–33.

Perlroth, D. J., Goldman, D. P., & Garber, A. M. (2010). The potential impact of comparative effectiveness research on US health care expenditures. *Demography, 47*(Suppl.), S173–S190.

Reddy, J. (2011). The physician value index: A tool for effective physician integration. *Healthcare Financial Management, 65*(2), 92–98.

Reschovsky, J. D., Hadley, J., & Landon, B. E. (2006). Effects of compensation methods and physician group structure on physicians' perceived incentives to alter services to patients. *Health Services Research, 41*(4 Pt 1), 1200–1220.

Rossiter, L. F. (1984). Prospects for medical group practice under competition. *Medical Care, 22,* 84–92.

Shields, M.C., Patel, P. H., Manning, M., & Sacks, L. (2011). A model for integrating independent physicians into accountable care organizations. *Health Affairs, 30*(1), 161–172.

Shrank, W. H., Liberman, J. N., Fischer, M. A, Girdish C., Brennan, T. A., & Choudhry, N., K. (2011). Physician perceptions about generic drugs. *Annals of Pharmacotherapy, 45*(1), 31–38.

Silversmith, J., MMA Work Group to Advance Health Care Reform. (2011). Five payment models: The pros, the cons, the potential. *Minnesota Medicine, 94*(2), 45–48.

Ubel, P. A., Angott, A. M., & Zikmund-Fisher, B. J. (2011). Physicians recommend different treatments for patients than they would choose for themselves. *Archives of Internal Medicine, 171*(7), 630–634.

Weil, T. P. (2002). Multispecialty physician practices: Fixed and variable costs, and economies of scale. *Journal of Ambulatory Care Management, 25*(3), 70–77.

Williams, T. E., Jr., Satiani, B., Thomas, A., & Ellison, E. C. (2009). The impending shortage and the estimated cost of training the future surgical workforce. *Annals of Surgery, 250*(4), 590–597.

Zilberberg, M. D., & Shorr, A. F. (2010). Understanding cost-effectiveness. *Clinical Microbiology & Infection, 16*(12), 1707–1712.

Costs: Long-Term Care

Bekele, G., & Holtmann, A. G. (1987). A cost function for nursing homes: Toward a system of diagnostic reimbursement groupings. *Eastern Economic Journal, 13,* 115–122.

Bishop, C. E. (1980). Nursing home cost studies and reimbursement issues. *Health Care Financing Review, 1,* 47–65.

Bishop, C. E. (1983). Nursing home cost studies. *Health Services Research, 18,* 383–386.

Candy, B., Holman, A., Leurent, B., Davis, S., & Jones L. (2011). Hospice care delivered at home, in nursing homes and in dedicated hospice facilities: A systematic review of quantitative and qualitative evidence. *International Journal of Nursing Studies, 48*(1), 121–133.

Chattopadhyay, S., & Hefley, D. (1994). Are for-profit nursing homes more efficient? *Eastern Economic Journal, 20,* 171–186.

Chattopadhyay, S., & Ray, S. C. (1996). Technical, scale, and size efficiency in nursing home care. *Health Economics, 5,* 363–374.

DaVanzo, J. E., El-Gamil, A. M., Dobson, A., & Sen, N. (2010). A retrospective comparison of clinical outcomes and medicare expenditures in skilled nursing facility residents with chronic wounds. *Ostomy Wound Management, 56*(9), 44–54.

Dudzinski, C. S., Erekson, O. H., & Ziegert A. (1998). Estimating a hedonic translog cost function for the home health care industry. *Applied Economics, 30,* 1259–1267.

Gonzales, T. I. (1997). An empirical study of economies of scope in home healthcare. *Health Services Research, 32*(3), 313–324.

Heinrich, S., Rapp, K., Rissman, U., Becker, C., & Konig, H. H. (2010). Cost of falls in old age: A systematic review. *Osteoporosis International, 21*(6), 891–902.

Helton, M. R., Cohen, L. W., Zimmerman, S., & van der Steen, J. T. (2011). The importance of physician presence in nursing homes for residents with dementia and pneumonia. *Journal of the American Medical Directors Association, 12*(1), 68–73.

Holahan, J., & Yemane, A. (2009). Enrollment is driving medicaid costs—But two targets can yield savings. *Health Affairs, 28*(5), 1453–1465.

Kass, D. I. (1987). Economies of scale and scope in the provision of nursing home services. *Journal of Health Economics, 6,* 129–146.

McKay, N. L. (1988). An econometric analysis of costs and scale economies in the nursing home industry. *Journal of Human Resources, 23,* 58–75.

Nyman, J. A. (1988a). Improving the quality of nursing home outcome. *Medical Care, 26,* 1158– 1171.

Nyman, J. A. (1988b). The marginal cost of nursing home care. *Journal of Health Economics, 7,* 393–412.

Nyman, J. A., & Conner, R. A. (1994). Do case mix adjusted nursing home reimbursements actually reflect costs? *Journal of Health Economics, 13,* 145–162.

Okunade, A. A. (1993). Production cost structure of U.S. hospital pharmacies: Time series, cross sectional bed size evidence. *Journal of Applied Econometrics, 8,* 277–294.

Qian, X., Russell, L. B., Vallyeva, E., & Miller, J. E. (2011). "Quicker and sicker" under Medicare's prospective payment system for hospitals: New evidence on an old issue from a national longitudinal survey. *Bulletin of Economic Research, 63*(1), 1–27.

Schlenker, R. E., & Shaughnessy, P. W. (1984). Case mix, quality, and cost relationships in Colorado nursing homes. *Health Care Financing Review, 6,* 61–71.

Schlenker, R. E., Shaughnessy, P. W., & Yslas I. (1985). Estimating patient level nursing home costs. *Health Services Research, 20,* 103–128.

Spector, W. D., Limcangco, M. R., Ladd, H., & Mukamel, D. (2011). Incremental cost of post acute care in nursing homes. *Health Services Research, 46*(1, Pt. 1), 105–119.

Trueman, P., Haynes, S. M., Felicity Lyons, G., McCombie, L., McQuigg, M. S., Mongia, S., Counterweight Project Team. (2010). Long-term cost effectiveness of weight management in primary care. *International Journal of Clinical Practice, 64*(6), 775–783.

Ullman, S. G. (1984). Cost analysis and facility reimbursement in the long-term health care industry. *Health Services Research, 19*, 83–102.

Ullman, S. G. (1986). Chain ownership and long-term health care facility performance. *Journal of Applied Gerontology, 5*, 51–63.

Van Lear, W., & Fowler, L. (1997). Efficiency and service in the group home industry. *Journal of Economic Issues, 31*, 1039–1051.

Vitaliano, D. F., & Toren, M. (1994). Cost and efficiency in nursing homes. *Journal of Health Economics, 13*, 281–300.

Costs: Other Areas

Blair, R. D., Ginsburg, P. B., & Vogel, R. J. (1975a). Blue Cross-Blue Shield administrative costs. *Economic Inquiry, 13*, 237–251.

Blair, R. D., Jackson, J. R., & Vogel, R. J. (1975b). Economies of scale in the administration of health insurance. *Review of Economics and Statistics, 57*, 185–189.

Cutler, D. M., & Ly, D. P. (2011). The (paper) work of medicine: Understanding international medical costs. *Journal of Economic Perspectives, 25*(2), 3–25.

Hay, J. W., & Mandes, G. (1984). Home health care cost-function analysis. *Health Care Financing Review, 5*, 111–116.

Kessler, D. P. (2011). Evaluating the medical malpractice system and options for reform. *Journal of Economic Perspectives, 25*(2), 93–110.

Sengupta, A. (2011). Medical tourism: Reverse subsidy for the elite. *Signs, 36*(2), 312–319.

Smith, T. J., & Hillner, B. E. (2011). Bending the cost curve in cancer care. *New England Journal of Medicine, 364*(21), 2060–2065.

Williams, T. E., Jr., Satiani, B., Thomas, A., & Ellison, E. C. (2009). The impending shortage and the estimated cost of training the future surgical workforce. *Annals of Surgery, 250*(4), 590–597.

Chapter 6

Behavior of Supply

OBJECTIVES

1. Define a supply curve in terms of the quantity of healthcare services supplied.

2. For a single investor-owned provider, describe a model that can be used to predict the quantity of healthcare services supplied.

3. Define a market, and describe and use a market model of healthcare supply.

4. For a single tax-exempt provider, describe an output-maximizing model to predict supplier behavior.

5. Describe the joint "quantity-quality" output-maximizing model to predict supplier behavior.

6. Describe the "administrator-as-agent" model to predict the effect of ownership status (investor-owned versus tax-exempt) on operating efficiency.

6.1 INTRODUCTION

This chapter is concerned with the determinants of the quantity and quality of output of various health-related products. Our approach is to consider the behavior of the organizations supplying these products. It provides hypotheses about what causes suppliers to produce particular quantities and qualities of output. These hypotheses are formulated in terms of models of supplier behavior, and they incorporate the key causes of such behavior. The goal is to isolate the direction in which individual factors cause supply to move while keeping in mind other factors that may also be influencing supply movements.

In presenting the hypotheses about supply behavior, a distinction is made between the supply of a single producer and the supply of all producers in the market (i.e., individual versus market supply). It should be pointed out that, like in our analyses of demand, our focus is on the behavior of a group of market participants in isolation—in this case, suppliers.

In this chapter, no single model of supplier behavior is presented as uniquely appropriate. The subject is complex, and our models offer suggestions rather than definitive answers. In particular, healthcare providers differ with regard to type of organization. Some organizations, such as investor-owned hospitals and nursing homes and physician practices, are profit-seeking institutions. Others, such as tax-exempt hospitals, the Red Cross, independent blood banks, and philanthropic organizations (e.g., the March of Dimes and the American Heart Association), operate under other legal and philosophical structures. This means that their "owners" (or, more appropriately, governors, boards, or trustees) can neither appropriate for themselves any profits that the organization might make nor sell the rights to the assets of the organization for personal gain. Separate hypotheses are discussed for both types of organizations.

We start off by developing a basic model of an individual profit-seeking supplier, then develop a model of the market supply behavior of a group of such firms. Because investor-owned and tax-exempt organizations can differ substantially, the following three sections focus on the effects that the tax-exempt organizational form has on the behavior of a tax-exempt organization. Much disagreement exists over the analysis of tax-exempt agency behavior. As a result, several alternative hypotheses about tax-exempt agency behavior need to be presented.

In Section 6.4, the tax-exempt agency is examined as if it were an output-maximizing agency. In the next section, we extend this analysis to incorporate the role of the agency in producing quality as well as quantity output, and we look at the organizational structure of the tax-exempt hospital, a peculiar type of tax-exempt organization. In Section 6.6, we develop a model in which the tax-exempt agency is regarded as an instrument used to the benefit of its managers.

6.2 A MODEL OF SUPPLY BEHAVIOR: AN INDIVIDUAL INVESTOR-OWNED COMPANY

As a review, please recall that supply reflects the quantity of a good or service that a producer is willing and able to supply in the market at a given price at a particular period of time. For a normal good or service, there is a direct relationship between price and quantity; that is, as price increases, the quantity a producer is willing and able to offer for sale in the market increases. This quantity offered for sale at various prices reflects the cost of resources required to produce the good or service and the profit required by the producer.

Price is the endogenous (internal) factor impacting the quantity offered in the market. A change in price will cause movement along a given supply curve. Other factors impacting supply will cause a shift in the entire supply curve, reflecting that a different quantity will be supplied at any price as a result of the change in these exogenous (external) factors. In general, the exogenous factors impacting the supply of a good or service are costs of production resulting from changes in the price of inputs; changes in the technologies used in the production of the good or service; changes in government taxes or subsidies associated with the production of the good or service; changes in the prices of substitutes and or complements; changes in the general environment (economic and/or physical); and changes in the opportunity costs of the alternative uses for the resources used by the supplier in the production process. A change in any of these exogenous factors will cause a shift, either outward or inward, of the entire supply curve. A shift outward in the supply curve reflects a greater quantity offered for sale at each price; an inward shift of the supply curve reflects a smaller quantity offered for sale at each price.

6.2.1 The Basic Model

The assumptions of our initial supply model fall into three categories: (1) revenue assumptions, (2) cost assumptions, and (3) assumptions about the objectives of the organization. In our analysis, we will use the example of a laboratory (ABC Labs) that is owned by a pathologist and produces blood tests of a given level of quality.

We will assume that ABC Labs' revenues can come from only two sources: payment for patient services (termed *patient* or *earned revenues*); and other sources (philanthropic or government grants, endowment funds, and other nonpatient-related sources). We will, initially, assume that all revenues come from payment for services provided (i.e., nonpatient-related revenues are zero). This assumption will be altered later in the analysis.

With regard to patient revenues, we make the assumption that ABC Labs is a "price taker," that is, ABC Labs is a supplier that has no influence on the price of its output. This may be because the price is set by an independent administrative agency or because the lab is operating in a competitive situation in which the best price it can get for its product is the price prevailing in the market. The charging of higher prices by one supplier in a highly competitive market will drive consumers to the lower priced competitors, and these lower prices will therefore not enable the higher priced supplier to achieve its goal of selling its product above the market price.

We will assume that ABC Labs receives \$14 for each test performed. Its marginal revenue (*MR*), defined as the addition to total revenue (*TR*) for one additional unit of output produced and sold ($\Delta TR/\Delta Q$), is \$14. The total and marginal revenues for output levels 0 to 10 are shown in Table 6-1, columns 9 and 10.

As for cost, we will assume that there are both fixed (cannot be changed in a single production cycle) and variable costs (changes with changes in quantity of output produced). Our assumption regarding fixed costs is that the lab spends \$7 monthly on equipment rental and mortgage payments. In addition, we assume that the pathologist-owner could earn a total of \$5 if she worked elsewhere. This sum is, at the same time, a fixed cost and an opportunity cost. That is, it incorporates a "normal" return on the investment of the owner's assets and efforts. The pathologist, once committed to work in the lab, gives up \$5 per period that could have been earned with alternative activities. The total fixed costs are thus, \$12, and being fixed, they do not vary as amount of output changes. The total fixed costs are shown in column 2 in

Table 6-1: Illustrative Data on Relationships Among Revenue, Costs, Profit, and Output

(1)	(2)	(3)	(4)	(5)	(6)	(7)	(8)	(9)	(10)	(11)
Quan-tity of Tests	Total Fixed Costs (TFC)	Total Variable Costs (TVC)	Total Costs (TC)	Average Fixed Costs (TFC/Q)	Average Variable Costs (TVC/Q)	Average Total Costs (TC/Q)	Marginal Costs (ΔTC/ΔQ)	Total Earned Revenue (TR = PXQ)	Marginal Revenue (ΔTR/ΔQ)	Profits (TR – TC)
0	12	0.00	12.00	—	—	—	—	—	—	–12.00
1	12	6.75	18.75	12.00	6.75	18.75	6.75	14.00	14	–4.75
2	12	10.50	22.50	6.00	5.25	11.25	3.75	28.00	14	5.50
3	12	13.25	25.25	4.00	4.42	8.42	2.75	42.00	14	16.75
4	12	17.00	29.00	3.00	4.25	7.25	3.75	56.00	14	27.00
5	12	23.75	35.75	2.40	4.75	7.15	6.75	70.00	14	34.25
6	12	35.50	47.50	2.00	5.92	7.92	11.75	84.00	14	36.50
7	12	54.25	66.25	1.71	7.75	9.46	18.75	98.00	14	31.75
8	12	82.00	94.00	1.50	10.25	11.75	27.75	112.00	14	18.00
9	12	120.75	132.75	1.33	13.42	14.75	38.75	126.00	14	–6.75
10	12	172.50	184.50	1.20	17.25	18.45	51.75	140.00	14	–44.50

Table 6-1; the associated average fixed costs (total fixed costs divided by total quantity produced) are shown in column 5.

Variable inputs are assumed to be employed in a least-cost manner (the total minimum variable cost for operating the lab at different levels of output is shown in column 3). The average variable cost initially falls, and then subsequently rises (column 6), and the marginal cost eventually rises (column 8). The figures for the total cost, the sum of the fixed and variable costs, are shown in columns 4 and 7 (total and average values, respectively). Therefore, the cost curves are shaped as hypothesized in the chapter on healthcare production and costs (see Figure 6-1). Whereas in Table 6-1 the values jump in discrete steps, the curves are drawn as smooth functions for geometric convenience.

These dollar figures are approximated in graph A of Figure 6-1 for total values and graph B for marginal revenue (MR), marginal cost (MC), average variable cost (AVC), and average total cost (ATC). Note that the TR curve rises at a rate of $14 per blood test and that MR is constant at $14. These are two different ways of saying the same thing: the revenue per unit of output sold is fixed at $12. This is a concrete expression of our assumption that ABC Labs is a price taker, because the lab can sell all desired products at that price but cannot sell any at a price above the market price of $14. Finally, because ABC Labs is an investor-owned company, it seems reasonable to assume that its main objective is to maximize profits (total revenues minus total costs).

We are now in a position to examine the conclusions of our model and answer the question that underlies our analysis: What will the quantity of

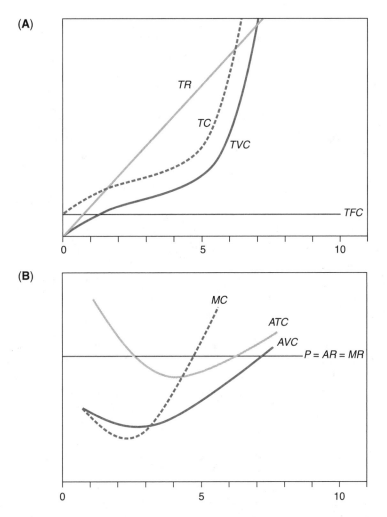

Figure 6-1 Supply Relationship for a Profit-maximizing Firm in Terms of Total Costs and Revenues (Graph A) and Average and Marginal Costs and Revenues (Graph B). In Graph A, the supplier produces where total profits, equal to the difference between total revenues (*TR*) and total costs (*TC*), are at a maximum. In Graph B, the same conclusion can be derived in terms of marginal costs and revenues. Here, the profit-maximizing point is where *MR* = *MC*. In the diagram, since the price per unit is constant, price and *MR* are the same.

output be? Our task is to present a hypothesis that will enable us to predict which quantity will be chosen to be produced and offered in the market and how this quantity will vary when some of the underlying variables in our model—prices and costs—themselves vary.

Referring to Table 6-1, we can now derive, from our model, a specific quantity of output that achieves ABC Labs' profit-maximizing objective: profits at a maximum at six units of output (here they amount to $36.50).

The reasoning used to obtain this conclusion can best be presented in marginal terms. Say that ABC Labs was initially supplying four units of output. Profits here, given the assumed revenue and cost conditions, equal $27.00. If ABC Labs produces and sells one more test, the additional revenue will be $14.00 (i.e., MR = $14.00), and the additional costs of production (MC) will be $6.75. The additional profit obtained by expanding output from four to five tests will be $7.25, bringing total profits to a new level of $34.25. ABC Labs, being profit maximizers, would expand production to at least five units. In fact, they will move beyond this amount because profits can be further increased by doing so. The best ABC Labs can do, at the given price and cost conditions, is produce six units of output. Expanding beyond six units still results in positive profits for a while, but these profits would be less than the profit at six units of output. According to our model, a profit-maximizing firm will continue to expand production as long as MR exceeds MC. If we were dealing with smooth, continuous changes, our conclusion would be that a profit-maximizing firm will expand output up to the point at which MR = MC, as long as MC is rising with output. At this point, the firm is maximizing its profits, and so the quantity at which MC = MR is the supply position for which the firm should be aiming.

This conclusion is shown diagrammatically in Figure 6-1. In Graph A, profits at each level of output are shown as the vertical distance between total revenues and total costs at that level of output. Because profits are defined as $TR - TC$, then where this vertical distance is at a maximum, profits are also at a maximum. This profit-maximizing point occurs at six units of output (allowing for small variations because we are dealing with continuous curves). In Graph B, the same conclusion is shown, but in terms of marginal costs and revenues. Here, the point at which MR = MC is the profit-maximizing quantity, that is, the quantity that will be supplied by a profit-maximizing producer. A movement in quantity supplied in either direction would detract from total profits and so would not be consistent with the profit-maximizing objective.

The first conclusion of our model then, is that, given revenue (i.e., price) and cost conditions, and given the profit-maximizing objective, a profit-maximizing firm will produce at the quantity at which MC = MR. Using this information, we can now derive a supply curve, or schedule, that shows what the quantity supplied will be at different prices. This analysis is shown diagrammatically in Figure 6-2. If the price rises from $14 to $15, the lab will add to its profits by expanding output to a sixth unit because, even though the cost of this unit is higher, the higher extra revenue will make it profitable to expand output. The same reasoning applies to additional price increases: higher prices will bring forth greater quantities supplied until MC = MR. It also applies to price declines, with one major exception: eventually, the price could become so low that the owner of the firm would be better off, from the point of view of profits (or losses), to shut down operations and produce nothing. For all prices below this level (represented by point j in Figure 6-2), the quantity supplied by the firm would be zero. Basically, the firm will continue to produce as long as the price covers variable costs and some of the fixed costs. If price falls below variable costs, then the producer will stop production.

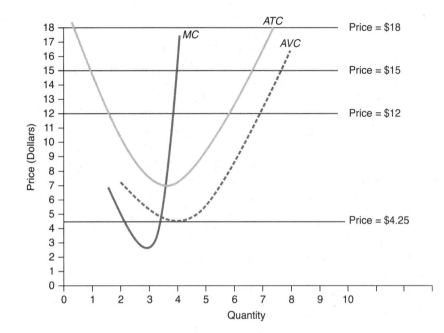

Figure 6-2   Profit-maximizing Supply Points at Alternative Prices. At each price above $4.25, the firm will maximize profits by supplying at the quantity where price = *MC*. If the price is at $4.25, the firm will just be meeting its variable costs. At any price below this, the firm's least unprofitable supply point will result in larger losses than if the firm shut down operations; therefore, the firm will not supply at any price below $4.25. For prices above $4.25, the firms supply curve and its *MC* curve are the same.

The critical price below which the firm will shut down depends on the variable costs of the firm. Recall that fixed costs are the same thing as "already committed" costs, while variable costs are those that can be avoided by not hiring the variable factors; total costs are the sum of the two at each output level. If the price falls sufficiently, it is possible that even at its best level of output (from the profitability standpoint), the firm will be incurring a loss. The criterion the firm would use in deciding whether to continue operating under such unfavorable circumstances is not whether the firm is incurring a loss but whether it is minimizing its losses. The importance of variable costs comes into play here. As long as the firm's revenues are exceeding its total variable costs, the firm will be adding to a surplus. In this case, $TR - TVC$ will be positive. Even though total profits $[TR - (TVC + TFC)]$ may be negative, sig-nifying a loss, the loss is less than it would be if the firm shut down entirely. For if the firm shuts down, both TR and TVC are zero, and the losses would equal TFC. In sum, as long as the firm is meeting its variable costs and adding something to cover some or all of its fixed costs, the firm should continue to operate; in this case, its supply curve is traced out by the MC curve. The quan-tity supplied will be where price equals marginal cost. Should the price fall so low that at no level of output could the firm meet all its variable costs, then it should shut down.

We can now present a complete analysis of the firm's supply behavior using the curves in Figure 6-2. If the price is equal to or greater than the lowest point on the AVC curve (point j), then at some level of output, all variable costs will be covered and the firm will produce some output. If the price is lower than this critical minimum price, the firm will shut down operations. If the price is above the critical minimum level, the firm will produce output at the quantity at which $MR = MC$ (i.e., when price $= MC$). The MC curve of the firm then is its supply curve, relating price to output.

In the context of this analysis, we can make some sense of the assumption that the costs of an investor-owned firm are at a minimum. It is shown in the chapter on healthcare and production costs that the producer has a choice of producing a given quantity of output at the lowest possible cost or above the lowest possible cost. By choosing the lowest possible cost method of production, the firm can achieve its greatest profits because profits are defined as the difference between total revenues and total costs. If costs were above the minimum, they would cut into profits, which is contrary to the assumed goal of the firm.

It should be noted that the supply relationship focuses on the behavior of suppliers in isolation. That is, the term *quantity supplied* refers to a distinct schedule—that of supplier responsiveness to price. As in the chapter on demand, in which we studied how demanders would respond to price while ignoring suppliers, in this chapter, we focus on supplier behavior in isolation from demanders. Before putting the separate forces, supply and demand, together, it is essential to understand how each operates on its own.

6.2.2 Nonpatient Revenues

Let us now introduce a new element into our analysis: nonpatient revenues. We will focus on a particular form of unearned revenue, a grant or subsidy, that is unrelated to output. Such a grant might be received from a donor, the government, or a foundation. Although nonmarket-related revenue occurs in many different markets, these are especially relevant for the healthcare industry. Many healthcare providers receive grants from different sources that are unrelated to quantity of the goods or services produced. These grants can be viewed as supplemental revenue that is independent from the costs of producing a good or service. Our analytical task is to determine how it might affect the provider's supply.

The economic significance of a grant unrelated to output is that it provides a set amount of money whether output expands or contracts. Such a grant can be treated analytically in one of two ways, either as a fixed addition to revenue or as a fixed reduction from total costs (a negative fixed cost). Although the rationale for the first option seems clear-cut, the rationale for the second requires some explanation. In a sense, a fixed subsidy reduces, by a fixed amount, the total costs that the provider must meet at each output level. Operationally, it will have the same impact on profits. We can therefore treat it as a reduction in total costs.

Let us say that ABC Labs received a fixed subsidy of $5. This would increase revenues in Table 6-1 by $5 at each and every level of output. Profits would also increase by $5 at each level of output. In Figure 6-1, the increase would appear as an upward parallel shift in the *TR* curve.

What is important from a supply standpoint is that neither patient revenues (including *MR*) nor variable costs are affected. Thus, while profits are higher by $5 at every output level, the maximum profitability level of output remains at six units. The fixed subsidy does not affect the most profitable level of output; it only affects the level of profits at that and every other level of output. The nonpatient revenue in this case can be viewed similarly to the impact that fixed costs have on the production side. It is the marginal costs and marginal revenue that are considered in determining the level of output to supply in the market.

This conclusion would not hold if the subsidy was related to output. For then, as output expanded, the marginal revenue would be the additional revenue from patient sources plus the additional (output-related) grant revenues. When estimating the most profitable output level, the firm would have to consider both sources of additional revenue and relate them to marginal cost.

The conclusion then is that a grant that is not output related will not influence the supply decisions of a profit-maximizing firm; the firm's supply position will still be where marginal patient revenue equals marginal cost. The firm simply receives a greater profit at that point.

6.2.3 Shifts in the Supply Curve

In this section, we consider what happens to the supply curve of the firm when factors that influence the position of the *MC* curve change. These factors are referred to as exogenous to the market and were reviewed at the beginning of this chapter. A supply schedule is a table, or listing, that provides varying values for the prices of a good or service and the corresponding quantities that the producer/seller would be willing and able to offer for sale at each price during a particular period of time. The supply schedule can reflect either the behavior propensities of a single producer or the aggregation of producers across the market. The values listed in the supply schedule, when plotted in a graph, become the supply curve. In general, as shown in Figure 6-3, any factor that causes the *MC* curve to shift upward from MC_1 to MC_2 will amount to a leftward shift in the supply schedule of the firm (a decrease in supply). The quantity supplied at any price will be reduced from Q_1 to Q_2. Such shifts might occur because of higher input prices or a higher quality of product being produced, to cite two of the factors discussed in Section 5.4 that might cause the firm's cost curve to shift. In the case of the production of a higher quality product, for example, the net result is that a lower quantity will be produced by the firm at any given price when producing the higher quality costs more. In the healthcare industry, it has been shown that higher quality care does not always increase costs (Rantz, Hicks, Petroski, Madsen, Alexander, Galambos,...& Greenwald, 2010). There are other times when higher quality does cost more (Auerbach, Maselli, Carter, Pekow, & Lindenauer, 2010).

The same reasoning, in reverse, holds for downward (to the right) shifts in the *MC* curve. For example, an increase in the capacity of the firm to produce

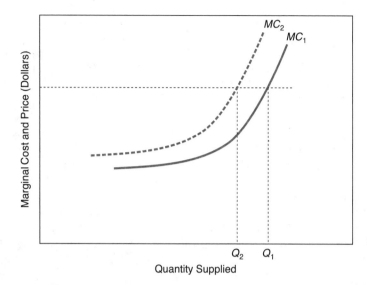

Figure 6-3   Shifts in the Marginal Cost Curve for a Profit-maximizing Supplier. An upward shift in the MC curve of a profit-maximizing firm will mean a lower quantity supplied at any price. In this figure, a shift from MC_1 to MC_2 means a decrease in supply level indicated by the dotted line (the quantity supplied decreases from Q_1 to Q_2).

output, caused by a technological advancement, will cause the MC, and thus the supply curve, to shift to the right, indicating a willingness on the part of the firm to supply more output at any given price. Such expansion in output is likely when the firm is operating on the downward-sloping part of its long-run average cost curve. An expansion in output would allow it to move to a lower point on the $LRAC$ curve (i.e., to a lower-cost short-run curve).

6.3 MARKET SUPPLY

We now demonstrate how the analysis of individual supply movements can be extended to form a hypothesis about movements in product supply in a specific market. To do this, we will add two new assumptions concerning individual supply behavior:

1. There is a set number of suppliers in the market.

2. There are no agreements on the part of suppliers to restrict supply.

In the present model, two groups of factors influence market supply: the number of suppliers and the factors that influence individual supplier behavior. In other words, the market supply schedule can be obtained once we know the number of suppliers and their individual supply schedules. Let us assume the market consists of three suppliers: ABC Labs, XYZ Labs, and GHI Labs (see Figure 6-4). Each lab has a given supply schedule. XYZ Labs supplies 5 tests at $1.00, a total of 10 tests at $1.50, a total of 15 at $2.00, and so on. GHI Labs supplies 3, 6, and 9 tests at these prices, respectively; and ABC Labs

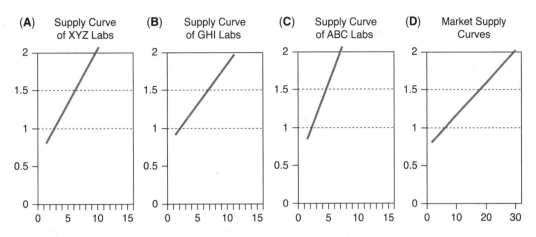

Figure 6-4 Derivation of the Market Supply Curve from Individual Supply Curves. The market supply shows the quantity supplied by all firms providing the product to the market at each price. It is obtained by summing individual suppliers' quantities at each price.

supplies 6, 9, and 12 tests. Given these schedules, and the fact that these three labs are the only ones in the market, the market supply curve is the sum of these individual supply curves at each price. At $1.00, the market supply of tests is 14 (5 + 3 + 6); at $1.50, a total of 25 tests are supplied; and at $2.00, a total of 36 tests are supplied. The market supply curve is shown as the horizontal sum of all individual supply curves. Given a particular price, our model predicts the quantity that will be supplied by all producers in the market.

The market supply curve will shift outward (to the right) if, given the number of producers, any factors cause the individual supply curves to shift outward or if the number of suppliers increases. In either case, more will be supplied at any given price. Our model has enabled us to classify these influences and separate their effects on supply. The same type of analysis applies to reductions in supply.

With regard to the number of suppliers, just as profits are the motivating force behind the expansion (or contraction) of output by an individual firm, so are they a driving force behind the expansion of firms in the market—the entry of new firms into the market. At any particular time there are a number of prospective suppliers capable of acquiring the techniques and equipment needed to supply a product (e.g., blood tests). If profits are high in the market, prospective suppliers will be motivated to enter the market and thus will shift the supply curve to the right. Of course, in real life, existing firms, protective of their high profits, may act to keep potential suppliers out, but this type of behavior is ruled out of the model discussed here.

6.4 SUPPLY BEHAVIOR OF TAX-EXEMPT AGENCIES: THE OUTPUT MAXIMIZATION HYPOTHESIS

Tax-exempt suppliers abound in the healthcare field. One reason appears to be the existence of external demands for healthcare products and services. These external demands may arise when people are concerned about, and willing to pay for, the health care of others. To satisfy these external demands, individuals may form tax-exempt agencies whose purpose is to provide products and services to those perceived to be needy, usually on a less-than-cost basis. Health-related philanthropies, such as the American Heart Association, give away educational services that are financed by donors who want others to consume the services. The Red Cross blood program exists because there is sufficient concern on the part of blood donors about the health of those requiring transfusions. Tax-exempt hospitals originally provided free and subsidized hospital care to the needy in substantial amounts; this care was financed largely through philanthropic donations, which can be regarded as payments to satisfy the donors' external demands for care of the needy. As the population grew, and the costs associated with hospital services increased, it became necessary for larger subsidies to be obtained for the hospital care provided to the needy. These subsidies tended to take the form of government-assistance programs supported through taxation. Public health departments attempt to satisfy external demands for health care through government-provided services.

There are, no doubt, other reasons for the formation of tax-exempt agencies. For example, these agencies may be formed as "captives" of other tax-exempt groups. During the 1930s and 1940s, Blue Cross plans began under the auspices of tax-exempt hospitals to ensure that hospitals were paid. The scope of our inquiry does not encompass the conditions under which health service agencies become organized on a tax-exempt basis (see Culyer, 1971). Rather, we will treat the existence of this type of organization as a given and restrict our attention to the supply behavior of these agencies once they are formed.

To ensure that the services offered by a tax-exempt agency are provided in a reasonable manner, a board of trustees is formed. The members of a board of trustees cannot gain direct financial benefit from the organization, either in the form of profits or of proceeds from the sale of the enterprise. Furthermore, they are frequently banned from garnering indirect gains, such as what might occur if a board member's law firm provided legal services to the organization. The board of trustees is primarily responsible for setting organizational policies, but many of their responsibilities are delegated to a full-time, salaried administrative (executive) staff. The actual responsibilities of each (the trustees and the staff), including the making of supply decisions, vary from organization to organization.

Several approaches can be taken in forming hypotheses about the supply behavior of tax-exempt agencies. One approach is to regard the trustees as being in charge. Following this approach, we would hypothesize goals the trustees are likely to pursue and then develop a model of the actions of the organization that incorporates these goals. Another approach is to regard the salaried executives as the people who maintain control, make hypotheses about their goals, and develop a model of organizational supply based on *these* goals. No doubt the supply behavior of a real tax-exempt firm is influenced by both trustees and staff, but to keep our analysis simple, we will pursue each approach separately. We begin with the trustee-dominance model. We will assume that the trustees' objective is to maximize the output of the agency, that is, to carry out their mandate to the fullest extent possible by maximizing the quantity of services provided by the agency.

Now let us imagine a tax-exempt lab initially financed by a public-spirited benefactor. Cost and revenue conditions are the same as in the ABC Labs example, with the exception that the pathologist is under contract and receives an explicit payment of $5 per month for her services. From the point of view of the lab, once the contractual commitment is made, this is a fixed cost, and so the total fixed costs of the laboratory are $12. The quality of the product is the same as in the previous example and is constant. Revenues are $14 per test, but now the reimbursement may be made by a third party. (Reimbursement may be collected through individual donations or from a united agency.) The major difference between the two examples is that the tax-exempt lab seeks to maximize output rather than profits.

According to our model, because revenues come only from reimbursement for services, output will be expanded to the point at which the firm breaks even, that is, when $TR = TC$. In Table 6-1, given a price of $14, output will be expanded to eight units. In graph A of Figure 6-1, the break-even point at eight units of output is shown in total terms. In graph B, the lab's operating point is where price per unit equals average total cost. The lab just covers costs for all units when it operates at this level.

Given our assumptions, output for an investor-owned firm will be lower than that for a tax-exempt firm that behaves as we have hypothesized (i.e., maximizes output). The supply curve for an output-maximizing firm is its *ATC* curve for prices above the minimum point on the curve. If the revenues do not total at least this minimum amount, the firm runs a deficit and must raise the funds from nonpatient sources. For the moment, we will assume that nonpatient revenues are zero and that the firm has no reserves to meet a deficit. If it does not meet all its obligations, it will go out of business.

As long as the price is above the minimum point on the *ATC* curve, the supply curve of the tax-exempt agency that maximizes output is the *ATC* curve. As the price rises, so will the supply. Any factor that shifts the *ATC* curve downward (lower unit costs at any level of output) will cause output to increase at any price.

The response of an output-maximizing tax-exempt firm to a fixed subsidy is very different from that of a profit-maximizing firm. Recall that a fixed subsidy will not influence a profit-maximizer's supply (Section 6.2). Let us assume that a donor gives our nonprofit lab a $25 subsidy unrelated to output. Analytically, we can treat this as an overall increase in total revenues or as an overall reduction in total costs (and a reduction in average fixed costs of $25/Q). In the former case, the analysis in Table 6-1 would be altered to show *TR* and profits higher at every level of output by $25. Whereas formerly, the output-maximizing output level was 8, with the subsidy, an output level of 9 will show an overall (operating and nonoperating) profit of $18.25 ($25.00 – $6.75). The lab would be losing money (in the red) at an output level of 10, but it could now meet all its costs at a level of 9, and this is when it would maximize output (subject to the fact that it must break even).

Graphically, if the fixed subsidy is treated as a reduction in fixed costs, it would appear as a downward shift in *AFC* and also *ATC* (because *AFC* is part of *ATC*). It will appear as an outward shift in the firm's supply curve, which is identical to the *ATC* curve. The conclusion in either case is the same: a non-output-related grant will shift the supply curve of the output-maximizing firm and thus will lead to increased output. In this respect, the output-maximizing firm is very unlike the profit-maximizing firm.

The market supply analysis in the case of tax-exempt organizations is some-what more complicated than in the case of investor-owned organizations. If we make the assumption that each separate tax-exempt supplier has a vested inter-est in providing output to the needy, the market supply curve will be made up of the sum of what all the individual suppliers would be willing to supply at each price or reimbursement rate. That is, the market supply curve is the sum of the individual producers' supply curves for prices above the minimum *ATC*.

Individual tax-exempt suppliers might act competitively if the trustees developed some sense of identification with the organizations of which they were board members. However, if this sense of identification did not develop, trustees would not care which organization supplied the output to the needy as long as it was supplied by someone. In this situation, market supply would consist of a far more complicated set of arrangements, because trustees would pull their organizations out of the market when other organizations supplying the same product appeared. We will assume that, in our example, organiza-tional pride develops to the point that the standard market supply model is appropriate.

6.5 SUPPLY DECISIONS INVOLVING QUALITY

Until now, we have assumed that quality of output was held constant and thus did not enter the supply decision. In fact, quality is an extremely impor-tant supply variable for suppliers, especially in the healthcare system. In par-ticular, it has frequently been asserted that hospitals seek to supply output of the highest quality. In this section, a model is developed to incorporate qual-ity of care into the supply picture.

To understand the bias of tax-exempt hospitals toward high-quality sup-ply, it is necessary to examine their unusual management structure. Like other tax-exempt firms, a tax-exempt hospital includes a board of trustees and a group of salaried administrators. However, physicians have a special relation-ship to the hospital: they are in charge of the medical activities of the hos-pital, and yet, for the most part, they are unsalaried staff members. Because their services are so crucial (indeed, the hospital's activities revolve around them), physicians have enormous influence over hospital supply decisions, and hospital supply policies are set by an informal arrangement among physi-cians, trustees, and administrators. This type of arrangement has been termed a "management triangle," depending on mutual accountability, interdepen-dence, and responsibility for appropriate performance of their respective obli-gations. Hospital activities are the result of directives (sometimes conflicting) issued by three lines of authority: medical, trustee, and administrative. In par-ticular, the medical influence in the decision-making process has been held to be responsible for the bias toward quality in hospital objectives, because physicians benefit considerably from high-quality inputs.

In most hospitals, the physicians form an organized medical staff, which is a self-governing organization that typically has the responsibility for determining the membership of the medical staff, performing credentialing of the members, granting privileges and peer-review activities, and providing timely oversight of the clinical quality of care provided and for patient safety. The medical staff seeks maximum physician autonomy with minimal interference in the practice of medicine from hospital procedures. These goals of the medical staff may come in conflict with the hospital's goals of increasing efficiency in the production of medical services in order to improve the financial bottom line of the hospital, creating tension in the relationship. In many cases, the hospital has been viewed as a "free" workshop for physicians to perform their activities of delivering patient care. In addition, because hospitals rely upon physicians for patients, and therefore financial resources, administration has attempted to create attractive practice environments for physicians. Because physicians are paid separately for their services from the hospital, the physicians have a financial interest in the facilities, technologies, and staff that can improve their personal productivity and increase ease of patient care, not necessarily what is best for the institution.

A supply model that is based on the preceding analysis, but incorporates the bias toward quality, can be developed. Assume a given level of reimbursement, say \$2,000 per patient day (see Figure 6-5). *ATC* curves are drawn for three different levels of quality of service; each higher level is produced with more resources. ATC_1 represents an *ATC* curve for a specific level of output

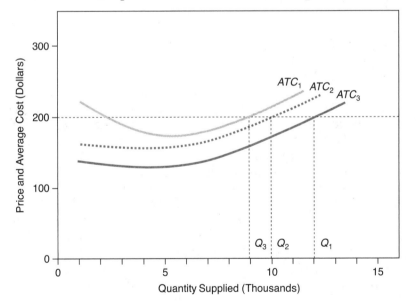

Figure 6-5 Alternative Quantities and Qualities Supply by a Tax-exempt Supplier. The *ATC* curves represent relationships between *ATC* and output at various quality levels. ATC_3 represents the highest level, ATC_2 the intermediate level, and ATC_1 the lowest level. A tax-exempt producer who maximizes the quantity of output (given the quality level) will produce where the unit payment rate, or price, equals *ATC*. For the lowest quality level, the output will be 12. Higher quality levels entail a reduction in the maximum output levels achievable given the payment rate.

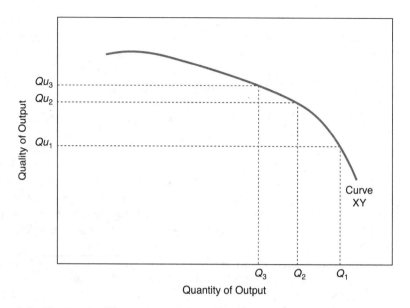

Figure 6-6   The Tradeoff Between Quality and Quantity. Based on Figure 6-5, for any given reimbursement rate, a higher quality level can be achieved only with a lower quantity of output. The curve shows alternative levels of quantity and quality that can be achieved at a given payment rate (or price).

and level of quality. ATC_2 and ATC_3 are similar curves for successively higher levels of quality.

An output-maximizing hospital will choose Q_1 (12,000) units of output at Quality Level 1; Q_2 (10,000) units at Quality Level 2; and Q_3 (9,000) units at Quality Level 3. Indeed, a trade-off between quality and quantity of care typically occurs. Such a trade-off is shown in Figure 6-6, with quality of care represented on the vertical axis and the quantity on the horizontal. Curve *XY* shows the maximum output that can be achieved for each level of quality given the reimbursement rate of $2,000 and thus reflects the constraints or the choices facing the hospital. The actual combination of quality and quantity supplied will depend on the hospital's policies. A highly-quality-oriented hospital will choose a quality level close to Qu_3, whereas an output-oriented hospital will choose a level closer to Qu_1. If the assertion that hospitals are quality oriented is correct, it might be expected that Qu_3 would be more frequently observed. That is, of the various output combinations that a tax-exempt hospital can choose, it will tend to provide care of a higher quality level. By itself, however, this does not mean that we will observe such high-quality care in the market, for it must be remembered that we are currently examining only the supply side of the market. The quality of care actually produced will be determined by what the suppliers are willing to supply and what the consumers are willing and able to purchase. Determining what output actually is produced and utilized requires that we examine the market in its entirety.

6.6 SUPPLY BEHAVIOR OF TAX-EXEMPT AGENCIES: THE ADMINISTRATOR-AS-AGENT MODEL

An alternative theory of resource allocation and product supply in tax-exempt agencies focuses on the behavior of the executive or administrator of the organization. The underlying assumption is that the administrator, even though just an agent of the trustees, has considerable control over the organization's resources. This seems a plausible assumption given that trustees of a tax-exempt agency typically can devote only a small portion of their time to trustee-related activities, whereas the administrator is usually a full-time employee. As part of this approach, a comparative analysis can be done that examines how the same administrator would behave if operating the same agency as an investor-owned enterprise and as a tax-exempt enterprise. The differences in behavior, which are due solely to the different incentive structures of the two types of organization, create differences in the use of the agency's resources and in the agency's output.

The theory can be viewed as simply an extension of the basic demand hypothesis presented in the chapter on the demand for medical care. According to this hypothesis, the lower the direct cost of a good or service or other benefit to an individual, the more the good or service will be demanded. The extension of the hypothesis involves identifying the goods and services that are desired by the administrator of an agency, as well as their relative prices or costs under varying institutional circumstances. Because we are focusing on the administrator's behavior, we will identify two types of benefits that can be obtained in the context of the job. First, there are the pecuniary (monetary) benefits, especially the administrator's salary. In addition, if the administrator is a part or full owner of the agency, the pecuniary benefits will encompass the profits that accrue. Benefits of the second type, sometimes called *on-the-job* benefits, or amenities, are nonpecuniary. These include high-grade office furniture, a relaxed work atmosphere, "business" trips to exotic places, and so on. Both types of benefits are wanted by the administrator, but because their supply is limited, the administrator cannot have everything he or she would like.

Before developing the hypothesis about how much of each type of benefit will be demanded, we will look at the implications for the resource use of obtaining the two types. First, when a smaller amount of resources is used to obtain a given output, an opportunity to increase profits is created. Nonpecuniary benefits also require the commitment of resources. Better office equipment, more liberal working conditions, better fringe benefits, and other on-the-job benefits are obtained from the expansion of the total resource commitment and result in an increase in costs and a contraction of profits. In a tax-exempt enterprise, this reduction in profits does not detract from the manager's pecuniary benefits, because he or she will not be rewarded on the basis of the profits the enterprise earns.

The hypothesis as to how the administrator will behave under these alternative incentive structures is based on the constraints facing the administrator in the two different environments. In a tax-exempt environment, because the administrator cannot convert profits into take-home pecuniary benefits (remember, the profits cannot be distributed to owners or stakeholders but must be reinvested in the organization), they must be converted into organizational resources if any benefit is to be obtained. On the other hand, the use of these extra resources in an investor-owned organization will detract from profits and hence from take-home pecuniary benefits, assuming these are related. The personal costs of on-the-job benefits are lower for the administrator of the tax-exempt agency, and we thus hypothesize that more will be demanded.

The implications of this hypothesis for tax-exempt resource allocation are considerable. The hypothesis implies that the tax-exempt agency will use more resources to get a given job done, and so its costs will be higher. The absence of incentives for efficiency has been the target of investigation, including its effect on tax-exempt agency operating costs, particularly in the case of tax-exempt health insurers (Frech, 1976), nursing homes (Borjas, Frech, Ginsburg, 1983; Frech, 1985), and dialysis units (Lowrie & Hampers, 1981). Similar analyses comparing tax-exempt and investor-owned hospital behavior have not been as conclusive for several reasons. First, to compare operating costs between tax-exempt and investor-owned hospitals, such variables as case mix, case severity, and quality must be used to adjust results. Assertions have been made that tax-exempt hospitals have a more complex case mix because investor-owned hospitals engage in "cream skimming" by encouraging the admission of low-cost cases. Evidence on this score seems mixed (Bays, 1979a, 1979b; Renn, Schramm, Watt, & Derzon, 1985; Schweitzer & Rafferty, 1976). Even more difficult to determine is whether quality differentials exist by ownership category. Tax-exempt managers do have an incentive to produce quality care (which will show up in higher costs). The role of quality in pushing costs higher has yet to be fully explored.

Another difference that has been uncovered when comparing tax-exempt and investor-owned hospital behavior lies in the pricing area. Charges are the prices set by the hospital for its services. Two California studies found that investor-owned hospitals had higher charges (relative to costs) for ancillary (lab, radiology, pharmacy) services (Eskoz & Peddecord, 1985; Pattison & Katz, 1983). Generally, markups (charge-to-cost ratios) for ancillary services were found to be higher than basic room charges. Investor-owned hospitals also provided more (high-profit) ancillary services per patient than tax-exempts in the studies and were more profitable, although cost levels were similar. One possible explanation of this finding is that tax-exempt managers (or trustees) can gain nonpecuniary benefits from encouraging the use of hospital services by keeping patient charges low (which may result in lower profits) as well as by providing more free care to indigents.

A RAND report by Shugarman, Nicosia, and Schuster (2007) reviewed literature between 1996 and 2006 regarding comparisons between tax-exempt and investor-owned healthcare organizations. This review provided conflicting evidence on the relationship between type of hospital ownership and costs but provided consistent evidence that investor-owned nursing homes had lower costs. A study by Wheeler, Burkhardt, Alexander, and Magnus (1999) found that investor-owned hospitals offered less sub-acute care than did tax-exempt hospitals. When examining the amount of uncompensated care provided, Cram, Bayman, Popescu, Vaughan-Sarrazin, Cai, & Rosenthal (2010) found that the percentage of admissions that were classified as uninsured was lower in tax-exempt hospitals than in either investor-owned or government hospitals.

However, relying solely on the incentives identified in the administrator-as-agent model to explain cost and price differences between investor-owned and tax-exempt hospitals would be a mistake. The incentive differences are but one factor operating to influence costs (and possible cost differences) in the two types of organization. The reimbursement system is another major influence on cost and supply behavior. Indeed, the absence of cost differences between tax-exempt and investor-owned hospitals that was uncovered by the investigators in California may have been partly due to the reimbursement system, which, at the time of the studies, encouraged cost inflation in all types of hospitals.

EXERCISES

1. Over 4,000 individuals called up Dr. Kalikorn and asked him to perform a new surgical procedure. Dr. Kalikorn booked 2,000 of these and told the rest to seek care from another physician. What is his quantity supplied?
2. Some 1,000 patients called up Dr. Kalikorn and asked him to perform a new surgical procedure. Dr. Kalikorn booked all 1,000 and told them that he could perform twice as many procedures if only he had more patients. What is his quantity supplied?
3. The state Medicaid agency sets the price for nursing home care. The unit price is $180 per day. This price is beyond the control of any nursing home. What is the marginal revenue for another patient day at Holly Head Nursing Home?
4. The following is a cost function for clinic visits in a small inner city clinic:

Quantity of Visits	Total Cost Per Week
0	$10
1	15
2	25
3	45
4	75
5	115
6	165

   a. Determine the marginal cost for each level of output.
   b. If the price per visit is given to be $25, at what level of visits will the maximum profit position be? What are the profits at this level? What is the quantity supplied?
   c. If the price per visit increases to $45, what will be the quantity supplied (assuming maximizing profits)?

5. Given the following data, answer questions (a) and (b). The total fixed cost for the Grand Forks Clinic is $30 per month. The total variable cost is given as follows:

Quantity of Visits	Total Cost Per Week
1	$10
2	25
3	45
4	70
5	105
6	145

   a. If the price per visit is $30, what is the quantity supplied?
   b. If the total fixed cost increases to $40 and the price per visit is $30, what is the quantity supplied?

6. Given the following cost schedule for a regional hospital that seeks to maximize its profits, answer the following three questions:

Days of Care	Supplied Total Cost
0	$100
1	200
2	400
3	700
4	1100
5	1600
6	2200

   a. If the price per day is $220, what is the quantity supplied?
   b. If the price per day increases to $320, what is the quantity supplied?
   c. If the price per day is $450, what is the quantity supplied?

7. Given the following cost schedule for a clinic, determine the quantity supplied at alternative prices of $10, $20, and $30 per visit.

Quantity of Visits	Total Cost	Marginal Cost
0	$10	
1	25	$15
2	43	18
3	75	32
4	125	50

8. The following is a marginal cost curve and an average variable cost curve for the White River Hospital. The government is considering setting prices for White River's output (days of care), but

it is unsure what per diem to set. It has asked you to evaluate the following per diem rates, assuming that the hospital has the objective of maximizing its profits.

a. What is the quantity supplied if the price per diem is $100?

b. If the price is $200?

c. If the price is $400?

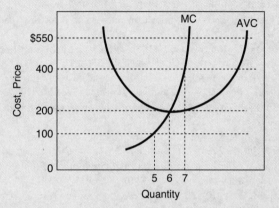

9. A clinic receives a per-visit payment of $20. It has an upward sloping supply curve. Indicate the net effect on the quantity of visits supplied if the following occur:

   a. The wage rates for the clinic nursing staff increase.

   b. The fixed overhead costs (rent, electricity) increase.

   c. The clinic patients become sicker.

   d. The clinic increases productivity.

   e. The clinic decides to increase "quality" (defined as a more thorough examination for each patient).

10. Given the supply curve for radiographs by a radiology practice, predict how this curve will shift (supply will increase or decrease) if the following occur:

    a. An increase in the wages of radiological technicians

    b. A reduction in productivity

    c. A decrease in the wages of technicians

    d. An increase in the price of radiographs

    e. An increase in the quality of services (radiologists spend more care in reading and interpreting radiographs)

    f. An increase in the price of film

    g. An increase in the number of patients with multiple and rare problems

BIBLIOGRAPHY

Supply Functions

Ananthakrishnan, A. N., Hoffmann, R. G., & Saelan, K. (2010). Higher physician density is associated with lower incidence of late-stage colorectal cancer. *Journal of General Internal Medicine, 25*(11), 1164–1171.

Fehring, T. K., Odum, S. M., Troyer, J. L., Iorio, R., Kurtz, S. M., & Lau, E. C. (2010). Joint replacement access in 2016: A supply side crisis. *Journal of Arthroplasty, 25*(8), 1175–1181.

Glied, S. (1998). Payment heterogeneity, physician practice, and access to care. *American Economic Review, 88*(2), 127–131.

Goldfarb, M., Hornbrook, M., & Rafferty, J. (1980). Behavior of the multi-product firm: A Model of the Nonprofit Hospital System. *Medical Care, 19,* 185–201.

Goodman, C. (2010). Graduate medical education: A brief history and its role in physician supply. *Journal—South Carolina Medical Association, 106*(7), 245–247.

Hornbrook, M., & Goldfarb, M. (1983). A partial test of a hospital behavior model. *Social Science and Medicine, 17,* 667–680.

Kahn, M. J., & Nelling, E. F. (2010). Estimating the value of medical education: A net present value approach. *Teaching & Learning in Medicine, 22*(3), 205–208.

Lupu, D. (2010). Estimate of current hospice and palliative medicine physician workforce shortage. *Journal of Pain & Symptom Management, 40*(6), 899–911.

Posey, L. M., & Tanzi, M. G. (2010). Diabetes care: Model for the future of primary care. *Journal of the American Pharmacists Association, 50*(5), 623–236.

Rabinowitz, H. K. (2011). AM last page. Truths about the rural physician supply. *Academic Medicine, 86*(2), 272.

Schneider, S. M., Gardner, A. F., Weiss, L. D., Wood, J. P. et al (2010). The future of emergency medicine. *Journal of Emergency Medicine, 39*(2), 210–215.

Shipman, S. A., Lan, J., Chang, C. H., & Goodman, D. C. (2011). Geographic maldistribution of primary care children. *Pediatrics, 127*(1), 19–27.

Simoens, S., & Giuffrida, A. (2004). The impact of physician payment methods on raising the efficiency of the health care system: An international comparison. *Applied Health Economics & Health Policy, 3*(1), 39–46.

Smith, B. D., Haffty, B. G., Wilson, L. D., Smith, G. L., Patel, A. N., & Buchholz, T. A. (2010). The future of radiation oncology in the United States from 2010 to 2020: Will supply keep pace with demand? *Journal of Clinical Oncology, 28*(35), 5160–5165.

Thornton, J., & Eakin, B. K. (1996). The utility-maximizing self-employed physician. *Journal of Human Resources, 32,* 98–127.

Not-for-Profit (Tax Exempt) Organization Behavior

Adams, K., & Martin, S. (2011). Ethical tissue: A not-for-profit model for human tissue supply. *Cell & Tissue Banking, 12*(1), 9–10.

Banks, D. A., Paterson, M., & Wendel, J. (1997). Uncompensated hospital care: Charitable mission or profitable business decision? *Health Economics, 6,* 133–144.

Berg, J. W. (2010). What is left of charity care after health reform? *Hastings Center Report, 40*(4), 12–13.

Bess, K. D., Perkins, D. D., & McCown, D. L. (2011). Testing a measure of organizational learning capacity and readiness for transformational change in human services. *Journal of Prevention & Intervention in the Community, 39*(1), 35–49.

Bjork, D. A. (2010). Regulation of executive compensation at nonprofit health care organizations: Coming changes? *Inquiry, 47*(1), 7–16.

Brown, D. S. (2010). The governance imperative for nonprofit hospitals. *Trustee, 6*(1), 30–32.

Cohen, J. R., Gerrish, W., & Galvin, J. R. (2010). Health care reform and Connecticut's non-profit hospitals. *Journal of Health Care Finance, 37*(2), 1–7.

Culyer, A. J. (1971). Medical care and the economics of giving. *Economica, 38*, 295–303.

Gaskin, D. J. (1997). Altruism and moral hazard: The impact of hospital uncompensated care pools. *Journal of Health Economics, 16*, 397–416.

Harris, J. F. (1977). The internal organization of hospitals. *Bell Journal of Economics, 8*, 647–682.

Lee, M. L. (1971). A conspicuous production theory of hospital behavior. *Southern Economic Journal, 38*, 48–58.

Luksetich, W., Edwards, M., & Carroll, T. M. (2000). Organizational form and nursing home behavior. *Nonprofit and Voluntary Sector Quarterly, 29*, 255–279.

McGuire, A. (1985). The theory of the hospital: A review of the models. *Social Science and Medicine, 20*, 1177–1184.

Pauly, M., & Redisch, M. (1973). The not-for-profit hospital as a physicians' cooperative. *American Economic Review, 63*, 87–100.

Rauscher, S., & Wheeler, J. R. (2010). Hospital revenue cycle management and payer mix: Do Medicare and Medicaid undermine hospitals' ability to generate and collect patient care revenue? *Journal of Health Care Finance, 37*(2), 81–96.

Rosenbaum, S., & Margulies, R. (2011). Tax-exempt hospitals and the Patient Protection and Affordable Care Act: Implications for public health policy and practice. *Public Health Reports, 126*(2), 283–286.

Smith, P. C. (2006). An evaluation of charity care for tax-exempt hospitals engaging in joint ventures. *Journal of Health Care Finance, 33*(1), 40–53.

Vaughan, S. K. (2010). The importance of performance assessment in local government decisions to fund health and human services nonprofit organizations. *Journal of Health & Human Services Administration, 32*(4), 486–512.

For-Profit (Investor-Owned) and Not-for-Profit (Tax Exempt) Comparisons (Dialogue)

Barsi, E., Jones, D., Kotsonis, D., Lowell, M., Paret, C., & McPherson, B. (2010). Community benefit: Overcoming organizational barriers and laying the foundation for success. *Inquiry, 47*(2), 103–109.

Bays, C. (1979a). Case-mix differences between nonprofit and for-profit hospitals. *Inquiry, 14*, 17–21.

Bays, C. (1979b). Cost comparisons of for-profit and nonprofit hospitals. *Social Science and Medicine, 13C*, 219–225.

Bogart, L. M., Howerton, D., Lange, J., Setodji, C. M., Becker, K., Klein, D. J., & Asch, S. M. (2010). Provider-related barriers to rapid HIV testing in US urban non-profit community clinics, community-based organizations (CBOs) and hospitals. *AIDS & Behavior, 14*(3), 697–707.

Borjas, G. J., Frech, H.E. III, & Ginsburg, P. B. (1983). Property rights and wages: The case of nursing homes. *Journal of Human Resources, 17*, 231–246.

Cherlin, E. J., Carlson, M. D., Herrin, J., Schulman-Green, D., Barry, C. L., McCorkle, R., ... & Bradley, E. H. (2010). Interdisciplinary staffing patterns: Do for-profit and nonprofit hospices differ? *Journal of Palliative Medicine, 13*(4), 389–394.

Clarkson, K. W. (1972). Some implications of property rights in hospital management. *Journal of Law and Economics, 15*, 363–384.

Comondore, V. R., Devereaux, P. J., Zhou, Q., Stone, S. B., Busse, J. W., Ravindran, N. C., ...& Guyatt, G. H. (2009). Quality of care in for-profit and not-for-profit nursing homes: Systematic review and meta-analysis. *British Medical Journal, 339*, b2732.

Cram, P., Bayman, L., Popescu, I., Vaughan-Sarrazin, M. S., Cai, X., & Rosenthal, G. E. (2010). Uncompensated care provided by for-profit, not-for-profit, and government-owned hospitals. *Health Services Research, 10*, 90.

DeCesare, E., & Narayan, M. (2010). When a for-proft acquires a nonprofit organization: Lessons learned from one home health/hospice's experience. *Home Healthcare Nurse, 28*(3), 147–153.

Decker, F. H. (2008). Nursing home performance in resident care in the United States: Is it only a matter of for-profit versus not-for-profit? *Health Economics, Policy, & Law, 3*(Pt 2), 115–140.

Eskoz, R., & Peddecord, K. M. (1985). The relationship of hospital ownership and service composition to hospital charges. *Health Care Financing Review, 6,* 51–58.

Frech, H. E. (1976). The property rights theory of the firm: Empirical results from a natural experiment. *Journal of Political Economy, 84,* 143–152.

Frech, H. E. (1985). The property rights theory of the firm: Some evidence from the U.S. nursing home industry. *Zeitschrift fur die Gestamte Staatswissenschaft, 141,* 146–166.

Grabowski, D. C., & Stevenson, D. G. (2008). Ownership conversions and nursing home performance. *Health Service Research, 43*(4), 1184–1203.

Haldiman, K. L., & Tzeng, H. M. (2010). A comparison of quality measures between for-profit and nonprofit medicare-certified home health agencies in Michigan. *Home Health Care Services Quarterly, 29*(2), 75–90.

Lewin, L. S., Derzon, R. A., & Marqulies, R. (1981). Investor-owneds and nonprofits differ in economic performance. *Hospitals, 1*(July), 52–58.

Lowrie, E. G., & Hampers, C. L. (1981). The success of Medicare's end-stage renal disease program. *New England Journal of Medicine, 305,* 434–438.

Pattison, R. V., & Katz, H. M. (1983). Investor-owned and not-for-profit hospitals. *New England Journal of Medicine, 309,* 347–353.

Relman, A. S. (1980). The new medical-industrial complex. *New England Journal of Medicine, 303,* 963–970.

Relman, A. S., & Reinhardt, U. E. (1986). Debating for-profit health care. *Health Affairs, 5*(2), 5–31.

Renn, S. C., Schramm, C. J., Watt, J. M., & Derzon, R. A. (1985). The effects of ownership and system affiliation on the economic performance of hospitals. *Inquiry, 22,* 219–236.

Rice, T., & Gabel, J. (1996). The internal economics of HMOs: A research agenda. *Medical Care Research and Review, 53*(Suppl.), S44–S64.

Ruchlin, H. S., Pointer, D. D., & Cannedy, L. L. (1976). A comparison of for-profit investor-owned chains and nonprofit hospitals. *Inquiry, 10,* 13–23.

Schweitzer, S. O., & Rafferty, J. (1976). Variations in hospital product: A comparative analysis of proprietary and voluntary hospitals. *Inquiry, 13,* 158–166.

Shugarman, I. R., Nicosia, N., & Schuster, C. R. (2007). *Comparing for-profit and not-for-profit health care providers: A review of the literature.* Santa Monica, CA: RAND.

Wheeler, J. R., Burkhardt, J., Alexander, J. A., & Magnus, S. A. (1999). Financial and organizational determinants of hospital diversification into subacute care. *Health Services Research, 34*(1, Pt 1), 61–81.

Provider Supply Under Managed Care Contracting

Albizu-Garcia, C. E., Rios, R., Juarbe, D., & Alegria, M. (2004). Provider turnover in public sector managed mental health care. *Journal of Behavioral Health Services & Research, 31*(3), 255–265.

Auerbach, A. D., Maselli, J., Carter, J., Pekow, P. S., & Lindenauer, P. K. (2010). The relationship between case volume, care quality, and outcomes of complex cancer surgery. *Journal of the American College of Surgeons, 211*(5), 601–608.

Bittinger, A. (2007). A strategic approach to managed care contracting. *JCR: Journal of Clinical Rheumatology, 13*(6), 346–349.

Debrock, A., & Arnould, R. J. (1992). Utilization control in HMOs. *Quarterly Review of Economics and Business, 32*(3), 31–53.

Elder, K., & Miller, N. (2006). Minority physicians and selective contracting in competitive market environments. *Journal of Health & Social Policy, 21*(4), 21–49.

Feldstein, P. J., Wickizer, T. M., & Wheeler, J. R. (1988). Private cost containment. The effects of utilization review programs on health care use and expenditures. *New England Journal of Medicine, 318,* 1310–1314.

Freed, G. L., Dunham, K. M., & Singer, D. (2009). Health plan use of board certification and recertification of surgeons and nonsurgical subspecialists in contracting policies. *Archives of Surgery, 144*(8), 753–758.

Garnick, D. W., Horgan, C. M., Reif, S., Merrick, E. L., & Hodgkin, D. (2008). Management of behavioral health provider networks in private health plans. *Journal of Ambulatory Care Management, 31*(4), 330–341.

Hansen-Turton, T., Ritter, A., & Torgan, R. (2008). Insurers' contracting policies on nurse practitioners as primary care providers: Two years later. *Policy, Politics, & Nursing Practice, 9*(4), 241–248.

Hillman, A. L. (1987). Financial incentives for physicians in HMOs. *New England Journal of Medicine, 317,* 1743–1748.

Hillman, A. L., Pauly, M. V., & Kerstein, J. J. (1989). How do financial incentives affect physicians' clinical decisions and the financial performance of health maintenance organizations? *New England Journal of Medicine, 321,* 86–92.

Mukamel, D. B., Weimer, D. L., Zwanziger, J., & Mushlin, A. I. (2002). Quality of cardiac surgeons and managed care contracting practices. *Health Services Research, 37*(5), 1129–1144.

Nugent, M. E. (2010). Managed care contracting and payment reform: Avoiding a showdown. *Healthcare Financial Management, 64*(7), 36–39.

Pauly, M. V., Hillman, A. L., & Kerstein, J. (1990). Managing physician incentives in managed care. *Medical Care, 28,* 1013–1024.

Rantz, M. J., Hicks, L, Grando, V. et al (2004). Nursing home quality, cost, staffing, and staff mix. *Gerontologist, 44*(1), 24–38.

Rantz, M. J., Hicks, L., Petroski, G. F., Madsen, R. W., Alexander, G., Galambos, C., ... & Greenwald, L. (2010). Cost, staffing, and quality impact of bedside electronic medical record (EMR) in nursing homes. *Journal of the American Medical Directors Association, 11*(7), 485–493.

Robinson, J. C. (1993). Payment mechanisms, nonprice incentives, and organizational innovations in health care. *Inquiry, 30,* 328–332.

Scheffler, R. M., Sullivan, S. D., & Ko, T. H. (1991). The impact of Blue Cross and Blue Shield plan utilization management programs, 1980–1988. *Inquiry, 28,* 276–287.

Scholle, S. H., Roski, J., Adams, J. L., Dunn, D. L., Kerr, E. A., Dugan, D. P., & Jensen, R. E. (2008). Benchmarking physician performance: Reliability of individual and composite measures. *American Journal of Managed Care, 14*(12), 833–838.

Ullmann, S. G. (2003). "Out of our crisis": The lack of long-term relationships in the provision of managed care. *Hospital Topics, 81*(2), 4–8.

Unruh, L., Lugo, N. R., White, S. V., & Byers, J. F. (2005). Managed care and patient safety: Risks and opportunities. *Health Care Manager, 24*(3), 245–256.

Wickizer, T. M., Wheeler, J. R. C., & Feldstein, P. J. (1989). Does utilization review reduce unnecessary hospital care and contain costs? *Medical Care, 27,* 632–647.

Zwanziger, J., & Khan, N. (2006). Safety-net activities and hospital contracting with managed care organizations. *Medical Care Research & Review, 63*(6 Suppl.), 90S–111S.

Chapter 7

Provider Payment

OBJECTIVES

1. Explain the principal-agent framework as it relates to provider payment in health care.

2. Identify the major types of physician payment and compare their incentives using the principal-agent framework.

3. Explain the Resource-Based Relative Value Scale as a fee-for-service funding instrument.

4. Identify the alternative bases for the payment of hospitals.

5. Using the principal-agent framework, explain the incentives associated with each of the major types of hospital payment.

6. Explain the diagnosis-related group payment system for Medicare.

7. Identify the major methods for reimbursing long-term care facilities.

8. Explain the method by which capitation rates are set for health maintenance organizations in Medicare.

9. Explain the impact of alternative provider payment methods on HMO performance.

10. Identify the different methods that can be used by payers to monitor and regulate provider behavior.

7.1 INTRODUCTION

In the healthcare field, there is a wide variety of services; the major services are hospital, physician, outpatient drug, long-term care facility, and home care services. In addition, there are combined service units, such as health maintenance organizations, medical homes, and accountable care organizations. For each of these types of services, there are alternative ways of paying the provider. For example, physicians can be paid on a fee-for-service basis, by capitation, per case, or by salary, and hospitals can be paid on the basis of a global budget, on a per-case basis, capitated, per diem basis, or for costs already incurred (retrospectively). Earlier, there was a swing toward prospective payment (that is, predetermined rates) for hospitals and away from retrospective payment.

In recent years, critical access hospitals have had retrospective payment reinstated. Critical Access Hospitals (CAHs) are acute care hospitals that have converted and received certification from the Centers for Medicare and Medicaid. They are eligible to receive cost-based payments plus 1% from Medicare, potentially increasing revenue and reducing the risk of closure. CAHs are limited to 25 acute care beds and must maintain an annual average length of stay of 96 hours or less for their acute care patients. In addition, CAHs must provide 24-hour emergency services with medical staff on-site or on-call available on-site within 30 minutes (the limit is 60 minutes if certain frontier area criteria are met). It was shown in the chapter on behavior of supply that the rate of payment will influence supplier behavior. In addition, payment bases are not neutral with respect to their impacts; that is, the basis of payment will have an impact on the quantity and quality of services provided. The theory of agency can shed light on the effect of the different types of payment. In this chapter, a description of the key forms of provider payment in the healthcare field is provided.

7.2 PRINCIPAL-AGENT RELATIONSHIPS AMONG PAYERS AND PROVIDERS

A principal-agent relationship or arrangement exists when one entity or individual (called the agent) acts on behalf of another individual or entity (called the principal). When the agent is an expert at making the necessary decisions that are in the best interest of the principal, and coincide with what the principal would do if he/she possessed sufficient information and expertise, the arrangement works well. However, if the interests of the agent and the principal differ substantially, or there is a conflict of interest in carrying out the conditions of the arrangement, then the arrangement will not work well.

In the area of provider payment, the provider, acting as an agent, faces two principals: the patients and, when there is health insurance, the insurers (Blomquist, 1991). Our primary focus is on the relationship between payers (insurers) and providers (physicians, hospitals, long-term care facilities, and home care agencies).

Insurers must pay providers a given amount when the providers render services to patients. The payments include the costs incurred by the providers and any profits they may make. In addition, as will be seen presently, some payment bases impose higher risks on the providers than others. Providers may demand a risk premium to compensate them for incurring these risks, and if they are risk averse, these risk premiums can be considerable, thus adding to the insurer's costs. In addition to the payment to providers, insurers and other payers will incur costs of transacting with the providers. These include the costs of searching for product availability, characteristics of the products, and prices; costs of negotiating and preparing contracts; costs of monitoring the providers' performance; and costs of enforcing the terms of the contracts. These transaction costs will vary according to the basis of payment. For example, if a particular payment basis encourages the provision of low-quality care or of excessive services, then additional monitoring and enforcement costs will be imposed on the insurer. In turn, the costs to the insurer are passed on to consumers in the form of premiums. The higher the insurers cost, the higher the premium the consumer (individually or through an employer) will have to pay. In this chapter, we will examine the economic implications of different payment systems in light of these concepts.

7.3 PHYSICIAN PAYMENT

There are four major types of physician payment: fee-for-service, per case, per capita, and salary payment. Oftentimes, the stated fee-for-service amount is discounted to physicians.

7.3.1 Fee-for-Service Payment

The fee-for-service method of payment is similar to a piece-rate method. The physician is paid a specific sum for each individual service he or she provides to the patient. The services are broken down into units, such as a complete physical exam, a follow-up visit, a tonsillectomy, and so on. Typically, the fee to be paid to the provider is set in advance (prospectively).

There are several ways in which the fees can be set by the third party. One, which most closely corresponds to the assumption of an absence of control by the provider over the fee, is the relative value scale (Carroll, 2011; Havighurst & Kissam, 1979; Hsiao & Stason, 1979; Malay, 2011). In this method, each category of service is assigned a relative value in accordance with some criterion (e.g., the number of minutes required to perform the procedure). For example, in the frequently used California Relative Value Scale (surgical component), a single coronary bypass operation would have an index number of 25. This relative value can be converted to fees by applying a conversion factor. If the conversion factor for surgery was $250 per point on the relative value scale, the surgeon would be paid $6,250 for the bypass operation. A recent version of this mode of payment is discussed in the next paragraph. In this instance, the physician is viewed as a price taker. The physician can determine the amount of services to provide at that price but cannot influence the price received for the service. The amount of services provided depends upon the marginal cost of production of the provider.

A second type of fee setting does not really correspond to the assumption that fees are beyond the control of the individual provider. This method is referred to as the UCR (usual, customary, and reasonable) form of payment. *Usual* refers to the usual or typical fee charged by the billing physician, *customary* refers to fees charged by all physicians in the community, and *reasonable* refers to allowances for particular circumstances (Epstein & Blumenthal, 1993). Suppose Dr. Welby performed 100 varicose vein injections and charged an average of $100. Her usual fee for the procedure would then be $100. The customary fee would be derived from the frequency distribution of the fees charged by all physicians in the community for the procedure (e.g., the physicians in the 10th percentile might charge an average of $55, those in the 20th percentile might charge $63, and so on). The insurer then decides which percentile to use to set an allowable maximum fee. If the payer used the 70th percentile, then the associated charge might be $87. Dr. Welby would then be paid her usual fee or the customary fee, whichever was lower (in her case, the customary fee of $89, because her usual fee is $100).

The reason why the provider is not a pure price taker in this approach is that the provider's fee partly determines the customary fee prevailing in the market. If all physicians (or even some) raise their fees, the customary fee will increase as well. Each physician thus exerts some degree of influence over the market's fees. When there are many physicians in the market, the degree of influence may be small, and for analytical purposes, the physicians might take the customary fee as a given fee. (Note that the fee, in this case, is also beyond the control of the insurer.) The use of the UCP payment method has often been viewed as inflationary (Miller, 2009; Simoens & Giuffrida, 2004). Because providers know that increasing fees charged in one year will impact the amount of the customary rate of fees charged the following year, the incentive provided is to increase the rate charged, creating a spirally inflationary result. Even though the higher rate charged will not impact the current customary fee in the market, it does influence future customary rates. The profit-maximizing model is useful for analyzing the effects of the level of rates in a fee-for-service payment system. Because the physician is paid a fixed rate per unit of service provided, the number of units produced will depend on what the payment rate is and on the physician's marginal costs for the specific service. If the marginal cost schedule slopes upward steeply, only a slight addition to supply will result from an increase in the fee (Chernew, Mechanic, Landon, & Safran, 2011; Miller, 2009; Phelps, 1976). Another important factor is the composition of fees. If surgical fees are high relative to general checkup fees, that is, surgical operations yield considerable profits relative to checkups, then surgeons will have an incentive to operate more. Physicians, on the other hand, will not have an incentive to perform checkups (which might be marginally profitable, if at all). Indeed, fee-for-service payment is believed to encourage physicians to provide more medical care or increase the volume of care provided. As we have just seen, however, the degree of encouragement, if any, will depend on the relation between the fee and the service's marginal cost. Some analysts have taken the argument one step further and claimed that fee-for-service payment encourages many medically unnecessary practices (Goodwin, Singh, Reddy, Riall, & Yong-Fang., 2011; Klarman, 1963; Swensen., Kaplan, Meyer, Nelson, Hunt, Pryor,.... & Chassin, 2011). In the context of the present analysis, we can only say whether additional services are likely to be offered; we cannot determine whether they would be medically necessary.

The fee schedule is a potentially powerful tool that third parties can use to influence both the type of practices performed and where they are performed. For example, tonsillectomies are thought to be unnecessary in many instances. If a third party wanted to discourage this procedure, it could lower the amount of payment. Also, if a third party wanted to encourage certain procedures to be performed on an outpatient rather than an inpatient basis, it could pay physicians differentially for the same procedure. For example, an insurance company could pay a provider $3,000 for a colonoscopy performed in an outpatient setting and $2,000 for the same procedure performed in a hospital.

The profit-maximizing hypothesis can be altered to take into account alternative possible behavior patterns of the physician-owners of medical practices. These behavior patterns are influenced by the payment method. When price is fixed externally, then the provider can impact the quantity of services provided, and that quantity is influenced by the marginal cost of production. Marginal costs to providers include not only the direct costs of supplies, labor, overhead, and such but also the mental (psychological costs associated with their behavior).

7.3.2 Per Case Payment

The second type of physician payment is on a per-case basis. In this type of payment, the physician is paid a fixed amount for each type of case treated, much like the DRG system. In fact, the DRG system is among the systems considered as a basis for per-case payment (Mitchell, 1985). In per-case payment, the physician bears the cost of any services he or she provides and is paid a sum for the entire case. If the physician reduces the number of services provided per case, more money will be left over as profit. Concern has been expressed that this payment method may lead to the underservice of patients.

Per-case payment for physicians is not widely being considered for all physicians at this time, in part because studies have indicated that there are wide variations in services for a single case type (DRG). This variation would result in difficulties in establishing rates, or fees, and would give providers greater leeway to select cases with potentially low costs and to refer potentially high-cost cases. Per-case payment has been used for obstetrical care by many insurers, in which a set fee is established for prenatal care and delivery. Per-case basis has also been applied to surgical cases for physicians.

The Patient Protection and Affordable Care Act in 2010 has become a catalyst for developing innovative models for delivering and paying for health care in an effort to improve the efficiency and effectiveness of health care. One program, the Medicare Shared Savings Program, establishes financial incentives for Accountable Care Organizations (ACOs) to provide coordinated, well-integrated care. Although the program is in its early stage, emphasis is being placed on moving away from the fee-for-service chassis and placing the provider at financial risk for a patient population. Limitations currently faced by providers, however, include lack of health information systems necessary to provide the clinical and financial data required to coordinate care among providers at different levels efficiently or effectively. ACOs intensify the incentives to improve quality and reduce costs in health care. Although a number of different financial models have been adopted by these early ACOs, increasing emphasis is being placed on bundled payments.

A bundled payment, also known as episode-based payment, case rate, package pricing, or global payment, is simply a single payment made for all healthcare services related to a specific course of treatment or condition over a period of time; the provider is not paid for each discrete service, interaction, or procedure. The single payment amount covers all providers and services performed for a clinically defined episode of care for a single patient, and that amount is then allocated among the providers involved in the care. This bundled payment system is expected to create financial incentives to provide better coordinated care across providers to achieve high-quality outcomes because each provider in the chain of care does not receive a separate payment for every service.

7.3.3 Per Capita and Salary Payment

The incentives for physicians who are paid on a per capita or a salary basis are decidedly different than the incentives in fee-for-service payment. In both cases, there is some incentive for physicians to provide no more than the basic minimum level of services. However, a physician who intends to remain in practice a long time could not afford to allow the quality of services to fall to a low level. Considerable evidence exists regarding the impact that the payment system has on physician practices. Reference has been made to the large difference in surgical operations in the United States and England, and the difference in general payment patterns is considered one underlying factor. In England, surgeons were, traditionally, paid on a salary basis, while in the United States, the usual payment basis is fee-for-service (Aaron & Schwartz, 1984), although the fee schedule has been changed considerably since the introduction of the Resource-Based Relative Value Scale (RBRVS).

In the United States, several payment experiments have been undertaken (Eisenberg & Williams, 1981; Myers & Schroeder, 1981). In one, primary care physicians were given financial responsibility for the entire healthcare expenditures of their patients (a global capitation system); they shared in any surpluses of premiums over total medical care costs (including hospitalization costs, laboratory fees, radiology fees, etc.), as well as in any deficits. The incentive was for them to reduce the expenditures paid out so that the surpluses would be greater. This experiment was based on a view of the physician as "gatekeeper" to the healthcare system, someone who has the ability to control a good deal of the patient's cost. The results showed a considerable reduction in overall expenses relative to a fee-for-service comparison group (Moore, 1979). Another study examined how physician prescribing behavior was affected by an ambulatory care center's introduction of monetary incentives to generate additional business. The findings showed there was a substantial increase in radiographs (Hemenway, Killen, Cashman, Parks, & Bicknell., 1990).

Briefly, capitation is a payment method by which a healthcare provider is paid a fixed amount of money for each individual enrolled in his/her member panel, usually on a monthly basis, regardless of whether or not the individual uses any services. The provider is placed at financial risk for all members in his/her panel. If the cost of services provided to the members of the panel is less than the fixed amount, then the provider retains the difference as additional income; if the costs are greater, then the provider suffers a loss in income. Capitation creates an incentive for providers to be efficient and effective in the provision of care in order to contain costs. A concern raised by capitation is that providers may in fact have an incentive to provide too few services to panel members or to limit members' access to services.

Salaried physicians, on the other hand, are paid a fixed amount (weekly or monthly usually), and the amount of the payment is not tied to the number of enrollees or the amount of services rendered, either in terms of services performed during each visit or the number of visits the member has. With a salary, the physician does not have a financial incentive to change treatment patterns because he/she does not face a financial risk, other than possible future salary increases.

7.3.4 Agency Theory and Physician Payment

Many investigators have linked the fee-for-service payment system with the generation of a high volume of services and consequently with high expenditure levels. Usually, fee-for-service is compared with capitation funding.

Under any payment system, the physician has the ability to generate additional services because of the information asymmetry between physician and patient. Information asymmetry occurs when at least some relevant information for the transaction is known to some, but not all, of the parties involved. This creates an imbalance of power in the decision-making process, potentially resulting in inefficiencies in market transactions. When acquiring information is expensive, such as a patient obtaining complete information regarding medical conditions and treatment options, then decisions may be informed or delegated to the "expert" physician. In health care, this delegation removes the independence between demand and supply because the physician is also the supplier.

Under fee-for-service, the physician has the incentive to generate more services, especially if the fee exceeds the marginal cost of the service. By comparison, the physician will not have such an incentive under capitation. If the physician is not concerned about repeat visits, then he or she will have an incentive to reduce the volume of visits. However, if the physician has a desire to encourage repeat visits by patients, then he or she will not want to reduce services to the point at which quality of care is compromised.

The capitation payment system imposes risks on the provider; the provider must incur the costs of all services for all patients, including the very high cost ones. In determining his or her capitation rates, the provider will add a risk premium that will vary with his or her degree of risk aversion. This will be very high if the provider is risk averse. A risk averse provider is cautious, and desires to minimize exposure to risk, even when the potential benefit of the activity is rather large. The risk averse provider, if given a choice, will select a guaranteed payoff rather than gamble that a payoff might be substantially larger. For example, if offered 50 cents guaranteed or offered a chance for a dollar with the flip of a coin, the risk averse individual will select the guaranteed 50 cents. A third-party payer will incur contract costs under both fee-for-service and capitation funding. Under fee-for-service funding, the insurer must monitor for excessive services, while under capitation funding, the insurer must monitor for low quality of care due to inadequate provision. There is no predetermined answer as to which funding system is more costly once societal costs are included, although most commentators would say that fee-for-service costs more.

7.3.5 A Resource-Based Relative Value Scale

Medicare adopted a variant of the UCR system called *customary, prevailing,* and *reasonable* (CPR), but it had regulated these fees since 1984. In 1992, a new fee schedule was adopted to replace the old fee system. The new schedule has fixed fees that are based on resource-use measures. This system, called RBRVS, attempts to classify the costs that would be incurred by physicians operating in a competitive environment. Based on the classification, a questionnaire was developed to capture the costs incurred in the classification scheme. The questionnaire was applied to national samples of physicians in 18 specialties to develop a relative cost schedule for physician procedures or services. The cost categories include costs related to actual work done by a physician, costs of operating practices, and practice liability insurance.

The national survey interviewed a sample of physicians about the time, mental effort and judgment, physical effort, technical skill, and stress associated with each procedure. These elements were combined into work indexes. For example, an office visit for internal medicine had a work index of 100, whereas a resection for rectal carcinoma had an index value of 445. To these work indexes were added practice cost factors and the professional liability insurance costs. Practice costs were determined by specialty based on a survey of costs and revenues by physicians in each specialty. On average, the physician work component accounts for 52% of the total relative value for each service, the practice expense component accounts for 44%, and the professional liability component accounts for 4%.

The results of the calculations indicate the value of the services relative to each other, not their value in dollars. The relative valuations must then be assigned a dollar value, the conversion rate, in order to be translated into a fee schedule. For example, if the dollar value assigned to the schedule was $1 per index point, then the physician would receive $445 for a resection for rectal carcinoma (which was given an index value of 445 points).

The relative value of each service is multiplied by Geographic Practice Cost Indices (GPCIs) to adjust for locality cost differences. Differences are also paid based on facility or nonfacility practice type. Because the physician work relative values are based on the CPT (Current Procedural Terminology) codes, new and revised codes necessitate annual revisions in the RBRVS. The CPT codes reflect tasks and services performed by a medical practitioner in the provision of medical, surgical, and diagnostic care. Medicare actually uses HCPCS codes (Healthcare Common Procedure Coding System); their Level I HCPCS codes are identical to CPT codes, and their Level II codes are additional codes typically associated with services provided outside the physician's office. CMS publishes information on RVUs for CPT codes in the Federal Register. The CY 2010 conversion factor was $36.0846. The effects of such changes can be analyzed in terms of the supply analysis presented in this chapter. An increase in the fee for a procedure should increase the quantity supplied of that procedure, and a reduction should reduce the quantity supplied. Thus, for those procedures whose fees are increased, the quantity supplied will increase. This is shown in Figure 7-1, in which S_1 is a supply curve for a single profit-maximizing

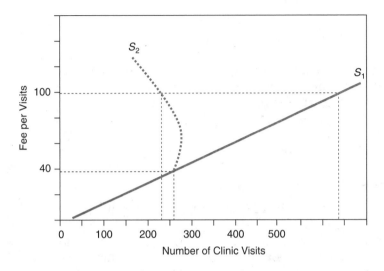

Figure 7-1 Supply Curves for Physician Services Under Two Sets of Assumptions. Curve S_1 shows a situation where higher fees result in more labor (and less leisure). Curve S_2 shows a case where higher fees result in physicians taking more leisure time and cutting back on work.

physician (ignore S_2 for the moment). Initially, the fee for an office visit is \$40, and at this level the physician will be willing to supply 210 office visits. An increase in the fee to \$100 will result in a supply of 500 visits. According to this analysis, a fee increase will increase the quantity of procedures and a fee reduction will reduce the quantity. We should note that this discussion is restricted to the issue of supply. The number of services actually provided will depend on the quantity of services *demanded*.

There are some other qualifications that should be kept in mind. The first is the appropriateness of this analysis for dealing with labor supply issues. After all, the physician's labor is a key factor in the supply of physician visits. Individual physicians have limitations on their work time, and the supply model needs to be modified to take this into account.

At lower income and wage levels, the propensity to substitute leisure for work may be strong enough to more than offset the income effect. An upward-sloping supply curve would result. However, at higher wage levels, the income effect may more than offset the substitution effect, and a backward-bending supply curve would result. Recall, the income effect reflects the change in the described hours of work resulting from a change in income when the wage is held constant. The substitution effect reflects the change in desired hours of work resulting from a change in the wage rate, holding income constant. Leisure is a normal good and so higher income implies a desire for more leisure and fewer hours of work (income effect), but a higher wage raises the relative price of leisure, implying a desire for more hours of work (substitution effect). The net effect will depend upon which of the two effects is stronger.

In Figure 7-1, the supply curve of S_2 begins to bend back just beyond 200 office visits. Up to the fee of \$40, the physician behaves as in curve S_1.

If the fee rises above $40 per visit, the physician's supply will increase in smaller amounts and eventually begin to decrease. If this is the way physicians behave, then raising fees above the maximum point will cause physicians to cut back on the number of services they are willing to provide. An increase in primary care fees, then, may not necessarily cause an increase in the quantity of primary care supplied. However, there is little evidence to support the notion of a backward sloping supply curve of labor.

7.4 HOSPITAL PAYMENT

7.4.1 Alternative Bases of Payment

Until the early 1980s, hospitals were paid on a retrospective basis. That is, a third-party insurer would pay a hospital for the expenses it had already incurred (if payment was on a cost basis) or the charges it had already billed (if payment was on a charge basis). There are numerous variations of retrospective payment. The third party can pay on a cost-plus basis, which means it can pay the hospital for its allowable operating costs plus a specified amount (say, 2% of costs) for capital equipment. In another method of payment, the third party pays the hospital whichever is lower, costs or charges. There is also considerable variation in how costs are defined. Allowable costs could exclude costs not directly related to patient care (e.g., teaching costs). Whatever the arrangement, retrospective payment has one overriding effect on supply and on costs: it encourages an organization to expand. Increases in both the scope and quality of services tend to occur, and if the provider is a maximizer of anything (e.g., profits or perquisites), retrospective payment can lead to higher costs, more services, and higher quality services.

In response to this recognized bias in retrospective payment, a number of prospective payment plans have been introduced. Prospective payment involves setting the basis of payment before the payment period. As a result, this sort of payment scheme puts the provider "at risk" for any excess of cost over revenue. There are many different bases for setting the rate of prospective payments and an infinite number of rate levels. We will examine several of the alternatives and their hypothesized effects on cost and quantity.

To help classify the effects of different types of payment, we will use the following formula to break out the components of total cost:

Total Cost = Cost per service × Services per Day × Days of Stay per Admission × Number of Admissions. Let us now explore the likely effect of three types of prospective payment—per service, per diem (per day), and per admission—on an output-maximizing hospital.

In per-service payment, the hospital will receive a fixed amount for each service performed (e.g., an operation, a radiograph, or kidney dialysis). The amount for each service is set in advance (e.g., $45 for a specific lab test, $300 for a complete CT scan, etc.). The second method of payment is per diem payment. Under this method, an amount is arrived at by multiplying the per diem cost for the particular service by the number of days of care provided. The third prospective payment method, per-admission payment, rewards the hospital only for adding more patients. Under the per-admission method, payers usually adjust the payment by a case mix or severity index because cases differ considerably by diagnosis and severity. For a discussion of a diagnosis-adjusted per-admission payment system, see the section entitled "Diagnosis-Related Groups." Even cases within a diagnosis group may differ from one another; in such circumstances, the per-admission and per diem bases of payment may be combined. This will be discussed next.

7.4.2 Agency Theory and Hospital Payment

We can use the agency framework to analyze the effects of the different hospital payment systems. As usual, the key issues include uncertainty, information asymmetry, and monitoring and other transactions costs.

7.4.2.1 Retrospective Payments

Retrospective payment is the funding of costs that were actually incurred. Under retrospective funding, the payer incurs all of the financial risks. The provider has an incentive to increase the quality and volume of services, as it will be paid for these; it bears no financial risks. In order to protect itself financially, the payer must incur expenses to set standards and monitor and enforce them. These contracting costs can be quite high because of the technical nature of medical care, including the wide variety of diagnoses and treatments; the complexity of the product leads to information asymmetries such that the provider may have considerably more technical and detailed knowledge of the patient than does the payer.

7.4.2.2 Prospective Fee-for-Service System

Prospective payment means the setting of the rate in advance of the service. Fee-for-service means that a fee for each service is set before the services are provided. Under this type of payment, almost all of the financial risk is imposed on the payer. This is because all services provided by the hospital will be paid for by the payer. As long as the per-service rate exceeds the hospital's marginal cost, the provider will have an incentive to add additional services. The payer would have to set standards and monitor and enforce them, thus incurring costs. The detailed knowledge possessed by the providers would create considerable information asymmetries. Information asymmetries would add considerably to the costs incurred by the payers.

7.4.2.3 Per Diem Fees

Under a flat per diem fee, there will be a sharing of financial risks between the payer and the hospital. The longer the hospital keeps the patient, the more it will be paid. Because the latter part of most hospital stays is less costly than the earlier portion, the per diem rates are likely to exceed the marginal costs of the latter part of a stay.

The actual rates paid in relation to cost will be very important incentives. The per diem cost of a case depends on the diagnosis. For example, a liver transplant case will have daily costs that are well above the average. A hospital that performs transplants could lose money on such operations. The provider would require a risk premium if a flat per diem payment system were implemented because the hospital might demand compensation if it treats high-cost cases. In addition, the payer would incur the cost of monitoring the stays. The hospital will have considerable leeway in extending stays; because the hospital has considerably more information on the patients and their conditions than the payers, information asymmetries will arise. One factor that must be kept in mind is that it is the physician who controls admission to and discharge from the hospital, not the hospital administrators. Although hospitals can influence physicians, they do not control the final decisions. The payer would have to develop standards, write contracts, monitor these, and enforce them. These costs could be substantial.

7.4.2.4 Per Case Payment

Because of the wide range of diagnoses and treatments, all per-case payment systems make use of case-mix groups. Each group contains cases that use roughly the same amount of resources, and payers pay the hospitals the same sum of money for all cases within each group. Under such a system, the risk to the payer is reduced considerably. However, there is still a wide range of costs within each diagnosis group; sometimes, the within-group variation in resource use is said to be due to "severity." Hospitals that attract higher severity cases, either because they are referral centers or inner city hospitals, may lose money due to the higher costs. They may, therefore, refuse to accept such cases without some kind of severity adjustment. In addition to these additional costs, a case-mix system contains considerable informational asymmetries. The providing hospitals have considerable discretion in assigning patients to diagnosis groups. In order to counteract this tendency, the payer will have to develop an adequate reporting system and ensure that it is being followed. The development and maintenance of such a system will impose considerable costs on the payer.

7.4.2.5 Per Case Payment with Adjustment for Outliers

In order to reduce the costs imposed on providers who accept more severe cases under a flat per-case payment system, payers have developed a two-part system. Cases within each diagnosis group are divided into two groups, typical cases and outliers. Using the distribution of stays within each diagnosis group, a trim point is established that separates long-stay outliers from typical cases. The actual setting of the trim point is arbitrary and depends on how much pressure the payer wants to impose on the provider to reduce its stays. Outliers are paid in two parts: a per-case portion to cover those days inside of the trim and an additional per diem payment to cover the additional days. Thus, the risk of very high cost cases due to very long stays will be borne, in a large part, by the payer. Such a system has been adopted by the Medicare payment system.

7.4.3 Other Hospital Payment Issues

When evaluating types of hospital payment, several things have to be kept in mind. First, one must distinguish between an all-payer system and a multipayer system. In an all-payer system, each payer pays the same rate. For example, assume that Medicare, Blue Cross, and commercial insurers each have one-third of the overall caseload of 300 cases in a hospital, and that the case mixes and severities of the patient groups are identical (so there is no objective basis for differential payments). Assume further that the regulatory authority in the state has determined that the hospital's allowable revenues should be $900,000. This means that each insurer "should" pay $300,000, and this is what it would pay in an all-payer system.

A multipayer system is more like a free-for-all, with each payer setting up its payment rules unilaterally or based on market principles. Let us say that, in the preceding example, the regulatory agency regulates only Medicare and Blue Cross rates and that it allows each to pay $270,000. The commercial group rates are unregulated. In this instance, the hospital must charge the commercials more to cover its deficit. Whether or not it collects all its bills is another issue. What is significant here is that the hospital is no longer a price taker, and so a more complex model that can incorporate the reaction by the hospital to the regulated rate is needed. A second important fact to keep in mind is that other parts of the healthcare system may be affected by the payment type and level. For example, if a system penalizes a hospital for keeping patients hospitalized for more than a specified time, this will most certainly reduce length of stay. It may have other effects as well. For instance, if home health care or long-term care facility care is paid separately, the hospital may open up a long-term care facility or begin a home healthcare program to which it could discharge its patients. A considerable number of experiments with prospective payment have been conducted at the state level (Bauer, 1977; Carter, Jacobson, Kominski, & Perry, 1994; Simoens & Giuffrida, 2004). Most of these have occurred in multipayer systems, and so their effects are harder to identify than they would be in an all-payer system. One such experiment, conducted by the New York State legislature, set rates on a per diem basis for Medicare- and Blue Cross-paid patients according to a preestablished formula beginning in 1970. This had the effect of rewarding hospitals for longer stays. In testing for the effect of this type of payment, a comparison was made between length of stay and occupancy rates after 1970 in New York State and those in several comparison states, where prospective per diem rates were not in force (Ohio and the New England states). Between 1970 and 1974, New York showed a slight increase in the average length of stay and no net change in the occupancy rate (i.e., the average percentage of beds filled). Both of these indicators of hospital supply decreased considerably in the control states during the same period of time. This suggests that the payment mechanism had its expected effect (Berry, 1976).

7.5 DIAGNOSIS-RELATED GROUPS

In 1983, the federal government introduced a new prospective payment system (PPS) for Medicare hospital patients. In this system, payment for all Medicare discharges is on a per-diagnosis basis. Here we review how diagnoses are grouped into separate DRGs and how rates are set for each DRG.

The DRG system is one of many possible ways of classifying patients according to common elements (Hornbrook, 1982). There is the presumption that, if the classification system is to be used for payment purposes, all cases in each group must be similar with regard to resource use. Based on several patient characteristics (the major diagnostic group, the presence of comorbid diagnoses, the presence of a surgical procedure, and discharge status), an algorithm was developed to assign individual cases to groupings that exhibit common resource-use tendencies (as measured by length of stay) (Fetter, Youngsoo, Freeman, Averill, & Thompson 1980). In 2007, the DRG system was substantially revised, and the newly resequenced DRGs are now known as MS-DRGs (Medicare Severity-Diagnosis Related Groups), and the numbering goes through 999, although gaps have been left throughout the sequence of numbers to allow for modifications and new MS-DRGs in the same body system to be located more closely in the numerical sequence. One additional modification in 2008 involved hospital-acquired conditions; these conditions are no longer considered to be complications if they were not present on admission, which will result in reduced payment from Medicare for conditions apparently caused by the hospital. Figure 7-2 provides the logic used in the development of Medicare Severity-Diagnosis Related Groups. In the MS-DRG system, there were a total of 746 DRGs in 2011, up from the earlier 538; and a total of 2,583 complications and comorbidities identified, down from 3,326 under the old DRG system. Under the new system, the age 0–17 category has been dropped. There are now three levels of severity: MCC—Major Complication/Comorbidity, which reflect the highest level of severity; CC—Complication/Comorbidity, which is the next level of severity; and Non-CC—Non-Complication/Comorbidity, which do not significantly affect severity of illness and resource use.

MS-DRGs were developed based on the major diagnostic groups the disorders fell into and on such factors as the need for surgery and the presence of complicating diagnoses. The criteria were selected so that cases in each category would use similar amounts of resources and thus could be paid with a single rate. There were 538 categories in the 2006 DRG classification system and 725 in the 2007 MS-DRG system.

Based on cross-hospital studies, an average cost for each DRG was estimated. Factors in the calculation included the lengths of stay (within the DRG) in routine and special care, per diem costs in routine and special care, and the estimated per-case cost of ancillary services (laboratory, radiology, drugs, medical supplies, anesthesia, and other services) (Pettengill & Vertrees, 1982). Each DRG was then assigned a relative weight intended to approximate the relative amount of resources used by an average case in the group. For example, a cardiac arrest unexplained with MCC (DRG 296) had an assigned weight of 1.665, and a coronary bypass with PTCA without MCC (DRG 232) had an assigned weight of 5.5589. This means that, in comparison to an "average" diagnostic group (with a weight set equal to 1), a typical case of DRG 296 uses 1.1665 times the amount of resources, and a case of DRG 232 uses 5.5589 times the amount.

Using these weights and the frequency of types of cases, a hospital can develop a case-mix-adjusted admissions measure. This measure would presumably be a better approximation of the resources required to serve the hospital's patient population than mere admissions or patient days (which have traditionally been used).

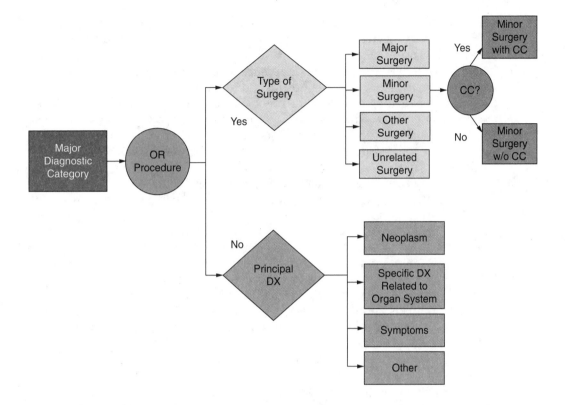

Figure 7-2   Logic Used in Determination of MS-DRGs. Once a major diagnostic category has been determined, then the first branch involves the performance of an operation procedure. If surgery was performed, then the type of surgery is determined. If no surgery, then the principle diagnosis is determined. For either surgery or no surgery, if applicable, then whether or not a complication or co-morbid condition occurred is determined.

For example, let us say that both Aiken and Bethesda General Hospitals treated 200 patients in 2010, with an average length of stay of six days. Both would have a measured output of 1,200 patient days. Let us say, however, that of Aiken's 200 cases, half were heart failure and shock without CC/MCC (MS-DRG 293, with a weight equal to 0.6940) and half were heart failure and shock with MCC (MS-DRG 291, with a weight equal to 1.4609). Then Aiken's case-mix-adjusted measure of admissions would be equal to 215.49 [(0.6940 × 100) + (1.4609 × 100)]. Bethesda's case mix included 100 cases of coronary bypass with PTCA with MCC (MS-DRG 231, with a weight equal to 7.6784) and 100 cases of coronary bypass without cardiac cath without MCC (MS-DRG 236, with a weight equal to 3.6128). Bethesda's adjusted output would be equal to 1,129.12 [(7.6784 × 100) + (3.6128 × 100)].

With the hospital's output being measured in terms of case-weighted admissions, a payment rate (called a standardized payment amount) must be set for each single point (relative weight = 1.00). Originally, this rate had national-, regional-, and hospital-specific components. Currently, the standardized amount includes a labor-related share and a nonlabor-related share. The labor-related share is adjusted by a wage index to reflect area differences in the cost of labor. The wage-adjusted standardized amount is multiplied by a relative weight for the DRG. If applicable, additional amounts are added to teaching medical residents, for hospitals that treat a disproportionate share of low-income patients, for cases that involve certain approved new technologies, and for high cost outlier cases. In FY 2011, the national operating base rate was $5,164.11, and the capital base rate (designed to cover costs for depreciation, interest, rent, and property-related insurance and taxes) was $420.01.

If the hospital was a teaching hospital, it would be entitled to an "indirect" teaching adjustment to pay for additional services (lab tests, radiographs, etc.) consumed in the process of teaching interns and residents. This additional amount is based on the hospital's intern-resident per-bed ratio (Lave, 1984). The indirect teaching adjustment equals a 5.5% increase in the basic rate for each 0.1 interns and residents per bed. A large teaching hospital with a ratio of 0.4 residents per bed would have a 22% increase added to its basic rate. In 2011, this hospital would receive $6,300 per point (1.22 × 5164.11). As an example, let us say that a typical teaching hospital, Denver City Hospital, with 200 beds and 0.4 residents per bed, had 24,000 admissions last year, one-quarter of which were Medicare patients. Assume further that one-half (3,000) of the Medicare cases fell into MS-DRG 114 (orbital procedure without CCI MCC, with a weight equal to 1.1843) and one-half into DRG 124 (other disorders of the eye with MCC, with a weight equal to 1.1843). The hospital would be paid at a rate of $6,300 per point (after the adjustment for its intern-resident population). Denver's receipts for its 6,000 Medicare patients would be about $39.1 million (3,000 cases with a weight equal to 0.8825 and 3,000 cases with a weight equal to 1.1843). The hospital would also receive capital payment of $420.01 per point.

Medicare also pays the hospitals for certain additional costs that fall outside of the basic case-mix formula: outlier-related costs, disproportionate share of low-income patients, and cases involving certain new technology.

Table 7-1:   Relative Weights for Selected MS-DRGs, 2011

MS-DRG	MDC	Type	MS-DRG TITLE (Description)	Relative Weight
332	06	Surg	Rectal Resection W MCC	4.8691
333	06	Surg	Rectal Resection W CC	2.4758
334	06	Surg	Rectal Resection W/O CC/MCC	1.6038
374	06	Med	Digestive Malignancy W MCC	2.0951
375	06	Med	Digestive Malignancy W CC	1.2851
376	06	Med	Digestive Malignancy W/O CC/MCC	0.8715

Source: Derived from information on CMS website. Accessed February 2, 2012 from https://www.cms.gov/acuteinpatientpps/downloads/FY_2011_FR_Table_5.zip.

An *outlier* is a case whose cost is sufficiently high that it falls outside certain predetermined limits. Originally, there were two kinds of outliers: day and cost outliers. A day outlier for a specific DRG was a case whose length of stay exceeded a preset number of days (e.g., 24 days); all days in excess of this trim point were called *outlying days*. For example, if the trim point for DRG 103 is 24 and a case has a stay of 32 days, then 8 of these days will be deemed outlying days. In 1997, Medicare stopped paying for long-stay outliers and provided extra funding only on the basis of high-cost cases. A high-cost outlier is one whose adjusted charges exceed the fixed loss threshold ($23,075 in FY 2011), and hospitals are paid 80% of costs above the fixed cost threshold. Outlier rules were developed to pay hospitals for cases that used an unusually high amount of resources. Rates for paying hospitals for outlying portions of cases are set by Congress. Outlier payments cover about 5.1% of total per-case payment, and their importance will vary depending on the degree of complexity of the hospital's cases.

7.6 LONG-TERM CARE FACILITY PAYMENT

Because there is such wide variability in long-term care facility lengths of stay, it is not feasible to pay long-term care facilities on a per-case basis. They are therefore funded on a per diem basis. Medicaid state agencies, being the largest third-party payers of long-term care facilities, have traditionally paid long-term care facilities in two different ways: with a flat per diem (per day) rate or with a facility-specific per diem rate. Facility-specific rates are largely retrospective and consequently result in high costs. In flat-rate payment, a single rate is paid to all long-term care facilities, regardless of patient characteristics, quality levels, and so on. Often, a separate rate will be paid by level of facility—SNF or ICF. One virtue of the flat rate is that, at least in the case of investor-owned long-term care facilities, the facilities have an incentive to minimize costs. This may lead to some problems, however. Long-term care facilities might seek to attract patients who are healthier or who need less care (and hence cost less to treat), or they might compromise on quality (which would also lower costs and increase profits). As long as long-term care facilities seek profits to some degree (they might also have other objectives), they will tend to lower costs when such a payment mechanism is in place. It is primarily to balance the incentive to select patients with fewer needs that case-mix measures have been introduced (Schlenker, 1986). The primary purpose of case-mix payment in long-term care is to relate payment rates to required levels of care and help ensure that patients receive appropriate care.

One case-mix measure that has been developed is called *Resource Utilization Groups* (RUGs) (Fries & Cooney, 1985). This measure has now been superseded by RUGs II (Micheletti & Shlala, 1986), RUGs III (Fries, Schneider, Foley, Gavazzi, Burke, & Gornelius, 1994), and RUGs IV (Urban Institute, 2007). The RUGs case-mix measure is based on a set of hierarchical groups related to levels and types of services (rehabilitation, extensive services, special care, clinically complex cases, impaired cognition, behavioral problems, and reduced physical functioning) and, within these hierarchical groups, scores on the activities of daily living (ADL) scale. The ADL scale assigns numerical scores according to the degree of physical functioning an individual can attain in each of six categories: bathing, dressing, toileting, feeding, transferring between locations, and continence (Katz, Ford, Moskowitz, Jackson, & Jaffe, 1963). RUGs III used four of these categories: eating, transferring, bed mobility, and toileting. Based on the points assigned to each of these, in combination with the hierarchical groups, the patient was assigned to 1 of 44 RUGs III categories. The RUGs IV system contains 53 categories. The categories are assigned weights according to their relative costs (see, e.g., Schlenker, Shaughnessy, & Yslas, 1985), and payment is made in accordance with these relative weights.

Such a system overcomes the first disadvantage mentioned: that case-mix selection creates a bias in favor of light-care patients. Indeed, if the weights of each category are in line with the relative costs of treating patients, then the selection bias should be removed. This does not mean that other selection biases do not exist. Indeed, three other types of biases that result from a RUGs type of payment system have been identified (Butler & Schlenker, 1989). The first of these is a bias against patient rehabilitation. If a patient improves, he or she moves into another payment category and the long-term care facility loses revenue. Particularly, if the case-mix-payment system is oriented toward patient condition rather than services, the long-term care facility will incur higher costs by rehabilitating patients. An incentive not to rehabilitate would therefore be present (Smits, 1984). To counteract this, a payment program might pay long-term care facilities on the basis of outcomes or pay at the higher payment level for a limited period even when the patient improves. A second bias in such a system involves the provision of unnecessary care. If the payment system pays more for certain services (e.g., rehabilitation), then this might give the long-term care facility an incentive to provide such services, sometimes unnecessarily. As for the third bias, the long-term care facility has a motive to misreport patient status thus acquiring a higher payment rate.

The best way to eliminate these biases may be to adopt regulations and institute a monitoring system. New York State, which adopted the RUGs II system, had a regulatory system to monitor the quality of care in long-term care facilities (Micheletti & Shlala, 1986). Such a monitoring system was developed because the payment system was not sufficient to achieve all of the public policy goals of the long-term care facility system.

RUGs IV was implemented in 2009, with the design such that the overall payment would be the same as under RUGs III. However, the distribution of the overall payment does change, with the payments for complex medical groups increasing substantially. There are now 66 RUGs, compared to 53 used by RUGs III. The RUGs system uses the Minimum Data Set (MDS) to calculate the group to which the resident is assigned.

The MDS is a standardized clinical assessment tool for facilitating care management in nursing homes because the assessment involves a comprehensive evaluation of the functional capabilities of the resident and enables staff to identify health problems. All residents in Medicare- or Medicaid-certified homes are assessed regardless of payment source of the individual. The MDS 3.0 contains 15 categories, designed to capture the physical and mental functioning capacity of residents and the rehabilitation and restorative services needed by the residents.

7.7 HEALTH MAINTENANCE ORGANIZATIONS

The major characteristics of an HMO from a supply standpoint are that it is simultaneously responsible for two types of services: health insurance and health care. Health insurance coverage is sold to customers on a per capita basis. The medical care itself is provided, or contracted for, by the HMO directly. The HMO assumes all the financial risk for providing this care. At the same time, its physicians act as gatekeepers and therefore have some degree of control over the patients' utilization of care. In discussing the supply incentives inherent in such an organization, we must recognize that an HMO can make a number of different types of arrangements with the physicians with which it contracts and the hospitals to which it sends its patients. The arrangement made impacts the relative risk of the HMO and the provider.

The per capita funding formula provides an incentive for any investor-owned HMO to minimize costs (all other factors being held constant). An HMO can reduce its costs by lowering the use of services by existing patients, encouraging the enrollment of members who are at low risk and disenrolling high-risk patients. Lower cost enrollees would include younger members, non-smokers, individuals who exercise, and so on. In order to encourage healthy enrollees to select it, the HMO can design a product with this end in mind. It might, for example, have more pediatricians and fewer gerontologists on staff, specialize in sports medicine, and open more branches in the suburbs and few or no branches in the inner city (Enthoven, 1988; Hellinger, 1995; Luft, 1986). Indeed, the likelihood of an HMO encouraging self-selection and thus having an enrollee mix that does not reflect the demographics of the general population has resulted in the development of adjustment formulas to compensate for potential differences in enrollee risk and the cost of utilization (Anderson, Steinberg, Holloway, & Canton, 1986). These formulas are used to calculate higher payment rates for higher risk individuals, thus inducing HMOs to enroll these individuals.

One such adjustment formula, Medicare's former average adjusted per capita cost (AAPCC) formula, was used to determine the rates at which Medicare pays HMOs. The rates are based on Medicare's own current payment rates for hospital and physician services in the fee-for-service system. AAPCCs were calculated for separate groups of patients (factors used in constructing the groups included gender, age bracket, county, welfare status, and institution-alization). For example, the monthly AAPCC for noninstitutionalized females aged 70–74 who were not on welfare in Washington County, Oregon, was $62 for hospital services and $30 for medical services. The Medicare rate to be paid to the HMOs for these individuals was 95% of the AAPCC of $92. The rationale behind this payment rate was that, for those individuals who did shift from fee-for-service coverage to HMO coverage, Medicare would save 5% of its average cost. The HMO would benefit if it could provide coverage at a cost lower than this.

One criticism of this payment system was that it did not pinpoint risk categories accurately enough and that HMO cream skimming was a distinct possibility, even with the AAPCC adjustments. For example, the AAPCC did not take into account the amount of prior health services used, which is a good indicator of future utilization of services. If an HMO could use this information to supply a product with characteristics that appeal to low-risk individuals, then it could obtain a large share of low-cost users, even allowing for AAPCC adjustments. The result could be costly to Medicare, whose 95% rule was designed to achieve savings for the program.

Assume that there are 100 individuals in Washington County who are enrolled in Medicare and who have the characteristics specified previously (70–74 years old, female, noninstitutionalized, nonwelfare). If they were in the fee-for-service program, Medicare would pay, on average, $92.00 a month for each. For each such individual attracted by an HMO, the HMO will receive 95% of the AAPCC, or $87.40 monthly. If the HMO is successful, through careful design of product characteristics, in drawing 10 very healthy, low-risk females from this group of 100, its average costs for these members will likely be below the $87.40 rate. The total cost to Medicare will be $87.40 times 10. The fee-for-service sector will now be left with a higher cost pool, having lost 10 lower-than-average-cost members, and its costs will rise. It is thus possible that this payment scheme could end up costing Medicare more money.

A second problem with this system was that it created a wide regional variation in rates. Medicare paid low rates for residents who lived in counties where costs were low, and HMOs would not offer services in counties with low AAPCC rates.

In order to address these problems, Medicare instituted a new risk-premium-setting mechanism in 2000. This system was called "Medicare + Choice" and was instituted under a new Part C of Medicare. The risk-adjustment factors included prior hospitalization and demographic factors. The demographic factors included age, gender, disability status, Medicaid eligibility, and institutional status. As an example, an HMO that newly enrolled a male aged 66 would receive a payment of $2,921 annually. If the person was also Medicaid eligible, the HMO would receive an additional $3,297.

If the individual had been hospitalized in the previous year, and if his or her diagnosis fell into a serious category, the HMO would receive an additional payment to cover a higher risk status. There are 15 illness categories that are based on reason for hospitalization. The new categorization system is called Principal Inpatient-Diagnostic Cost Group (PIP-DCG). As an example, PIP-DCG 8 is asthma, and if a person has been hospitalized for asthma, Medicare will add an additional $4,192 annually onto its rate (Health Care Financing Administration, 1999).

In developing a single rate, Congress hopes that HMOs will increase supply in areas currently underserved because of low rates. The new system seems to address risk factors better, but it may overserve low-cost areas and underserve areas where costs are high.

7.8 PROVIDER SUPPLY UNDER MANAGED CARE

7.8.1 Agency Theory and Incentive Contracts

The quantity and quality of services that an HMO supplies to its members are determined, to a large extent, by the healthcare providers with whom the

HMO contracts. The HMO is reliant on these providers to assess the HMO members' conditions and to provide appropriate levels of care. The manner in which the HMO compensates these providers will affect their supply behavior.

The HMO management does not usually know its members' health status or what treatments are appropriate. The providers have the best information about these matters, and so there is an "information asymmetry" between the two groups. Consequently, it is possible for the providers to act strictly in their own interest. In order to encourage the providers to act in the interest of the HMO, the HMO management can design a compensation scheme for the providers. Agency models can be used to analyze such compensation schemes. The two contracting bodies in such models are the *principals* (HMOs) and their *agents* (providers). We will set out a model in this section to examine how alternative compensation schemes influence the supply behavior of providers.

The principal, or HMO, contracts with its members (on a per capita payment basis) to provide them with care.

- *HMO objectives.* We assume that the HMO's objectives are to maximize profits. However, we also assume that there is a minimum profit level that is acceptable to the HMO; in our example, this will be $1 million. Profits are equal to total revenue minus total cost.

- *HMO revenues.* The HMO's revenues depend on the capitation rate applied to its members and the number of members who join the HMO. In our model, we will hold the capitation rate constant.

- *HMO costs.* The HMO's costs include those that are incurred in treating the HMO members who become patients.

- *HMO-provider interaction.* In many respects, the HMO is dependent on its agents, the providers of care (physicians, physical therapists, hospitals, etc.), for the achievement of its profit targets. Providers can influence HMO profits by varying their levels of effort. If providers function at very low effort levels, patients will be dissatisfied with the heath care they receive and will switch to other health plans. As a result, HMO profits will be low. As physician efforts increase, quality of care will improve and more members will join. However, additional physician effort means more lab tests, more procedures, and so on. Although this will bring in more members to the HMO, it will also increase costs. Eventually, the additional effort will work against profitability, and profits will fall. Graph A of Figure 7-3 shows the relationship between the HMO's profits and the effort of the agents. At some effort level (E_3), profits will be at a maximum level. At other effort levels (E_1 and E_4), profits will be at minimally acceptable levels. HMO profits, then, are directly tied to the efforts of its contracting physicians. The physicians know how much effort they are providing and how much is required to treat their patients. The HMO cannot directly observe this effort. This is another way of saying that there is an information asymmetry between the principal and its agents. Although the HMO cannot directly observe physician efforts, it can observe its profits. This performance indicator will come in useful when the HMO sets compensation policies for the physicians.

- *Physician objectives.* We turn now to the assumptions about the behavior of the physicians. The objective of each physician is to maximize net income (profits), which is equal to revenues from the HMO minus the personal costs of supplying care (or exerting effort). With a rising marginal cost curve for effort, the maximization point (which indicates

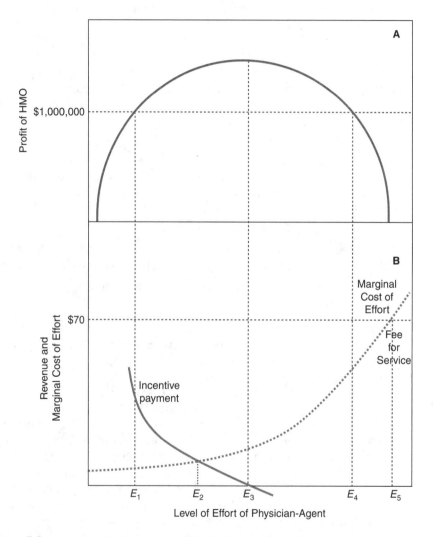

Figure 7-3 Optimal Compensation of Healthcare Providers by an HMO. Graph A, the top diagram, shows the relationship between the providers' average effort and the HMO's profit. The minimum acceptable profit level for the HMO is $1,000,000. Graph B indicates each provider's level of effort under alternative payment schemes. The MC of additional effort is the same under all payment schemes. Under a straight salary payment scheme, the provider will supply the minimum level of effort acceptable to the HMO, E_1. Under a fee-for-service system, at the assumed wage of $70, the provider will supply up to E_5, but only E_4 is acceptable. Under a profit incentive arrangement, E_2 will be provided. This is slightly less than the HMO's maximum profit, because the incentive system is not "perfect."

what level of effort will be chosen by the physician) occurs where the marginal revenue (MR) equals the marginal cost (MC) for the physician.

- *Physician costs.* We will assume that all provider revenues come from the HMO (i.e., that each provider has no additional source of revenue). The relationship between alternative payment schemes that the HMO can institute and physician revenues will be discussed later. The physician costs in this model are the opportunity costs to the physician of engaging in productive practices. The physician places a value on his or her time, and this value is based on alternative uses of the time spent on care. We assume that the marginal cost to the physician of time spent on patient care increases as more time is spent. Put another way, as more time is taken away from leisure activities, the value of the last unit of time increases. This rising marginal cost curve of effort is shown in graph B of Figure 7-3.

- *Physician revenues.* The proposition being established in this section is that the level of effort selected by the physician will be influenced by the basis and level of payment. We will now examine three alternative forms of compensation: salary, fee-for-service payment, and incentive compensation based on the HMO's profits.

If the physician is paid a straight salary, any additional effort by the physician results in costs but yields no extra revenue. There is a minimum acceptable level of effort that the physician must put in—the level that corresponds to the minimum profit target of the HMO (level E_1). The physician will provide this level but no more. We will now assume the physician is paid a fee of $70 per service. Extra effort on the part of the physician will result in extra services provided. These extra services result in marginal revenues of $70 per service (see the straight line at $70 in Figure 7-3). The physician would maximize net income at a level of effort of E5. However, because the HMO's profits are below those that are acceptable to the HMO, the physician will reduce his or her effort level to E_4. If the fee falls below $70, then the physician will choose an effort level below E_5. If the fee level increases, then the effort level will also increase. It is quite possible therefore to have a low effort level under fee-for-service payment if the fee levels are low enough.

The HMO can set a contract that provides specific incentives. Recall that the HMO does not know how much effort is provided by the physician. The HMO only has a proxy for this, mainly HMO performance (in this case, HMO profits). The HMO can pay the physician a fixed percentage of HMO profits. The MR curve for the physician will appear like that in any demand situation—it will decline to a level of zero as profits increase to their maximum. Beyond this point, the MR to the physician will be negative because HMO profits are falling. However, in these circumstances, the physician will not choose the level of effort that corresponds to maximum HMO profits but will choose instead level E_2, where the MR and marginal cost curves intersect. This will provide the HMO with lower than maximum profits but more profits than under a salary compensation scheme. There are numerous other compensation schemes that can be selected, some of which are more complicated, but may motivate the physician to supply an effort close to the optimal level from the point of view of the HMO.

7.8.2 Management of Provider Behavior

In addition to setting contracts, insurers can engage in the direct management of provider supply behavior with the objective of influencing utilization patterns. The direct management of providers is an activity that is most closely associated with HMOs because of their close association with physicians. However, in recent years, the management of care has become widespread under all types of payment arrangements. Most of these practices have been focused on the use of inpatient care, primarily because of the expense of this mode of care.

There are a number of different measures that insurers can use to influence providers' supply of hospital care (Scheffler, Sullivan, & Ko, 1991). They include overall case management, preadmission management (e.g., second opinions and preadmission testing), concurrent management (e.g., concurrent review and discharge planning), and posthospital review (e.g., retrospective review and claims denials). Figure 7-4 indicates where the measures are applied. Each measure involves the setting of standards and the review of patients in accordance with these standards.

Many of the regulations set by HMOs carry financial penalties, such as nonpayment for a claim. For example, if a second opinion is required for surgery, payment might be denied if the surgeon operated without a confirming opinion. Probably for this reason, the private regulation of providers has been quite successful in containing utilization and costs. One study indicated savings of about 7% overall (Feldstein, Wickizer, & Wheeler, 1988; Wickizer, Wheeler, & Feldstein., 1989), although the savings will depend on the type of program and types of penalties imposed (Scheffler, Sullivan, & Ko, 1991).

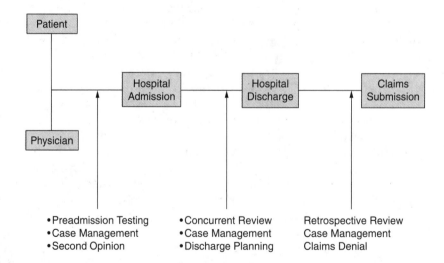

Figure 7-4 Techniques for Managing Provider Behavior. Provider behavior can be regulated before, during, or after hospital admission, or with a combination of these three time periods. Prior to hospitalization, insurers can require providers to seek permission (pre-authorization); during hospitalization, insurers can monitor length of stay or use of procedures (concurrent review); and following hospitalization, insurers can conduct reviews and deny claims (retrospective review).

EXERCISES

1. Which costs are incurred by insurers when there is information asymmetry between payer/insurer and provider?
2. What are four different methods for reimbursing physicians?
3. How will each of these methods of paying physicians influence the volume of services supplied?
4. What "perverse" incentives must an insurer guard against in fee-for-service and per capita funding?
5. What is the Resource-Based Relative Value System, and how were fees set in order to influence the volume of surgical and medical services?
6. What is retrospective hospital payment, and what incentives are created by this type of payment?
7. What is prospective payment? List three alternative bases of prospective hospital payment.
8. How will each of the following bases for hospital payment affect the number of admissions, the average length of stay, the volume of services per day, and the unit cost of services (cost per service):
   a. Fee-for-service payment
   b. Per diem payment
   c. Fixed-fee per admission
9. Indicate the effect of each of the following hospital payment systems on the relative risks of the insurer and the hospital:
   a. Retrospective payment
   b. Prospective fee-for-service payment
   c. Per diem fees
   d. Per case payment
   e. Per case payment plus outlier adjustments
10. What is the benefit of a diagnosis-related grouping system over a flat per diem payment system?
11. If DRG001 (craniotomy) had a weight of 3.0970, how much would the hospital receive for a craniotomy case if the hospital was a teaching hospital in a large urban area?
12. How can a hospital influence its case mix?
13. What methods can be used to fund a long-term care facility on a prospective basis?
14. What indicators are used to place long-term care facility patients in a RUGs group?
15. If a single rate is set for all HMO members, what basis can the HMO use to recruit less costly members?
16. What criteria can be used to develop groups for HMOs who are paid for by Medicare?
17. What incentives do HMOs have with regard to
    a. Recruiting members
    b. Providing services to its members

BIBLIOGRAPHY

Per Capita Payment

Anderson, G. F., & Knickman, J. (1984). Adverse selection under a voucher system: Grouping Medicare recipients by level of expenditure. *Inquiry, 21,* 135–143.

Anderson, G., Steinberg, E. P., Holloway, J., & Canton, J. C. (1986). Paying for HMO care: Issues and options in setting capitation rates. *Milbank Quarterly, 64,* 548–565.

Anderson, G. F., Steinberg, E. P., Powe, N. R., Antebi, S., Whittle, J., Horn, S., & Herbert, R. (1990). Setting payment rates for capitated systems: A comparison of various alternatives. *Inquiry, 27,* 225–233.

Beebe, J. A. (1992). Outlier pools for Medicare HMO payments. *Health Care Financing Review, 14*(Fall), 59–63.

Chernew, M. E., Mechanic, R. E., Landon, B. E., & Safran, D. G. (2011). Private-payer innovation in Massachusetts: The "alternative quality contract." *Health Affairs, 30* (1), 51–61.

Choi, S., & Davitt, J. K. (2009). Changes in the Medicare home health care market: The impact of reimbursement policy. *Medical Care, 47*(3), 302–309.

Ellwood, P. (1972). Models for organizing health services and implications for legislative proposals. *Milbank Quarterly, 50,* 73–100.

Enthoven, A. (1988). *Theory and practice of managed competition in health care finance.* Amsterdam, The Netherlands: North-Holland.

Giacomini, M., Luft, H. S., & Robinson, J. C. (1995). Risk adjusting community rated health plan premiums. *Annual Review of Public Health, 16,* 401–430.

Goodwin, J. S., Singh, A., Reddy, N., Riall, T. S., & Yong-Fang, K. (2011). Overuse of Screening Colonoscopy in the Medicare Population. *Archives of Internal Medicine 171*(15): 1335–1343.

Hellinger, F. J. (1995). Selection bias in HMOs and PPOs: A review of the evidence. *Inquiry, 32,* 135–142.

Hornbrook, M. C. (1984). Examination of the AAPCC methodology in an HMO prospective payment demonstration experiment. *Group Health Journal, 5*(Spring), 13–21.

Hornbrook, M. C. (1995). Assessing relative health plan risk with the RAND-36 Health Survey. *Inquiry, 32,* 56–74.

Hornbrook, M. C., & Berki, S. E. (1985). Practice mode and payment method. *Medical Care, 23,* 484–511.

Hornbrook, M. C., & Goodman, M. J. (1991). Health plan case mix: Definition, measurement, use. *Advances in Health Economics and Health Services Research, 12,* 111–148.

Klarman, H. E. (1963). The effect of prepaid group practice on hospital use. *Public Health Reports, 78,* 955–965.

Luft, H. S. (1978a). How do health maintenance organizations achieve their "savings?" *New England Journal of Medicine, 298,* 1336–1343.

Luft, H. S. (1978b). Why do HMOs seem to provide more health maintenance services? *Milbank Quarterly, 56,* 140–168.

Luft, H. S. (1981). *Health maintenance organizations.* New York, NY: John Wiley.

Luft, H. S. (1986). Compensating for biased selection in health insurance. *Milbank Quarterly, 64,* 566–591.

Luft, H. S. (1995). Potential methods to reduce risk selection and its effects. *Inquiry, 32,* 23–32.

Manton, K.G., & Stallard, E. (1992). Analysis of underwriting factors for AAPCC. *Health Care Financing Review, 14*(Fall), 117–132.

Miller, H. D. (2009). From volume to value: Better ways to pay for health care. *Health Affairs, 28*(5), 1418–1428.

Newhouse, J. P., Manning, W. G., Keeler, E. B., & Sloss, E. M. (1989). Adjusting capitation rates using objective health measures and prior utilization. *Health Care Financing Review, 10*(Spring), 41–54.

Smith, C. T. (1986). Hospital management strategies for fixed-price payment. *Health Care Management Review, 11*(1), 21–26.

Stafford, R. S., Li, D., Davis, R. B., & Iezzoni, L. I. (2004). Modelling the ability of risk adjusters to reduce adverse selection in managed care. *Applied Health Economics & Health Policy, 3*(2), 107–114.

Swensen, S. J., Kaplan, G. S., Meyer, G. S., Nelson, E. E., Hunt, G. C., Pryor, D. B., … & Chassin, M. R. (2011). Controlling Healthcare Costs by Removing Waste: What American Doctors Can Do Now. *BMJ Quality & Safety 20*(6): 534–537.

Van de Ven, W. P. M. M., van Vliet, R. C. J. A., van Barneveld, E. M., & Lamers, L. M. (1994). Risk adjusted capitation: Recent experiences in the Netherlands. *Health Affairs, 13,* 120–126.

Van Kleef, R. C., & Van Vliet, R. C. (2011). Prior use of durable medical equipment as a risk adjuster for health-based capitation. *Inquiry, 47*(4), 343–358.

Yu, H., & Dick, A. W. (2010). Risk-adjusted capitation rates for children: How useful are the survey-based measures? *Health Services Research, 45*(6, Pt. 2), 1948–1962.

Payment and Supply: Physicians

Aaron, H., & Schwartz, W. B. (1984). *The painful prescription.* Washington, DC: Brookings Institution.

Blomquist, A. (1991). The doctor as double agent: Information asymmetry, health insurance, and medical care. *Journal of Health Economics, 10,* 411–432.

Burney, I. L. Schieber, G. J., Blaxall, M. O., & Gabel, J. R. (1978). Geographic variation in physicians' fees. *JAMA, 240,* 1368–1371.

Carroll, J. (2011). Changing payment methodologies force physicians into larger groups. *Managed Care, 20*(2), 14–16.

Clark, D., & Olsen, J. A. (1994). Agency in health care with an endogenous budget constraint. *Journal of Health Economics, 13,* 231–251.

Cromwell, J., Dayhoff, D. A., & Thoumaian, A. H. (1997). Cost savings and physician responses to global bundled payments for Medicare heart bypass surgery. *Health Care Financing Review, 19*(Fall), 41–57.

Culler, S., & Ehrenfried, D. (1986). On the feasibility and usefulness of physician DRGs. *Inquiry, 23*(1), 40–55.

Eisenberg, J. M., & Williams, S. V. (1981). Cost containment and changing physicians' practice behavior. *JAMA, 246,* 2195–2201.

Epstein, A. M., & Blumenthal, D. (1993). Physician payment reform: Past and future. *Milbank Quarterly, 71,* 193–215.

Feldstein, M. (1970). The rising price of physicians' services. *Review of Economics and Statistics, 52,* 121–133.

Gabel, J. R., & Redisch, M. A. (1979). Alternative physician payment mechanisms. *Milbank Quarterly, 57,* 38–59.

Gruber, J., Kim, J., & Mayzlin, D. (1999). Physician fees and procedure intensity: The case of cesarean delivery. *Journal of Health Economics, 18,* 473–490.

Havighurst, C. C., & Kissam, P. (1979). The antitrust implications of relative value studies in medicine. *Journal of Health Politics, Policy and Law, 4,* 48.

Hemenway, D., Killen, A., Cashman, S. B., Parks, C. L., & Bicknell, W. J. (1990). Physicians' responses to financial incentives. *New England Journal of Medicine, 322,* 1059–1063.

Holahan, J. (1989). The potential effects of an RBRVS-based payment system on health care costs and hospitals. *Frontiers of Health Services Management, 6,* 3–37.

Hornbrook, M. C. (1983). Allocative medicine: Efficiency, disease severity and the payment mechanism. *Annals of the AAPSS, 468,* 12–29.

Hsiao, W. C., & Stason, W. B. (1979). Toward developing a relative value scale for medical and surgical services. *Health Care Financing Review, 1,* 23–39.

Hsiao, W. C., Braun, P., Becker, E. R., & Thomas, S. R. (1987). The resource based relative value scale: Toward the development of an alternative physician payment system. *JAMA, 258,* 799–802.

Hsiao, W. C., Braun, P., Dunn, D., Becker, E. R., DeNicola, M., & Ketcham, T. R. (1988a). Results and policy implications of the resource based relative value study. *New England Journal of Medicine, 319,* 881–888.

Hsiao, W. C., Braun, P., Dunn, D., & Becker, E. R. (1988b). Resource based relative values: An overview. *JAMA, 260,* 2347–2353.

Hsiao, W. C., Braun, P., Yntema, D., & Becker, E. R. (1988c). Estimating physicians' work for a resource based relative value scale. *New England Journal of Medicine, 319,* 835–841.

Levy, J. M., Borowitz, M. J., Jencks, S. F., Kay, T. L., & Williams, D., K. (1990). Impact of the Medicare fee schedule on payments to physicians. *JAMA, 264,* 717–722.

Lowenstein, S. R., Iezzoni, L. I., & Moskowitz, M. A. (1985). Prospective payment for physician services. *JAMA, 254,* 2632–2637.

Lu, M., & Donaldson, C. (2000). Performance-based contracts and provider efficiency. *Disease Management and Health Outcomes, 7,* 127–137.

Ma, A., & McGuire, T. G. (1997). Optimal health insurance and provider payment. *American Economic Review, 87,* 685–704.

Malay, D. S. (2011). Payments for surgical services and the medical inflation rate. *Journal of Foot & Ankle Surgery, 50*(1), 74–76.

Mitchell, J. B. (1985). Physician DRG's. *New England Journal of Medicine, 313,* 670–675.

Monsma, G. (1970). Marginal revenue and the demand for physicians' services. In H. F. Klarman (Ed.), *Empirical studies in health economics.* Baltimore, MD: Johns Hopkins University Press.

Moore, S. (1979). Cost containment through risk sharing of primary-care physicians. *New England Journal of Medicine, 300,* 1359–1362.

Myers, L. P., & Schroeder, S. A. (1981). Physician use of services for the hospitalized patient. *Milbank Quarterly, 59,* 481–507.

Phelps, C. E. (1976). Public sector medicine. In C. M. Lindsay (Ed.), *New directions in public health care.* San Francisco, CA: Institute for Contemporary Studies.

Saultz, J. W., Brown, D., Stenberg, S, Rdesinski, R. E., Tillotson, C. J., Eigner, D., & DeVoe, J. (2010). Access assured: A pilot program to finance primary care for uninsured patients using a monthly enrollment fee. *Journal of the American Board of Family Medicine, 23*(3), 393–401.

Schreiber, G. I., Burney, I. L., Golden, J. B., & Knaus, W. A. (1976). Physician fee patterns under Medicare: A descriptive analysis. *New England Journal of Medicine, 294,* 1089–1093.

Showstack, J. A., Blumberg, B. D., Schwartz, J., & Schroeder, S. A. (1979). Fee-for-service payment: Analysis of current methods and their development. *Inquiry, 16,* 230–246.

Siddel, K. (2011). Is there a standard surgical supply markup? *OR Manager, 27*(3), 24–25.

Simoens, S., & Giuffrida, A. (2004). The impact of physician payment methods on raising the efficiency of the healthcare system: An international comparison. *Applied Health Economics and Health Policy, 3*(1), 39–46.

Sisk, J., McMenamin, P., Ruby, G., & Smith, E. S. (1987). Analysis of methods to reform Medicare payment for physician services. *Inquiry, 24,* 36–47.

Sloan, F. A. (1975). Physician supply behavior in the short run. *Industrial and Labor Relations Review, 28,* 549–569.

Sloan, F. A., & Hay, J. W. (1986). Medicare pricing mechanisms for physician services. *Medical Care Review, 43,* 59–100.

Stano, M., Cromwell, J., Velky, J., & Saad, A. (1983). Fee or use? What's responsible for rising health care costs? *Michigan Medicine, 82,* 228–234.

Wilensky, G. R., & Rossiter, L. F. (1986). Alternative units of payment for physician services. *Medical Care Review, 43,* 133–156.

Yip, W. C. (1998). Physician response to Medicare fee reductions. *Journal of Health Economics, 17,* 679–699.

Payment and Supply: Long-Term Care Facilities

Adams, E. K., & Schlenker, R. E. (1986). Case-mix reimbursement for nursing home services. *Health Care Financing Review, 8*(Fall), 35–45.

Butler, P. A., & Schlenker, R. E. (1989). Case-mix reimbursement for nursing homes. *Milbank Quarterly, 67,* 103–136.

Doty, P., Cohen, M. A., Miller, J., & Shi, X. (2010). Private long-term care insurance: Value to claimants and implications for long-term care financing. *Gerontologist, 50*(5), 613–622.

Fries, B. E., & Cooney, L. M. (1985). Resource utilization groups. *Medical Care, 23,* 110–122.

Fries, B. E., Schneider, D. P., Foley, W. J., Gavazzi, M., Burke, R., & Cornelius, E. (1994). Refining a case mix measure for nursing homes: Resource utilization groups (RUG-III). *Medical Care, 32,* 668–685.

Holahan, J., & Cohen, J. (1987). Nursing home reimbursement. *Milbank Quarterly, 65,* 112–147.

Iwasaki, M., McCurry, S. M., Borson, S., & Jones, J. A. (2010). The future of financing for long-term care: The own your future campaign. *Journal of Aging & Social Policy, 22*(4), 379–93.

Katz, S., Ford, A. B., Moskowitz, R. W., Jackson, B. A., & Jaffe, M. W. (1963). Studies of illness in the aged. *JAMA, 185,* 914–919.

Micheletti, J., & Shlala, T. J. (1986). RUGs II: Implications for management and quality in long-term care. *Quality Review Bulletin, 12,* 236–242.

Miller, E. A., Mor, V., & Clark, M. (2010). Weighing public and private options for reforming long-term care financing: Findings from a national survey of specialists. *Medical Care Research & Review, 67*(4 Suppl.), 16S–37S.

Rosko, M. D., Broyles, R. W., & Aaronson, W. E. (1987). Prospective payment based on case-mix: Will it work in nursing homes? *Journal of Health Politics, Policy and Law, 12,* 683–701.

Schlenker, R. E. (1986). Case-mix reimbursement for nursing homes. *Journal of Health Politics, Policy and Law, 11,* 445–461.

Schlenker, R. E., Shaughnessy, P. W., & Yslas, I. (1985). Estimating patient level nursing home costs. *Health Services Research, 20,* 103–128.

Simon, G. A. (2010). Can long-term care insurance be fixed? *Journal of Health Care Finance, 37*(1), 51–77.

Smits, H. L. (1984). Incentives in case-mix measures for long-term care. *Health Care Financing Review, 6*(Winter), 53–59.

Wiener, J. M. (2010). Long-term care: Getting on the agenda and knowing what to purpose. *Medical Care Research & Review, 67*(4 Suppl.), 126S–140S.

Payment and Supply: Hospitals

Averill, R. F., Vertrees, J. C., McCullough, E. C., Hughes, J. S., & Goldfield, N. I. (2006). Redesigning Medicare inpatient PPS to adjust payment for post-admission complications. *Health Care Financing Review, 27*(3), 83–93.

Bauer, K. (1977). Hospital rate setting—this way to salvation? *Milbank Quarterly, 55,* 117–118.

Berry, R. E. (1976). Prospective reimbursement and cost containment. *Inquiry, 13,* 288–301.

Bradford, W. D., & Craycraft, C. (1996). Prospective payments and hospital efficiency. *Review of Industrial Organization, 11,* 791–809.

Capps, C., Dranove, D., & Lindrooth, R. C. (2010). Hospital closure and economic efficiency. *Journal of Health Economics, 29*(1), 87–109.

Clyde, A. T., Bockstedt, L., Farkas, J. A., & Jackson, C. (2008). Experience with Medicare's new technology add-on payment program. *Health Affairs, 27*(6), 1632–1641.

Dowling, W. L. (1974). Prospective reimbursement of hospitals. *Inquiry, 11,* 163–180.

Dranove, D., & White, W. D. (1987). Agency and the organization of health care delivery. *Inquiry, 24,* 405–415.

Draper, A. (2011). Managing bundled payments. *Healthcare Financial Management, 65*(4), 110–116.

Eby, C. L., & Cohodes, D. R. (1985). What do we know about rate setting. *Journal of Health Politics, Policy and Law, 10,* 299–323.

Feldman, R., & Lobo, F. (19970. Global budgets and excess demand for hospital care. *Health Economics, 6,* 187–196.

Foster, R. W. (1982). Cost-based reimbursement and prospective payment: Reassessing the incentives. *Journal of Health Politics, Policy and Law, 7,* 407–420.

Holmes, G. M., Slifkin, R. T., Randolph, R. K., & Poley, S. (2006). The effect of rural hospital closures on community economic health. *Health Services Research, 41*(2), 467–485.

Horn, S. D., & Sharkey, P. D. (1983). Measuring severity of illness to predict patient resource use within DRGs. *Inquiry, 20,* 314–321.

Hornbrook, M. (1982). Hospital case mix: Its definition, measurement, and use. Parts 1, 2. *Medical Care Review, 39,* 1–43, 73–123.

Ligon, J. A. (1997). The capital structure of hospitals and reimbursement policy. *Quarterly Review of Economics and Business, 37,* 59–77.

Ona, L., & Davis, A. (2011). Economic impact of the critical access hospital program on Kentucky's communities. *Journal of Rural Health, 27*(1), 21–28.

Preyra, C., & Pink, G. (2006). Scale and scope efficiencies through hospital consolidations. *Journal of Health Economics, 25*(6), 1049–1068.

Prince, T. R., & Sullivan, J. A. (2000). Financial viability, medical technology, and hospital closures. *Journal of Health Care Finance, 26*(4), 1–18.

Stensland J., Moscovice, I., & Christianson, J. (2002). Future financial viability of rural hospitals. *Health Care Financing Review, 23*(4), 175–188.

Zuckerman, S., Becker, E. R., Adams, K., Musacchio, R. A., & Streckovich, C. (1984). Physician practice patterns under hospital rate-setting programs. *JAMA, 252,* 2589–2592.

Payment and Supply: Pharmacies

Brooks, J. M., Sorofman, B., & Doucette, W. (1999). Varying health care provider objectives and cost-shifting: The case of retail pharmacies in the U.S. *Health Economics, 8,* 127–150.

Chalkidou, K., Anderson, G. F., & Faden, R. (2011). Eliminating drug price differentials across government programmes in the USA. *Health Economics, Policy, & Law, 6*(1), 43–64.

Winkelmayer, W. C. (2011). Potential effects of the new Medicare prospective payment system on drug prescription in end-stage renal disease care. *Blood Purification, 31*(1–3), 66–69.

Zaric, G. S., & Xie, B. (2009). The impact of two pharmaceutical risk-sharing agreements on pricing, promotion, and net health benefits. *Value in Health, 12*(5), 838–845.

Diagnosis-Related Groups and Case Mix

Agarwal, R., Bergey, M., Sonnad, S., Butowsky, H., Bharqavan, M., & Bleshman, M. H. (2010). Inpatient CT and MRI utilization: Trends in the academic hospital setting. *Journal of the American College of Radiology, 7*(12), 949–955.

Anderson, G., & Ginsburg, P. B. (1983). Prospective capital payment to hospitals. *Health Affairs, 2,* 52–63.

Aronow, D. (1988). Severity of illness measurement. *Medical Care Review, 45,* 339–366.

Broyles, W. W., & Rosko, M. D. (1985). A qualitative assessment of the Medicare prospective payment system. *Social Science and Medicine, 20,* 1185–1190.

Carter, G. M., Jacobson, P. D., Kominski, G. F., & Perry, M. J. (1994). Use of diagnosis-related groups by non-Medicare payers. *Health Care Financing Review, 16*(Winter), 127–158.

Cleverley,W. O., & Cleverley, J. O. (2011). Is there a cost associated with higher quality? *Healthcare Financial Management, 65*(1), 96–102.

Conrad, D. A. (1984). Returns on equity to not-for-profit hospitals. *Health Services Research, 19,* 41–63.

Cotterill, P. G. (1991). Prospective payment for Medicare hospital capital. *Health Care Financing Review,* (Annual suppl.), 79–86.

Donaldson, C. (1991). Minding our Ps and Qs: Financial incentives for efficient hospital behavior. *Health Policy, 17,* 51–76.

Donaldson, C., & Magnusson, J. (1992). DRGs: The road to hospital efficiency. *Health Policy, 21,* 47–64.

Ellis, R. P. (1988). Insurance principles and the design of prospective payment systems. *Journal of Health Economics, 7,* 215–237.

Ellis, R. P., & McGuire, T. G. (1986). Provider behavior under prospective reimbursement. *Journal of Health Economics, 5,* 129–151.

Ellis, R. P., & Ruhm, C. J. (1988). Incentives to transfer patients under alternative reimbursement mechanisms. *Journal of Public Economics, 37,* 381–394.

Fetter, R. B., Youngsoo, S., Freeman, J. L., Averill, R. F., & Thompson, J. D. (1980). Case mix definition by diagnosis-related groups. *Medical Care, 18*(Suppl 2), 1–53.

Fitzgerald, J. F., Fagan, L. F., Tierney, W. M., & Dittus, R. S. (1987). Changing patterns of hip fracture before and after implementation of the prospective payment system. *JAMA, 258,* 218–221.

Fitzgerald, J. F., Moore, P. S., & Dittus, R. S. (1988). The care of elderly patients with hip fracture. Changes since implementation of the prospective payment system. *New England Journal of Medicine, 319,* 1392–1397.

Gilman, B. H. (2000). Hospital response to DRG refinements: The impact of multiple reimbursement incentives on inpatient length of stay. *Health Economics, 9,* 277–294.

Hart, A. C., & Richards, B. (Eds.). (2000). *DRG guidebook: A comprehensive resource to the DRG classification system, 2001* (17th ed.). Reston, VA: Ingenix.

Hsiao, W. C., & Dunn, D. L. (1987). The impact of DRG payments on New Jersey hospitals. *Inquiry, 24,* 212–220.

Lave, J. R. (1984). Hospital reimbursement under Medicare. *Milbank Quarterly, 62,* 251–268.

Lave, J. R. (1985). *The Medicare adjustment for the indirect costs of medical education.* Washington, DC: Association of American Medical Colleges.

Lave, J. R. (1989). The effect of the Medicare prospective payment system. *Annual Review of Public Health, 10,* 141–161.

Lavoie-Tremblay, M., Bonin, J. P., Lesage, A., Lavigne, G. L., & Trudel, J. (2011). Implementation of diagnosis-related mental health programs: Impact on health care providers. *Health Care Manager, 30*(1), 4–14.

Long, M. J., Chesney, J. D., Ament, R. P., Desharnais, S. I., Fleming, S. T., Kobrinski, E. J., & Marshall, B. S. (1987). The effects of PPS on hospital product and productivity. *Medical Care, 25,* 528–538.

Mark, B. A., & Harless, D.W. (2011). Adjusting for patient acuity in measurement of nurse staffing: Two approaches. *Nursing Research, 60*(2), 107–114.

Matheny, M. E., Miller, R. A., Ikizler, T. A., Waltman, L. R., Denny, J. C., Schildcrout, J. S., Dittus, R. S., & Peterson, J. F. (2010). Development of inpatient risk stratification models of acute kidney injury for use in electronic health records. *Medical Decision Making, 30*(6), 639–650.

McCarthy, C. (1988). DRGs—five years later. *New England Journal of Medicine, 318,* 1683–1686.

Mitchell, K. C. (2007, November). Understanding the financial impact of MS-DRGs. *Health Care Financial Management, 61*(11), 56–48.

Morrisey, M., Sloan, F. A., & Valvona, J. (1988). Medicare prospective payment and post-hospital transfers to subacute care. *Medical Care, 26,* 685–698.

Muller, A. (1993). Medicare prospective payment reforms and hospital utilization. *Medical Care, 31,* 296–308.

Mullin, R. L. (1985). Diagnosis-related groups and severity. *JAMA, 253,* 1208–1210.

Neumann, B. R., & Kelly, J. V. (1984). *Prospective reimbursement for hospital capital costs.* Chicago, IL: Healthcare Financial Management Association.

Omenn, G. S., & Conrad, D. A. (1984). Implications of DRG's for clinicians. *New England Journal of Medicine, 311,* 1314–1317.

Pettengill, J., & Vertrees, J. (1982). Reliability and validity in hospital case-mix measurement. *Health Care Financing Review, 4*(December), 101–128.

Russell, L. (1989). *Medicare's new hospital payment system.* Washington, DC: Brookings Institution.

Sloan, F. A., Valvona, J., Hassan, M., & Morrisey, M. A. (1988). Cost of capital to the hospital sector. *Journal of Health Economics, 7,* 25–45.

Tillett, J., & Senger, P. (2011). Determining the value of nursing care. *Journal of Perinatal & Neonatal Nursing, 25*(1), 6–7.

Vertrees, J. C., & Manton, K. G. (1986). A multivariate approach for classifying hospitals and computing blended payment rates. *Medical Care, 24*(4), 283–300.

Vladeck, B. C. (1984). Medicare hospital payment by diagnosis-related group. *Annals of Internal Medicine, 100,* 576–591.

Vladeck, B. C. (1988). Hospital prospective payment and the quality of care. *New England Journal of Medicine, 319,* 1411–1413.

Wennberg, J. E., McPherson, K., & Caper, P. (1984). Will payment based on diagnosis-related groups control hospital costs? *New England Journal of Medicine, 311,* 295–300.

Young, D. W., & Saltman, R. B. (1982). Medical practice, case mix, and cost containment. *JAMA, 247,* 801–805.

Other Case Mix Classification Systems

Arling, G., & Williams, A. R. (2003). Cognitive impairment and resource use of nursing home residents: A structural equation model. *Medical Care, 41*(7), 802–812.

Atkinson, G., & Murray, R. (2008). The use of ambulatory patient groups for regulation of hospital ambulatory surgery revenue in Maryland. *Journal of Ambulatory Care Management, 31*(1), 17–23.

Berlowitz, D. R., & Stineman, M. (2010). Risk adjustment in rehabilitation quality improvement. *Topics in Stroke Rehabilitation, 17*(4), 252–261.

DeJong, G. (2010). Bundling acute and postacute payment: From a culture of compliance to a culture of innovation and best practice. *Physical Therapy, 90*(5), 658–662.

Fries, B. E., Mehr, D. R., Schneider, D., Foley, W. J., & Burke, R. (1993). Mental dysfunction and resource use in nursing homes. *Medical Care, 31*(10), 898–920.

Fries, B. E., Schneider, D. P., Foley, W. J., Gavazzi, M., Burke, R., & Cornelius, E. (1994). Refining a case-mix measure for nursing homes: Resource utilization groups (RUG-III). *Medical Care, 32*(7), 668–685.

Iglesias, C., & Alonso, V. M. J. (2005). A system of patient classification in long-term psychiatric inpatients: Resource utilization groups T-18 (RUG T-18). *Journal of Psychiatric & Mental Health Nursing, 12*(1), 33–37.

Kelly, W. P., Fillmore, H., Tenan, P. M., & Miller, H. C. (1990). The classification of resource use in ambulatory surgery. *Journal of Ambulatory Care Management, 13*(1), 55–63.

Kerber, C. S., Dyck, M. J., Culp, K. R., & Buckwalter, K. (2005). Comparing the geriatric depression scale, minimum data set, and primary care provider diagnosis for depression in rural nursing home residents. *Journal of the American Psychiatric Nurse Association, 11*(5), 269–275.

Optenberg, S. A., Coventry, J. A., & Baker, S. W. (1990). A specialty-based ambulatory workload classification system. *Journal of Ambulatory Care Management, 13*(3), 29–38.

Rawlings, D., Hendry, K., Mylne, S., Banfield, M., & Yates, P. (2011). Using palliative care assessment tools to influence and enhance clinical practice. *Home Healthcare Nurse, 29*(3), 139–145.

Starfield, B., Weiner, J., Mumford, L., & Steinwachs, D. (1991). Ambulatory care groups: A categorization of diagnoses for research and management. *Health Services Research, 26,* 53–74.

Stineman, M. G., Escarce, J. J., Goin, J. E., Hamilton, B. B., Granger, C. V., & Williams, S. V. (1994). A case-mix classification system for medical rehabilitation. *Medical Care, 32,* 366–379.

Tenan, P. M., Fillmore, H. H., Caress, B., Kelly, W. P., Nelson, H., Graziano, D., & Johnson, S. C. (1988). PACs: Classifying ambulatory care patients and services for clinical and financial management. *Journal of Ambulatory Care Management, 11*(3), 36–53.

Urban Institute (2007). *Final Report to CMS Options for Improving Medicare Payment for SNFs.* Washington DC: Author.

Weiner, D. E. (2011). The 2011 ESRD prospective payment system: Welcome to the bundle. *American Journal of Kidney Diseases, 57*(4), 539–541.

Weiner, J. P., Starfield, B. H., Steinwachs, D. M., & Mumford, L. M. (1991). Development and application of a population-oriented measure of ambulatory care-mix. *Medical Care, 29,* 452–472.

Provider Supply under Managed Care Contracting

Albizu-Garcia, C. E., Rios, R., Juarbe, D., & Alegria, M. (2004). Provider turnover in public sector managed mental health care. *Journal of Behavioral Health Services & Research, 31*(3), 255–265.

Blough, D. K., Madden, C. W., & Hornbrook, M. C. (1999). Modeling risk using generalized linear models. *Journal of Health Economics, 18,* 153–171.

Burgess, J. F., Christiansen, C. L., Michalak, S. E., & Morris, C. N. (2000). Medical profiling: Improving standards and risk adjustments using hierarchical models. *Journal of Health Economics, 19,* 291–309.

Debrock, A., & Arnould, R. J. (1992). Utilization control in HMOs. *Quarterly Review of Economics and Business, 32*(3), 31–53.

Elder, K., & Miller, N. (2006). Minority physicians and selective contracting in competitive market environments. *Journal of Health & Social Policy, 21*(4), 21–49.

Feldstein, P. Jl, Wickizer, T. M., & Wheeler, J. R. (1988). Private cost containment. The effects of utilization review programs on health care use and expenditures. *New England Journal of Medicine, 318,* 1310–1314.

Freed, G. L., Dunham, K. M., & Singer, D. (2009). Health plan use of board certification and recertification of surgeons and nonsurgical subspecialists in contracting policies. *Archives of Surgery, 144*(8), 753–758.

Hansen-Turton, T., Ritter, A., & Torgan, R. (2008). Insurers' contracting policies on nurse practitioners as primary care providers: Two years later. *Policy, Politics, & Nursing Practice, 9*(4), 241–248.

Health Care Financing Administration. (1999). *Medicare + Choice rates—45 day notice.* Baltimore, MD: Health Care Financing Administration. Retrieved from http://www.hcfa.gov/stats/hmorates/45d02.htm

Hillman, A. L. (1987). Financial incentives for physicians in HMOs. *New England Journal of Medicine, 317,* 1743–1748.

Hillman, A. L., Pauly, M. V., & Kerstein, J. J. (1989). How do financial incentives affect physicians' clinical decisions and the financial performance of health maintenance organizations? *New England Journal of Medicine, 321,* 86–92.

Hirth, R. A., & Chernew, M. E. (1999). The physician labor market in a managed care–dominated environment. *Economic Inquiry, 37,* 282–294.

Keeler, E. B., Carter, G., & Newhouse, J. P. (1998). A model of the impact of reimbursement schemes on health plan choice. *Journal of Health Economics, 17,* 297–320.

Mukamel, D. B., Weimer, D. L., Zwanziger, J., & Mushlin, A. I. (2002). Quality of cardiac surgeons and managed care contracting practices. *Health Services Research, 37*(5), 1129–1144.

Nas, N., & Seinfeld, J. (2008). Is managed care restraining the adoption of technology by hospitals? *Journal of Health Economics, 27*(4), 1026–1045.

Pauly, M. V., Hillman, A. L., & Kerstein, J. (1990). Managing physician incentives in managed care. *Medical Care, 28,* 1013–1024.

Robinson, J. C. (1993). Payment mechanisms, nonprice incentives, and organizational innovations in health care. *Inquiry, 30,* 328–332.

Robinson, J. C. (1996). Decline in hospital utilization and cost inflation under managed care in California. *JAMA, 276*(13), 1060–1064.

Rubin, P. H., & Schrag, J. L. (1999). Mitigating agency problems by advertising, with special reference to managed health care. *Southern Economic Journal, 66,* 39–60.

Scheffler, R. M., Sullivan, S. D., & Ko, T. H. (1991). The impact of Blue Cross and Blue Shield plan utilization management programs, 1980–1988. *Inquiry, 28,* 276–287.

Ullmann, S. G. (2003). "Out of our crisis:" The lack of long-term relationships in the provision of managed care. *Hospital Topics, 81*(2), 4–8.

Wickizer, T. M., Wheeler, J. R. C., & Feldstein, P. J. (1989). Does utilization review reduce unnecessary hospital care and contain costs? *Medical Care, 27,* 632–647.

Worzala, C., Zhang, N., & Anderson, G. F. (2000). The effect of HMOs on hospital capacity, 1982–1996. *Managed Care Interface, 13*(2), 51–61.

Zwanziger, J., & Khan, N. (2006). Safety-net activities and hospital contracting with managed care organizations. *Medical Care Research & Review, 63*(6 Suppl.), 90S–111S.

Chapter 8

Competitive Markets

OBJECTIVES

1. Specify the assumptions of a competitive market model.

2. Use the competitive model to predict movements in price and utilization due to changes in factors that influence supply and demand for health services.

3. Use the supply-demand framework to predict the factors that influence shortages and surpluses.

4. Identify the evidence for and against the competitive model.

5. Describe the factors that influence how the competitive bidder sets the price for a contract.

6. Define the concept of supplier-induced demand, and describe the influence of supply on price in a market in which supplier-induced demand exists.

8.1 INTRODUCTION

In other chapters, a number of hypotheses about the behavior of demanding and supplying units were developed. These hypotheses that dealt with demand behavior and supply behavior were examined in isolation. As a result, although we developed a way of predicting what quantity would be demanded (supplied) at any price, our model did not incorporate simultaneous consideration of the behavior of the supplying and demanding units and thus could not tell us whether the same quantity would be both demanded and supplied.

In this chapter, we focus on models in which demanders and suppliers interact. The setting in which this interaction occurs is called a *market*. A market in economics should not be thought of as a physical location; rather, the term *market* denotes the web of interactions among those who have commercial relationships or the potential to have such relationships with other buyers and sellers of similar commodities. For example, we can think of a market for psychiatric services as consisting of a group of consumers and a group of providers who have the potential to enter into business relationships with all members of the other group. Central to the analysis of the functioning of a market is the price that the buyer pays and the seller receives. In expositions elsewhere, the price was taken as given for both groups; variations in price were beyond the control of any one buyer or seller. Yet, as a consequence of the related interactions of these groups, prices are set; as a result of some change in demand or supply behavior, prices change.

The market analyses that we will examine involve two categories of concepts:

1. *Phenomena to be explained.* These are objective events, such as changes in the price or the quantity of medical care utilized. The phenomenon of interest might be a rise in prices, and our models would be used to explain why the phenomenon occurred.
2. *Behavioral relationships.* The economic "forces" influencing these phenomena have been referred to as *demand* and *supply*. The strength of these forces can be increased or decreased by individual factors, such as incomes and tastes on the demand side, and input prices on the supply side. Demand can be increased, for example, by higher consumer incomes, and supply can be decreased by higher input costs. As a consequence of changes in causal factors, demand or supply will change, as will price and quantity. Our models should be able to predict such causal chains of events.

In this chapter, one particular market model is developed and used to explain the outcome of price and quantity in the medical care market. This is the competitive market model, which treats the market as an interactive mechanism with many suppliers competing for consumer business. Such a model is helpful in explaining a broad range of phenomena. It offers hypotheses to explain rising prices; increasing or decreasing utilization; shortages in such commodities as physicians' services, nursing services, and blood; and surpluses in such commodities as hospital beds. Thus, it is a valuable starting point for any analysis of markets. The competitive market model is presented in Section 8.2, and the predictions of the model are discussed in Section 8.3. Although the competitive model is able to generate a large number of predictions, not all the predictions are borne out by actual events. Indeed, several events are either at odds with, or fail to corroborate, the predictions of the competitive model. Because accurate prediction is the bottom line of explanatory economics, Section 8.4 is devoted to a discussion of corroborating evidence relating to the competitive hypothesis. Section 8.5 discusses a recent application of the competitive hypothesis in the healthcare field, in particular, the use of the model to explain selective contracting. Section 8.6 concerns a deviation from the competitive market that involves the notion of supplier-induced demand.

8.2 THE COMPETITIVE MODEL: ASSUMPTIONS

In our exposition of the competitive model, we will use a market for physician services as our example. The product is physician visits, which we will assume to be of constant quality, each characterized by the same accuracy of diagnosis, effectiveness of treatment, and personal attentiveness.

- *Individual demand.* Our initial demand assumption is that each consumer has a normal demand curve. This includes the stipulation that consumers are fully informed about the nature of the services they require and the benefits that they can obtain. This stipulation implies that physicians cannot *directly* influence consumer demand for medical care.

- *Market demand.* We further assume that there are many consumers in the market and that they are competing for physician services. This assumption rules out the possibility that buyers are large enough, or can join together, to have any influence over price. The market demand curve (*D*) in our model is shown in Figure 8-1. Here conditions

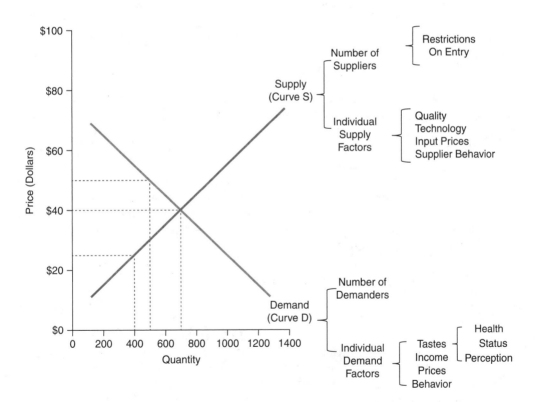

Figure 8-1 Interaction of Behavioral Relationships. The phenomena, price and quantity, are influenced by supply and demand. These, in turn, are affected by a number of individual causal factors (listed in the diagram). The positions of the supply and demand curves have been set based on the assumption that supply and demand are at given levels. Changes in the magnitude of any of the underlying factors will cause a shift in supply or demand (or both).

are assumed to be such that, at a price of $50 per visit, the quantity demanded is 500 visits: at $45, the quantity demanded is 600 units; at $25, the quantity demanded is 1,000 units; and so on. Curve *D* traces out this relationship. Any change in the underlying causal factors (tastes, for example) will shift demand. These causal factors are listed in the diagram for the purpose of reminding the reader of the underlying assumptions of the model.

- *Individual supply.* Our supply assumptions can similarly be separated into assumptions about individual suppliers and about the supplier group. Individually, each supplier has an upward-sloping marginal cost curve. Assuming supplier profit maximization and no supplier influence over price (a market assumption), the marginal cost curve is the supply curve.

- *Market supply.* With regard to the supplier group, we assume there are many suppliers, they do not collude with each other to influence price, and none is large enough by itself to influence price.

Consumers are assumed to be aware of the price offers of alternative suppliers and so can compare prices when making purchase decisions. Because of consumer knowledge, any supplier charging a higher price than what would prevail in a competitive situation will sell no units. Charging a lower price will mean forgoing some intramarginal profits. And so, in such a market, each supplier will take the price as given and supply the quantity at which price equals *MC*. The market supply will be the summed individual suppliers' marginal cost curves. Market supply is shown in Figure 8-1 as curve *S*, with a total of 700 units supplied at $40, a total of 800 at $45, a total of 1,000 at $55, and so on. The factors influencing the position of the supply curve are also shown.

Under these conditions of supply and demand, bargaining occurs between consumers and producers. An equilibrium is reached when the quantity demanded equals the quantity supplied. The next section is devoted to the predictions of the model. That is, it presents what we would expect the market outcome to be (in terms of prices and quantities) if such conditions were approximated in reality.

8.3 THE COMPETITIVE MODEL: PREDICTIONS

8.3.1 Overview

Several important groups of conclusions can be drawn from the competitive model regarding how resources are allocated in the healthcare sector. These conclusions are presented next. Keep in mind that these conclusions are presented as possible explanations whose usefulness is determined by how well they conform to actual experience.

8.3.2 Market Price

In a competitive market, a single price will emerge that clears the market. Competitive bidding will lower the price if a surplus of output exists (i.e., if there is unsold output or excess capacity) and will raise the price in the case of a shortage. Only when buyers are satisfied with the quantities they purchase at the established price and sellers are making maximum profits will market equilibrium be established (i.e., quantity supplied equals quantity demanded). In our example, equilibrium will be reached at a price of $40 and a supply of 700 visits.

If the price is higher, say, $50, then 500 units of service will be demanded, whereas the suppliers will be prepared to supply 900. To eliminate this excess capacity, physicians will lower prices and the amounts supplied. The quantity demanded will increase at the same time. The process goes on until both groups are simultaneously satisfied. The quantity supplied will just equal the quantity that consumers demand. The same process will occur in reverse if the price is below $40, in which case prices will be driven up to the equilibrium point.

It can be shown that the end result of this process is a single price charged by all producers. If any single physician charged more than the equilibrium price per visit, then his or her patients, who we assume to possess full knowledge of prices charged by other physicians, would obtain medical care elsewhere. The physician would be forced to bring his or her price down to the price other physicians are charging. On the other hand, if a physician sets fees below the equilibrium level, patients will flock to this physician, creating an overload of work. Given a rising *MC* schedule for this physician, if he provides service for the additional patients, the profits gained from the sale of each additional unit will in fact be negative. The physician with such an *MC* schedule would have been better off profitwise to accept the highest price, which is the market price. That a single market-clearing price will emerge is thus one conclusion of the competitive model.

8.3.3 Price and Quantity Movements Caused by Demand Shifts

Additional conclusions based on the competitive model can be drawn regarding price and quantity movements when there is a change in any of the factors that influence demand. This set of conclusions is illustrated in Figure 8-2. Assume D_1 to be the demand curve consistent with given initial values of underlying causal factors of demand. Let S be the supply curve, which remains stable because all supply shift factors are assumed constant. The equilibrium price for these conditions is P_1 ($40), and the equilibrium quantity for the market is Q_1 (700 visits). If any of the initial conditions that influence demand change, causing an increase in demand to D_2, for example, there will be a new equilibrium price ($45) and a new quantity (800 units). The willingness of consumers to buy more at each price allows the producers to increase profits by producing more output (up to 800 units). Such a shift in demand can be caused by higher consumer incomes or a greater degree of illness in the population. Or it can be caused by an increase in the amount of health insurance purchased, which also causes demand to shift out. In either case, the result is the same—higher prices and quantities. The opposite situation, lower prices and quantities, would be the consequence of factors shifting demand downward.

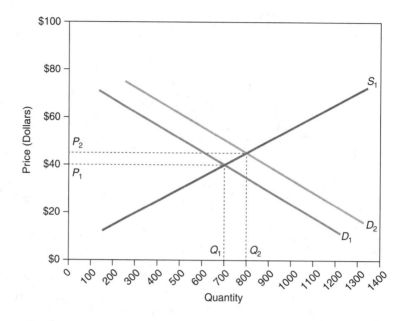

Figure 8-2   Shift in Demand with Stable Supply. An initial set of supply and demand forces, characterized by D_1 and S_1 will produce given price and output levels. An increase in demand to D_2, with a stable S, will cause price and output to increase.

If the quantity utilized is to increase, additional quantity must be available. *Utilization* refers to the actual quantity traded in the market. This should not be confused with the amount demanded because when there is disequilibrium, more (or less) might be demanded than is supplied. Nor should it be confused with the quantity offered by the supplier because at any one price more (or less) might be supplied than consumers are willing to take at that price. Disequilibrium situations occur when the price does not adjust to allow the quantity demanded and the quantity supplied to equalize.

8.3.4 Price and Quantity Movements Caused by Supply Shifts

Another set of conclusions based on the model concern changes in factors that cause the supply to shift. What occurs if there is an increase in supply is shown in Figure 8-3. In this example, the commodity becomes less scarce and the supply shifts from S_1 to S_2. If the demand remains the same, the supply increases relative to the demand and the price falls. As a result, a new lower price ($35) and a higher level of utilization (800 units) are predicted. Of course, a factor that causes a reduction in supply will have the opposite effect on the price and the quantity utilized.

Changes in supply can occur because of changes in circumstances that are beyond the control of supplying firms (and to which they react) or because of changes that the present or potential suppliers themselves initiate. For example, if hospitals or public health departments decide to hire medical technicians, they will enter the market and bid for the existing supply of

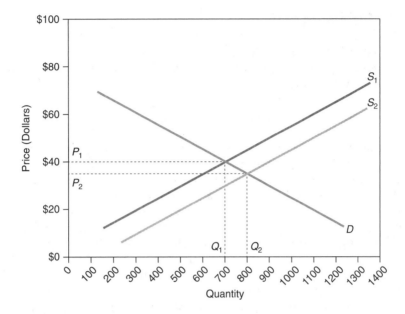

Figure 8-3 Shift in Supply with Stable Demand. Beginning with initial demand and supply levels D and S_1, and resulting price and output levels, an increase in supply to S_2 will cause output to increase and price to fall.

technicians. This will raise the price of technicians that all market participants have to pay because the supply will initially remain relatively stable while the demand will increase. An increase in the price of technician services (or for that matter of any input) will shift to the left the supply curve of all producers who use this input. Thus, the market supply curve will shift leftward as well, and the price of physician services will increase.

Provider-initiated changes in supply will be undertaken by for-profit suppliers when these changes have the potential to add to profits. Three types of situations are discussed here:

1. A change in input combinations brought about by existing suppliers,
2. An increase in the capital stock of existing suppliers,
3. Entry into the market by new suppliers.

An example of the first situation, a change in input combinations, might occur if physicians were to hire nurse practitioners to perform, at a lower cost, services previously performed by the physicians themselves. Such a change might be the result of the passage of a law allowing such substitution to occur. The effect would be to shift the average total cost curve downward and the marginal cost curve to the right. In a competitive market, one supplier making such a change would not cause a large shift in the market supply curve. Prices would remain about the same, and that one supplier would reap an increase in profits. However, if all suppliers made a change, the market supply curve would shift to the right considerably, and the price of medical care would then fall. Consumers would reap the benefits from such actions.

The net profit position of each provider after all suppliers have acted may not be any greater than before because the price of output has fallen; but it is important to note that the providers make their decisions to undertake cost-reducing activities based on preexisting prices. Providers do not collude with their fellow suppliers, and they do not always anticipate that prices will fall as a consequence of their concerted actions. The end result of their actions, however, is lower prices and greater utilization.

The same process occurs when existing suppliers invest in plants and equipment. Additions to capital are often made in anticipation of additions to profits because of lower unit costs. If these investments cut costs, and if they are sufficiently widespread in the industry, the net effect will be to lower prices and raise utilization. As a result, after these effects have worked themselves out, profits may be no greater than before (they may even be less). These effects are presented in a before-after manner here. In actuality, they take a considerable time to occur. The potential for profits must first be realized, then planning for the additions and financing them, and the additional capital equipment and plant must be constructed and put into use. As a result, the increase in supply and the fall in price may take months and even years. For this reason, the analysis of provider behavior involving capital additions, with resulting shifts in average and marginal cost curves, has been referred to as *long-run analysis*. (It is generally difficult to decide when a change in supply conditions is long run and when it is short run. Short-run changes are usually taken to be changes in quantity supplied that occur without changes in capital equipment.)

The third type of variation in supply occurs when new (profit-seeking) suppliers enter an industry or a market in response to high profits. Such a movement results in an increase in supply and a consequent fall in price and an increase in utilization. In this instance, because the cost conditions of existing suppliers remain the same, the profit levels must fall for all existing suppliers.

The conditions that determine how easily potential providers can actually enter the industry and place their products on the market are referred to as *conditions of entry*. These conditions depend on existing productive techniques as well as on legal impediments. In some industries, extensive capital requirements preclude many firms from entering because of the large financial commitment necessary to undertake the capital investment and commence production. Such requirements may exist for some types of medical care, such as intensive surgery, although the financial impediments are not nearly as great as they are, for example, in the automobile industry. For many types of medical care, financial impediments are not relevant to entry. More relevant are the legal impediments, such as the licensing requirements for medical personnel and facilities. Licensing regulations frequently amount to restrictions placed on potential entrants into an industry.

8.3.5 Simultaneous Demand and Supply Shifts

In addition to creating movements in either demand or supply alone, in which the effects are readily predictable, underlying factors may cause shifts in both demand and supply at the same time. We must be careful at this stage of the analysis to specify that we are referring to separate factors causing changes in demand and supply. That is, an increase in the number of ill people occurring at the same time as an influx of physicians into the market will cause both demand and supply curves to shift; the increase in the illness level will cause demand to increase, and the increase in the number of physicians will cause supply to increase. In Figure 8-4, this is shown as a shift in demand from D_1 to D_2 and, at the same time, a shift in supply from S_1 to S_2. Although quantity increases, the net effect on price is ambiguous and will depend on how much each curve shifts, that is, on the changes in the values of the causal variables and the degree to which they cause demand and supply to shift. In the specific case illustrated in Figure 8-4, price will remain constant. But if we do not know the extent to which both curves are shifted, our model fails us as a predictive device.

A second type of simultaneous shift may occur when the same factor that causes demand to shift independently causes supply to shift. An increase in quality, for example, will cause supply to decrease and demand to increase. When demand increases and supply decreases, price will increase, but quantity will increase, fall, or remain the same, depending on the extent of the shifts. (Another type of simultaneous shift that does *not* belong in this

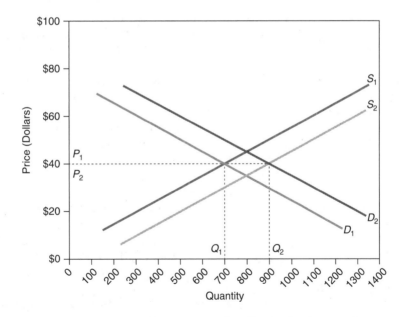

Figure 8-4 Simultaneous Shift in Demand and Supply Curves. Beginning with initial demand and supply levels D_1 and S_1, and resulting price and output levels, a simultaneous shift in demand and supply curves (to D_2 and S_2) will have an ambiguous effect on price and will increase output. The extent of both shifts determines the effects on price and quantity. Some directional shifts, such as a decrease in demand and a simultaneous increase in supply, will lower the price, but have an ambiguous effect on quantity traded.

category is when the factors affecting supply and demand are not independent, such as when physicians can induce consumer demand. This phenomenon is discussed in Section 8.6.)

8.3.6 Shortages

Our predictions so far have been concerned with what happens to the equilibrium price when one or several factors change. Not all situations are such that the quantity demanded is the quantity supplied. The medical care market often experiences shortages. A shortage occurs when the quantity demanded exceeds the quantity supplied at the current price. Our model shows that in a competitive market with free bidding, a shortage will cause the price to rise. Then the suppliers will offer more services and the consumers will reduce their demand, making the shortage disappear. That is the theory, although persistent shortages have been observed in the blood market, the market for nurses, the physician services market, and, in some countries, the hospital market. A slight modification of the competitive model allows us to predict why these shortages occur and how they can be eliminated.

Refer to the example in Figure 8-1. Assume that, because of a government regulation, the price cannot rise above $30 per visit. Perhaps the regulation is passed and enforced to help low-income consumers who may go without medical services if the price is $40. The consequences of the passage of the regulation can be determined using the competitive model. At $30, consumers will be more willing to visit their physicians and, according to our figures, 900 will call for appointments. But at this price, it would be unprofitable for physicians to see 900 patients. Indeed, they will reduce quantity supplied and will see only 500 patients. A queue of untreated patients will form; in this case, 400 patients who want treatment will be untreated. Some shortages are the result of such price ceilings. In a competitive market, a shortage can persist only if the price is somehow administered to remain below the market-clearing price. This will usually be done by an official or semiofficial agency that can overrule the price that market forces set.

A shortage can also occur when insurance is purchased or when a government program "guaranteeing" medical care is instituted. In such situations, the consumers may face a zero money price, which will mean a high quantity demanded (e.g., 1200 units, as shown in Figure 8-5). The reimbursed price to the provider may be only $20 per unit, and at this price, 700 units are provided. In our example, it would take a price of $60 to bring forth a supply of 1,200 units. At the administered reimbursement rate of $20, there is a shortage of 500 units.

The situation requires a mechanism to ration the 700 available units, assuming that the quality produced remains the same. One tactic is to make the prospective patients wait in line; those who are willing to pay the "time costs" will receive the service (Buchanan, 1965; Culyer & Cullis, 1976; Drumm, Arkins, & Dayan, 2010; Sloan & Lorant, 1976;). Another possibility is for the providers to lower the quality of their product, for example, by reducing the time devoted to providing the service. This action would reduce demand because the service would not have the same worth as before and it would increase supply. As a result, the shortage would be reduced and perhaps even eliminated.

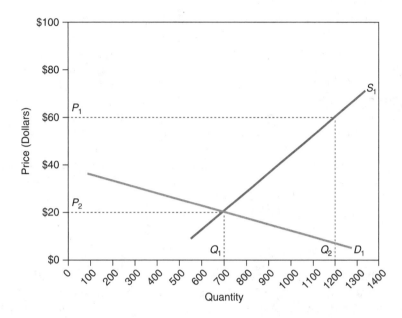

Figure 8-5 Supply and Demand Forces Under Full-Service Coverage by Third-party Insurer. Full-service coverage (zero out-of-pocket price) with a reimbursement rate of $20 will lead to a quantity demanded of 1,200 and a quantity supplied of 700. To reach a quantity supplied of 1,200, the payment rate would have to be $60 (curve S_1).

8.3.7 Surpluses

The usual definition of a surplus is an excess of quantity supplied over quantity demanded at a given price. For a surplus to persist, some factor must keep quantity supplied above quantity demanded. If the price in the market was kept permanently above the equilibrium price, a surplus would persist: Suppliers would be willing to provide more units than consumers would be willing to purchase. In Figure 8-1, if the suppliers' reimbursed price and the consumers' out-of-pocket price were both $45 and could not be lowered, a surplus would appear. In this case, suppliers would be willing to supply more units at that price than demanders would want, and the suppliers would find themselves with excess capacity.

For a surplus to persist, something must prevent the market price from falling because in a normal competitive situation an excess supply would induce suppliers to lower their prices to induce demanders to buy more. If the government pegged or supported an above-equilibrium price in the market, a surplus would occur. In the case of health care, where insurance exists, a surplus can occur if the reimbursement rate suppliers receive induces a greater quantity supplied than the quantity demanded by consumers at the price they have to pay out of pocket. In Figure 8-1, if the reimbursement rate was $50 and the out-of-pocket price was $30, a surplus would exist.

In the early 1990s, there was much talk of a "physician surplus" (Burns, 2009; Otari, Waterman, Faulkner, Boslaugh, Burroughs, & Dunagan, 2009; Schwartz & Mendelson, 1990). In discussions of this topic, one heard talk of falling physicians' fees and incomes (although this not always borne out by the data). To the extent that the fees and incomes of physicians were falling during that period, this situation was not a surplus in the technical sense. Falling fees are characteristic of prices responding to a shift in supply en route to a new equilibrium point. For a surplus to develop, the market cannot be allowed to move to a new equilibrium; it must remain in *dis*equilibrium.

The surplus in hospital beds is more likely a case of permanent disequilibrium. High hospital reimbursement rates have induced a large quantity supplied; at given out-of-pocket prices, there has not been enough quantity demanded to clear the market.

8.3.8 Multimarket Analyses

The competitive model is well suited to making predictions about the effect of supply and/or demand changes in one market on price and quantity in a related market. Let us take an example of two substitute services, inpatient and outpatient surgical care. Because of the development of quicker acting anesthetics, outpatient surgery has become more feasible. Further, the total cost of outpatient surgery is much less than inpatient surgery for most cases, and outpatient surgery, for many procedures, is now covered.

Analytically, the impact of moving from no outpatient coverage for a procedure (e.g., tonsillectomy) to outpatient coverage is shown in Figure 8-6. The pre-outpatient coverage market for inpatient procedures is characterized in graph A. Here, S is the inpatient supply curve and D_i is the inpatient demand

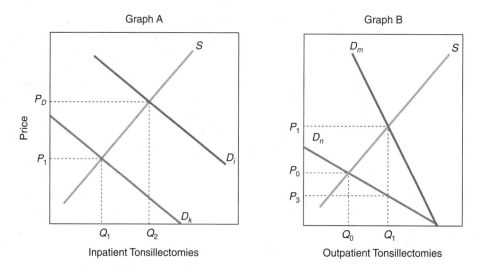

Figure 8-6 Multimarket Analysis. Demand curves in inpatient and outpatient markets are related (the services can be substitutes). When the out-of-pocket price in the outpatient market falls (because of an increase in insurance coverage), the demand curve in the inpatient market shifts inward and price and quantity falls.

curve. In graph B, D_n is the demand curve for outpatient tonsillectomies (without insurance) and S is the supply curve. Note that the demand function for *inpatient* care is dependent on the out-of-pocket price for *outpatient* surgery because the two are substitutes.

Initially, there is no insurance coverage for outpatient tonsillectomies, and P_0 is the prevailing price. An increase in outpatient coverage will shift the market curve for outpatient care outward (to D_m in graph B) and simultaneously lower the out-of-pocket price of outpatient care from P_0 to a point such as P_3. This will result in an inward shift in the D_i curve for inpatient care to D_k The inpatient price will fall and the quantity of inpatient procedures will be reduced. Note also that the outpatient procedures will be increased.

Similar types of analyses can be conducted for other types of substitute procedures. It can also be conducted for complements, such as film and radiologist services. In some cases, it is not clear whether two services are substitutes or complements. For example, it is not clear whether nursing home care replaces hospital care or is used in conjunction with it. The same holds for home health care and hospital care. In these instances, the model cannot provide unambiguous conclusions.

8.4 EVIDENCE FOR AND AGAINST THE COMPETITIVE MODEL

8.4.1 Overview

There has been some use of the competitive model in explaining resource allocation trends in medical care markets. In the physician services market, the phenomenon of rapidly rising physician fees, both before and after the watershed year of 1966, when Medicare and Medicaid were instituted, was explained using the competitive model by hypothesizing that the rapid increase in medical care insurance caused demand shifts and consequent rising prices. In this market, the length of time required to train new physicians means a slow supply response, even in a competitive market, and prices would be expected to rise (Garbarino, 1959; Ginsburg, 2010; Newhouse, Phelps, & Schwartz., 1977). In the hospital care market, the same type of explanation can be made for rising hospital costs, with one modification. Although insurance was increasing during this time period, hospital input prices, notably employee wages, were also rapidly rising. This latter phenomenon would shift the supply curve inward. Couple this with a rapidly outward-shifting demand curve for hospital care, and the net effect would be a larger price increase. Whether utilization would increase or decrease would depend on the magnitude of both shifts. As seen in the chapter on economic dimensions, hospital utilization increased. Our "after the fact" explanation would state that the supply and demand shifts were such that the increase in utilization was likely to occur. (An application of the competitive model to the hospital field is found in Ro [1977].)

The competitive model has also been used to explain the persisting queues and unmet demands that have resulted from the institution of the National Health Service (NHS) in Great Britain in 1946. The NHS is characterized by a zero money price paid by consumers, per capita remuneration for general practitioners, and salaried remuneration for surgeons. The competitive model applied to this type of healthcare system would predict large increases in quantity demanded following the lowering of the price to zero. Supply decisions passed into the hands of the central government, and large increases in supply did not materialize. As a result, persistent shortages occurred, particularly in hospital care (Culyer & Cullis, 1976).

Although the competitive model is a useful device for explaining price and quantity movements and uncovering the causes of shortages of medical care, much attention has focused on the shortcomings of the model. Evidence of the existence of shortcomings might be obtained in three ways. First, we might examine data on market outcomes, such as profits and prices. If such outcomes are not what we would expect in a competitive market (i.e., not what the competitive model predicts would happen), we could infer that the model does not explain what we have observed and seek alternative models to explain the data better. Second, we might observe some conditions and characteristics of a market, such as consumer ignorance or product quality-level differences. If the observed characteristics are at odds with the competitive model's assumptions, we should consider seeking a different model that incorporates realistic assumptions. Third, we might observe direct actions on the part of providers that suggest the prevalence of noncompetitive practices. These might include constraints on certain activities usually thought of as competitive, such as entry into the market. We now turn to some of the evidence that the competitive model has serious flaws as a model of the healthcare market.

8.4.2 Excessive Profits

Studies made of the profits accruing from medical practice have shown these profits to be persistent and considerable. These profits, which are the net incomes of the physicians operating the practices, must be adjusted for the costs incurred in medical training, including fees paid and earnings forgone while practicing medicine or during internship and residency. Even after adjusting for these costs, the net present value of medical practice indicates the existence of persistently high profits (i.e., earnings in excess of normal returns) (Cooper, 2011; Lindsay, 1976; Sloan, 1976). Generally, the competitive model predicts that such excess profits would eventually be bid away by new providers entering the industry to take advantage of the high returns. This has not occurred in medical practice.

8.4.3 Fee Differences Among Patients

The competitive model predicts that one price will prevail in the market for all suppliers and demanders. Before the spread of health insurance, physician pricing was characterized by a sliding scale of fees, with high-income patients paying higher prices than low-income patients. This phenomenon has led economists to reject the competitive model as inappropriate for the physician services market and to substitute a monopoly model (De Jaegher & Jegers, 2001; Kessell, 1958; Leonard, Stordeur, & Roberfroid, 2009; Newhouse, 1970; Wu & Masson, 1974; see chapter on Market Power in Health Care).

8.4.4 Quality of Care

The competitive model assumes that a homogeneous service is being bought and sold and that competition is based on price. Yet product quality is a major element of a hospital's output, and health insurance companies often offer different types of policies in terms of coverage (viewed as differences in the quality of the policy as well as differences in service).

When a supplier can vary its quality, it can attract consumers on the basis of its quality. It follows that some "brand loyalty" may ensue, and buyers will not switch brands easily (because of a slight increase in price, for example). This phenomenon is called *product differentiation*, and it implies that each supplier then faces a downward-sloping demand curve, not a horizontal one (as is the case in perfect competition), and can choose to compete with other providers on the basis of price or product quality. The competitive model is not equipped to handle this feature of the healthcare market, which requires a somewhat more complex model.

8.4.5 Restricting Competitive Behavior

Additional evidence of anticompetitive control mechanisms is found by examining the behavior of physicians when confronted with potentially competitive colleagues. Two practices, historically, have been restricted by physician associations: the advertising of physician fees and the participation by physicians in prepayment group practices. In an ideal world, such as that set out in the model in Section 8.2, advertising is unnecessary because consumers know all about physician fees. But in the real world, considerable consumer ignorance exists, and advertising would reduce ignorance about alternative physician prices (and perhaps qualifications). Coupled with fee cutting (price reductions), advertising would result in more business for the fee-cutting advertiser, but in generally lower prices and profits in the industry.

Advertising bans have been enforced by state medical societies (Kessell, 1958), and although such bans are no longer legally enforceable, their existence in the past was evidence that physicians were able to intervene in the market on behalf of themselves and eliminate some degree of competition in the market. Bans on advertising (and other competitive practices) have been used as evidence of the availability of mechanisms to restrict competition.

8.4.6 Consumer Ignorance and Supplier-Induced Demand

The competitive model operates under the assumption that consumers possess a considerable degree of information about their condition, the products they need, and the outcomes of using the products. In fact, consumers appear to operate under a considerable degree of ignorance in this area, which has led some commentators to view physicians as essentially agents acting on behalf of consumers (Calcott, 1999; Carlsen & Grytten, 2000; Feldstein, 1974). If physicians do behave as agents for their patients, the implicit assumption that suppliers and demanders are acting independently must be rejected. Demand is subject to direct supplier influence.

Nor can we assume that, if they do act as agents for their patients, physicians always behave in the patients' best interests. Because of information asymmetry, the possibility exists that physicians can use their influence to further their own interests. Consumer demands can be shifted by the suppliers through the provision of biased information.

Demand shifting can be detected in market outcome statistics in some circumstances. According to the competitive theory, an increase in the per capita supply of physicians results in an increase in market supply. With everything else held constant, this should bring down the price of health care. Yet it has been alleged that the relationship between physician per capita supply and price is exactly opposite to that predicted by the model; that is, the more physicians per capita in an area, the higher the observed price (Evans, 1974; Fuchs & Kramer, 1972). The reason why this phenomenon is not considered proven is that a number of intervening factors exist that may cause demand to rise at the same time as physician supply increases.

Let us make a simple comparison of two hypothetical medical markets, one in a small town and one in a large metropolitan center with several medical schools. The large city may have more physicians per capita than the small town, and yet the price for a visit to a physician may be greater. This "raw" relationship by itself does not mean that the higher supply has caused the higher price. Many other intervening variables must also be taken into account, among them insurance, the health status of the two populations, and the quality of care provided. The third factor, the quality of care, is especially important in making comparisons, mainly because it is such a difficult variable to measure and thus may be ignored. It may well be that the quality of care in the city is higher than in the town. If all factors other than the quality of care were adjusted for, we might still observe a positive relationship between physician density and price. Until quality has been adjusted for, however, we cannot be certain that the higher price is not due to the fact that a better quality of service is being provided.

Another factor to take into consideration when comparing urban and rural physician-to-population ratios is the role of specialists and the critical mass of population required to support specialists. Because, for example, fewer people require the services of an oncologist than a general internist, the population base required to support the oncologist is larger, making direct comparison of physician-to-population ratios difficult (Stensland & Stinson, 2002).

This type of confounding relationship has caused controversy regarding the observed relationship between price and physician density (Sloan & Feldman, 1978). Some commentators have proceeded as if it were true and have constructed alternative supplier-induced demand models.

8.5 COMPETITIVE BIDDING

The competitive market has often been held up as an ideal, a standard in the light of which other allocative arrangements might be judged. One mechanism that has been put forward as potentially providing a competitive-style outcome for public programs is competitive bidding. Competitive bidding occurs when a purchaser (e.g., a government agency) requests bids from alternative competing providers and allocates the right to treat patients based on the bids. The object of this practice is to have the patients treated for the least cost.

One approach to developing a model of the competitive bidding process is to examine the behavior of an individual supplier who is facing a single paying agency and who is competing with other providers for the right to provide the services. In constructing such a model, it is essential to recognize that the bids are made under conditions of risk. When they submit their bids, the bidders do not know for certain whether or not they will be selected as providers. Their behavior can be modeled in a manner similar to that of consumers who are faced with risky medical expenses.

The bidder faces two possible outcomes: the bid is accepted, or the bid is rejected. To simplify matters, let us assume that no losses are associated with an unsuccessful bid (i.e., the bidder is no worse off than if he or she did not bid). What the bidder must do is compare the outcomes of the various bids to assess which will prove the most satisfactory.

Our simplified model is presented in numerical form in Table 8-1. We make the following assumptions. First, a request is put out calling for providers to bid for the right to serve a given number of patients in a public program. The bids are to be expressed in per capita terms for a certain set of services (physician care, hospital care, and drugs). Second, five options (labeled A through E) are open to the bidder: bids of $100, $95, $90, $85, and $80. Third, as the bidder lowers his or her bid, the probability of having the bid accepted increases. At a bid of $100, there is a 20% chance of the bid being accepted. This rises to 90% with a bid of $80. Fourth, the bidder's profits, if the bid is accepted, are equal to the revenues less the costs of serving the designated number of patients. Given the number of patients (Q) and the costs per patient (C), the higher the accepted bid, the higher will be the profits [equal to $(B \times Q) - (C \times Q)$]. Fifth, we translate the profitability situation of the bidder into a wealth level. We assume that, without a contract, the bidder's wealth would be $200. A successful bid, thus, adds to the successful bidder's wealth level by the level of the bidder's profits.

Table 8-1: Hypothetical Bidding Data

Option	Bid Price	Probability of Acceptance	Profits (if bid accepted)	Wealth Level (if bid accepted)	Utility Levels	
					Risk Averter	Risk Taker
A	$100	0.2	$800	$1,000	126	2,000
B	95	0.4	400	600	122	800
C	90	0.6	200	400	118	400
D	85	0.8	100	300	110	200
E	80	0.9	50	250	100	100

The bidder is thus faced with a trade-off between profits (and hence wealth) and the probability of a successful bid. The individual bidder can increase the likelihood of success but only by lowering the bid and thus lowering the profits. Given the range of alternatives, which option will the bidder choose? As set up now, our model is incomplete; it does not incorporate the objectives of the bidders or the bidding rules set up by the contracting agency.

With regard to bidder's objectives, let us assume first that the bidder is extremely risk averse. He or she puts a high personal value on small gains and successively lower additional values on larger gains (i.e., wealth, for the bidder, has a diminishing marginal utility). Under this assumption, reflected in column 6 of Table 8-1, the bidder will choose the option that maximizes his or her *expected* utility, measured as the product of the probability of success (3) and the utility associated (6) or (7) with the wealth level of that option. In our example, the risk averse bidder will choose Option E, which yields an expected utility of 90 (0.9 × 100). Option D, for example, would yield an expected utility of 88 (0.8 × 110). Although the profits for this option are greater, the bidder prefers to select a very safe but relatively unprofitable option.

A risk taker, whose tastes might be like those summarized in column 7, considers high levels of wealth to be of the utmost importance, which is shown by the sharply increasing utilities of wealth. To this bidder, substantial profits are so important that they overshadow the very small chances of attaining them. To the risk taker, Option E has an expected utility of 90 (0.9 × 100), whereas Option A has an expected utility of 400 (2,000 × 0.2). Option A is the one to be selected by the risk-taking bidder.

Competitive bidding does not automatically lead to a low-price bid. Much of the outcome depends on the bidders' costs and goals, but there are several other factors as well. First, an increase in the number of bidders will reduce the probability of any single bidder being successful. Depending on the bidders' utility schedules, a larger number of competitive bidders may cause each bidder to reduce his or her bid. Second, there are a number of selection and reimbursement methods to which a contracting agency can resort. These may influence the bidding strategies of the bidders (Christianson, Smith, & Hillman, 1984; Miller, Rossiter, & Nuttall, 2002; Town, Feldman, & Kralewski, 2011). One method is to reimburse each winning bidder (more than one provider in an area may be chosen as a winner) at the level of the bid he or she submitted. Thus, if Bidder 1 submitted a bid of $95; Bidder 2, a bid of $90; and Bidder 3, a bid of $85, and if Bidders 2 and 3 are selected as providers, then Bidder 2 would be reimbursed at $90 and Bidder 3 at $85. This method tends to encourage bidding providers to gamble and seek a higher price because there is a potential reward to them for doing so (they are reimbursed at the price they bid if their bid is accepted). An alternative method will check this tendency to gamble. If the set of rules entailed that all winning bidders would be reimbursed at the rate bid by the lowest winning bidder, there would be no benefit to a winner making a higher bid if he or she deems that some other winner will bid lower. Indeed, raising the bid merely reduces the chances of being successful.

Competitive bidding rules may lead to a competitive market-type outcome. Whether it does will depend on a number of factors, including the number of bidders, their attitudes toward risk, and the bidding rules set up by the agency. In 1982, the California legislative assembly passed a law allowing selective contracting by third-party payers with hospitals and physicians. Previously, third-party payers in California could not exclude any providers from the group they were obligated to reimburse for services provided.

In the 1990s, managed care grew rapidly as a tool for reducing the rate of increase in healthcare costs. One mechanism used by managed care companies to restrain costs was to limit the providers included in the plan, selecting the lowest cost providers. However in many states, opponents were successful in getting "any willing provider" laws passed, which required plans to accept any provider into the plan that was willing to accept the terms of the plan. This effectively removed the ability of managed care plans to limit provider participation and control costs.

8.6 SUPPLIER-INDUCED DEMAND

8.6.1 A Pedagogic Model

In the chapter on Additional Topics in the Demand for Health and Medical Care, we focused on the asymmetry of information between consumers and providers in the medical care market. We raised the possibility that consumers may not have good information about their health status or the probable effect of medical care on their health. Although consumers are not likely to be completely ignorant, they often rely on physicians to act as agents and inform them about these variables. Physicians can, in many instances, provide information that will allow patients to form a demand curve, but this information may not be fully correct. Physicians can affect the demand curve for medical care by providing information that is inaccurate or incomplete. If physicians do induce demand unnecessarily, perhaps in response to the excess capacities of their practices, then when the ratio of physicians to population is high, demand will be shifted out more. Ultimately, the extent of unnecessary inducement of demand is an empirical question—and a difficult one to answer.

A large number of studies have been developed that attempt to incorporate supplier-induced demand into the framework of medical markets. Many of these models focus on the provider (physician) and assume implicitly that the ability to shift demand is unlimited. Because consumers have access to information about the quality of advice they receive from their physicians, it is more realistic to recognize that limitations to demand generation may exist. We present a simple model of medical care markets that brings out some of their more important features (Cooper, 2011; Leonard, Stordeur, & Roberfroid., 2009; Pauly, 1980; Peacock & Richardson, 2007).

We assume that consumers' "taste" for medical care depends on information about initial health status (H_0); the effect of medical care on health ($\Delta H/\Delta M$, in which M stands for medical care); and the impact of health on utility, incomes, and prices. It also depends on the number of physicians in the market. In particular, a lower physician (DOC) to population ratio (shortened to *DOCPOP*) will lead to a higher demand for each physician in the market.

For each patient, we suppose there is a "true" level of H and $\Delta H/\Delta M$ that can be determined by the patient's physician. If the physician is fully truthful with the patient, a demand curve for the patient can be derived (D_{true} in Figure 8-7). This demand curve is downward sloping, which means that, for any given level of belief about H and $\Delta H/\Delta M$, the quantity demanded will be responsive to out-of-pocket price.

Of course, the physician can tell the patient that H and $\Delta H/\Delta M$ have values other than the actual ones. If the patient believes the physician, the patient's demand curve will shift outward (i.e., at any price, the quantity demanded will be greater). But the physician is only one source of information, and the patient can get information elsewhere if he or she questions the physician's assessment. It is therefore likely that there is an upper limit to the physician's ability to generate demand that is not grounded in reality. We will call the demand curve at this upper limit D_{limit}.

8.6.2 Supply

Having specified the demand characteristics of the model, we now turn to the supply side of the market. With regard to physician behavior, the following assumptions are made:

- Each physician has an upward-sloping marginal cost (MC) curve (i.e., as more services are provided, marginal costs increase).

- The price of services is fixed by a fee schedule and so fees are beyond physician control.

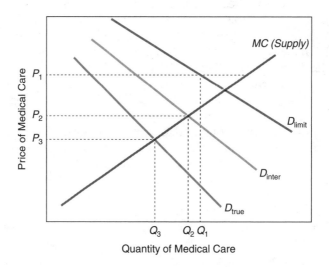

Figure 8-7   Supplier-induced Demand. The three demand curves, D_{true}, D_{inter}, D_{limit}, represent the demand of three successive levels of supplier inducement; no unnecessary inducement (D_{true}), an intermediate level of inducement (D_{inter}), and the maximum level of inducement possible (D_{limit}). The physician's marginal cost is MC. Three alternative fee levels, P_1, P_2, and P_3, are shown. The quantity of medical care "induced" will depend on the fee level, the degree of inducement, and the physician's MC. However, at high fee levels, patient-influenced limitations may be a factor in determining utilization.

8.6.3 Objectives

A number of studies have identified many possible physician objectives, ranging from healing patients to maximizing profits. We will assume each physician's goal is profit maximization for the sake of convenience, not because it is the most realistic assumption. It also elucidates the "worst case" scenario and shows how the most selfish physicians will behave under specified conditions.

The model has been designed to predict the quantity of medical care provided. We will now show that this quantity will depend on the specific price received by the physician. Let us start with a high price, such as P_1 in Figure 8-7. At this price, the physician will generate demand to the limit and provide services at level Q_1. At this point, marginal revenue (MR) is greater than MC, and the physician would be able to earn additional profits if demand could be generated beyond D_{limit}. But the patient cannot be pushed further, and so this is the best the physician can do.

If the price were lower, at P_2, the physician would generate demand up to some intermediate point D_{inter} and would provide Q_2 units of service. Beyond this point, MC would exceed MR, and the physician would reduce profits by inducing further demand. At an even lower price, P_3, the physician would not generate any unnecessary demand and would provide Q_3 units of service. The conclusions of even this simple model are that, with the most selfish of physicians, the quantity demanded—and the degree of demand generation—will depend on the given price.

What about an increase in the supply of physicians (i.e., an increase in the *DOCPOP*)? From the viewpoint of the individual physician, such an increase would lead to a reduction in each demand curve (D_{true}, D_{inter}, and D_{limit}), because these curves are the individual physician's demand curves and each physician will have a smaller market. In these circumstances, each physician's quantity of services supplied will be reduced. Overall demand cannot be generated beyond the maximum, and at a price such as P_3, there is not likely to be any change in overall services.

As pointed out earlier, there are a number of reasons why consumers might not be totally gullible and vulnerable to demand-generating tactics. First, consumers can obtain information from sources other than their physicians, especially given access to the Internet today. Second, a number of studies have suggested that there is a limit to the willingness of physicians to generate demand (Rossiter & Wilensky, 1984; Stano, 1987a, 1987b; Xirasagar & Lin, 2006), although the nature of this reticence has not been spelled out. Analysts have alternatively modeled the generation of ungrounded demand as a cost to physicians and as a cause of disutility (perhaps as a result of feelings of guilt). In either case, generating too much unnecessary demand will make the physicians (as well as the patients) worse off.

As has been hypothesized, the generation of ungrounded demand will result in higher marginal costs to the physician and depending on revenues, may yield more profits. But what if the physician's objectives included patient well-being? The impact of this goal will be to reduce the degree to which the physician would be willing to generate demand.

This model has dealt with demand generation and patient utilization at given prices. It presents a pedagogic treatment of the issue of demand generation and its likely degree of restriction. But it ignores the fact that, contrary to what might be expected, higher physician fees have been associated with an increase in *DOCPOP*. We turn now to possible explanations of this surprising relationship between fees and supply.

8.6.4 DOCPOP and Physician Fees: A Positive Relationship?

One hypothesis concerning price formation in the physician services market is that when supply shifts out, price increases (Evans, 1974). This prediction is contrary to that of the competitive model, which predicts that price will fall when supply increases. The standard competitive model discussed in this chapter is represented geometrically in Figure 8-8. In this figure, D_1 represents an initial demand level and S_1 an initial supply level. The initial supply level corresponds to an initial supply of physicians (an initial level of *DOCPOP*). Let us now increase the level of *DOCPOP* to the point at which the supply shifts out to S_2. According to this theory, physicians will offer more services and as supply shifts out, prices will fall and utilization will increase. This prediction does not square with the alleged empirical fact that increases in price accompany increases in physician supply (*DOCPOP*). In order to fit the theory to the facts, a number of observers have contended that suppliers can shift out demand. For example, suppose the suppliers in our example could push the demand curve out to D_2. Even if the supply was to increase from S_1 to S_2, the equilibrium price would increase to P_3. Of course, supplier-induced demand

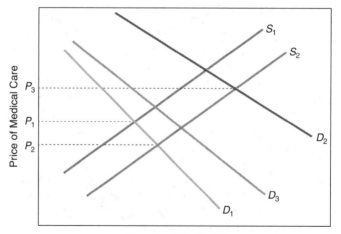

Quantity of Medical Care

Figure 8-8 Difficulties in Identifying Supplier-induced Demand Based on Actual Market Data. An increase in the physician population will result in an increase in supply from S_1 to S_2. Absence of supplier-induced demand, this will cause a fall in price from P_3 to P_1, a result of a movement along demand curve D_1. However, supplier-induced demand is consistent with both an increase in price (if demand shifts to D_2) and a reduction in price (if demand shifts, but only to D_3).

can also occur when prices *fall* after an outward shift in supply. If, following an increase in supply to S_2, suppliers were only successful in shifting the demand to D_3, the price would fall, even though suppliers had been successful in shifting the demand. Thus, a fall in price when supply increases is consistent with both the competitive and the supplier-induced demand theories! This makes it impossible to distinguish between them. Only when prices are observed to rise following an increase in *DOCPOP* and all else stays the same can we be sure that the supplier-induced demand model is the appropriate model.

The major problem in verifying the existence of supplier-induced demand lies in the fact that other demand- and supply-influencing variables are changing along with *DOCPOP*. Let us say that supply shifts from S_1 to S_2 and we observe a price increase from P_1 to P_3. In order to be sure that we are actually observing supplier-induced demand, we must be sure that we have controlled for all other variables that could affect demand and supply. For example, if S_1 represents supply conditions in Salt Lake City and S_2 conditions in San Antonio, the demand differences between the two markets may have occurred because of supplier-induced demand or myriad other demand-influencing factors, such as health status, quality of care, insurance coverage, and so on. Further, even if we have controlled for differences in *DOCPOP* between the two markets, we must be sure that other intervening supply variables have not resulted in greater increases (or decreases).

A number of statistical studies have been undertaken to estimate the extent of supplier-induced demand. The majority of these have focused their attention on *utilization* of medical care and how it has been influenced by *DOCPOP*. For example, Rossiter and Wilensky (1984) studied data obtained from a national sample survey of families (known as the National Medical Care Cost and Expenditure Survey) to determine the effect of a number of variables, such as direct price, travel time, health status, and the physician-to-population ratio, on the number of physician-initiated visits. Physician-initiated visits, although suggested by physicians, are not the same as physician-induced visits because the term *inducement* connotes lack of necessity. There is no way of telling from a dataset such as that used by the authors the degree to which physician-initiated visits were unnecessary and induced by physicians for their own benefit. The results of the study indicated a very small effect of *DOCPOP* on ambulatory care utilization: An increase in the ratio by one physician per 100,000 population resulted in an increase in expenditures on physician-initiated visits of only seven cents. However, the authors did not directly test the supplier-induced demand hypothesis.

Cromwell and Mitchell (1986) and Fuchs (1978), on the other hand, did directly test for the effect of supplier-induced demand in the market for surgery by examining the effect of surgeon population ratios on surgery utilization and surgeons' fees. The dataset in the Cromwell–Mitchell study consisted of metropolitan area statistics on families' characteristics and surgical utilization obtained from the Health Interview Survey of the National Center for Health Statistics coupled with Medicare surgical fee data. The authors studied how both surgical fees and surgery utilization rates differed among markets (metropolitan areas) when variables, such as age distribution, education level, average coinsurance rate, the number of general practitioners per 1,000 population, and the number of surgeons per 1,000 population, varied. They also controlled for the supply effect of higher fees causing more surgeons to locate in the area.

Their results indicated a price elasticity for surgical operations of −0.15, when all identified demand-shifting variables were held constant. With regard to the variable *DOCPOP* for surgeons, they identified a considerable effect of this variable on surgical utilization and on surgical fees. In the case of utilization, the magnitude of the relationship was such that a 10% increase in surgeons in the population resulted in a 9% increase in surgical operations. With regard to fee increases, a 1% increase in surgeons in the population resulted in a 0.9% increase in surgeons' fees. The authors presented these results as indicative of a significant supplier-induced demand effect in the market for surgery. However, because of the many variables influencing supply and demand and the difficulty of controlling for these in statistical tests, there is controversy surrounding any results in this area (Cooper, 2011; Dranove & Wehner, 1994; Feldman & Sloan, 1988; Mulley, 2009; Peacock & Richardson, 2007).

EXERCISES

1. Predict the effect of the following changes on the market price and quantity utilized of eye examinations conducted by ophthalmologists:
   a. An increase in the degree of insurance coverage for eye exams (i.e., lower insurance copayments by the patients)
   b. An increase in the number of ophthalmologists
   c. An increase in the average age of the population
   d. A reduction in the price of optometry services (which are substitute services)
   e. An increase in the price of eyeglasses, which are complementary goods
2. Given the initial demand and supply curves for prescription drugs and an equilibrium price and quantity, predict the direction of change of the equilibrium price and quantity if the following occur:
   a. More consumers enter the market
   b. The price of nonprescription drugs, which are substitutes, falls
   c. The price of bottled water, a complement, falls
   d. Consumers become more enamored with the wonders of modern drugs
   e. Consumers become better educated about the dangers of taking excess drugs
3. Given an initial equilibrium in the market for clinical care, predict the effect of the following changes on equilibrium price and quantity:
   a. An increase in nurses' wages in the clinic market
   b. An increase in the number of clinics
   c. An increase in clinic productivity
   d. A reduction in supply costs for clinics

4. Beginning with an initial equilibrium in the market for private, noninsured dermatology services, predict the effect on price and quantity for the following changes:
   a. An increase in consumer tastes for cosmetic dermatological services
   b. An increase in nurses' wages
   c. An increase in the severity of patient illness
   d. A reduced quality of care offered by dermatologists
5. For-Profit Labs, Inc. (FPL) is a private laboratory that does only routine blood counts. With total assets of $8 million last year, FPL took in $3 million in revenues and had expenses of $200,000. The average firms in other industries make a return of 10% on their assets. The market for lab services is potentially competitive, but right now there are only a few firms in the industry. However, lab technicians are free to enter the industry if they wish. Firms in the industry charge $300 for blood counts and their costs are $20. What do you expect will happen in the long run?
6. The market for physiotherapists is competitive. Chiropractic services and physiotherapy services are substitutes. Currently, the price per visit is $40 and the quantity utilized is 30,000 visits annually. Physiotherapists face stiff competition from chiropractors. Currently, chiropractors charge $35 per visit and there are 15,000 visits annually in the region. The chiropractic association has decided to license another 20 practitioners in the region. This will lower the price to $25 per visit. There is no change in the supply of physiotherapists. What will be the direction of the effect of the change in chiropractors on the price and quantity utilized for physiotherapy services?
7. The market for physiotherapist visits is shown in the accompanying diagram. The current equilibrium price is $30 and the equilibrium quantity is 150 visits. The healthcare authorities are concerned that the price is too high and so have proposed lowering the price to $10 per visit. They contend that at a lower price more people will get to use these services. Predict the effect on quantities demanded and supplied and on quantity of services actually utilized as a result of such an intervention.

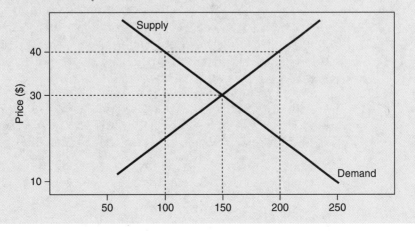

8. The equilibrium price for physiotherapy visits is $30 and the quantity utilized is 150 visits as a result of the demand and supply conditions in this diagram. The state legislature is concerned that the current price does not give the physiotherapists enough incentive to produce a high volume of services. A proposal has been made to increase the price paid by the consumers to the suppliers to $40. What will the resulting quantities demanded and supplied and the resulting utilization be?

9. The demand and supply for hospital care in the Garden State is given in the following diagram. Currently, the state legislature has mandated that all hospital care must be free and that providers will be reimbursed at a rate of $450 per day. The Hospital Association has expressed its concern that at this reimbursement rate, there will not be enough hospital care to "go around" and meet all the demands. It is proposed that the reimbursement rate be increased to $600 a day. What is the quantity demanded and supplied and the quantity utilized at the two rates? What is the total amount funded at the two rates?

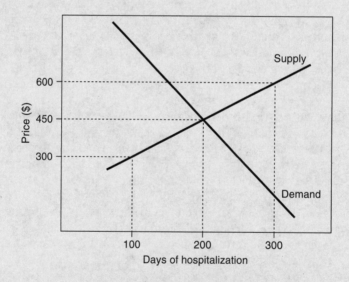

10. The state healthcare commission is planning to put out bids for hospital care. Key Hospital is considering making a bid but is unsure how much to bid. The hospital's actuary has developed four options: bid a price per case of $1,000, $800, $600, or $400. The hospital currently has a wealth level of $1,000. Added profits associated with each level are provided in the accompanying table. Also provided in this table are the estimated probabilities of each

of the four bids being accepted and the hospital board's utility of each wealth level. Given that the hospital is a risk averse, utility-maximizing entity, what bid should it make?

Option	Bid Price	Probability of Bid Being Accepted	Added Profits if Bid Accepted	Wealth Level if Bid is Accepted	Utility of a Given Level of Wealth
A	$1,000	0.2	$4,000	$5,000	380
B	800	0.4	3,000	4,000	340
C	600	0.6	2,000	3,000	280
D	400	0.8	1,000	2,000	200
No bid				1,000	100

BIBLIOGRAPHY

On the Competitive Market Model

Brameld, K., Holman, D., & Moorin, R. (2006). Possession of health insurance in Australia—How does it affect hospital use and outcomes? *Journal of Health Services & Research Policy, 11*(2), 94–100.

Buchanan, J. M. (1965). *The inconsistencies of the National Health Service.* Occasional paper 7. London, England: Institute of Economic Affairs.

Burns, J. (2009). Is the doctor in? Proven strategies for physician recruitment and retention. *Journal of Medical Practice Management, 24*(6), 344–346.

Christianson, J. B., & McClure, W. (1979). Competition in the delivery of medical care. *New England Journal of Medicine, 301,* 812–818.

Culyer, A. J., & Cullis, J. G. (1976). Some economics of hospital waiting lists in the NHS. *Social Policy, 5,* 239–264.

Drumm, T. L., Arkins, J. P., & Dayan, S. H. (2010). Retailicine, somewhere between retail and medicine. *Facial Plastic Surgery Clinics of North America, 18*(4), 491–498.

Evans, R. G. (1974). Supplier-induced demand. In M. Pearlman (Ed.), *The economics of health and medical care.* London, England: MacMillan.

Feldstein, M. S. (1970). The rising price of physicians' services. *Review of Economics and Statistics, 52,* 121–133.

Feldstein, M. S. (1974). Econometric studies in health economics. In M. Intriligator & S. Kendrick (Eds.), *Frontiers in quantitative economics.* Amsterdam, The Netherlands: North-Holland.

Frank, R. G., & Welch, W. P. (1985). The competitive effects of HMOs: A review of the evidence. *Inquiry, 22,* 148–161.

Friedman, M. (1962). *Capitalism and freedom.* Chicago, IL: University of Chicago Press.

Fuchs, V. R., & Kramer, M. (1972). *Determinants of expenditures for physicians' services in the United States, 1948–1968.* Publication no. HSM 73–3013. Washington, DC: National Center for Health Services Research.

Garbarino, J. W. (1959). Price behavior and productivity in the medical market. *Industrial and Labor Relations Review, 13,* 3–15.

Ginsburg, P. B. (2010). Wide variation in hospital and physician payment rates evidence of provider market power. *Research Briefs, 16,* 1–11.

Greene, V. L., Lovely, M. E., & Ondrich, J. I. (1993). Do community-based long-term care services reduce nursing home use? *Journal of Human Resources, 28,* 297–317.

Hay, J. W., & Leahy, M. J. (1984). Competition among health plans. *Southern Economic Journal, 50,* 831–846.

Kessell, R. (1958). Price discrimination in medicine. *Journal of Law and Economics, 1,* 20–53.

Lindsay, C. M. (1976). More real returns to medical education. *Journal of Human Resources, 11,* 127–129.

Mwabu, G., Ainsworth, M., & Nyamete, A. (1993). Quality of medical care and choice of treatment in Kenya. *Journal of Human Resources, 28,* 838–862.

Newhouse, J. P. (1970). A model of physician pricing. *Southern Economic Journal, 37,* 147–183.

Newhouse, J. P., Phelps, C. E., & Schwartz, W. B. (1977). Policy options and the impact of national health insurance revisited. *International Journal of Health Services, 7,* 503–509.

Otari, K., Waterman, B., Faulkner, K. M., Boslaugh, S., Burroughs, T. E., & Dunagan, W. C. (2009). Patient satisfaction: Focusing on "excellent." *Journal of Healthcare Management, 54*(2), 93–102.

Pauly, M. V., & Langwell, K. M. (1983). Research on competition in the market for health services. *Inquiry, 20,* 142–161.

Reschovsky, J. D., Hadley, J., Saiontz-Martinez, C. B., & Boukus. E. R. (2011). Following the money: Factors associated with the cost of treating high-cost Medicare beneficiaries. *Health Services Research, 46*(4), 997–1021.

Rizzo, J. A., & Zeckhauser, R. J. (1992). Advertising and the price, quantity, and quality of primary care physicians' services. *Journal of Human Resources, 28,* 387–421.

Ro, K. K. (1977). Anatomy of hospital cost inflation. *Hospitals and Health Services Administration, 22,* 78–88.

Salkever, D. (1978). Competition among hospitals. In W. Greenberg (Ed.), *Competition in the health care sector.* Washington, DC: Federal Trade Commission, Bureau of Economics.

Schwartz, W. B., & Mendelson, D. N. (1990). No evidence of an emerging physician surplus. *JAMA, 263,* 557–560.

Scott, A., & Shiell, A. (1997). Analysing the effect of competition on general practitioners' behavior using a multilevel modeling framework. *Health Economics, 6*(6), 577–588.

Shields, M. (2011). From clinical integration to accountable care. *Annals of Health Law, 20*(2), 151–164.

Sinanan, M., Wicks, K., Peccoud, M., Canfield, J., Poser, L., Sailer, L....Edwards, D. (2000). Formula for surgical practice resuscitation in an academic medical center. *American Journal of Surgery, 179*(5), 417–421.

Sloan, F. A. (1976). Real returns to medical education. *Journal of Human Resources, 11,* 118–126.

Sloan, F. A., & Feldman, R. (1978). Competition among physicians. In W. Greenberg (Ed.), *Competition in the health care sector.* Washington, DC: Federal Trade Commission, Bureau of Economics.

Sloan, F. A., & Lorant, J. H. (1976). The allocation of physicians' services. *Quarterly Review of Economics and Business, 16,* 86–103.

Soleimani, F., & Zenois, S. (2011). Disrupting incrementalism in health care innovation. *Annals of Surgery, 254*(2), 203–208.

Stensland, J., & Stinson, T. (2002). Successful physician-hospital integration in rural areas. *Medical Care, 40*(10), 908–917.

Stoeckle, J. D. (2000). From service to commodity: Corporization, competition, commodification, and customer culture transforms health care. *Croatian Medical Journal, 41*(2), 141–143.

Wu, W. S., & Masson, R. (1974). Price discrimination for physicians' services. *Journal of Human Resources, 9,* 63–79.

Zuckerman, A. M. (2011). How should the medical staff and hospital be aligned in a post-reform market? *Healthcare Financial Management, 65*(8), 134–135.

Zwanzinger, J., Melnick, G. A., & Mann, J. M. (1990). Measures of hospital market structure: A review of the alternatives and a proposed approach. *Socio-Economic Planning Sciences, 24*, 81–95.

Zwanzinger, J., Melnick, G. A., & Bamezaf, A. (2000). Can cost shifting continue in a price competitive environment? *Health Economics, 9*, 211–226.

Competitive Bidding

Benson, S. (2006). Is there life left in non-competes? Part 1. Physician non-compete agreements in contract negotiations. *Tennessee Medicine, 99*(11), 37–39.

Brown, E. R., Cousineau, M. R., & Price, W. T. (1985). Competing for Medi-cal business: why hospitals did, and did not, get contracts. *Inquiry, 22*, 237–250.

Christianson, J. B. (1984). Provider participation in competitive bidding for indigent patients. *Inquiry, 21*, 161–177.

Christianson, J. B. (1985). The challenge of competitive bidding. *Health Care Management Review, 10*(2), 39–54.

Christianson, J. B., Hillman, D. G., & Smith, K. R.. (1983). The Arizona experiment: Competitive bidding for indigent medical care. *Health Affairs, 2*, 87–103.

Christianson, J. B., Smith, K. R., & Hillman, D. G.. (1984). A comparison of existing and alternative competitive bidding systems for indigent medical care. *Social Science and Medicine, 18*, 599–604.

Davis, J. M. (2007). Non-acute care facility ownership: If not you, who? *Journal of Medical Practice Management, 22*(6), 346–347.

De Jaegher, K., & Jegers, M. (2001). The physician-patient relationship as a game of strategic information transmission. *Health Economics, 10*(7), 651–668.

Dranove, D., Shanley, M., & Simon, C. (1992). Is hospital competition wasteful? *Rand Journal of Economics, 23*, 247–262.

Elder, K., & Miller, N. (2006). Minority physicians and selective contracting in competitive market environments. *Journal of Health & Social Policy, 21*(4), 21–49.

Freeland, M. S., Hunt, S. S., & Luft, H. S. (1987). Selective contracting for hospital care based on volume, quality, and price. *Journal of Health Politics, Policy and Law, 12*, 409–426.

Gleicher, N. (2000). The consumer and provider: Pillars of the new health care system. *Physician Executive, 26*(2), 38–43.

Hoerger, T. J., & Meadow, A. (1997). Developing Medicare competitive bidding: A study of clinical laboratories. *Health Care Financing Review, 19*, 59–85.

Johns, L. (1989). Selective contracting in California: An update. *Inquiry, 26*, 345–353.

Johns, L., Derzon, R. A., & Anderson, M. D. (1985). Selective contracting in California: Early effects and policy implications. *Inquiry, 22*, 24–32.

Katz, H. S., & Knight, C. C. (1999). Selecting an MSO. How to assess options and compatibility. *Medical Group Management Journal, 46*(1), 29–34.

Keijser, G. M., & Kirkman-Liff, B. L. (1992). Competitive bidding for health insurance contracts. *Health Policy, 21*, 35–46.

Kirkman-Liff, B. L., Christianson, J. B., & Hillman, D. G. (1985). An analysis of competitive bidding by providers for indigent medical care contracts. *Health Services Research, 20*, 549–577.

McCall, N., Henton, D., Crane, M., Haber, S., Freund, D., & Wrightson, W. (1985). Evaluation of the Arizona health care cost containment system. *Health Care Financing Review, 7*, 77–88.

McCombs, J. S. (1989). A competitive bidding approach to physician payment. *Health Affairs, 8*(1), 50–64.

Melia, E. P., Aucoin, L. M., Duhl, L. J., & Kurokawa, P. D. (1983). Competition in the health care marketplace. A beginning in California *New England Journal of Medicine, 308*, 788–792.

Melnick, G. A., & Zwanzinger, J. (1988). Hospital behavior under competition and cost containment policies. *JAMA, 260,* 2669–2681.

Melnick, G. A., Zwanziger, J., Bamezal, A., & Pattison, R. (1992). The effects of market structure and bargaining position on hospital prices. *Journal of Health Economics, 11,* 217–233.

Miller, P., Rossiter, P., & Nuttall, D. (2002). Demonstrating the economic value of occupational health services. *Occupational Medicine, 52*(8), 477–483.

Mobley, L. R. (1998). Effects of selective contracting on hospital efficiency, costs and accessibility. *Health Economics, 7,* 247–262.

Pauly, M. V. (2011). Analysis & commentary: The trade-off among quality, quantity, and cost: How to make it—if we must. *Health Affairs, 30*(4), 574–580.

Robinson, J. C., & Luft, H. S. (1988). Competition, regulation, and hospital costs, 1982 to 1986. *JAMA, 260,* 2676–2681.

Robinson, J. C., & Phibbs, C. S. (1989). An evaluation of selective contracting in California. *Journal of Health Economics, 8,* 437–455.

Town, R., Feldman, R., & Kralewski, J. (2011). Market power and contract form: Evidence from physician group practices. *International Journal of Health Care Finance & Economics, 11*(2), 115–132.

Vaitkus, P. T., & Senesac, D. L. (1996). A two-step program of competitive bidding and physician feedback to reduce coronary angioplasty equipment costs. *American Journal of Cardiology, 78*(7), 829–832.

Zwanzinger, J., & Melnyck, G. A. (1988). The effects of hospital competition and the Medicare PPS program on hospital cost behavior in Ontario. *Journal of Health Economics, 7,* 301–320.

Supplier-Induced Demand

Auster, R. D., & Oxaca, R. L. (1981). The identification of supplier-induced demand in the health care sector. *Journal of Human Resources, 16,* 327–342.

Blackstone, E. A. (1980). Market power and resource misallocation in neurosurgery. *Journal of Health Politics, Policy and Law, 3,* 345–360.

Calcott, P. (1999). Demand inducement as cheap talk. *Health Economics, 8*(8), 721–733.

Carlsen, F., & Grytten, J. (1998). More physicians: Improved availability or induced demand? *Health Economics, 7,* 495–508.

Carlsen, F., & Grytten, J. (2000). Consumer satisfaction and supplier-induced demand. *Journal of Health Economics, 19*(5), 731–753.

Cooper, R. A. (2011). Geographic variation in health care and affluence-poverty nexus. *Advances in Surgery, 45,* 63–82.

Cromwell, J., & Mitchell, J. B. (1986). Physician-induced demand for surgery. *Journal of Health Economics, 5,* 293–313.

De Jaegher, K., & Jegers, M. (2000). A model of physician behavior with demand inducement. *Journal of Health Economics, 19*(2), 231–258.

Dranove, D. (1988). Demand inducement and the physician-patient relationship. *Economic Inquiry, 26,* 281–298.

Dranove, D., & Wehner, P. (1994). Physician-induced demand for childbirths. *Journal of Health Economics, 13,* 61–73.

Evans, R. G. (1974). Supplier-induced demand. In M. Perlman (Ed.), *The economics of health and medical care.* London, England: Macmillan.

Feldman, R., & Sloan, F. (1988). Competition among physicians. *Journal of Health Politics, Policy, and Law, 13,* 239–264.

Fuchs, V. (1978). The supply of surgeons and the demand for operations. *Journal of Human Resources, 13*(Suppl.), 35–55.

Hay, J. L., & Leahy, M. J. (1982). Physician-induced demand. *Journal of Health Economics, 1,* 231–244.

Hemenway, D., & Fallon, D. (1985). Testing for physician-induced demand with hypothetical cases. *Medical Care, 23,* 344–349.

Labelle, R., Stoddart, G., & Rice, T. (1994). A re-examination of the meaning and importance of supplier-induced demand. *Journal of Health Economics, 13,* 347–368.

Leonard, C., Stordeur, S., & Roberfroid, D. (2009). Association between physician density and health care consumption: A systematic review of the evidence. *Health Policy, 91*(2), 121–134.

Mulley, A. G. (2009). Inconvenient truths about supplier-induced demand and unwarranted variation in medical practice. *BMJ, 339,* b4073.

Pauly, M. V. (1979). What is unnecessary surgery? *Milbank Quarterly, 57,* 95–117.

Pauly, M. V. (1980). *Doctors and their workshops.* Chicago, IL: University of Chicago Press.

Pauly, M. V., & Satterthwaite, M. A. (1980). The pricing of primary care physicians' services. *Bell Journal of Economics, 12,* 488–506.

Peacock, S. J., & Richardson, J. R. (2007). Supplier-induced demand: Re-examining identification and misspecification in cross-sectional analysis. *European Journal of Health Economics, 8*(3), 267–277.

Reinhardt, U. (1978). Comment. In W. Greenberg (Ed.), *Competition in the health care sector.* Washington, DC: Federal Trade Commission.

Reinhardt, U. (1983). The theory of physician-induced demand and its implications for public policy. *Beitrage zur Gesundheitsökonomie, 4,* 153–172.

Rice, T. H. (1983). The impact of changing Medicare reimbursement rates on physician-induced demand. *Medical Care, 21,* 803–815.

Richardson, J. R., & Peacock, S. J. (2006). Supplier-induced demand: Reconsidering the theories and new Australian evidence. *Applied Health Economics & Health Policy, 5*(2), 87–98.

Rizzo, J. A., & Blumenthal, D. (1996). Is the target income hypothesis an economic heresy? *Medical Care Research and Review, 53,* 243–266.

Rossiter, L. F., &. Wilensky, G. R. (1983). A reexamination of the use of physician services. *Inquiry, 20,* 162–172.

Rossiter, L. F., & Wilensky, G. R. (1984). Identification of physician-induced demand. *Journal of Human Resources, 19,* 231–244.

Rossiter, L. F., & Wilensky, G. R. (1987). Health economist-induced demand for theories of physician-induced demand. *Journal of Human Resources, 12,* 624–626.

Smith, R. (2010). Why medicine is overweight. Don't forget inconvenient truth of supplier-induced demand. *BMJ, 340,* c3334.

Sorensen, R. J., & Grytten, J. (1999). Competition and supplier-induced demand in a health care system with fixed fees. *Health Economics, 8*(6), 497–508.

Stano, M. (1987a). A further analysis of the physician inducement controversy. *Journal of Health Economics 6*(3), 228–237.

Stano, M. (1987b). A further analysis of the "variations in practice style" phenomenon. *Inquiry, 23*(2), 176–182.

Van de Voorde, C., Van Doorslaer, E., & Schokkaert, E. (2001). Effects of cost sharing on physician utilization under favourable conditions for supplier-induced demand. *Health Economics, 10*(5), 457–471.

Xirasagar, S., & Lin, H. C. (2006). Physician supply, supplier-induced demand, and competition: Empirical evidence from a single-payer system. *International Journal of Health Planning & Management, 21*(2), 117–131.

Chapter 9

Market Power in Health Care

OBJECTIVES

1. Use the monopoly model to predict the price charged or quantity of services utilized.

2. Use the monopoly model to explain how providers are able to charge different groups of patients different prices.

3. Describe the functioning of a market in which the buyers have market power.

4. Describe a measure of market power and demonstrate how it can be applied in a market situation.

5. Describe the determinants of market power.

6. Explain the concept of nonprice competition and describe a model with market power and nonprice competition.

7. Demonstrate how the monopoly model can be used to predict resource allocation in markets with preferred provider organizations.

9.1 INTRODUCTION

Market power refers to the ability of one participant in a market to influence the terms by which he or she makes an exchange. Market power can be wielded by either buyers or sellers. For example, a heart surgeon can be in a position to influence the fee that patients or insurers pay. Similarly, an insurance company, or government health insurance program, can be in a position to influence the rate at which it pays providers for supplying services to its members.

Essential ingredients of market power are the limited availability of viable substitutes for the service and the ease with which buyers and sellers can weigh these alternatives. A hospital may be the only hospital for hundreds of miles, in which case, it possesses some degree of market power (i.e., it has some leeway in setting prices and other terms for the services it provides). On the other hand, a large number of HMOs may be vying to become providers for a firm's employees; in this case, the HMOs have little or no market power, although the firm may possess some.

Market power is important because, if possessed by buyers or sellers, it might allow them to wield influence over the use of resources to their benefit and to the detriment of the other bargaining parties. In this chapter, an analysis of how market power influences market outcomes (i.e., prices, quantities, and quality) is developed. The analysis is "explanatory," in the sense that the question being asked is how one set of factors (related to market power) influences specific phenomena. Discussion of the desirability (or undesirability) of market power must wait until yardsticks with which to gauge actual market conduct is discussed.

Several models are examined that explain resource allocation when either buyers or sellers possess some degree of market power. In Section 9.2, two models of the behavior of the ultimate wielder of market power—the monopolist—are examined that offer predictions about how monopolistic suppliers and demanders set price and quantity. All suppliers and demanders would benefit if they possessed market power, and so a pertinent question is, how does one obtain it? In Section 9.3, the determinants of market power are considered. This section includes a general discussion of market power, as well as an account of how providers in one market possessing many of the preconditions of a competitive market, the physician services market, were nevertheless able to develop and maintain a considerable degree of market power and use it to bolster their incomes.

The monopoly model and the competitive model are two polar extremes of models of market power. In many (perhaps most) markets, market power and competition are mixed to varying degrees. In Section 9.4, several models of incomplete market power are discussed that elucidate how product quality can be an important outcome in provider competition.

9.2 MONOPOLISTIC MARKETS

9.2.1 Simple Monopoly

A supplier has monopoly in a market when it is the sole source of supply in that market. In a monopolistic market, the demanders do not have any close substitutes for the service, and there are barriers to the entry of new sellers. Of course, some substitutability usually exists. For example, in health care, an alternative to treatment usually exists, even if that alternative is to do nothing.

The monopoly model will be developed in the context of a supposed monopolistic market, the market for pediatric ambulatory services. It is assumed that, in this market, there is a single group practice. The product is defined as quality-constant pediatric visits. The simple monopoly model consists of demand, cost, and behavioral assumptions.

9.2.2 Demand

With regard to demand, it is assumed that the pediatric group faces a single market demand curve (see Table 9-1 and Figure 9-1). Note that there is a price ($100) at which patients will abstain from making any visits. As one

Table 9-1   Revenue and Cost in a Hypothetical Monopolistic Market

(1)	(2)	(3)	(4)	(5)	(6)	(7)
Price	Units of Output	Total Revenue (TR)	Marginal Revenue (MR)	Total Cost (TC)	Marginal Cost (MC)	Profits (TR – TC)
$100	0	$0	$—	$30	$—	$–30
90	1	90	90	40	10	50
80	2	160	70	60	20	100
70	3	210	50	90	30	120
60	4	240	30	130	40	110
50	5	250	10	180	50	70
40	6	240	–10	240	60	0
30	7	210	–30	310	70	–100

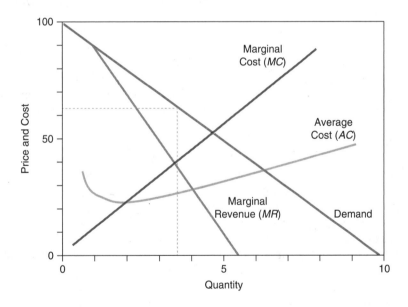

Figure 9-1   Equilibrium Price (P) and Output (Q) in a Monopolistic (Single Seller) Market. The monopolist faces a given demand curve for the service, and from this curve is derived its marginal revenue (MR) curve. The monopolist's cost conditions are presented in marginal (MC) and average (AC) terms. The profit-maximizing monopolist will set price and quantity such that its MR = MC. Equilibrium price is between $60 and $70, and equilibrium quantity is between 3 and 4 units. (This graph is based on data in Table 9-1).

moves down the demand curve, one moves through elastic, unit elastic, and inelastic portions of the demand curve, and the total revenue (*TR*) will increase, level off, and decrease. The marginal revenue (*MR*) is falling throughout, although it is positive when it is associated with the elastic portion of the demand curve and zero at the unit elastic point on the demand curve. For the provider, the *MR* represents the additional *TR* that it will receive by lowering the price enough to sell one more visit. Note that as the provider lowers its price, it sells more units, but all of them are sold at the new, lower price. The *MR* is the net change in *TR* and is equal to the difference in the two *TR*s at the two quantity levels.

The monopolist has the ability to set prices at any level it wishes. This ability represents the ultimate degree in market power. (Of course, the price it sets will influence the quantity demanded, something the monopolist will want to keep in mind when setting the price.)

9.2.3 Cost

Our cost assumptions are that the total fixed cost (*TFC*) is $30 and that the total variable cost (*TVC*) is increasing in such a way that marginal cost (*MC*) increases as output expands (see Table 9-1, column 6). The total cost (*TC*) is the sum of *TVC* and *TFC*.

9.2.4 Objectives

Profits (column 7) are equal to *TR* − *TC*, and they initially increase and then decrease as output expands. But what price will be charged and what output (and profit) levels will be attained cannot be determined until we know what objectives the provider is pursuing. It is initially assumed that the provider's objective is to maximize profits.

The analysis of the model is as follows. First, the price will be set at that point on the demand curve at which *MR* comes closest to (or equals) *MC* (without *MC* exceeding *MR*). Assume that the monopolist initially sets its price at $100 per visit. It would have no buyers at such a price (see Table 9-1), and its losses would be confined to its fixed costs because it would have no variable costs at zero output. If price was lowered to $90, one visit would be sold and the *MR* would be $90. One additional visit would cost only $10 extra (*MC* = $10) and would add $80 to the previous output level's profits. Total profit would therefore be $50. This is certainly better than not operating at all, but not as good as lowering the price to $80, selling two units in total and deriving an additional $70 in revenue in the process (*MR* = $70). For then it would cost the pediatricians only $20 more to provide this added visit, and they would be adding another $50 (*MR* − *MC*) to the previous profit level, making the profits $100 in total. Indeed, the practice would lower its price to $70, selling three visits. It would stop there because beyond this level of output, *TC* increases more than *TR* increases, and as a result *MR* − *MC* becomes negative. Any further increase in output would detract from total profits.

This analysis is shown graphically in Figure 9-1, which has smoothed-out revenue and cost functions. Here it is seen that the *MR* and *MC* curves intersect (meaning *MR* = MC) at a quantity of between 3 and 4 (because of our smoothed-out values). This corresponds to a price on the demand curve of between $60 and $70. Profitability cannot be increased by raising or lowering the price.

Let us now see what the model implies. First, the provider will set the price at that point on the demand curve above where the *MR* and *MC* curves intersect. Because *MC* is positive, *MR* must also be positive (because *MR* = *MC* at the profit-maximizing point). It should be noted that *MR* is positive only at those quantities that correspond to the *elastic* portion of the demand curve. Therefore, a monopolist will set the price only on the elastic portion of its demand curve. Indeed, if the price was set on the inelastic portion of the curve, say at $30, *MR* would be negative, meaning that a reduction in output coming from a price increase would raise total revenues. At the same time, a reduction in output would reduce *TC*. Profits would therefore always be greater at a higher price (one on the elastic portion of the demand curve). See Table 9-2 for a further explanation of the relationship between price elasticity and total revenue.

In addition, because the most profitable level of output is determined by *MR* and *MC* alone, and because *MC* is unaffected by fixed costs, the profit-maximizing price will similarly be unaffected by changes in fixed costs. Let us say that fixed costs in the example increase to $50. Profits would be lower by $20 at every level of output. But the maximum profit level of output would still be the same (at Q = 3), only now the provider would be earning less profit. This important result implies that if the provider's fixed costs increase (e.g., because of an increase in mortgage rates), it cannot do anything about it. If it tries to pass on these added fixed costs to the consumer by raising the price, it will only be moving away from the profit-maximizing position; in raising the price, it will sell less, and total revenue will decrease more than total cost. This of course is not true for an increase in variable costs (i.e., *MC*).

In a similar vein, if the profit-maximizing monopolist received a fixed subsidy (i.e., one unrelated to output) of $20 to treat poor patients, *TR* would be increased at every level of output by $20, but *MR* would not be affected. The monopolist's profit-maximizing price will not change. That is, the profit-maximizing monopolist will not lower the price to induce people to demand more.

Understanding price elasticity is very important because of the relationship between price elasticity and total revenue. If demand is price elastic, then an increase in price will cause total revenue to decrease, because the percent change in quantity demanded is greater than the percent change in price.

Table 9-2 Total Revenue (TR) Resulting from Elasticity.

(1)	(2)	(3)
Elasticity	*Price Increase*	*Price Decrease*
Inelastic (<1)	TR Increases	TR Decreases
Elastic (>1)	TR Decreases	TR Decreases
Unitary (=1)	TR the Same	TR the Same

One outcome of the monopoly model is that the firm could be persistently earning excess profits. Because the *AC* curve incorporates all the monopolist's costs, including opportunity costs, the monopolist's profits in this analysis are equal to *TR* − *TC* or, using average terms, the product of the unit margin (*P* − *AC*) and output (*Q*). These profits are true economic profits. That is, they are profits over and above all the costs required to operate the enterprise, including a normal return for the owner's efforts and capital. Furthermore, nothing in the model will allow the monopolist's profits to be bid away. There are no potential entrants into the market who can charge a lower price. As a result, the monopolist can earn above-normal profits that persist over time. Note the contrast with the competitive market model, in which entry is inexpensive and any excess profits will attract new entrants who will expand supply and lower price and profits.

9.2.5 Price Discrimination

Under some conditions, a monopolist can further increase its profits by charging different prices for the same product to different buyers. This is called *price discrimination*, which can be practiced only when there is market segmentation and the product or service in the lower price market cannot be resold (a secondary exchange) in the higher price market. In addition, the demand elasticities in the two markets have to be different to make the practice worthwhile.

Now, assume that a pediatric practice can separate its patients into two distinct markets according to patient income. Assume further that demand elasticity is influenced by income so that each market will have a different demand curve. Thus, one of the preconditions for price discrimination is met. The product sold is patient visits. These can hardly be sold in one market and resold in the other, so the other precondition is met as well. The demand curves for the two separate markets, "rich" and "poor," are shown in Figure 9-2, graphs A and B. The cost assumption is that the *MC* eventually rises, as shown in graph C. Note that there is one *MC* for the entire operation; production is not separated. The behavioral assumption is that the pediatric practice seeks to maximize its profits.

Given these assumptions, the monopolistic model can be used to elucidate the monopolist's pricing policy. In doing so, we must rely on the equimarginal principle of maximization. To maximize profits, the provider will set the price (and therefore the quantity) in each market, so that (1) the *MR* earned by lowering (raising) the price in all markets is the same; and (2) overall the *MR* in each market is equal to the *MC* of producing that total level of output.

The derivation of the profit-maximizing prices is shown in Figure 9-2. The curve *MC* shows the provider's marginal cost for all units provided (it does not have a separate cost for each market), and the curve *SMR* shows the quantity that would be supplied overall, when the firm allocated output to each market according to the specific level of *MR*. *SMR* is thus the sum of quantities in both markets at a given level of *MR*. Given the *MR* curves for the poor and the rich markets (MR_p and MR_r) at an *MR* level in both markets

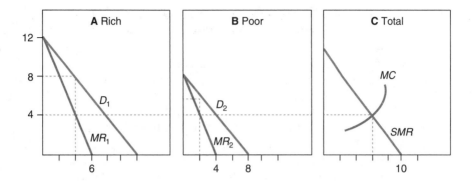

Figure 9-2 Price Setting by Discriminating Monopolist. If the monopolist can separate its market into two submarkets, "rich" and "poor," the price charged in each submarket will be derived from firm-level conditions, and will occur where the *MR* in the submarket equals the overall *MC* to the firm. The curve *SMR* in Graph *C* shows the total quantity in all submarkets at each level of *MR*. Note that the equilibrium occurs in each market at the same value of *MR*.

of \$40, the corresponding quantities in the markets are 4 and 2, respectively. The *SMR* curve for those quantities will be at a quantity of 6, in which $Q_m = Q_p + Q_r$.

The firm's maximum profit position will be determined by equating *MC* with the *MR* in each market. Overall, this occurs when *MC* = *SMR* (at quantity 6). The corresponding outputs in each market are 4 and 2, and the prices in the two markets that equate the *MR*s are \$80 and \$60, respectively. Profits, which are equal to the sum of *TR* in each market less *TC*, will be greater than if the same price was set in all markets.

Price discrimination such as this cannot exist in a competitive market, and this is one reason why physician pricing has been characterized as monopolistic. In a competitive market, if two submarkets had different prices, "traders" would buy goods in the low price market and resell them (at a higher price, but below the market price) in the second market. For many years, physicians, particularly specialists, resorted to a sliding scale of fees when setting prices, charging the richer patients more than the poorer ones (Kessell, 1958). By the 1970s, physician services became more highly insured, and the sliding scale all but disappeared by that time (Filler, 2007; Gattuso, 1997; Greenberg, Peiser, Peterburg, & Pliskin, 2001; Newhouse, 1970).

9.2.6 Physician Pricing and Supply in Public Programs

A variant of the two-payer monopoly model outlined in Section 9.2.5 has been used to explain physician pricing and supply in relation to the payment policies of Blue Shield (Sloan & Steinwald, 1978), Medicare (Paringer, 1980; Rice, 1984), and Medicaid (Cromwell & Mitchell, 1984; Hadley, 1979; Kushman, 1977) and the 1972–1975 price limitations set by the Economic Stabilization Program (Hadley & Lee, 1978/1979).

The Medicare studies examined the effect of Medicare payment levels (80% of the reasonable charges) on the assignment decision—the decision of physicians to accept the Medicare-determined fee as full payment for their services. On an individual-case basis, physicians were allowed to accept Medicare assignment of their patients. A physician who accepted the reasonable fee in full (i.e., who accepted assignment) for a specific patient receives 80% of the fee directly from Medicare and could bill the patient for the copayment. If the physician did not accept assignment for that patient, he or she could bill the patient whatever fee he or she chose. In this case, Medicare would reimburse the patient directly for 80% of its reasonable fee, and the physician would collect the entire charge from the patient. The acceptance by physicians of assignment relieves patients from the financial risks associated with higher physician fees. Currently, physicians can no longer decide to accept assignment on a case-by-case basis. Instead, the physician must choose to accept the Medicare-approved amount as payment in full on all claims or none. When the physician agrees to accept assignment, then the patient may only be billed for the deductible and coinsurance amounts.

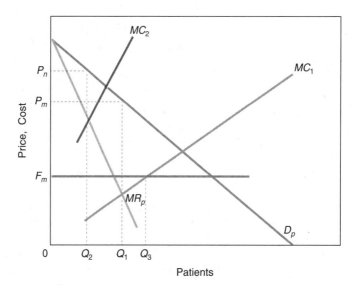

Figure 9-3 Price Setting by Monopolist Facing Private Market and a Publicly Financed Market. In this market, demand is represented by D_p, marginal revenue by MR_p, and with the publicly financed market having a set fee, marginal revenue is represented by F_m. With a marginal cost of MC_1, the monopolist will set the price to equate the MR in both markets. In this case, the price in the private market is set at P_m. The marginal revenue for public and private patients will be the same, MR_p. Total output supplied is Q_3, with $Q_3 - Q_1$ going to public patients. With an MC such as MC_2, the monopolist would not supply any output to the public patients; the price and output levels in the private market would be P_n and Q_2.

The analysis is set out graphically in Figure 9-3. The physician is assumed to be a monopolist facing two submarkets: one with private patients and one with patients in a public program. (The extra billing is ignored in this analysis.) The output is defined as patients served. D_p is the demand curve for private patients, and MR_p is the related MR curve. The public agency reimburses the physicians for its patients at a fee level of F_m; because the fee level is fixed, F_m is also the physician's MR for public patients. Assume that the physician's MC curve is at MC_1. Finally, assume that the physician is a profit maximizer.

According to the equimarginal principle, the physician will supply services to Q private and $(Q_3 - Q_1)$ public patients because at this output $MR_p = F_m$ and both are equal to MC_1. The private patients will be charged a price of Pm. To attract any additional private patients, the physician would have to lower the price to private patients below P_m, which would imply an MR for private patients below that for public patients. A profit-maximizing physician will thus prefer to serve additional public patients for which the MR is constant at a level F_m rather than lower his or her price and have a marginal revenue below F_m.

A lower public fee would lower the supply to the public patients (it would also cause the physician to lower his or her private fee because the physician will now move down the MR_p curve). A physician facing the same demand curve, but with a higher MC (say, MC_2), will not supply any services to public patients and will set a private fee of P_n. This analysis demonstrates that the public and private sectors are interdependent. A public program that lowers fees will reduce the supply to the public market and will also affect the private market.

A model similar to the one discussed in the previous section has been used to explain hospital cost shifting, a tactic purportedly used by hospitals to raise fees on self-pay and commercially insured patients in response to low payment levels by Medicare, Medicaid, and in some instances, Blue Cross (Danzon, 1982; Dobson, Davanzo, & Sen, 2006; Dowless, 2007; Frakt, 2011; Sloan & Becker, 1984; Sloan & Ginsburg, 1984; Zimmerman, 2011).

9.2.7 Nursing Home Markets and Public Rates

The two-payer monopoly model is also suited to analyzing economic behavior in the nursing home market. Care provided in nursing homes generally enhances quality of life rather than curing a particular problem. The demand for long-term care reflects a basic demand rather than a derived demand. Generally in this market, there are two major groups of payers: self-pay (relatively uninsured) patients and state Medicaid agencies. Many Medicaid agencies pay nursing homes a flat rate, whereas self-pay patients are charged according to market conditions. With Medicaid agencies being economy minded and having the power to set rates, one option they have in pursuing the goal of budget containment is to set low rates. In doing so, they must recognize the tradeoffs involved.

Because the nursing homes can differentiate their products, they can develop some form of "brand loyalty" on the part of patients and prospective patients. When they have patients with some degree of preference, nursing homes will face demand curves that have some elasticity (i.e., are downward sloping). The more loyal their patients are, the more inelastic their demand curves will be.

Figure 9-3 can therefore be interpreted as pertaining to nursing home markets. In this diagram, assume that F_m is the rate that Medicaid pays to nursing homes, D_p is the demand of private-pay patients, and MC_1 is a nursing home's marginal cost. At the fee level (and marginal revenue) of F_m, the nursing home will equate its marginal cost so that it is equal to the MR for each class of patients. It will therefore serve Q_3 patients, with Q_1 of these being private and $Q_3 - Q_1$ being Medicaid. If the Medicaid agency lowered its rates below F_m, fewer Medicaid patients (and more private-pay patients) would be served. Shortages of Medicaid patient nursing home beds would therefore appear (Grabowski, 2002; Gulley & Santerre, 2007; Paringer 1980).

From a structural perspective, nursing home markets resemble a monopolistically competitive industry. The nursing home provider basically faces three market segments. One segment reflects the private-pay market for residents paying more than the state-set Medicaid rate. This segment faces a downward-sloping demand curve. The second segment is the Medicaid-eligible people in the market, and because Medicaid pays a single rate, the demand curve is horizontal. The nursing home cannot impact the price received for these residents. The remaining supply is provided to private-pay residents who pay less than the Medicaid rate. As long as the nursing home has excess capacity and the price received covers fixed costs and some variable costs, nursing homes will sell services to this downward-sloping demand.

9.3 MONOPSONY—BUYERS' MARKET POWER

A large buyer that faces many small sellers may be in a position to exert market power. Market power possessed by buyers is referred to as *monopsony*. In the healthcare sector, the monopsony model has been applied to situations as diverse as the labor market for nurses, the purchase of hospital services by such big insurers such as Blue Cross plans (Foreman, Wilson, & Scheffler, 1996; Staten, Dunkelbert, & Umbeck, 1987), the purchase of specialized medical services by managed care plans (Pauly, 1998), and the procurement of organs for transplant (Barnett, Beard, & Kaserman, 1993).

The basic monopsony model can be illustrated by the example of a large hospital chain that is a purchaser of aspirin. The supply curve faced by the monopsonist is the result of many small sellers' willingness to produce and sell aspirin at any given price. Higher prices result in a greater quantity supplied, so the supply curve looks like S in Figure 9-4.

For the monopsonist, however, the supply price associated with any quantity of aspirin does not give a true indication of the cost to it of expanding its purchases. In order to induce suppliers to sell added quantities, it must offer a higher price. Of course, it must pay this higher price, not just on the

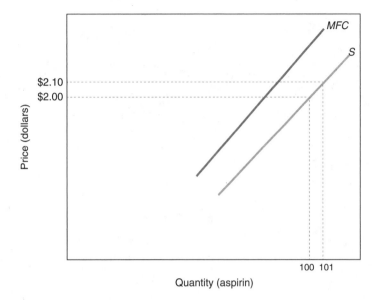

Figure 9-4 Supply and Marginal Factor Costs (*MFC*) for Buyer with Market Power. The *MFC* curve is derived from the supply curve (*S*).

added purchases, but on all its purchases. This means that for the monopsonist, the marginal cost of an additional unit of aspirin is higher than its price. This is illustrated in Figure 9-4. Initially, the buyer is purchasing 100 units at a price of $2, spending a total of $200. To induce sellers to supply 101 units, the price offered must rise to $2.10. The new total spending on aspirin is thus $2.10 × 101 = $212.10. So the added expense is not just the $2.10 price for the 101st unit, but also the additional $10 paid on the initial 100 units. The expense of adding another unit of an input for a monopsonist is called the *marginal factor cost* (*MFC*), and it will be higher than the supply price, as shown by the *MFC* curve.

Because there are many substitutes for aspirin, the hospital chain will have a somewhat elastic demand curve, indicating its marginal benefit for any quantity (based on increased revenue the input will enable it to earn). In making a purchase decision, it will weigh this marginal benefit against the *MFC* and buy the quantity at which these two are equal. At any quantity less than this, there would be increased profit as a result of expanding purchases. At any higher quantity, profit would be enhanced by a reduction in quantity purchased.

The result is shown in Figure 9-5. A total of Q_0 units will be purchased at a price of P_0 per unit. The contrast of this result with the result that would occur in perfect competition is noteworthy. If the demand curve had represented the total demand of many small buyers, equilibrium would have been at P_cQ_c. So the effect of monopsony is to decrease price and quantity compared to what would occur in perfect competition.

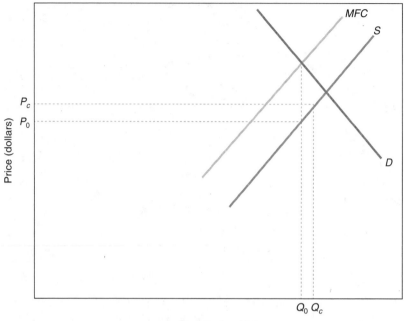

Figure 9-5   Price Setting with Buying Power. *D* is the monopsonist's demand curve and indicates marginal benefit to the monopsonist of an additional unit purchased. To maximize profit, the monopsonist would purchase the quantity at which marginal benefit (*MB*) equals *MFC* (Q_0 in this case). The price paid for this amount is P_0. Under monopsony, price and quantity (P_0, Q_0) are lower than they would be under perfect competition (P_c, Q_c).

9.4 MARKET STRUCTURE AND ITS DETERMINANTS

9.4.1 Measuring Market Concentration

Market structure has a major influence on market power. Structure is usually presented in terms of an index, or percentage, representing the size of the largest firm (or four firms or eight firms) relative to the overall market's output, or else measuring the distribution of firm size in the market. A four-firm concentration ratio shows the percentage of the total market (in terms of sales, assets, or some other indicator of firm size) represented by the largest four firms. For example, a completely monopolized market has a concentration ratio of 100%; a market with 20 firms, total sales of $1 billion, and combined sales for the largest four firms of $500 million would have a four-firm concentration ratio of 50%. The choice of four or eight firms is arbitrary and does not indicate the concentration of the remainder of the market. A more general measure of concentration, which incorporates all firms in the market, is the Herfindahl (*H*) index. According to this index, concentration is measured as

$$H = \Sigma(S/M)^2 \times 10,000$$

in which S is the size of each firm and M is the size of the total market. The figure 10,000 is used as a multiplier because H is usually presented as a sum of percentages expressed in absolute terms. The summation sign (Σ) indicates summation over all firms. Thus, if a monopolist with sales of $200 is the only firm in the market, its H index is (200/200) $\times$ 10,000, or 10,000. If there were three hospitals, each with sales of $100, the H index for that market would be 3,300 [$\Sigma(100/300)^2 \times 10,000$].

There is no true cutoff point for a concentrated versus a nonconcentrated market, although a figure of about 1,800 is sometimes used (Wilder & Jacobs, 1986). Generally, it is thought that the greater the degree of concentration, the greater will be the ability of the leading firms to influence price, quantity, and other characteristics of output.

9.4.2 Determinants of Market Structure

Market structure can be thought of as having market and governmentally imposed (regulatory) determinants. Let us examine these in the context of the health insurance market. In the United States, the health insurance market is largely a localized market; in part because each state requires operating licenses for any insurance company operating within the state and also because of unique relationships between local providers and some insurers (primarily the Blues). Aside from government insurance, health insurance has been broken down into two categories of operators: the Blues and the commercial insurance companies. The Blues comprise Blue Cross (for hospitalization insurance) and Blue Shield (for medical and other insurance). In some states, the two plans are combined. Originally, the Blues were tax exempt in terms of organization. Commercial insurers include a large number of mutual (member owned) and commercial (investor owned) firms, none of which has a substantial share of the healthcare market. Blue Cross and Blue Shield collects about one-quarter of the total health insurance premiums nationally, although their share of the private insurance market varies considerably by state. Currently, the Blues have converted from tax-exempt organizations to investor-owned organizations.

9.4.3 Economies of Scale

Among the most important market determinants of market power are economies of scale, which reflect an increase in efficiency of production as the number of goods or services produced increases. Usually, the average cost per unit of output decreases when economies of scale are achieved because fixed costs are shared over an increased number of units of output, and usage level of inputs increases more slowly than usage level of outputs.

Now assume that the market demand for private health insurance is D_m in Figure 9-6, and that the long-run average cost curve for a state-of-the-art insurance company is LAC. Two things should be noted in the example. First, the long-run average cost incorporates capital and other fixed setup costs, as well as current operating costs; if there are high start-up costs for the industry, the LAC at low output levels will be quite high. Second, the LAC, in the

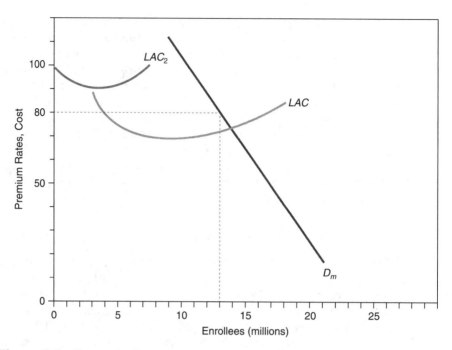

Figure 9-6 Output in Insurance Market Under Alternative Cost Conditions. D_m represents market demand for insurance coverage. If the cost conditions are represented by cost curve *LAC*, one firm can capture a substantial portion of the market by virtue of its economies of scale and pricing policies. A producer with the cost conditions represented by *LAC* could set a price of $80; if it did so and chose to supply 13 million policies (as shown by the dashed lines), another producer with the same cost conditions could not reach a large enough scale of output to match the first producer's cost (and price). If the cost conditions were represented by LAC_2, no producer could dominate the market in this way.

example, includes insurance administration costs and the amount the insurance company reimburses the providers. In the example, the shape of the *LAC* curve is such that the minimum cost is reached at a large scale of output (about 12 million subscribers).

9.4.4 Pricing Policies

Given certain cost conditions, one firm could capture a considerable portion of the market. To do so however, it must resort to a second, and related, market share determinant: pricing policy. If the insurance company sets a very low price relative to costs of other insurers (represented by the curve LAC_2), say, $80 per subscriber per month, market demand would be quite large (20 million subscribers). In this case, the insurance company would have considerable discretion in choosing its own output level; the level chosen would depend of course on its objectives. If it provided services for 13 million subscribers at this price, there would be an excess demand of

7 million potential subscribers. If the technology of insurance provision was known to other potential entrants, a second firm could provide insurance on a cost basis like that represented by the *LAC* curve. However, to reach a unit cost of $80, it would need to operate at a scale of 8 million subscribers. Because the potential entrant could not obtain such a volume, it might simply produce at a higher cost, charge a higher price, and obtain a smaller share of the residual market.

The final distribution of market shares will thus depend on the size of potential economies of scale relative to the potential market and also on the pricing policies of the larger firms. As seen in Figure 9-6, if the initial insurance company charged a higher price, say, $90 or $100, potential entrants would have less problem gaining an entry to the market.

On the other hand, if the state-of-the-art cost curve was like LAC_2 (with no substantial economies of scale), no firm could obtain a substantial share of the market, and a concentration of firms would be unlikely. There is some evidence economies of scale exist in health insurance operations, but these economies are not of the magnitude that would permit a single firm to dominate the health insurance market (Beaulieu, 2004; Blair, Jackson, & Vogel, 1975; Carroll, 2011; Town, Feldman, & Kralewski, 2011).

9.4.5 Input Prices and Taxes

A third cause of market concentration relates not to the cost-scale relation, but to the potentially different levels of cost curves for different providers. If, for example, one provider could obtain its inputs (workers, materials, etc.) at a lower cost than a second provider, its cost curve would be lower at all scales of output than the cost curve of the second provider. The first firm could capture a larger share of the market by turning its cost advantage into a price differential. One such input price differential is the discount that many Blue Cross plans receive from hospitals (Feldman & Greenberg, 1981a, 1981b; Goldberg & Greenberg, 1985), which is perhaps partly due to the special traditional relationship between Blue Cross and hospitals (Blue Cross was founded by hospitals). Whereas commercial insurance companies typically have paid hospitals for close to full charges, about half of the Blue Cross plans have received discounts ranging from 2 to 30% and averaging from 8 to 15%. These discounts have the effect of lowering the *LAC* curves of the Blue Cross plans relative to the commercial ones, allowing Blue Cross to gain an increased market share by charging lower premium rates. One earlier estimate attributed 7% of Blue Cross's market share to this cost differential (Feldman & Greenberg, 1981a, 1981b).

9.4.6 Regulation

There might also be regulatory causes of market concentration. Like the Blue Cross discount, discriminatory regulations can give one firm, or type of firm, a cost advantage that allows it to lower price and increase market share. One such regulation was the tax on health insurance premiums, which was imposed on commercial insurance companies in all states; in some states, the

Blue plans were exempt from such a tax, which was about 2% of premiums. In addition, the Blue plans, being nonprofit, were exempt from income taxes and in some states, from property taxes. Such exemptions lowered the Blues' total costs, giving them a cost advantage. This cost advantage was lost when the Blues lost their tax-exempt status and were forced to convert to investor-owned status.

However, these advantages need not always result in a larger market share. Firms can incur costs providing on-the-job benefits for the managers. This is particularly true for nonprofit firms, whose profits cannot be directly shared by the managers. Thus, any cost advantage possessed by a nonprofit firm can be appropriated by the managers rather than be passed on to consumers in the form of lower premiums. On-the-job amenities have been hypothesized to be a factor in the behavior of Blue Shield plans that were not "controlled" by physicians. Blue Shield plans deemed to be physician controlled were found to have lower operating costs. One possible explanation is that the physician-controlled plans passed on surpluses to the physicians in the form of payments. Nonphysician-controlled plans could appropriate potential surpluses and in the process, generate higher operating costs (Clark & Thurston, 2000; Einav & Finkelstein, 2011; Eisenstadt & Kennedy, 1981; Enders, 1995).

9.4.7 Market Power in the Market for Physicians' Services

Market structure and market power are not always equivalent. In the physician services market, there are a number of manifestations of market power, and yet the market structure does not have a high degree of provider concentration. For instance, for many years, physicians were able to maintain a sliding scale of fees (charging different prices for the same services), indicating price discrimination. Also, their incomes have been well above normal, even allowing for the high cost of medical training. Yet significant economies of scale in medical practice are not present, and there is a very low degree of market concentration, conditions that normally accompany monopolistic pricing and profit levels.

The explanation of this paradox is that the medical profession developed a mechanism of control to police its members and prevent them from engaging in such competitive practices as price cutting (Kessell, 1958; Rayack, 1970). This control mechanism was basically in the hands of organized medical associations at the county, state, and national levels.

The key players were the teaching hospitals, the American Medical Association (AMA), the local medical associations, and practicing physicians, especially specialists (see Figure 9-7). The operation of the mechanism depended on the fact that it benefited several of the key groups: (1) residents were an important (and low-cost) input in the operation of teaching hospitals, and (2) physicians, especially specialists, needed membership on hospital medical staffs to make a good, secure living.

The basis of the mechanism was a convention developed by the AMA regarding the certification of teaching hospitals. According to this convention, known as the Mundt Resolution, hospitals that were certified as teaching hospitals were advised that their medical staffs should be composed only

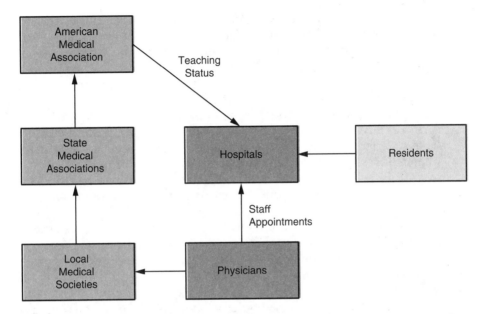

Figure 9-7 Control Mechanisms that Exist in the Medical Profession. Key players include hospitals with teaching programs that require accreditation from the Council on Teaching Hospitals (AMA associated) and physicians (who benefit from staff appointments in hospitals). Membership in local medical societies was required for a staff appointment to a hospital, a regulation enforced by the AMA through its control over hospital accreditation. Local medical societies could enforce regulations (regarding pricing policies, for example) through their control over membership.

of physicians who were members of local medical societies. Because the AMA certified teaching hospitals, the resolution carried great weight.

Here is an example of how the resolution helped to limit competitive behavior on the part of physicians. County medical association members generally disapproved of price cutting and other competitive practices. One target of disapprobation was prepaid group medicine. Prepaid group practices (proto-HMOs) charged a single fee for all members, thus undermining the price discrimination system that had become prevalent. The expulsion of physicians who joined prepaid group practice staffs from county medical societies occurred in several instances (Kessell, 1958), and the threat of expulsion was sufficient to make physician recruitment difficult for these practices. In addition, other competitive activities, such as advertising, were also discouraged by the organized medical profession.

The control of competitive practices by the medical profession at-large has not relied solely on such formal mechanisms. With the growth of specialization, physicians have become increasingly dependent on referrals from colleagues. Physicians who engaged in competitive practices could be "controlled" to some degree if they lost referrals from colleagues (Cooper & Kramer, 2010; Havighurst, 1978; Trunkey, 2011).

In recent years, there has been a considerable amount of regulatory activity, especially on the part of the federal government, to contain anticompetitive practices on the part of physicians and other healthcare providers. One such activity is the Stark Law, which prohibits referring patients to an entity in which the physician or a family member has a financial relationship. This law provides significant civil penalties, but not criminal penalties, substantially affecting costs of providing services. Mergers and acquisitions in health care also receive careful scrutiny to ensure that the resulting entity does not have sufficient market power to provide fewer choices for consumers, charge higher prices, and/or provide worse service. In addition, attention is given to ensure healthcare providers don't establish "destroyer prices" to prevent entry into the market or bankrupt existing providers to reduce competition in the area.

The number of acquisitions in the healthcare industry, especially among hospitals and hospital systems, has been intense in recent years. Although these activities are often presented as enabling the resulting organization to improve efficiency in the delivery of care, reduce the amount of excess capacity in the market, increase the ability of the organization to accept risk-based payment because of increased volume, and to reduce transaction costs in the market, these activities are being carefully evaluated to ensure the market isn't becoming so concentrated that the resulting organization has sufficient market power to prevent efforts to contain costs and to enable the organization to increase the price of services in the market.

Most antitrust evaluations consider horizontal consolidation (e.g., hospitals merging with or acquiring another hospital) in measuring the concentration of market share and its potential impact on market prices. In determining the acceptability of proposed mergers, courts are increasingly considering the balance between the enhanced consumer welfare by the consolidation and the increased potential ability of the organization to control price. This consideration of social welfare has allowed some mergers to occur that did give an organization a majority of the market share in an area when the court determined that the reduction in costs to the consumer or the improvement in quality outweighed the costs of increased market power of the organization in the community.

In addition to the horizontal consolidation of organizations, there has also been an increase in activity in the vertical consolidation of organizations. In a vertical consolidation, there is an increase in the amount of factors of production and distribution under the control of a single organization. For example, in health care, hospitals have been acquiring physician practices as a way of gaining more control over the referral of patients to their hospital, or they have acquired nursing homes and/or home health agencies as a way of gaining more control over the placement of patients once the need for the acute care services provided in the hospital has been met. The hospital may also acquire other suppliers of inputs into the production process, such as laundry services, pharmacies, medical supplies and equipment, and so on.

There has been some speculation that as large healthcare systems form Accountable Care Organizations (ACOs), they will also absorb the financing component or insurance functions as well. Accountable Care Organizations, or similar organizational structures, are viewed as having the potential to improve the quality of health care and slow the rate of growth in healthcare expenditures.

The foundation of ACOs is the reorganization of healthcare services around a team of providers, technology, and knowledge that is focused on the needs of the patient population. The ACO expands the patient-centered medical home concept beyond just the primary care relationships to include the entire continuum of health care. This horizontal consolidation of the healthcare system is being viewed as allowing better cost control and higher quality of care because it enables better overall cost management, less variation within the population served, and an improved ability to track quality because the system is not so fragmented and data are available in a single location for the patient.

In an Accountable Care Organization, not only do providers—primary care physicians, specialists, hospitals, home health agencies—work collaboratively, they also accept collective accountability for the cost and quality of care delivered and the outcomes achieved by the patients in a defined population. For ACOs to achieve these anticipated results, there must be clinical and financial alignment as well as systematic consistency of quality. Efforts to align the goals and incentives of all participants in the healthcare system face many barriers and challenges. In the current healthcare system, there are wide disparities in the incomes of the different specialties and in the methods by which the providers are paid. Given the current fragmented system, it is difficult to determine the size of the patient population that will be necessary to enable the ACO to operate efficiently and to have sufficient data available to produce meaningful outcome results.

There are also inconsistencies currently in how outcomes are measured, making it difficult to arrive at consensus on a single, consistent set of measures for accountability. If these large, integrated organizations are formed, issues involving antitrust laws, antikickback laws, and the physician self-referral Stark Laws will also need to be considered. The integration of clinical and financial processes will also require significant amounts of resources to ensure sufficient capacity is available to the ACO.

The ACO model is also viewed as having a potential to reduce the number and consequences of medical errors in the United States. Because the foundation of the ACOs is the coordination of care through collaboration among healthcare providers, the expectation is that the team approach inherent in the ACO will decrease the errors occurring in the system. Because many current errors occur during the handoff of the patients among providers in different settings, the reduction in the fragmentation in the system is expected to reduce errors and to reduce duplication of care, which can also result in fewer errors and better outcomes.

In addition to the direct costs associated with medical errors that typically result in additional services being provided and longer lengths of stay in hospitals, in admissions and readmissions to hospitals, and therefore higher costs, errors also result in indirect or social costs to patients and the economy. The value of the lost lives due to medical errors and the disabilities caused by these errors adds substantially to the cost of the healthcare system. One study (Van Den Bos, Rustagi, Gray, Halford, Ziemkiewicz, & Shreve, 2011) puts the annual cost of measurable medical errors that harm patients at $17.1 billion in 2008. A second study (Goodman, Villareal, & Jones, 2011) found that in addition to the direct costs of medical errors, the social costs ranged from $393 to $958 billion due to premature deaths and disabilities in 2008. Improvements in the quality of care that reduce the occurrence of adverse events could have a significant impact on controlling the rate of increase in healthcare costs.

9.5 NONPRICE COMPETITION AND MARKET POWER

9.5.1 Overview

The vast majority of healthcare markets are neither perfectly competitive nor completely monopolistic. Consumers develop some loyalty, or attachment, to specific providers, but this loyalty is not total. Furthermore, product quality or attributes other than price play a key role in the output of most healthcare providers; therefore quality has a key role to play in the competitive process as well. In this section, we discuss market power and the role of nonprice competition.

In addition to price, there are many product attributes that have the potential to attract patients. Providers can increase convenience by adding office hours in order to reduce their patients' waiting time. They can build satellite facilities and clinics to cut down on their patients' travel time. Pharmacists can initiate delivery services, emergency services, family prescription-monitoring records, and prescription waiting areas. Insurance companies and HMOs have a wide variety of services that might be covered, and they can also vary the degree to which these services can be covered (e.g., through the use of copayments, deductibles, and treatment limitations). Note, however, that in all such instances, additional quality is expensive to provide. There are three relevant varieties of price-quality competition: (1) price competition alone, (2) quality competition alone, and (3) joint price and quality competition. Price competition simply involves the direct use of monetary incentives/disincentives to allocate goods and services in the market. Quality competition uses nonmonetary incentives/disincentives to allocate goods and services, while the price-quality joint model uses a combination of both to allocate resources.

9.5.2 Monopolistic Competition

Competition in both price and quality is called *monopolistic competition*. In a monopolistic competition model, we assume that there are many competitors and potential competitors (i.e., there is low-cost entry). Each firm can vary its product quality (e.g., location of facilities, operating hours, etc.), and in the process will develop some consumer loyalty (and hence market power). That is, consumers will not be as willing to change suppliers at the drop of a price as in the quality-constant perfect competition case.

Let us develop the model using the example of an HMO. Assume that Palmedico HMO is one among a number of alternative providers (some of who might offer more traditional insurance and fee-for-service options). Also assume Palmedico is a provider of average efficiency, and the partial loyalty of its subscribers can be characterized by means of a downward-sloping demand curve (*D* in Figure 9-8, graph A). Associated with this demand curve is an *MR* curve. Palmedico's cost curve will depend on the characteristics of its product: the extent of coverage, the credentials of its staff, its operating hours, the number of satellite clinics it operates, and so on. Initially, assume that Palmedico is a profit-maximizing institution. Given these conditions, it will set its price at the quantity wherein *MR = MC*. Hence, the price will be around $750 per subscriber and the enrollment will be 5,000.

At this price, Palmedico is earning excess profits, and because it is a representative firm in the industry, presumably others are earning excess profits as well. Because entry is inexpensive, other potential entrants will be attracted by the prospect of high profits. To gain enrollees, they may reduce price, and they may also offer potential enrollees a higher quality product (longer clinic hours or more clinic sites, for example). Palmedico's demand curve will shift to the left unless it responds with an increase in quality and a decrease in price, which assume it does. As a consequence, its costs increase (because of the higher quality). The same forces will affect all firms in the market.

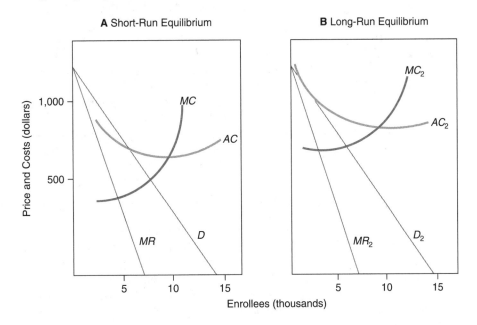

Figure 9-8 Equilibrium in Monopolistic Competition. In the short run (Graph **A**), the provider's equilibrium price and quantity are set where *MC = MR* (at about $750 and 5,000 enrollees). In the long run (Graph **B**), competitive responses, including increases in quality, lead to an equilibrium where no excess profits are made (price equals average cost).

As long as there are any excess profits to be made, this process will continue, and the quality of each firm's product will continue to rise. For each firm, demand will first shift outward in response to its higher quality and then inward in response to the quality and price changes instituted by its competitors. Profit margins (the excess of price over average cost) will continually be lowered as a result of the competition. For any firm, it cannot be predicted whether price will ultimately increase or decrease (i.e., the net result of the competitive process cannot be predicted), because demand has shifted in both directions and costs have changed as well. For the same reason, the direction of enrollment cannot be predicted. However, the final equilibrium will appear as in Figure 9-8, graph B, where AC_2 just touches the firm's demand curve D_2. The equilibrium quantity is at the point where $MC = MR$ (i.e., it is the most profitable position Palmedico can have); in this case, Palmedico is just breaking even. All that can be said for certain about this equilibrium is that AC_2 represents a higher quality level; it cannot be said for certain whether price and enrollment are higher or lower. For this reason, the monopolistic competition model has been criticized as being incomplete: It fails to make predictions about the direction of some key variables—price and quantity.

Competition between nonprofit firms would have a similar outcome. If the behavioral assumption was that the firm wants to maximize enrollees, for example, quality and price competition would still prevail, and the final result would be that each provider breaks even. Models similar to the monopolistic competition model in this section have been used to explain resource-allocation decisions in markets containing numerous HMOs (Christianson & McClure, 1979; Goldberg & Greenberg, 1980) and numerous retail drugstores (Cady, 1976). The importance of nonprice factors (including quality) in these markets has been stressed. Similar models have also been used to explain the diffusion of (high-quality) technological developments in the hospital industry, such as the use of radioisotopes and intensive care units (Baler, Messmer, Gyunko, Domagala, Conly, Eads, Harshman, & Layne, 2000; Harrison, 2007; Lee & Waldman, 1985; Rapoport, 1978).

9.5.3 Monopolistic Competition and Preferred Provider Organizations

The monopolistic competition model has been used to analyze how PPOs affect hospital price and quality behavior (Dranove, Satterthwaite, & Sindelar, 1986). The basic model is applied to interhospital competition, and the impact of PPOs on each individual hospital's demand curve is predicted.

A PPO is a subscription-based organization that has been formed to contract with providers in order to obtain discounted prices. The PPO shops around among providers (hospitals and physicians) for lower prices and then contracts with the providers who offer better terms on behalf of insurers and/ or employers. The medical providers accept the fee schedule established by the PPO and the guidelines established by the PPO for the provision of care. (The PPO might also institute utilization review.) The discounts are passed on in the form of lower copayments for insureds who choose the preferred providers. In effect, consumers are given incentives to choose providers on the basis of price. This increases the elasticity of demand facing any individual hospital because consumers lose some of their loyalty to "their" hospital.

The enrollees in the PPO have considerable flexibility when seeking care. Unlike a restrictive HMO, individuals enrolled in the PPO can decide to use an in-network or out-of-network provider each time they access the healthcare system. Typically, the fees (prices) paid for services are less when an in-network provider is selected. The providers join a PPO in hopes of gaining access to a larger population base.

Using the monopolistic competition model to analyze this phenomenon, the beginning assumption is that there are many differentiated firms, each facing a downward-sloping demand curve (D_1 in Figure 9-9). Assume that each firm has the same demand conditions, and that each firm's demand curve is elastic (although the market curve can be inelastic). The implications of this will be seen in the following paragraphs. Also, each firm has the cost conditions shown in Figure 9-9: marginal cost is constant up to a point, then it starts to increase. The corresponding ATC curve is U-shaped. Initially, assume that short-run equilibrium is at point A, with a price P_0 and quantity Q_0. This is based on the firm's cost conditions, demand conditions, and profit-maximizing objectives.

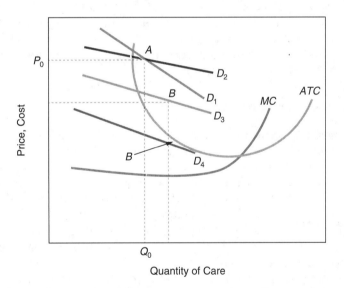

Figure 9-9 Effect of a PPO on Typical Hospital's Behavior. The initial demand curve facing the hospital (prior to the introduction of the PPO) is D_1, and the cost conditions of the hospital are represented by ATC and MC. The introduction of the PPO will initially increase the elasticity of the hospital's demand curve (to D_2). In response, the hospital will lower its price. All other hospitals are facing the same situation and will do the same. As they do so, each hospital's demand curve will shift inwards. The result of these cuts is uncertain, but the demand curve could end up at D_3 (in which case each would operate at a loss). In the latter case, some hospitals would have to cut costs or shut down operations entirely.

The change in demand conditions is the crux of this model. The introduction of a PPO will have the effect of increasing the elasticity of each individual hospital's demand (to D_2). That is, the effect of the PPO is to make each hospital more vulnerable to price changes instituted by other hospitals. With its demand elasticity increased, each hospital, assuming it acts as if all else is held constant, will lower its price to increase revenues and profits (this would be a profit-maximizing response of a firm facing an elastic demand curve). However, if all hospitals do the same, each hospital's demand curve will shift down (to D_3), and the new equilibrium will be at a point such as B (in which each hospital shares in the larger market demand, which has expanded because of the lower price charged by all hospitals). Initially, price will fall, but hospitals in such a market may respond further. If B (on a curve such as D_3) is above the ATC curve, then the hospitals will still be making a profit after the price cut, and no further change will result. On the other hand, if the collective price cuts drive the new demand curve down to D_4 (so that the equilibrium point is at B), the hospitals will all be suffering a loss, and they will have to cut costs (by reducing services, downsizing, etc.) or some will have to leave the market. Cost cutting will shift the cost curves downward, while abandonment of the market by a few hospitals will result in a greater market share for the remaining ones. The final result will be the same: The PPO will have had an impact on hospital services ("quality") and market share.

Note that if the hospitals are operating on the constant portion of their marginal cost curves and no hospitals exit (each hospital's demand thereby remaining the same), then "downsizing" (a reduction in services and thus "quality") will be the outcome.

9.5.4 Increased Concentration

When concentration increases and providers are fewer in number, the probability of price collusion increases. Price collusion involves an explicit agreement or implicit understanding among competitors in a market to limit price competition. If there are only a few suppliers in a market and each understands that the ultimate outcome of price competition is lower prices and profits for all, the likelihood of suppliers refraining from price competition increases.

Explicit agreements to restrict price competition are illegal, but cautious pricing behavior directed at avoiding conflicts in pricing policies among competitors is not. Such cautious behavior is more likely to be found when a market contains a small number of competitors because as the number of competitors increases, "cheating" is more likely. With fewer suppliers, the cost of detecting cheating is lower. Also, the impact of one supplier's price cuts is less dispersed; that is, each supplier's demand curve is shifted inward more when there are only a few suppliers.

Markets with a small number of suppliers and a significant degree of provider interdependence are called *oligopolistic*. Although vigorous price competition is not usually a characteristic of an oligopolistic market, quality competition is. In providing higher quality to attract and retain patients, the costs of oligopolistic competitors increase and profits are reduced.

Oligopolistic competition might occur when there are a few HMOs and traditional insurers in a market competing for the business of a large number of enrollees. In this case, rising quality would be expected, but not much price competition (Hay & Leahy, 1984). However, for an oligopolistic market to persist, entry by new competitors must be difficult, and the start-up costs for an HMO may be low enough to make entry easy and attractive. The eventual result might be price competition. Also, buying power may discourage providers from engaging in oligopolistic behavior. In many markets, businesses play a considerable role in selecting which insurers (including HMOs) will insure their employees. If the buyer's side of the market is dominated by a few large businesses, price competition may become important, despite the low number of providers.

9.5.5 Nonprice Competition

Price competition is sometimes not relevant. When patients are fully or substantially insured for a service and have a free choice among suppliers, they will choose suppliers based strictly on nonprice or quality considerations. Quality competition then becomes the only form of competition, and if the supply side of the market is competitive, costs will increase in response to quality improvements until the suppliers reach the break-even point or the limits placed by third-party payers are reached. Analyses of this type of competitive process have been done for hospital markets (Farley, 1985; Joskow, 1980) and dialysis markets (Held & Pauly, 1983). Studies across hospital markets have shown that, in market areas with greater degrees of competition (measured by the number of hospitals), hospitals are more likely to offer specialized heart surgery (Robinson, Garnick, & McPhee, 1987) and specialized clinical services (Luft, Robinson, Garnick, Maerki, & McPhee, 1986). Although these studies focused strictly on quality measures of output, there is some evidence that quality competition among hospitals is more prevalent than price competition (Noether, 1988).

EXERCISES

1. Given the following demand and cost conditions for a monopolistic medical practice, predict the profit-maximizing price and quantity of services utilized.

Price	Quantity of Visits Demanded
$100	0
90	1
80	2
70	3
60	4
50	5
40	6

Cost conditions: fixed costs are $50 and marginal cost is $35 per visit.

2. The state Medicaid agency has set a rate of $55 per visit for all Medicaid enrollees who visit a physician. Each physician also has private paying patients. The demand curve for each physician can be characterized as follows, and physicians can be regarded as individual monopolists.

Out of Pocket Price	Quantity of Visits Demanded
$80	0
70	1
60	2
50	3
40	4
30	5
20	6
10	7

Each physician also has a cost schedule that can be characterized as follows:

Quantity of Visits Provided	Total Cost
0	$50
1	70
2	110
3	170
4	250
5	350
6	470

a. If each physician is a profit maximizing provider, how many visits will he/she provide to public and private patients?

b. What will the number of visits provided be if the Medicaid Agency lowers its rate to $30 per visit but the demand remains the same?

3. A physician practice serves two groups of patients. One group, with limited insurance, has demand represented by Demand Schedule A; the other, with extensive insurance, has demand represented by Demand Schedule B. The cost to produce a visit is $75. The practice wishes to price discriminate in order to maximize revenue. What price should it charge each patient group?

Demand Schedule A		Demand Schedule B	
Price ($)	No. of Visits	Price ($)	No. of Visits
100	1	100	5
90	2	90	6
80	3	80	7
70	4	70	8
60	5	60	9

4. The following table shows the hospitals operating in two cities and their annual patient days:

City 1		City 2	
Hospital	Patient Days (000)	Hospital	Patient Days (000)
A	15	H	60
B	85	I	60
C	110	J	54
D	45	K	48
E	70	L	39
F	25	M	39

Compare the concentration of the markets in the two cities using the four-firm concentration ratio and the Herfindahl (H) index.

5. Following is the supply schedule faced by a monopsonist and its demand schedule for the goods. Determine how much will be bought and what price will be paid by the monopsonist.

Price ($)	Units Supplied	Price ($)	Units Demanded (nurse)
10	1	100	1
20	2	90	2
30	3	80	3
40	4	70	4
50	5	60	5
60	6	50	6
		40	7
		30	8

6. What characteristics of market structure make quality competition more likely than price competition? Which type of competition is more desirable from the viewpoint of the consumer? Discuss.
7. Explain why the market for physician services might exhibit some of the behavior of a monopoly market despite an apparently competitive structure.

BIBLIOGRAPHY

Monopoly and Physicians

Califano J. A., Jr. (1995). Busting the physicians' monopoly. As I see it. *American Nurse, 27*(4), 5, 7.

Cruess, S. R., Johnston, S., & Cruess, R. L. (2002). Professionalism for medicine: Opportunities and obligations. *Medical Journal of Australia, 177*(4), 208–211.

Cruess, S. R., Johnston, S., & Cruess, R. L. (2004). Professionalism for medicine: Opportunities and obligations. *Iowa Orthopaedic Journal, 24*, 9–14.

Ellerin, B. E. (2007). Debt, demographics, and dual degrees: American medicine at the crossroads: Part 2: External and internal threats to the monopoly model. *Journal of the American College of Radiology, 4*(7), 479–486.

Feldman, R., & Sloan, F. (1988). Competition among physicians, revisited. *Journal of Health Politics, Policy & Law, 13*(2), 239–261.

Gaynor, M. (2006). Why don't courts treat hospitals like tanks for liquefied gases? Some reflections on health care antitrust enforcement. *Journal of Health Politics, Policy & Law, 31*(3), 497–510.

Greenberg, W. (1998). Marshfield clinic, physician networks, and the exercise of monopoly power. *Health Services Research*, 33(5, Pt. 2), 1461–1476.

Grytten, J., & Sorensen, R. (2000). Competition and dental services. *Health Economics, 9*(5), 447–461.

Haug, M. R. (1988). A re-examination of the hypothesis of physician deprofessionalization. *Milbank Quarterly, 66*(Suppl. 2), 48–56.

Havighurst, C. C. (1978). Professional restraints on innovation in health care financing. *Duke Law Journal, 1978*, 303–388.

Kessell, R. (1958). Price discrimination in medicine. *Journal of Law and Economics, 1*, 20–53.

Kluge, E. H. (1993). Medicine as a service-provider monopoly: Implications for equitable access to health care. *Professional Ethics, 2*(3/4), 127–148.

Leffler, K. B. (1978). Physician licensure: Competition and monopoly in American medicine. *Journal of Law and Economics, 21*, 165–186.

Newhouse, J. P. (1970). A model of physician pricing. *Southern Economic Journal, 37*, 147–183.

Rabinowitz, A., & Laugesen, M. (2010). Niche players in health policy: Medical specialty societies in Congress 1969–2002. *Social Science & Medicine, 71*(7), 1341–1348.

Rayack, E. (1964). The supply of physicians' services. *Industrial and Labor Relations Review, 17*, 221–237.

Rayack, E. (1970). *Professional power and American medicine.* Cleveland, OH: World.

Wong, H. S. (1996). Market structure and the role of consumer information in the physician services industry: An empirical test. *Journal of Health Economics, 15*(2), 139–160.

Profits in Medicine

Adams, J. R., Ali, S., & Bennett, C. L. (2001). Pricing, profits and pharmacoeconomics—For whose benefit? *Expert Opinion on Pharmacotherapy, 2*(3), 377–383.

Bauer, M., Bach, A., Martin, E., & Bottiger, B. W. (2001). Cost optimization in anaesthesia. *Minerva Anestesiologica, 67*(4), 284–289.

Brekke, K. R., & Sorgard, L. (2007). Public versus private health care in a national health service. *Health Economics, 16*(6), 579–601.

Cooper, R., & Kramer, T. R. (2010). Revenue-based cost assignment: A potent but hidden threat to the survival of the multispecialty medical practice. *Academic Medicine, 85*(3), 538–547.

Deitch, C., Sunshine, J. H., & Bansal, S. (1995). Outside financial interests in radiology offices: Prevalence, payment, and practice patterns in involved offices. *AJR. American Journal of Roentgenology, 165*(6), 1331–1335.

Egan, M., Petticrew, M., Ogilvie, D., Hamilton, V., & Drever F. (2007). "Profits before people"? A systematic review of the health and safety impacts of privatising public utilities and industries in developed countries. *Journal of Epidemiology & Community Health, 61*(10), 862–870.

Gattuso, C. F. (1997). Negotiating managed care and capitated contracts to minimize risks. *Annals of Thoracic Surgery, 64*(Suppl. 6), S73–S75; discussion S80–S82.

Hoey, J. (2003). Profits, pressure, and perception: Expensive research collides with medicine. *Journal of Rheumatology, 30*(8), 1661–1662.

Klein, M. (2006). Profits and rewards—Why don't midwives earn high salaries? *Midwifery Today with International Midwife,* (79), 15–17.

Lindsay, C. M. (1973). Real returns to medical education. *Journal of Human Resources, 8,*331–348.

Lindsay, C. M. (1976). More real returns to medical education. *Journal of Human Resources, 11,* 127–129.

Matthews, M., Jr. (2004). Medicine as a business. *Mount Sinai Journal of Medicine, 71*(4), 225–230.

Rock, P., & Lubarsky, D. A. (2000). The business of perioperative medicine. *Anesthesiology Clinics of North America, 18*(3), 677–698.

Sloan, F. A. (1976). Real returns to medical education. *Journal of Human Resources, 11,* 118–126.

Price Discrimination and Physician Reimbursement

Adams, E. K. (1986). Implications of physician reimbursement reform: Patient access and physicians' practice. *Journal of Medical Practice Management, 2*(1), 19–23.

Cromwell, J., & Mitchell, J. (1984). An economic model of large Medicaid practices. *Health Services Research, 19,* 197–218.

Filler, B. C. (2007). Coding basics for orthopaedic surgeons. *Clinical Orthopaedics & Related Research, 457,* 105–113.

Gerbarg, Z. (2002). Physician leaders of medical groups face increasing challenges. *Journal of Ambulatory Care Management, 25*(4), 1–6.

Greenberg, D., Peiser, J. G., Peterburg, Y., & Pliskin, J. S. (2001). Reimbursement policies, incentives and disincentives to perform laparoscopic surgery in Israel. *Health Policy, 56*(1), 49–63.

Gabel, J. R., & Rice, T. H. (1985). Reducing public expenditures for physician services. *Journal of Health Politics, Policy, and Law, 9,* 595–609.

Hadley, J. (1979). Physician participation in Medicaid: Evidence from California. *Health Services Research, 14,* 266–280.

Hadley, J., & Lee, R. (1978/1979). Toward a physician payment policy: Evidence from the economic stabilization program. *Policy Sciences, 10,* 105–120.

Held, P. J., & Holahan, J. (1985). Containing Medicaid costs in an era of growing physician supply. *Health Care Financing Review, 7*(1), 49–60.

Kushman, J. E. (1977). Physician participation in Medicaid. *Western Journal of Agricultural Economics, 2,* 22–33.

Mayes, R., & Hurley, R. E. (2006). Pursuing cost containment in a pluralistic payer environment: From the aftermath of Clinton's failure at health care reform to the Balanced Budget Act of 1997. *Health Economics, Policy, & Law, 1*(Pt. 3), 237–261.

Muller, C., & Ostelberg, J. (1979). Carrier discretionary practices and physician payment under Medicare Part B. *Medical Care, 17,* 650–666.

Paringer, L. (1980). Medicare assignment rates of physicians: Their responses to changes in reimbursement policy. *Health Care Financing Review, 1*(Summer), 75–89.

Pourat, N., Rice, T., Tai-Seale, M., Bolan, G., & Nihalani, J. (2005). Association between physician compensation methods and delivery of guideline-concordant STD care: Is there a link? *American Journal of Managed Care, 11*(7), 426–432.

Rice, T. (1984). Determinants of physician assignment rates by type of service. *Health Care Financing Review, 5*(Summer), 33–42.

Seldon, B. J., Jung, C., & Cavazos, R. J. (1998). Market power among physicians in the U.S., 1983–1991. *Quarterly Review of Economics and Finance, 38*, 799–824.

Sloan, F. A., & Steinwald, B. (1978). Physician participation in health insurance plans. *Journal of Human Resources, 13*, 237–263.

Sorbero, M. E., Dick, A.W., Zwanziger, J., Mukamel, D., & Weyl, N. (2003). The effect of capitation on switching primary care physicians. *Health Services Research, 38*(1, Pt 1), 191–209.

Hospital and Nonprofit Agency Pricing

Baler, C. M., Messmer, P.L, Gyurko, C. C., Domagala, S. E., Conly, F. M., Eads, T. S., Harshman, K. S., & Layne, M. K. (2000). Hospital ownership, performance, and outcomes: Assessing the state-of-the-science. *Journal of Nursing Administration, 30*(5), 227–240.

Barnett, A. H., Beard, T. R., & Kaserman, D. L. (1993). Inefficient pricing can kill: The case of dialysis industry regulation. *Southern Economic Journal, 60*, 393–404.

Bauerschmidt, A. D., & Jacobs, P. (1985). Pricing objectives in non-profit hospitals. *Health Services Research, 20*(2), 153–162.

Bishop, C. E. (1988). Competition in the market for nursing home care. *Journal of Health Politics, Policy, and Law, 13*, 341–360.

Brooks, J. M., Dor, A., & Wong, H. S. (1997). Hospital-insurer bargaining: An empirical investigation of appendectomy pricing. *Journal of Health Economics, 16*, 417–434.

Danzon, P. M. (1982). Hospital "profits." *Journal of Health Economics, 1*, 29–52.

Dowless, R. M. (2007). The health care cost-shifting debate: Could both sides be right? *Journal of Health Care Finance, 34*(1), 64–71.

Harrison, T. D. (2007). Consolidations and closures: An empirical analysis of exits from the hospital industry. *Health Economics, 16*(5), 457–474.

Hay, J. W. (1983). The impact of public health care financing policies on private sector hospital costs. *Journal of Health Politics, Policy, and Law, 7*, 945–952.

Jacobs, P., & Wilder, R. P. (1984). Pricing behavior of non-profit agencies. *Journal of Health Economics, 3*, 49–61.

Johnston, W. P., Jacobs, P., & Dickson, M. (1985). Interhospital variations in hospital pharmacy markups. *American Journal of Hospital Pharmacy, 42*, 2492–2495.

Keeler, E. B., Melnick, G., & Zwanziger, J. (1999). The changing effects of competition on non-profit and for-profit hospital pricing behavior. *Health Economics, 18*, 69–86.

Mayes, R., & Lee, J. (2004). Medicare payment policy and the controversy over hospital cost shifting. *Applied Health Economic & Health Policy, 3*(3), 153–159.

Melnick, G., Keeler, E., & Zwanziger, J. (1999). Market power and hospital pricing: Are nonprofits different? *Health Affairs, 18*(3), 167–173.

Reeves, T. C., & Ford, E. W. (2004). Strategic management and performance differences: Nonprofit versus for-profit health organizations. *Health Care Management Review, 29*(4), 298–308.

Rotarius, T., & Trujillo A. J. (2005). Not-for-profit versus for-profit health care providers: Part 1: Comparing and contrasting their records. *Health Care Manager, 24*(4), 296–310.

Sloan, F. A., & Becker, E. (1984). Cross subsidies and payment for hospital care. *Journal of Health Politics, Policy, and Law, 8*, 660–685.

Sloan, F. A., & Ginsburg, P. B. (1984). Hospital cost shifting. *New England Journal of Medicine, 310*, 893–898.

Wilder, R. P., & Jacobs, P. (1986). Antitrust considerations for hospital mergers: Market definition and market concentration. *Advances in Health Economics, 7*, 245–262.

Market Power and Health Insurance

Adamache, K. W., & Sloan, F. A. (1983). Competition between non-profit and for-profit health insurers. *Journal of Health Economics, 2,* 225–244.

Beaulieu, N. D. (2004). An economic analysis of health plan conversions: Are they in the public interest? *Frontiers in Health Policy Research, 7,* 129–177.

Beazoglou, T., & Heffley, D. (1994). Reevaluating the "procompetitive" effects of HMOs: A spatial equilibrium approach. *Journal of Regional Science, 34,* 39–55.

Blair, R. D., Jackson, J. R., & Vogel, R. J. (1975). Economies of scale in the administration of health insurance. *Review of Economic Statistics, 57,* 185–189.

Bloch, R. E., & Falk, D. M. (1994). Antitrust, competition, and health care reform. *Health Affairs, 13*(1), 206–223.

Bundorf, M. K., Schulman, K. A., Stafford, J. A., Gaskin, D., Jollis, J. G., & Escarce, J. J. (2004). Impact of managed care on the treatment, costs, and outcomes of fee-for-service Medicare patients with acute myocardial infarction. *Health Services Research, 39*(1), 131–152.

Burns, L. R. (2000). Physician responses to the marketplace: Group practices and hospital alliances. *LDI Issue Brief, 5*(8), 1–4.

Capps, C., Dranove, D., & Satterthwaite, M. (2003). Competition and market power in option demand markets. *Rand Journal of Economics, 34*(4), 737–763.

Carroll, J. (2011). FTC antitrust rules offer hope of limiting ACO market power. *Managed Care, 20*(5), 5–7.

Clark, R., & Thurston, N. K. (2000). The future of orthopaedics in the United States: An analysis of the effects of managed care in the face of an excess supply of orthopaedic surgeons. *Arthroscopy, 16*(2), 116–120.

Costello, M. M. (2008). After the fact: The case for posttransaction antitrust review of health plan mergers. *Hospital Topics, 86*(3), 11–4.

Dobson A., Davanzo, J., & Sen, N. (2006). The cost-shift payment "hydralic": foundation, history, and implications. *Health Affairs, 25*(1), 22–33.

Dor, A., Koroukian, S. M., & Grossman M. (2004). Managed care discounting: Evidence from the MarketScan database. *Inquiry, 41*(2), 159–169.

Dranove, D., Satterthwaite, M., & Sindelar, J. (1986). The effect of injecting price competition into the hospital market: The case of Preferred Provider Organizations. *Inquiry, 23,* 419–431.

Eisenstadt, D., & Kennedy, T. E. (1981). Control and behavior of nonprofit firms: The case of Blue Shield. *Southern Economic Journal, 48,* 26–36.

Enders, R. J. (1995). Special report on antitrust. Antitrust implications of physician practice affiliations and acquisitions: A question of market power, Part I. *Health Care Law Newsletter, 10*(6), 9–12.

Feldman, R., & Greenberg, W. (1981a). Blue Cross market share, economies of scale and cost containment efforts. *Health Services Research, 16,* 175–183.

Feldman, R., & Greenberg, W. (1981b). The relation between Blue Cross market share and the Blue Cross "discount" on hospital charges. *Journal of Risk and Insurance, 48,* 235–246.

Frakt, A. B. (2011). How much do hospitals cost shift? A review of the evidence. *Milbank Quarterly, 89,* 90–130.

Frank, R. G., & Welch, W. P. (1985). The competitive effects of HMOs: A review of the evidence. *Inquiry, 22,* 148–161.

Frech, H. E. (1988). Competition among health insurers revisited. *Journal of Health Politics, Policy, and Law, 13,* 279–291.

Frech, H. E., & Ginsburg, P. B. (1978). Competition among health insurers. In W. Greenberg (Ed.), *Competition in the health care sector.* Washington, DC: Federal Trade Commission.

Ginsburg, P. B. (1997). The dynamics of market-level change. *Journal of Health Politics, Policy & Law, 22*(2), 363–82.

Goldberg, L. G., & Greenberg, W. (1977). The effect of physician-controlled health insurance. *Journal of Health Politics, Policy, and Law, 2,* 48–78.

Goldberg, L. G., & Greenberg, W. (1985). The dominant firm in health insurance. *Social Science and Medicine, 20*, 719–724.

Goodman, J. C., Villarreal, P., & Jones, B. (2011). The social cost of adverse medical events and what we can do about it. *Health Affairs, 30*(4), 590–595.

Kopit, W. G. (2002). Price competition in hospital markets: The significance of managed care. *Journal of Health Law, 35*(3), 291–326.

Lynk, W. L. (1981). Regulatory control of the membership of corporate boards of directors: The Blue Shield case. *Journal of Law and Economics, 24*, 159–174.

Marsteller, J. A., Bovbjerg, R. R., Nichols, L. M., & Verrilli, D. K. (1997). The resurgence of selective contracting restrictions. *Journal of Health Politics, Policy & Law, 22*(5), 1133–89.

Pauly, M. V. (1998). Managed care, market power, and monopsony. *Health Services Research, 33*(5, Pt. 2), 1439–1460.

Robinson, J. C. (2003). Hospital tiers in health insurance: Balancing consumer choice with financial incentives. *Health Affairs*, (Suppl. Web Exclusives), W3-135–W3-146.

Rosenthal, M. B., Landon, B. E., & Huskamp, H. A. (2001). Managed care and market power: Physician organizations in four markets. *Health Affairs, 20*(5), 187–193.

Steren, E. J., & Stewart, B. R. (1996). Antitrust implications of alternative delivery systems. *Clinical Laboratory Management Review, 10*(5), 561–567.

Town, R., Feldman, R., & Kralewski, J. (2011). Market power and contract form: Evidence from physician group practices. *International Journal of Health Care Finance & Economics, 11*(2), 115–132.

Van Den Bos, J., Rustagi, K., Gray T., Halford, M., Ziemkiewicz, E., & Shreve, J. (2011). The $17.1 billion problem: The annual cost of measurable medical errors. *Health Affairs, 30*(4), 596–603

White, J. (2007). Markets and medical care: The United States, 1993–2005. *Milbank Quarterly, 85*(3), 395–448.

Wholey, D. R., & Christianson, J. B. (1994). Price differentiation among health maintenance organizations: Causes and consequences of open-ended products. *Inquiry, 31*, 25–39.

Zimmerman, C. (2011). A review of the evidence on hospital cost-shifting. *Findings Bried Health Can Financing & Organization, 14(3)*, 1–3.

Monopsony

Barnett, A. H., Beard, T. R., & Kaserman, D. L. (1993). The medical community's opposition to organ markets: Ethics or economics? *Review of Industrial Organization, 8*, 669–678.

Bowblis, J. R., & North, P. (2011). Geographic market definition: The case of Medicare-reimbursed skilled nursing facility care. *Inquiry, 48*(2), 138–154.

Calhoun, J. G., Banaszak-Holl, J., & Hearld, L. R. (2006). Current marketing practices in the nursing home sector. *Journal of Healthcare Management, 51*(3), 185–200; discussion 201–202.

Castle, N. G. (2002). Low-care residents in nursing homes: The impact of market characteristics. *Journal of Health & Social Policy, 14*(3), 41–58.

Castle, N. G. (2005). Nursing home closures, changes in ownership, and competition. *Inquiry, 42*(3), 281–292.

Castle, N. G., & Ferguson, J. C. (2010). What is nursing home quality and how is it measured?. *Gerontologist, 50*(4), 426–442.

Cawley, J., Grabowski, D. C., & Hirth, R. A. (2006). Factor substitution in nursing homes. *Journal of Health Economics, 25*(2), 234–247.

Foreman, S. E., Wilson, J. A., & Scheffler, R. M. (1996). Monopoly, monopsony and contestability in health insurance: A study of Blue Cross plans. *Economic Inquiry, 34*, 662–677.

Grabowski, D. C. (2002). The economic implications of case-mix Medicaid reimbursement for nursing home care. *Inquiry, 39*(3), 258–278.

Grabowski, D. C., & Hirth, R. A. (2003). Competitive spillovers across non-profit and for-profit nursing homes. *Journal of Health Economics, 22*(1), 1–22.

Gruneir, A., Lapane, K. L., Miller, S. C., & Mor, V. (2007). Long-term care market competition and nursing home dementia special care units. *Medical Care, 45*(8), 739–745.

Gulley, O. D., & Santerre, R. E. (2007). Market structure elements: The case of California nursing homes. *Journal of Health Care Finance, 33*(4), 1–16.

Kash, B. A., & Miller, T. R. (2009). The relationship between advertising, price, and nursing home quality. *Health Care Management Review, 34*(3), 242–250.

Miller, E. A., & Weissert, W. G. (2003). Models, measures, and methods: Variability in aging research. *Home Health Care Services Quarterly, 22*(2), 43–67.

Netten, A., Darton, R., & Williams, J. (2003). Nursing home closures: Effects on capacity and reasons for closure. *Age & Ageing, 32*(3), 332–337.

Pauly, M. V. (1987). Monopsony power in health insurance: Thinking straight while standing on your head. *Journal of Health Economics, 6,* 73–81.

Pauly, M. V. (1988). Market power, monopsony, and health insurance markets. *Journal of Health Economics, 7,* 111–128.

Pauly, M. V. (1998). Managed care, market power and monopsony. *Health Services Research, 33,* 1439–1460.

Starkey, K. B., Weech-Maldonado, R., & Mor, V. (2005). Market competition and quality of care in the nursing home industry. *Journal of Health Care Finance, 32*(1), 67–81.

Staten, M., Dunkelberg, W., & Umbeck, J. (1987). Market share and the illusion of power: Can Blue Cross force hospitals to discount? *Journal of Health Economics, 6,* 43–58.

Monopoly and Monopolistic Competition

Almond, D., Currie, J., & Simeonova, E. (2011). Public vs. private provision of charity care? Evidence from the expiration of Hill-Burton requirements in Florida. *Journal of Health Economics, 30(1),* 189–199.

Bamezai, A. et.al. (1999). Price competition and hospital cost growth in the United States. *Health Economics, 8,* 233–244.

Barr, P. (2011). Insurance nor'easter. Thanks to merger, hospitals see benefits from competition with Blues. *Modern Healthcare, 41*(5), 14–15.

Bewley, L. W. (2010). Evaluating the impact of investments in information technology on structural inertia in health organizations. *US Army Medical Department Journal,* 58–63

Bojke, L., Claxton, K., Sculpher, M., & Palmer, S. (2009). Characterizing structural uncertainty in decision analytic models: A review and application of methods. *Value in Health, 12*(5), 739–749.

Burns, L. R., David, G., & Helmchen, L. A. (2011). Strategic response by providers to specialty hospitals, ambulatory surgery centers, and retail clinics. *Population Health Management, 14*(2), 69–77.

Cady, J. F. (1976). *Restricted advertising and competition.* Washington, DC: American Enterprise Institute.

Carey, K., Burgess, J. F., Jr., & Young, G. J. (2011). Hospital competition and financial performance: The effects of ambulatory surgery centers. *Health Economics, 20,* 571–581.

Christianson, J. B., & McClure, W. (1979). Competition in the delivery of medical care. *New England Journal of Medicine, 301,* 812–818.

Coller, B. S. (2011). Realigning incentives to achieve health care reform. *JAMA, 306*(2), 204–205.

Douven, R. C., & Schut, F. T. (2011). Pricing behaviour of nonprofit insurers in a weakly competitive social health insurance market. *Journal of Health Economics, 30*(2), 439–449.

Dowler, C. (2011). Private sector complains brakes have been put on competition too fiercely. *Health Service Journal, 121*(6261), 6–7.

Eichmann, T. L., & Santerre, R. E. (2011). Do hospital chief executive officers extract rents from Certificate of Need laws? *Journal of Health Care Finance, 37*(4), 1–14.

Einav, L., & Finkelstein, A. (2011). Selection in insurance markets: Theory and empirics in pictures. *Journal of Economic Perspectives, 25*(1), 115–138.

Enthoven, A. C. (2011). Reforming Medicare by reforming incentives. *New England Journal of Medicine, 364*(21),

Farley, D. E. (1985). *Competition among hospitals: Market structure and its relation to utilization, costs and financial position.* Hospital Studies Program, Research Note 7. DHHS publication no. PHS 85–3353. Washington, DC: U.S. Department of Health and Human Services, National Center for Health Services Research and Health Care Technology Assessment.

Fuller, R. L., McCullough, E. C., & Averill, R. F. (1984). A "brand name" theory of medical group practice. *Journal of Industrial Economics, 33,* 199–217.

Fuller, R. L., McCullough, E. C., & Averill, R. F. (2011). A new approach to reducing payments made to hospitals with high complication rates. *Inquiry, 48*(1), 68–83.

Getzen, T. E. (1983). The market and evaluation in quality assurance. *Evaluation and the Health Professions, 6,* 299–310.

Gilmer, T. (2011). Costs of chronic disease management for newly insured adults. *Medical Care, 49*(9), e22–e27.

Goldberg, L. G., & Greenberg, W. (1979). The competitive response of Blue Cross and Blue Shield to the health maintenance organizations in Northern California and Hawaii. *Medical Care, 17,* 1019–1028.

Goldberg, L. G., & Greenberg, W. (1980). The competitive response of Blue Cross to the health maintenance organization. *Economic Inquiry, 18,* 55–68.

Groves, K. S. (2011). Talent management best practices: How exemplary health care organizations create value in a down economy. *Health Care Management Review, 36,* 227–240.

Hay, J. W., & Leahy, M. J. (1984). Competition among health plans: Some preliminary evidence. *Southern Economic Journal, 50,* 831–846.

Held, P. J., & Pauly, M. V. (1983). Competition and efficiency in the end stage renal disease program. *Journal of Health Economics, 2,* 95–118.

Joskow, P. L. (1980). The effects of competition and regulation on hospital bed supply and the reservation quality of the hospital. *Bell Journal of Economics, 11,* 421–447.

Kaarboe, O., & Siciliani, L. (2011). Multi-tasking, quality and pay for performance. *Health Economics, 20*(2), 225–238.

Kelly, E. T., Rodowskas, C. A. Jr., & Gagnon, J. P. (1975). An examination of the effect of market demographic and competitive characteristics on gross margins of prescription drugs. *Medical Care, 12,* 956–965.

Lee, J. (2011). Competitive flaws. Bidding program expansion draws complaints. *Modern Healthcare, 41*(35), 12–13.

Lee, R. H., & Waldman, D. M. (1985). The diffusion of innovations in hospitals. *Journal of Health Economics, 12,* 371–380.

Luft, H. S., Robinson, J. C., Garnick, D. W., Maerki, S. C., & McPhee, S. J. (1986). The role of specialized clinical services in competition among hospitals. *Inquiry, 23,* 83–94.

Mobley, L. R. (1996). Tacit collusion among hospitals in price-competitive markets. *Health Economics, 5,* 183–194.

Mobley, L. R. (1997). Multiple hospital chain acquisitions and competition in local health care markets. *Review of Industrial Organization, 12,* 185–202.

Morrisey, M. A., & Ashby, C. S. (1982). An empirical analysis of HMO market share. *Inquiry, 19,* 136–149.

Moscone, F., & Vittadini, G. (2011). New evidence in health economics. *Expert Review of Pharmacoeconomics & Outcomes Research, 11*(1), 45–46.

Noether, M. (1988). Competition among hospitals. *Journal of Health Economics, 7,* 259–284.

Nyman, J. (1987). Prospective and "cost-plus" Medicaid reimbursement, excess Medicaid demand, and the quality of nursing home care. *Journal of Health Economics, 6,* 129–146.

Rapoport, J. (1978). Diffusion of technological innovations among non-profit firms. *Journal of Economics and Business, 30,* 108–118.

Robinson, J. C. (1988). Hospital competition and hospital nursing. *Nursing Economics, 6,* 116–124.

Robinson, J. C., & Luft, H. S. (1987). Competition and the cost of hospital care, 1972 to 1982. *JAMA, 257,* 3241–3245.

Robinson, J. C., Garnick, D. W., & McPhee, S. J. (1987). Market and regulatory influences on the availability of coronary angioplasty and bypass surgery in U.S. hospitals. *New England Journal of Medicine, 317,* 85–90.

Robinson, J. C., Luft, H. S., McPhee, S. J., & Hunt, S. S. (1988). Hospital competition and surgical length of stay. *JAMA, 259,* 696–700.

Scurlock, C., Dexter, F., Reich, D. L., & Galati, M. (2011). Needs assessment for business strategies of anesthesiology groups' practices. *Anesthesia & Analgesia, 113*(1), 170–174.

Scurlock, C., Raikhelkar, J., & Nierman, D. M. (2011). Targeting value in health care: How intensivists can use business principles to make strategic decisions. *Physician Executive, 37*(2), 18–20, 22, 24.

Stock, G. N., & McDermott, C. (2011). Operational and contextual drivers of hospital costs. *Journal of Health Organization & Management, 25*(2), 142–158.

Trunkey, D. D. (2011). The impact of health care reform on surgery. *Advances in Surgery, 45,* 177–185.

Winterhalter, S. J. (2011). Economic factors converge: Force hospitals to review pricing strategies. *Journal of Health Care Finance, 37*(4), 15–35.

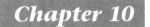

Health Insurance

10.1 INTRODUCTION

Health insurance has a significant influence on markets for medical care. In this chapter, the focus is on the market for health insurance itself. The first step is to explain briefly the theory and conditions necessary for an efficiently functioning insurance market. The analytical basis for the discussion of the health insurance market is a theory of decision making in the presence of risk. First, a model of demand for health insurance is developed. Then the supply behavior of insurance providers is considered. Finally, a model of a competitive market for health insurance is presented. Although much of the chapter applies the basic supply-demand framework to a new context, it also introduces some concepts that are unique to insurance markets, specifically moral hazard and adverse selection.

10.2 ROLE OF INSURANCE

Insurance exists because of risk and risk aversion. Risk involves uncertainty regarding an event or a state of being. A risk averse individual will prefer events, or states of being, that involve less uncertainty (more certainty). Insurance enables an individual to manage risk by substituting a known (certain) amount of loss, the insurance premium, for a potential but unknown occurrence of a large loss. Insurance transfers the risk associated with the possibility of a loss from one individual to a group of individuals through pooling. For example, if 10 individuals in a group know that one individual will suffer a $10,000 loss, but not which one, risk averse individuals will be willing to pay $1,000 (plus a small administrative cost) into a pool to be used to compensate the individual that actually incurred the loss. Each individual has a 1-in-10 chance of suffering the loss (9-in-10 of not), but doesn't want to take the risk of suffering a $10,000 loss if the event occurs to him or her. Insurance, then, is a method of pooling resources to mitigate the effects associated with the occurrence of a large, uncertain event. An implied condition in the pooling of risks is that the event being insured against is outside the control of the individuals; it is a random event.

In order for the market for insurance to perform efficiently, certain conditions must be met. First, the event being insured against must occur often enough to cause concern, but not occur so often that it becomes routine. It must be possible to determine, with relative accuracy and ease, the probability of the event occurring among the group covered by the insurance. Because the collection of premiums and the payment of benefits involve administrative costs, insurance premiums needed to cover routine events would exceed the utility derived from purchasing insurance. Second, the event being insured against must be identifiable and well defined to minimize transaction costs associated with determining the occurrence of the event. In addition, the event must have well-established boundaries with ownership able to be easily defined and observable; that is, it must also be possible to establish the value of the loss that will be suffered if the event occurs. Third, the occurrence of the event must be outside the control of the insured individuals; that is, the behavior of the insured regarding the event does not change just because the event is now covered by insurance.

These market conditions become very important as the market for health insurance is examined and analyzed. As the health insurance market is evaluated, adherence to, or violation of, these conditions are critical in determining the efficiency and effectiveness of market performance.

10.3 DEMAND FOR HEALTH INSURANCE

10.3.1 Individual Demand for Insurance

The simple analysis of demand for medical care is based on the condition that the consumer knows with certainty what his or her state of health will be during the relevant time period. This underlying assumption is not plausible for many medical problems. In these cases, a consumer cannot be certain whether or not a problem will occur. The consumer does know, however, that he or she *might* be sick during a particular period and might have to visit a physician and even be hospitalized.

In this type of situation, a consumer faces the choice of whether or not to prepare financially for medical contingencies. The individual can prepare by purchasing insurance. This action entails an increased outlay (the premium) at the outset, followed by reduced outlays should an illness occur. The basic theory of the demand for insurance presents a systematic view of how certain underlying variables—tastes, wealth, price, the likelihood of an illness, and the loss resulting from the illness—can influence the decision to buy insurance. Following is a presentation of the basic assumptions of the model:

- *Consumer tastes.* To characterize consumer tastes with regard to the alternative situations resulting from an illness, assume that when an illness occurs, it leads to medical care expenses that constitute a loss of wealth. To specify what this loss means to the individual, a concept to characterize the individual's well-being at alternative levels of wealth—the concept of *utility*—must be introduced. One hypothetical individual's taste for wealth is presented in the form of an index of utility in Table 10-1. This index shows what level of utility is associated with each specific level of wealth. Thus, a level of wealth of $10,000 is associated with a level of utility of 100; a level of wealth of $9,900 is associated with a level of utility of 99.8; and so on. The size of the specific numbers in the utility index are arbitrary. What is important is that higher wealth gives higher utility (i.e., increased wealth makes the individual "better off"). A further assumption is that the function is characterized by diminishing marginal utility. That is, each additional $100 of wealth results in less additional utility than the previous $100. For example, at $8,500, an extra $100 of wealth will yield three extra units of utility; at $8,600, an extra $100 of wealth will yield 2.8 extra units; and so on.

If wealth has diminishing marginal utility for an individual, that individual is said to be *risk averse*. The basic idea of being risk averse is that, for a given wealth level, a loss of a given amount is of greater subjective importance (utility) to the person than would be a gain of an equal amount. Utility is the subjective index of the relative importance of wealth.

In this model, a utility function is unique to an individual. Thus, it does not imply that additional wealth means less to a rich person than it does to a poor person. This kind of comparison, called *interpersonal comparison*, would involve specifying different people's utilities on the same scale.

Table 10-1   Relationship Between Wealth and Utility

Wealth	Total Utility	Marginal Utility
$8,000	57.0	4.2
8,100	61.2	4.0
8,200	65.2	3.8
8,300	69.0	3.6
8,400	72.6	3.4
8,500	76.0	3.2
8,600	79.0	3.0
8,700	81.8	2.8
8,800	84.4	2.6
8,900	86.8	2.4
9,000	89.0	2.2
9,100	91.0	2.0
9,200	92.8	1.8
9,300	94.4	1.6
9,400	95.8	1.4
9,500	97.0	1.2
9,600	98.0	1.0
9,700	98.8	0.8
9,800	99.4	0.6
9,900	99.8	0.4
10,000	100.0	0.2

- *Level of wealth.* The second assumption is that the individual has an initial level of wealth of $10,000.

- *Medical expenses in the event of illness.* The third assumption is that if the individual becomes sick, medical expenses of $1,000 will be incurred. This expenditure is assumed to restore the loss in health fully.

- *Likelihood of illness.* A fourth assumption concerns the element of uncertainty. The assumption is that probabilities can be assigned to the various possible health states the individual may experience. Assuming there is a 0.1 probability of illness (i.e., of 10 people in similar circumstances, 1 will become ill) and a 0.9 probability the individual will remain well and will not incur any medical costs. These are the only two possibilities, so the sum of the probabilities equals 1.

- *Price of insurance.* The individual can shift the risk of loss on to an insurer but will have to pay a premium to do so. In exchange for this premium, the insurer assumes the risk (i.e., the insurer will fully pay the $1,000, if the person should get sick).

- *Behavioral assumption.* The sixth assumption is that the individual wants to maximize the expected value of his or her utility. Thus, the individual will choose that course of action from which the highest level of utility can be expected to be achieved.

The model's conclusions are obtained by determining how, under these assumed conditions, the individual will behave so as to maximize expected utility (i.e., which of the two options, buy insurance or do not buy insurance, the individual will chose). The model predicts that if health insurance is available on the right terms, the individual will buy it to reduce risk (and hence increase expected utility). To see how this conclusion is derived, examine how much wealth and utility the individual would expect to have with and without insurance.

The decision problem is summarized in Table 10-2. Without insurance, the individual has a 90% chance of having $10,000 in wealth and a 10% chance of having only $9,000 because of the payout for medical care. The expected value of wealth will be 90% of $10,000 plus 10% of 9,000, or $9,900. This is the sum of the amounts the individual expects to receive under various conditions adjusted for the probabilities that those conditions will arise. If $10,000 is the level of wealth, the utility is 100 units. If $9,000 is available, the utility is 89 units. But the individual has only a 90% chance of having 100 units of utility and a 10% chance of having 89 units. The expected value of the utility achieved will be 90% of 100 plus 10% of 89, or 98.9.

So without insurance, the expected value of income is $9,900, and the expected value of utility is 98.9 units. The utility associated with a *certain* wealth of $9,900 is 99.8. So a certain wealth of $990 would be more desirable to the individual than the risky situation (because 99.8 > 98.9). A certain wealth of $9,900 could be obtained by buying an insurance policy costing $100. Payment of the $100 premium would reduce the initial $10,000 wealth to $9,900, but there is then no risk of further loss because even if illness occurs, the insurance would cover the costs. Thus, the individual in this model would have a demand for insurance at a premium of $100. Note that the premium of $100 here is called the actuarially fair premium or pure premium. It is the amount an insurer would have to charge to break even when insuring a large number of people, assuming no administrative costs of

Table 10-2   Comparison of Buy Insurance and Do Not Buy Insurance Options

Price of Insurance	Wealth after Insurance Purchase	Utility after Insurance Purchase	Expected Utility with No Insurance	Decision
$100	$9,990	99.8	98.9	Buy
200	9,800	99.4	98.9	Buy
300	9,700	98.8	98.9	Do not buy
400	9,600	98.0	98.9	Do not buy

operation. The costs associated with the administrative activities involved in managing the insurance process are known as loading fees.

In fact, the person in this example would be willing to pay considerably more than $100 for insurance. Suppose that for $200, the individual could buy insurance coverage against the $1,000 loss. By buying the insurance, the individual would be certain of having $9,800. This is because the individual's wealth would be reduced by the amount of the premium ($200), and if the individual then became ill, the insurer would pay the cost. Certainty of having $9,800 would yield 99.4 units of utility, which is a higher expected utility than that in the "no insurance" situation. Being a utility maximizer, the individual would buy the insurance on these terms. Indeed, the individual would pay up to roughly $300 to avoid the risk of losing wealth due to illness because at that price, the expected utility with no insurance is approximately equal to the utility of the certain wealth after the purchase of insurance.

Of course, the individual would not buy insurance "at any price." For example, if the premium were $400, the expected utility in the risky situation (98.9) is greater than the utility associated with a certain wealth of $9,600 (98.0), and the "do not buy insurance" option would be the more attractive one. Insurance demand also depends of course on the size of the possible loss. Suppose, for example, that the possible medical expense is not $1,000, but rather is $1,500, either because the illness is more serious or because the price of medical care is higher. In this situation, the individual faces an expected loss of $1,500 if illness occurs. The individual would have an expected utility of 97.6 units (10% of 76 plus 90% of 100) in the "no insurance" situation. If the individual was certain of having $9,600, he or she would be certain of receiving 98 units of utility. Therefore, in this case, the individual would be willing to pay something over $400 for insurance.

The conclusion is that, as the possible loss increases, the amount of money the individual is willing to pay to avert the possible loss increases as well, and the individual will be willing to buy additional insurance coverage if the terms are right. The size of the financial loss in relation to the individual's wealth and the associated utilities is called the *financial vulnerability factor*. A second factor, which is related to the probability of illness, is referred to as the *risk perception factor* (Berki & Ashcraft, 1980). In our example, if the probability of becoming ill increased from 10 to 20%, the expected utility in the "no insurance" situation would fall to 97.8 (80% of 100 plus 20% of 89). This is associated with a wealth level of close to $9,600, indicating that the individual would be willing to pay up to about $400 to avoid the risk of a $1,000 loss.

The amount an individual is willing to pay for insurance depends on the specific extent of his or her risk aversion. This is represented by the rate at which marginal utility diminishes with increasing wealth. An individual with constant marginal utility would be risk neutral. For such a person, insurance at the actuarially fair premium would be no more desirable than the "no insurance" option. The greater the rate of decrease of marginal utility for a person, the more risk averse the individual is and the more willing the individual is to pay premiums above the actuarially fair premium.

10.3.2 Limitations of the Theory

The theory of insurance demand has the virtue of explicitly organizing some of the variables that are central to the decision to purchase insurance. As presented, however, it has important limitations. The following observations may be of help in understanding what these limitations are.

First, the reader may find it strange that the utility function, which is supposed to measure satisfaction, does not include medical care. This is, indeed, a shortcoming of the model because well-being can depend on appropriate care. The model looks only at financial aspects of the situation, in effect assuming that the care, fully and instantly, restores health, with no utility implications of either the illness or the process of getting care. Clearly, this is an unrealistic assumption. Including medical care, however, creates a model that is much more complicated and more difficult to apply, and while it is important to understand that the model has been abstracted from reality, this should not detract from the value of the model. The present model has the virtue of focusing on the benefits of risk shifting, which is an economic good distinct from medical care.

Second, insurance has the effect of lowering the direct price of medical care. One would expect the demand for medical care to increase under these circumstances, yet in the basic insurance model, it has been assumed that medical care demand does not change with the lower, postinsurance price. That is, the model implies that, if an individual becomes ill, he or she will demand the same amount of medical care with or without insurance. This means that the elasticity of demand for medical care is zero, an unlikely scenario for most types of medical care. Again, such an assumption was necessary to simplify the model. If in fact the demand for medical care is affected by the existence of insurance, it violates one of the fundamental principles of the market for insurance.

Third, we have assumed that the individual pays the full amount of the premium. In fact, often a consumer's out-of-pocket premium is substantially less than the total premium. The consumer might receive insurance through his or her employer, who pays part, or all, of the premium. This is not to say that the consumer receives "free" insurance. The consumer, through a bargaining unit or via an employer's policy, negotiates for or receives a total compensation package that includes wages (a direct money component) and benefits (e.g., pension rights and health insurance). The individual pays taxes on the money portion of compensation, and with after-tax wages, directly pays his or her share of the premiums. Under the Internal Revenue Code, many nonwage benefits received through the employer, including health insurance, are not taxed. Therefore, insurance has a lower price when purchased through employment benefits than directly by the consumer.

This point is illustrated numerically in Table 10-3. In the example, the marginal tax rate of the individual or family is 20%, which means that for each $100 in taxable income the employee receives, he or she pays $20 in taxes and takes home $80. Now, if $625 of additional compensation is made in the form of wages, and there are no deductible expenses, the individual will pay $125 (20% of $625) in taxes and will have $500 left over to purchase

Table 10-3 Comparison of Health Insurance When Purchased by Employer and Employee

	Purchased by Employee	Purchased by Employer
Compensation	$625	$625
Tax	125	0
After-tax money available for purchasing premiums	500	625

goods or services, including health insurance. On the other hand, if the $625 in compensation is in the form of employer-provided health insurance, then this compensation is not taxed, and $625 in insurance coverage can be received. A dollar's worth of coverage purchased with after-tax wages is thus worth $(1 - T)$ times the value of the coverage received via employer benefits, in which T is the marginal tax rate. Thus, $(1 - T) \times \$1$ is sometimes called the price of $1 of employer-provided premiums (Taylor & Wilensky, 1983). In terms of this demand model, such tax benefits will lower the cost of health insurance to the individual and thus will increase demand.

10.3.3 The Market Demand for Insurance

Insurance availability requires the existence of at least one organization willing to accept the risks and pay the costs when they arise. To determine under which market conditions this will occur, assume an insurance company is being formed to cover the risks of 1,000 people with tastes, incomes, and health experience exactly like those of the representative individual in Section 10.3.1. A more definite meaning can now be given to the "probabilities" assigned to the alternative health states. Assume that the insurance company can be almost certain that 100 of the 1,000 consumers will become ill and require medical care during the month. Because pooling a large number of risks yields a considerable degree of certainty, it becomes possible to assign a risk to each consumer and evaluate his or her expected loss experience in terms of the group.

The insurance company knows that, in a group of 1,000 consumers, 100 will most likely become ill and will require $1,000 worth of medical care. The expected medical expenses total $100,000 for the group. As seen, the actuarially fair rate (the expected loss per individual consumer) is $100. If each consumer pays a premium of $100, the expected losses of the group will just be covered. According to the analyis in Section 10.3.1, every consumer would be willing to pay a premium equal to the actuarially fair rate to reduce the risk of large losses. Indeed, with diminishing marginal utility, they would be willing to pay somewhat more.

The insurance company cannot charge the actuarially fair rate because resources are necessary to administer an insurance business and some level of profit or surplus must be earned. The insurance company must charge more to cover these administrative costs and profits. The additional fee charged by the insurance company is called the *loading fee*. The premium each individual pays is thus made up of two components: the fee for benefits received and the loading fee. In this example, let us assume that the insurer has administrative expenses of $7,500 in total and desires a profit of $2,500; the total load is thus $10,000. The insurance company must charge premiums of $110,000, of which $100,000 will be paid out in benefits. With premiums spread over 1,000 consumers, if all pay the same premium rate, the rate will be $110 per consumer.

Strictly speaking, the price of insurance is the loading fee, not the premium. In this case, the price of insurance is $10 per insurance consumer. This price can be expressed in several ways, including as a ratio of premiums to benefits ($110/$100 or 1.1), as a cost per policy ($10), or as a ratio of the loading fee to benefits (0.10). The reason the loading fee is the price of insurance is that the product is insurance—the protection from risk—not the provision of medical care. The gains the consumer receives from insurance coverage are the utility gains from the risk reduction. The price of this risk reduction is the loading fee. It is the level of this fee that will determine whether or not the individual will purchase insurance.

The overall market demand will thus depend on the various factors that influence individual demand and the number of individuals in the market. If all individuals have exactly the same tastes, incomes, sickness profiles, and so on, then they will have the same demand for insurance. In actuality, this is unlikely to be the case. Individuals will differ by illness level, wealth, and degree of risk aversion. Their gains from risk reduction will therefore differ and as the price of *insurance* (the loading fee) increases, some individuals will drop their coverage and market demand will fall off.

10.3.4 Moral Hazard

Once an individual has purchased medical insurance, the direct price the individual pays for medical care decreases. If the individual has purchased full-coverage insurance, this price is zero. However, when the direct price of medical care decreases for any reason (including as a result of buying insurance), the quantity demanded will increase (i.e., the absolute value of the elasticity of demand is greater than zero). This phenomenon—the existence of an elasticity of demand for medical care in response to insurance—is known in the insurance industry as *moral hazard*. The term suggests that individuals "shirk" their responsibilities and consume recklessly when they are insured. From the point of view of economics, they are simply behaving in accordance with the principle expressed by the downward-sloping demand curve.

The existence of moral hazard has been used to explain why individuals only partially insure against healthcare risks; that is, why they accept copayments and deductibles rather than full insurance coverage (Feldstein & Friedman, 1977; Friedman, 1974; Kelly & Markowitz, 2009/2010; Pylypchuk, 2010; Steinorth, 2011). Such analyses are more complicated than the basic insurance models, but the essentials can be presented in a simple fashion.

Assume that an individual has the same utility function as in the model discussed in Section 10.3.1. Other basic assumptions are as follows:

- The probability of being sick is 0.2 and of being well is 0.8. That is, out of each 100 consumers, 20 will get sick.

- If a consumer gets sick, the price of each unit of medical care is $50.

- The individual's initial level of wealth is $10,000.

As in the previous model, utility received directly from medical care and health is initially ignored. Now, three options are distinguished: in Option 1, the individual has no insurance, but pays the market price ($50) per unit of medical care used; in Option 2, the individual is fully insured and pays a zero price for medical care; and in Option 3, there is a 10% coinsurance and thus a direct price to the individual of $5 per unit of medical care.

Because demand varies with price, the quantity of medical care demanded will vary in the three situations. Assume that in Option 1, in which the direct price is $50, there will be 10 units of medical care demanded. In Option 2, in which the price is 0, there will be 30 units demanded. In Option 3, where the price is $5, there will be 12 units demanded. Now the focus is on the demand for insurance. To simplify the analysis, specify a loading fee of zero (no load), which means that the premium rate will equal the expected loss to the individual. The information for this example is summarized in Table 10-4.

First, consider Options 1 and 2. Compare the expected utilities, $E(U)$, to determine which provides the highest utility level (and hence which is preferred). If the expected utility in Option 1 is greater than that in Option 2, then the individual will not buy insurance because having no insurance yields a higher expected utility than having full insurance. In fact, under Option 1, the individual faces a 20% chance of becoming sick, paying the full $50 per unit for a total of $500 in medical costs, and having $9,500 left over. The utility of $9,500 in wealth is 97 (see Table 10-1). On the other hand, the individual has

Table 10-4 Example of the Effects of Moral Hazard

	Situation 1 (No insurance)	Situation 2 (Full insurance)	Situation 3 (10% copayment)
Price paid by individual for one unit of care	$50	$0	$5
Units of care demanded	10	30	12
Amount paid by insurance company for care	$0	$1,500	$540
Pure premium	–	$300	$108
Expected utility	99.4	98.8	99.6

an 80% chance of not getting sick, in which case the level of wealth remains at $10,000 and the utility is 100. The $E(U)$ for this situation is 99.4 (80% of 100 plus 20% of 97). The $E(U)$ under Option 2 is equal to the utility of the original level of wealth minus the premium (i.e., the utility of $9,700). This amounts to 98.8. And because "no insurance" has greater expected utility than full insurance, the individual will demand "no insurance" under these conditions.

Now, bring Option 3 into the picture. First, note that the premium is less than under full insurance, in which 30 units of medical care were demanded. Under Option 3, there will be 12 units demanded, but because of the 10% coinsurance rate, the insurance company pays only $45 per unit, or $540 in total. The individual, having a 20% probability of becoming sick, will pay a premium of $108. In addition, if the individual is sick, he or she pays a copayment of $5 per unit, or $60 overall. The $E(U)$ for this situation is roughly 99.6 [20% of (10,000 − 108 − 60.00) plus 80% of (10,000 − 108)]. This is greater than the expected utility of not buying insurance. Now the individual will buy insurance.

However, this may not be the preferred option. Other copayment rates will have other expected utilities. What is important to note is that the individual will, in some circumstances, prefer insurance with a copayment to that with full coverage (or no coverage) if the moral hazard is great enough.

One shortcoming of this model should be mentioned. Medical care has utility, as does insurance. This fact has been ignored. Indeed, the extra units of medical care consumed in Options 2 and 3 yield extra utility in their own right. It may well be that the marginal utility of these units would make the full coverage option preferable to one of lesser coverage. Although this may be the case, the point of this discussion is that, if the conditions are right, insurance with a copayment may be preferred to all other options.

The typical insurance model views the increase in the demand for medical care by an insured individual as a welfare loss to society. This welfare loss occurs because decisions made by individuals are based on the price paid out of pocket for the service and not on the price the provider receives for the service. As a result, more services are purchased than would be purchased at the full price in the market. Basically, the effect is the same as would occur with an outward shift in the demand curve rather than a movement down the original demand curve—a larger quantity is now demanded at the original price. The traditional model views the difference between what the consumer would demand at the original price and the quantity demanded with insurance as a welfare loss to society because the true marginal costs now exceed marginal benefits. The additional medical services consumed by the insured individual are considered to be an inefficient use of society's scarce resources, generating more costs than benefits. If the consumer had to pay full price for these additional services, they would not be consumed.

Nyman (1999a, 2004) offers a different view, proposing that not all the increase in demand by insured individuals results in welfare loss to society. Nyman (2004) argues that acquiring insurance enables individuals to purchase medical care they could not afford previously, and that much of the increased utilization of services has a substantial impact on the health status of the individual. Because at least some of the increased utilization of services, especially among the vulnerable populations, has a positive benefit, it should not be viewed as a welfare loss to society. Under this model, it is important to separate services into those that have marginal benefits greater than their marginal costs and those that don't. Under Nyman's model, insurance should be viewed as a transfer of income at time of illness and that the increase in income shifts the demand curve to the right. This shift of the demand curve, rather than a movement down the demand curve because of reduced price, results in much less inefficiency in the market. Although Nyman's model doesn't maintain that moral hazard is efficient, it does require a separation of the effects into efficient and inefficient categories. In practice, the difficulty is determining when marginal costs exceed marginal benefits in health care.

10.3.5 Demand Responsiveness to the Price of Health Insurance

Remember the concept of the elasticity of demand for medical care, which is a measure of how responsive the quantity of medical care is to out-of-pocket price changes. In a similar vein, an elasticity of demand for health insurance showing how buyers will respond to changes in the price of insurance can be estimated. The formula for point elasticity can be written as follows:

$$E_d = \frac{(PREM_2 - PREM_1) / (PREM_1)}{(P_2 - P_1) / P_1}$$

in which E_d is the elasticity of demand for insurance coverage, PREM is the dollar amount of premiums demanded (with subscripts 1 and 2 referring to situations 1 and 2), and P is the price of insurance (with subscripts 1 and 2 referring to situations 1 and 2). Note that the price of insurance is the loading fee, as discussed in the previous section. Assume that the loading fee increases from $800 per policy to $1,000 and that as a result, consumers reduce their demand for insurance, and therefore their premiums from $10,050 to $9,500. Then the elasticity of demand is

$$\frac{(9,500 - 10,050) / 10,050}{(1,000 - 800) / 800}$$

It is very important to know the magnitude of this variable for policy purposes. The exemption from income tax of health insurance benefits is equivalent to a reduction in the price of health insurance. This exemption has the effect of increasing the demand for health insurance benefits, such as reductions in the coinsurance. Lower coinsurance rates increase the quantity of medical care demanded. In the immediate post–World War II era, when the government was trying to encourage the consumption of medical care, this increase in demand was not regarded as a problem. In current times, with the concern over rising medical care costs, the issue has grown in importance.

Several studies have been undertaken to establish the responsiveness of the demand for insurance to changes in the price of insurance. Taylor and Wilensky (1983) examined how premiums increase as the variable tax rate (1 – marginal tax rate) falls. (This variable was taken to be a proxy for the after-tax price of employer-provided health insurance.) They found the elasticity to be –0.2. In other studies, the value has ranged from –0.2 to –1.

There is considerable uncertainty, then, as to the value of this variable. If we accept −0.2 as the correct figure, then an individual in the 20% marginal tax bracket who received $10,000 in employer-provided premiums has been able to buy $1 in premiums for 80 cents. If the government eliminated this subsidy, the price would rise to $1, and the quantity of insurance demanded (premiums) would fall to about $9,550.

Such a reduction in benefits would mean higher coinsurance and would subsequently translate into less medical care demanded and, with an elastic demand for medical care, into lower medical expenditures. It is important to be aware of the interaction between insurance and medical care markets. What happens in one market influences what happens in the other.

10.3.6 Choice of Health Plan

The purchase of a particular health insurance policy through employment-based insurance requires two decisions, one by the employer and one by the employee. Many employers provide their employees with a selection of health plans and allow them to make their own decisions about the types of coverage and service they will obtain. The plans with more complete coverage will cost more, and for each of these, the insurer will charge a higher premium. Often the employer will pay a fixed contribution toward the premium regardless of the plan chosen, and the employee will pay out of pocket the difference between the premium and the employer's contribution. In such cases, the employee has a choice among alternative types of healthcare coverage. From an economic standpoint, the concern involves discovering what factors influence consumer demand for alternative plans.

Which economic determinants influence the choice of health plan is a topic of considerable importance. If individuals or families with specific characteristics (e.g., sick people, young couples with families) prefer one type of plan over another on economic grounds, selection is said to be *biased*, which means that these individuals or families will demand one particular plan systematically. Often the basis for the selection of a plan is economic. In such cases, the selection is a manifestation of demand behavior.

The economic significance of this lies in the fact that, as a result of these selections, different health plans will have different populations with different experiences of healthcare utilization. One plan (e.g., a traditional plan) may appear to be expensive relative to another (e.g., an HMO). Some of the difference in price may be due to the enrollment of families with different characteristics in the plan (e.g., older people may tend to enroll in the traditional plan). Any comparison of the cost of the two plans that *did not account for these differences* would be misleading. Thus, these factors and their causes must be considered.

To demonstrate the concept of biased selection, the insurance demand model is applied to two alternative situations. In both, there is an employer with 2,000 employees. Each employee has one chance in five (i.e., a probability of 0.2) of becoming sick. However, the employees can be divided into two groups of 1,000 each. Those in the "unhealthy" group will require $200 in medical care if they become sick; those in the "healthy" group will require only $100 of medical care. Individuals in both groups have an initial wealth level of $1,000 and the utility function shown in Table 10-1.

The insurance plan in situation 1 is a "high-option" plan, in that it covers all expenses in the event of illness. Assume, for simplicity's sake, that the insurance company has no loading fee. The premium is thus equal to the expected loss for the employee. The total payout will be $40,000 ($200 × 0.2 × 1,000) for the unhealthy employees and $20,000 for the healthy employees. On average, the payout is $30 per employee. Assume that all consumers pay according to a *community rating*; that is, each pays the same premium regardless of his or her experience. The full premium is $30. The employer's contribution is assumed to be $20 per employee, and the employee's contribution is $10. It should be remembered that the employer's $20 contribution is employee compensation, and normally there would be tax advantages in receiving compensation in this way. To keep the example uncomplicated, these benefits will be ignored for now.

With these assumptions specified, the demand for the high-option plan can now be examined. This is done using the utility model of insurance demand that was introduced in previous sections. According to this model, individuals will demand an insurance plan if the expected utility associated with the plan is greater than the expected utility in the absence of the plan. Consider first the unhealthy group. The expected loss for a person in this group, if he or she became sick and had no insurance, would be $200. The person would be left with $800 in wealth (yielding a utility of 57.1). However, 80% of the individuals in this group will remain healthy, and each of these individuals will be left with $1,000 and have an associated utility level of 100. The average expected utility for the entire group would be 91.4 (80% of 100 and 20% of 57.1). Similarly, the average expected utility of the healthy group would be 97.8 (20% of the utility of $900 plus 80% of the utility of $1,000), because their costs are only $100.

To determine the situation of these groups when they have insurance, the premium must be known. In this case, it is $30. This amount is treated as a reduction in employee's wealth, even though some of it may be employer paid, because more nonwage benefits would mean less wages (and so in the absence of tax considerations, these can be regarded as equivalent). If each employee incurs a premium cost of $30, he or she will be left with wealth of $970 and have a utility level of 98.8. Because utility with insurance for both groups is greater than utility with no insurance, both groups would demand insurance coverage.

Now, consider situation 2, in which there is a low-option plan with the following characteristics. First, there is a limit on the benefits of $100. That is, if anyone becomes sick, the insurance company would cover the first $100 of expenses, but beyond that, the individual would be responsible. The premium of such a plan would be lower because the insurance company's payout would be limited to only $100 per episode of illness. In fact, it would be $20 (0.2 × $100).

The utility model can again shed light on the choice of plan. First of all, if they joined such a plan, the unhealthy group members would pay the $20 premium plus the excess of illness expenses ($200) over covered expenses

($100), or $100 per illness. Their wealth would be $880 if they were sick and $980 if they were well, and their expected utility would be 96.4 (20% of 84.4 plus 80% of 99.4). Utility theory predicts that these individuals would be better off joining the high-option plan (in which the expected utility is 98.8) and so would choose the high-option plan. On the other hand, the healthy group would spend $20 on premiums for the low-option plan and would have no additional out-of-pocket expenses. They would retain $980 whether or not they were sick, and their expected utility would be 99.4. This is greater than under the high-option plan, and so they would choose the low-option plan.

This model thus shows that the characteristics of a group partially dictate the choice of plan. An unhealthy group uses more care and will demand higher coverage. There are a number of reasons why one group might consist of high-cost users: the individuals might be older, have special health problems, be more likely to have children, and so on. For whatever reason, if the group members have higher expected costs, then they will *systematically* select a plan with a higher degree of coverage.

Of course, when biased selection occurs, the rejection of the high-option plan by the healthy group would leave relatively more unhealthy people in that plan, and so the average cost of that plan would increase. This is an example of what is called *adverse selection*, and has implications for the functioning of the insurance market, which are discussed next.

There is a very important issue on which the model throws light. As shown earlier, different benefit plans will attract different types of consumers. For example, a high-option plan will attract individuals who are less healthy and tend to use more care. In a previous section, it was established that individuals with more complete coverage will demand more medical care (because of lower out-of-pocket costs) whatever their health status. If actual data comparing plans are reviewed and it is found that individuals in the higher option plan use more care than in the lower option plan, what can be concluded? In fact, it could be both the lower out-of-pocket price and the difference in health status that contributed to differences in utilization. This confounding of causal factors in healthcare demand has been a source of bias in many studies comparing utilization among plans. For example, a number of studies have compared utilization between enrollees in HMOs and conventional insurance plans. The general conclusion has been that hospital utilization under HMO coverage is lower than under conventional coverage (Herring & Adams, 2011; Miller & Luft, 1995; Pauly & Herring, 2007). But the issue has been somewhat clouded by the lack of clear evidence that the groups being compared were similar in terms of health status.

10.4 SUPPLY OF HEALTH INSURANCE

10.4.1 Supplier Behavior

The product of insurers is the assumption of risks initially borne by consumers, including the risk of heavy medical costs. An insurer has the choice of accepting or not accepting risks on behalf of consumers, and there are a number of factors that will induce any insurer not to accept certain risks. Not only consumers have preferences regarding risk; owners and managers of insurance companies react to risk as well. The insurer is in business to earn profits, which yield utility for its shareholders. Its tastes reflect those of its shareholders. The insurer's wealth (and hence utility) depends on the revenues collected by the insurer and on the insurer's costs, including its payout.

10.4.2 Risk and Size of the Insured Population

The degree of risk of most interest to the insurer is not that faced by any specific individual, but rather the mean (average) risk for the insured population. This is what determines the claims with which the insurer can expect to be faced. However, because the insurers are dealing with random events, in any given round of insuring, the actual value of claims the insurer experiences will almost always differ from the mean. Thus, the insurer is concerned with the variability of the insured population's risk; that is, the likelihood that in any given year, it will be very far above or below the mean value. Because of such variability, insurers must hold contingency reserves (i.e., funds available for covering claims in years when claims are unusually large).

An important thing to note is that this variability is inversely related to the number of people insured. As additional insured consumers are added, the insurer is less likely to experience a loss for the insured consumer group that is very different from the expected value. In other words, the insurer's risk of large losses is reduced as the size of the insurance pool increases, assuming the loss experiences of individuals are independent. So even if all the consumers face a high degree of risk (i.e., a big spread between financial outcomes), the variability faced by the insurance company can be much smaller because of the effect of big numbers on variation. In statistics, this effect is referred to as the *law of large numbers*.

The actual computation of this effect is beyond the scope of this book. However, the very powerful effect of the number of people insured can be illustrated using a simple example. Suppose each person has a risk function as follows: there is a 25% probability of an $800 loss, a 50% probability of a $700 loss, and a 25% probability of a $600 loss. The expected mean loss is thus $700. In any given year, the actually realized mean of a group's loss will not be exactly $700, but if the group is large, it won't be very far away from that.

The likelihood of extreme losses for the group as a whole is less than for any individual. For example, for any *one person*, the probability of a loss of $800 is 0.25. However, for a group of 100 such people with independent loss experiences, it is very unlikely that the *mean* loss would be $800. Such a result would imply that all 100 people experienced an $800 loss! Much more likely is the result that some will experience that loss and others will lose $700 or $600. The relevant computation shows that for this group, the mean loss with 25% probability is $704.70 or more. If the group size were 1,000, a mean loss of $704.70 or more would have a probability of only 0.018, and for a group of 10,000, the probability of a mean loss as large as $704.70 is virtually zero.

10.4.3 Insurer Costs

The calculation of expected costs involves two components: claims paid out and the insurer's administrative expenses. The administrative expenses are incurred in the selling of insurance policies and the administration of claims. Economies of scale may play a role in determining administrative costs. If that is the case, larger insurers will have lower per-member administrative costs than smaller insurers. Claims paid out are determined by the price of medical care and the quantity of medical care used by the consumers. To some extent, both of these are outside the control of the insurer. Prices of medical care are determined in the market for such care, and medical care consumed depends largely on the health status of the insured population. However, an analysis that assumed that both of these are taken as given by the insurer would be seriously flawed for two reasons. First, insurers often have some market power and play a very active role in setting the price of medical care; sophisticated bargaining arrangements (many covered in other chapters) exist under ordinary insurance arrangements, as well as under preferred provider and managed care arrangements. Second, utilization of care is also subject to a host of forces, including the moral hazard phenomenon and direct insurer-provider relationships under managed care.

10.4.4 Insurer Revenues

The insurer's revenues are the premiums it receives from the consumers. There are two basic ways in which premiums can be set: through experience rating or through community rating. *Experience rating* involves the setting of premiums for individuals or groups according to their risk of loss. Healthy, low-risk individuals will be charged lower premiums than unhealthy, high-risk individuals. In *community rating*, a single rate is set for the entire insured population based on the average experience of that population. High-risk individuals and low-risk individuals all pay the same rate, regardless of their expected loss.

10.4.5 Predictions about Supply

A simple supply model would show a typical positive relationship between price and quantity supplied. At higher premiums, an insurer would be more willing to take on additional risks. Conclusions can also be drawn about the effect of changes in other variables on the supply schedule of the insurer. Increases in the supply schedule (more risks accepted at a given premium rate) will be induced by the following: a less risk averse utility function on the part of the insurer, a greater initial level of reserves, a reduction in administrative costs, and a drop in the losses that may be experienced by the consumers. Several additional aspects of supply behavior are worthy of emphasis.

First, if all consumers do not have the same risk function and the insurer can choose between experience rating and community rating, the analysis becomes more complex. Suppose there are two groups, one high risk and the other low risk. With experience rating, a premium would be set that reflected each group's loss experience. The insurer would then have to decide for each group whether to supply insurance, a decision that would be based on the premium rate, marginal costs, and so on, for that particular group. Use of community rating would create a different situation. Again, there would be two groups, each with its own marginal costs. But now there would be a single premium rate, which would fall somewhere between those of the high-risk and low-risk groups. An investor-owned insurer would have an incentive to develop criteria to distinguish between high-risk and low-risk individuals and refuse to insure the former (i.e., it would engage in so-called preferred risk selection). In fact, community rating began and evolved as a method in the tax-exempt (not-for-profit) sector, wherein firms follow different objectives. A tax-exempt firm may have as an objective increasing the availability of insurance coverage for higher risk groups. If it did have this objective, its behavior would differ from the behavior of an investor-owned firm.

Second, insurers can lower their costs (and increase their profits) by reducing the consumers' utilization of insured healthcare services and by lowering the amounts they pay the providers of care. Indemnity insurers have developed a number of utilization-reducing instruments, including preadmission review and rules requiring second opinions for surgery. Indeed, HMOs were developed as a means of controlling the intensity of medical care provided to patients. However, even indemnity insurers have become active in the managed care arena and have resorted to utilization-reducing mechanisms.

Third, whereas previously insurers had played a passive role in the setting of prices, they have become increasingly active in contracting with providers and pushing for favorable terms. For example, in a preferred provider arrangement, insurers seek specified prices from providers. Insurers have sought to gain a market advantage over providers, so they can either pass the lower prices on to consumers or else can capture the gains for themselves.

10.5 ADVERSE SELECTION IN HEALTH INSURANCE MARKETS

In Section 10.2, the concept of self-selection in insurance coverage was introduced. Insurance plans with specific types of coverage will attract consumers who will benefit the most from the coverage. In the presence of information asymmetry, this can create a situation called *adverse selection*, which could damage an insurance market to such a degree that it ceases to exist. Whereas, in practice, economists have questioned whether this phenomenon is an empirically important one, it has drawn considerable attention in the literature (Buchmueller, 2009; Hirth, Baughman, Chernew, & Shelton, 2006; Jack, 2006; Marquis, Buntin, Escarce, & Kapur, 2007; Pauly, 1986).

In this insurance model, assume that there are three separate groups of 100 individuals with the following demand conditions:

- In group 1, the healthiest, each individual has a 10% probability of becoming ill and requiring medical care; in group 2, the intermediate group, the probability is 40%; and in group 3 it is 80%.

- The cost of medical treatment for an individual in any group (i.e., the total amount of the loss in the event of illness) is $100.

- Individuals have the utility function presented in Table 10-1.

Based on these assumptions, the expected utility of being uninsured for any individual will be the weighted average of the utility of $1,000 (which is 100.0, according to Table 10-1) if the individual stays healthy and the utility of $900 (which is 89.0) if he or she becomes sick. For group 1 individuals, this is $(0.9 \times 100) + (0.1 \times 89.0)$, or 98.9. The expected utilities for groups 2 and 3 are 95.6 and 91.2, respectively. Each member of group 1 would pay, at most, a premium of approximately $30 (resulting in a utility of 98.9) to be insured. For any premium above this amount, the members would accept the risk and not buy insurance. For any premium lower, they would demand insurance coverage. The indifference premium is approximately $60 for group 2 and approximately $90 for group 3.

Now, turn to the supply side of the market. The relevant assumptions are as follows:

- The insurance company's administrative costs are $2,000.

- Total insurance company expenses consist of the administrative costs plus the amount the insurer reimburses for medical care.

- The insurance company merely wants to break even, so revenues will just equal costs. As for the pricing policy of the insurance company, which is a critical element in the model, there are a number of alternatives the company could choose. For example, it could employ an experience-rating methodology, which involves dividing the total pool into subgroups and setting rates according to each subgroup's expected loss. In an experience-rating pricing scheme, groups 1, 2, and 3 would all pay different premiums because they have different levels of expected loss.

The second type of pricing policy is community rating. In a community-rating scheme, all individuals pay the same rate. Community rating would probably be the method chosen if the insurer were not able to distinguish between individuals in the three groups. It could not then charge a different premium based on expected loss.

Assume that an information asymmetry does exist. That is, the consumers know which group they fall into, but the insurer does not have that health status information. Under this condition, a single community rate is charged to all individuals. Now determine how the market might operate over time. Initially, the insurance company, wanting to break even, will charge a rate high enough to cover all the reimbursements for the three groups ($13,000) plus the administrative costs ($2,000). Over the 300 individuals, this rate amounts to $50 per individual. This rate exceeds group 1's indifference premium, and so members of group 1 will choose not to insure. Members of groups 2 and 3, on the other hand, will insure. With group 1 dropping out of the market, total expenses for groups 2 and 3 are $14,000. Again, the insurance company cannot distinguish between them and so it must charge a single community rate, this time of $70 per individual. But this rate will be above the amount members of group 2 are willing to pay, and they will drop out of the market, leaving only group 3. The rate will be raised to $100, but this will exceed group 3's indifference premium. The members of group 3 will drop out of the market as well, causing the market to collapse. This phenomenon is a joint result of adverse selection (those with the highest risks remain in the market) and community rating (chosen as a method because of the information asymmetry).

The popularity of this model might be attributable to its doom-and-gloom prediction of market disappearance, but there is some question as to how well it fits the present market for health insurance. There is scant empirical evidence to decide its applicability, but it has drawn attention to the phenomenon of community rating and its potential role in market failure. And in fact, in the present model, the market would perform differently if experience rating was used. To see this, assume that for each group, a premium is set equal to its expected medical costs plus $666 (which is one-third of the total administrative expenses). Then each group would pay a premium that was less than what it would be willing to pay. For example, group 1 individuals would be charged $16.66 in premiums ($1,000 + $666 divided by 100 people). This is below what they would be willing to pay for insurance coverage. Thus, it is the community rating pricing policy that caused the market to disappear.

There have been questions raised as to whether community rating results from informational asymmetry or other factors. Insurance companies have, or can get, considerable amounts of information about potential consumers by looking at age and medical history and by conducting medical exams. In fact, insurance companies use experience rating for pricing individual policies. This being the case, it may not be informational asymmetry that leads to community rating (Feldman, 1987) but other causes. For example, employers may want to be equitable to all employees and so offer a single (community) rate for all—the young, the old, the sick, and so on. Employees, including low-risk employees, may accept this, in part because they are happy with the idea that when they become unhealthy later in life their premiums will be community rated as well.

10.6 VIOLATIONS OF INSURANCE CONDITIONS

As was discussed at the beginning of this chapter, certain conditions must occur for an insurance market to function effectively. Here, a brief assessment of those conditions in the health insurance market will be conducted. As discussed, one condition for assessing risk for insurance coverage is that the event being insured against is outside the control of the covered individual—it is a random event. In health care, however, while becoming ill may be considered a random event, outside the immediate control of the individual, how the individual reacts to its occurrence is not independent. If the individual has health insurance, then that individual may be more likely to demand a covered service than if the service is not covered. As a consequence, the existence of insurance coverage may change not only the amount of care utilized but also the type of care used (prescription drugs vs. over-the-counter drugs, inpatient care vs. outpatient care).

A second condition is that the event must occur often enough to raise concern but not often enough to become routine—there needs to be an element of unpredictability to its occurrence. In health care, however, most policies now cover an annual prevention examination, which is routine and totally predictable—the probability of occurring is 100%, and so the insurance premium covers not only the medical expense but also a loading fee. This makes the cost of the coverage higher than if the individual had self-insured and saved the money necessary to pay for the known event.

A third condition is that the event being insured against must be identifiable and well defined to minimize transaction costs associated with determining the occurrence of the event. Although it may be relatively easy to determine when a certain type of illness or injury occurs after the treatment has occurred, it is often not easy to establish its occurrence earlier. Although an X-ray may determine whether or not a bone is broken and therefore establish the boundaries for treatment, such certainty is not known for many other illnesses, especially for early onset, and establishing a definition of an episode is difficult, especially for chronic conditions. The ambiguity in health and health care makes defining a covered event very difficult.

Another condition inherent in the market for insurance is the ability to establish a value for the loss associated with the event being insured. In health care, there is wide variability in approaches to treating an illness or injury, in the prices charged, and in the providers involved in providing the care. Also, because individuals are not standardized, it is very difficult to establish a value for the loss associated with the event.

As this discussion indicates, health insurance is different for insurance purchased for most other events—home, automobile, life, and such. The deviations do not imply that a market for health insurance does not exist, only that the conditions must be incorporated into an assessment of the efficiency of the health insurance market and how the violations impact decision making.

EXERCISES

1. Mrs. Smith's utility function is the same as that shown in Table 10-1. Her initial level of wealth is $1,000. Her annual medical expenses if she got sick would be $120. Her probability of getting sick (and thus incurring the medical expenses) is 0.2. The price of an insurance policy is $30.
   a. If Mrs. Smith were a utility maximizer, should she purchase insurance?
   b. Should she purchase insurance if the price were $60?
   c. Would Mrs. Smith purchase insurance at $60 if her medical expenses, in case she got sick, were $200?
   d. Is Mrs. Smith risk averse, risk neutral, or a risk taker?
2. Mrs. Rosen has a utility function like that in Table 10-1. There is a 0.5 probability that she will incur medical expenses of $200. What is the most she would pay for insurance?

3. Health insurance premiums obtained through an employer are deductible from income tax. An individual health insurance policy costs $500. The personal income tax rate is 30%. An employer provides premiums as a benefit. What is the price to the employee of the insurance?

4. An insurance company has a payout of health benefits of $100,000. Administrative expenses on top of that are $30,000 and profits are $10,000. What is the ratio of premiums to benefits? If there are 100 insureds, what is the premium rate each would pay?

5. A survey of insured persons indicates that, when the loading charge paid by each was $80, the premium was $2,000. When the loading charge was increased to $120, each person was willing to spend only $1,600 on insurance. What is the elasticity of demand for insurance?

6. The elasticity of an individual's demand for insurance is −0.2. When the loading fee was $100, the person purchased $3,000 in insurance premiums. The loading fee is increased to $120. How much insurance will the person purchase?

7. Buffalo Systems has 1,000 employees, all of whom are insured in the company plan. There are two groups of employees, healthy and unhealthy. Half of the employees are in each category. Persons in both groups have an equal probability of being sick of −0.2, an initial wealth level of $1,000, and the utility function shown in Table 10-1. When a healthy person gets sick, the cost of care is $100. The cost of care for an unhealthy person is $150.
   a. If the company plan is community-rated, such that each person pays $25, would both groups choose to insure?
   b. Assume that the company introduces a low-cost plan. Those in the plan pay $20. The plan insures up to only $100. Persons pay any excess out of pocket. Which group would purchase insurance? What would be the total expenditure of each group, including out-of-pocket expenses?

9. How will each of the following affect the supply for insurance:
   a. A larger pool of insured persons
   b. Lower administration costs for insurance companies
   c. Higher premiums (with no change in risk experience)
   d. A greater degree of risk aversion on the part of insurers

10. What is the effect of utilization management on insurance company expenses? Consider both administrative expense and claims expense.

11. What are community rating and experience rating?

12. What is information asymmetry in health insurance? How would information asymmetry result in a single rate for all persons, even if their expected losses differ?

13. What mechanisms are available to insurers to allow them to charge premiums by risk category?

BIBLIOGRAPHY

Health Insurance Market

Abraham, J. M., & Karaca-Mandic, P. (2011). Regulating the medical loss ratio: Implications for the individual market. *American Journal of Managed Care, 17*(3), 211–218.

Abraham, K. S. (1985). Efficiency and fairness in insurance risk classification. *Virginia Law Review, 71*, 403–451.

Altman, D., Cutler, D. M., & Zeckhauser, R. J. (1998). Adverse selection and adverse retention. *American Economic Review, 88*, 122–126.

Anderson, G., & Knickman, J. (1984). Adverse selection under a voucher system: Grouping Medicare recipients by level of expenditure. *Inquiry, 21*, 135–143.

Antos, J., Bertko, J., Chernew, M., Cutler, D., de Brantes, F., Goldman, D., … Shortell, S. (2010). Bending the curve through health reform implementation. *American Journal of Managed Care, 16*(11), 804–812.

Axelrod, D. A., Millman, D., & Abecassis, D. D. (2010). US health care reform and transplantation. Part I: Overview and impact on access and reimbursement in the private sector. *American Journal of Transplantation, 10*(10), 2197–2202.

Baker, L. C., & Corts, K. S. (1996). HMO penetration and the cost of health care: Market discipline or market segmentation? *American Economic Review, 86*, 389–394.

Bakker, F. M., van Vliet, R. C., & van de Ven, W. P. (2000). Deductibles in health insurance: Can the actuarially fair premium reduction exceed the deductible? *Health Policy, 53*(2), 123–141.

Barros, P. P., Machado, M. P., & Sanz-de-Galdeano, A. (2008). Moral hazard and the demand for health services: A matching estimator approach. *Journal of Health Economics, 27*(4), 1006–1025.

Bentley, T. G., Effros, R. M., Palar, K., & Keeler, E. B. (2008). Waste in the U.S. health care system: A conceptual framework. *Milbank Quarterly, 86*(4), 629–659.

Berki, S. E., & Ashcraft, M. (1980). HMO enrollment: Who joins what and why: A review of the literature. *Milbank Memorial Fund Quarterly, 58*, 588–632.

Berki, S. E., Ashcraft, M., & Penchansky, R. (1977). Enrollment choice in a multi-HMO setting: The roles of health risk, financial vulnerability, and access to care. *Medical Care, 15*, 95–114.

Bhattacharya, J., & Bundorf, M. K. (2009). The incidence of the healthcare costs of obesity. *Journal of Health Economics, 28*(3), 649–658.

Blomqvist, A. (2001). Does the economics of moral hazard need to be revisited? A comment on the paper by John Nyman. *Journal of Health Economics, 20*(2), 283–288.

Bolin, J. N. (2007). How well are we doing addressing disability in America? Examining the status of adults with chronic disabling conditions, 1995 and 2005. *Journal of Health & Human Services Administration, 30*(3), 306–326.

Bradford, D. B. (1996). Efficiency in employment-based health insurance: The potential for supra-marginal cost pricing. *Economic Inquiry, 34*, 341–356.

Buchmueller, T. C. (2009). Consumer-oriented health care reform strategies: A review of the evidence on managed competition and consumer-directed health insurance. *Milbank Quarterly, 87*(4), 820–841.

Buchmueller, T. C., & Feldstein, P. J. (1997). The effect of price on switching among health plans. *Journal of Health Economics, 16*, 231–247.

Buchmueller, T. C., & Liu, S. (2005). Health insurance reform and HMO penetration in the small group market. *Inquiry, 42*(4), 367–380.

Cannon, M. F., & Tanner, M. (2006). Healthy competition: What's holding back health care and how to free it. *AHIP Coverage, 47*(3), 44–46, 49–50, 52

Carande-Kulis, V. G., Getzen, T. E., & Thacker, S. B. (2007). Public goods and externalities: A research agenda for public health economics. *Journal of Public Health Management & Practice, 13*(2), 227–232

Chernick, H. A. (1987). Tax policy toward health insurance and the demand for medical services. *Journal of Health Economics, 6*, 1–25.

Cleeton, D. (1989). The medical uninsured: A case of market failure? *Public Finance Quarterly, 17*, 55–83.

Collins, S. R., Davis, K., Nicholson, J. L., & Stremikis, K. (2010). Realizing health reform's potential: Small businesses and the Affordable Care Act of 2010. *Issue Brief (Commonwealth Fund), 97*, 1–18.

Cuellar, A. E., & Gertler, P. J. (2006). Strategic integration of hospitals and physicians. *Journal of Health Economics, 25*(1), 1–28.

Cutler, D. M., & Reber, S. J. (1998). Paying for health insurance: The trade-off between competition and adverse selection. *Quarterly Journal of Economics, 112*, 433–466.

Doonan, M. T., & Tull, K. R. (2010). Health care reform in Massachusetts: Implementation of coverage expansions and a health insurance mandate. *Milbank Quarterly, 88*(1), 54–80.

Doty, M. M., Collins, S. R., Nicholson, J. L., and Rustgi, S. D. (2009). Failure to protect: Why the individual insurance market is not a viable option for most U.S. families: Findings from the Commonwealth Fund Biennial Health Insurance Survey, 2007. *Issue Brief (Commonwealth Fund), 62*, 1–16.

Douven, R. C., & Schut, F. T. (2011). Pricing behaviour of nonprofit insurers in a weakly competitive social health insurance market. *Journal of Health Economics, 30*(2), 439–449.

Dranove, D., Spier, K. E., & Baker, L. (2000). Competition among employers offering health insurance. *Journal of Health Economics, 19*, 121–140.

Dunn A. (2010). The value of coverage in the Medicare advantage insurance market. *Journal of Health Economics, 29*(6), 839–855.

Eisenhauer, J. G. (2006). Severity of illness and the welfare effects of moral hazard. *International Journal of Health Care Finance & Economics, 6*(4), 290–299.

Enthoven, A. (2006). Connecting consumer choice to the healthcare system. *Journal of Health Law, 39*(3), 289–305.

Farber, H. S., & Levy, H. (2000). Recent trends in employer-sponsored health insurance coverage: Are bad jobs getting worse? *Journal of Health Economics, 19*, 93–119.

Feldman, R. (1987). Health insurance in the United States: Is market failure avoidable? *Journal of Risk and Insurance, 54*, 298–313.

Feldman, R., & Dowd, B. (2000). Risk segmentation: Goal or problem? *Journal of Health Economics, 19*, 499–512.

Feldman, R., Dowd, B., Finch, M., & Cassou, S. (1989). *Employer based health insurance.* Publication no. PHS-89-3434. Rockville, MD: U.S. Department of Health and Human Services, National Center for Health Services Research and Health Care Technology.

Feldstein, M., & Friedman, B. (1977). Tax subsidies, the rational demand for insurance and the health care crisis. *Journal of Public Economics, 7*, 155–178.

Foreman, S. E., Wilson, J. A., & Scheffler, R. M. (1996). Monopoly, monopsony and contestability in health insurance: A study of Blue Cross plans. *Economic Inquiry, 34*, 662–677.

Fox, M. H. (2008). Who speaks for the health consumer? *Journal of Health Care for the Poor & Underserved, 19*(3), 671–676.

Frank, R. G., McGuire, T. G., Bae, J. P., & Rupp, A. (1997). Solutions for adverse selection in behavioral health care. *Health Care Financing Review, 18*, 109–122.

Frick, K. D., & Chernew, M. E. (2009). Beneficial moral hazard and the theory of the second best. *Inquiry, 46*(2), 229–240.

Friedman, B. (1974). Risk aversion and the consumer choice of health insurance option. *Review of Economics and Statistics, 56*, 209–214.

Fronstin, P. (2009). Findings from the 2009 EBRI/MGA Consumer Engagement in Health Care Survey. *EBRI Issue Brief,* (337), 1–42.

Gavin, J. N., Goodman, G., & Goroff, D. B. (2007). The transfer of a health insurance/managed care business. *Journal of Health Care Finance, 34*(2), 10–37.

Geyman, J. P. (2007). Moral hazard and consumer-driven health care: A fundamentally flawed concept. *International Journal of Health Services, 37*(2), 333–351.

Glied, S., & Gould, D. (2005). Variations in the impact of health coverage expansion proposals across states. *Health Affairs,* (Suppl. Web Exclusives), W5-259–W5-271.

Gould, E. (2009). The erosion of employer-sponsored health insurance: Declines continue for the seventh year running. *International Journal of Health Services, 39*(4), 669–697.

Gresenz, C. R., Rogowski, J., & Escarce, J. J. (2006). Dimensions of the local health care environment and use of care by uninsured children in rural and urban areas. *Pediatrics, 117*(3), e509–e517.

Haas, J., & Swartz, K. (2007). The relative importance of worker, firm, and market characteristics for racial/ethnic disparities in employer-sponsored health insurance. *Inquiry, 44*(3), 280–302.

Hall, M. A. (2010). Government-sponsored reinsurance. *Annals of Health Law, 19*(3), 465–478,

Hansen, R. A., Schommer, J. C., Cline, R. R., Hadsall, R. S., Schondelmeyer, S. W., & Nyman. J. A. (2005). The association of consumer cost-sharing and direct-to-consumer advertising with prescription drug use. *Research in Social & Administrative Pharmacy, 1*(2), 139–157.

Havighurst, C. C. (2005). Monopoly is not the answer. *Health Affairs,* (Suppl. Web Exclusives), W5-373–W5-375.

Heffley, D. R., & Miceli, T. J. (1998). The economics of incentive-based health care plans. *Journal of Risk and Insurance, 65,* 445–465.

Hemenway, D. (1990). Propitious selection. *Quarterly Journal of Economics, 104,* 1063–1069.

Hemenway, D. (1992). Propitious selection in insurance. *Journal of Risk and Uncertainty, 5,* 247–251.

Herring, B., & Adams, E. K. (2011). Using HMOs to serve the Medicaid population: What are the effects on utilization and does the type of HMO matter? *Health Economics, 20*(4), 446–460.

Himmelstein, D. U., & Woolhandler, S. (2009). US health care: Single-payer or market reform. *Urologic Clinics of North America, 36*(1), 57–62.

Hirth, R. A., Baughman, R. A., Chernew, M. E., & Shelton, E. C. (2006). Worker preferences, sorting and aggregate patterns of health insurance coverage. *International Journal of Health Care Finance & Economics, 6*(4), 259–277.

Huang, L. F., Cartwright, W. S., & Hu, T. W. (1989). Demand for Medigap insurance by the elderly. *Applied Economics, 21,* 1325–1339.

Jack, W. (2006). Optimal risk adjustment with adverse selection and spatial competition. *Journal of Health Economics, 25*(5), 908–926.

Jensen, G. R., Feldman, R., & Dowd, B. (1984). Corporate-benefit policies and health insurance costs. *Journal of Health Economics, 3,* 275–296.

Kaplan, R. M., & Babad, Y. M. (2011). Balancing influence between actors in healthcare decision making. *BMC Health Services Research, 11,* 85.

Kelly, I. R., & Markowitz, S. (2009/2010). Incentives in obesity and health insurance. *Inquiry, 46*(4), 418–432.

Kolstad, J. T., & Chernew, M. E. (2009). Quality and consumer decision making in the market for health insurance and health care services. *Medical Care Research & Review, 66*(1 Suppl.), 28S–52S.

Kuttner, R. (2008). Market-based failure—A second opinion on U.S. health care costs. *New England Journal of Medicine, 358*(6), 549–551.

Leidl, R. (2008). A model to decompose the performance of supplementary private health insurance markets. *International Journal of Health Care Finance & Economics, 8*(3), 193–208.

Linehan, K. (2010a). Keeping health insurance after a job loss: COBRA continuation coverage and subsidies. *Issue Brief/National Health Policy Forum,* (837), 1–9.

Linehan, K. (2010b). Self-insurance and the potential effects of health reform on the small-group market. *Issue Brief/National Health Policy Forum,* (840), 1–14.

Linehan, K. (2011). Individual and small-group market health insurance rate review and disclosure: State and federal roles after PPACA. *Issue Brief/National Health Policy Forum,* (844), 1–13.

Liu, H., Phelps, C. E., Veazie, P. J., Dick, A. W., Klein, J. D., Shone, L. P., Noyes, K., & Szilagyi, P. G. (2009). Managed care, quality of care and plan choice in New York SCHIP. *Health Services Research, 44*(3), 843–861.

Liu, L., Rettenmaier, A. J., & Saving, T. R. (2011). The welfare gain from replacing the health insurance tax exclusion with lump-sum tax credits. *International Journal of Health Care Finance & Economics, 11*(2), 101–113.

Long, S. H., Marquis, M. S., & Rodgers, J. (1998). Do people shift their use of health services over time to take advantage of insurance? *Journal of Health Economics, 17*, 105–115.

Marquis, M. S., & Buntin, M. B. (2006). How much risk pooling is there in the individual insurance market? *Health Services Research, 41*(5), 1782–1800.

Marquis, M. S., Buntin, M. B., Escarce, J. J., & Kapur, K. (2007). The role of product design in consumers' choices in the individual insurance market. *Health Services Research, 42*(6, Pt. 1), 2194–2223; discussion 2294–2323.

Marquis, M. S., Buntin, M. B., Escarce, J. J., Kapur, K., Louis, T. A., & Yegian, J. M. (2006). Consumer decision making in the individual health insurance market. *Health Affairs, 25*(3), w226–w234.

Marquis, M. S., & Long, S. H. (1995). Worker demand for health insurance in the non-group market. *Journal of Health Economics, 14*, 47–63.

Merlis, M. (2009). A health insurance exchange: Prototypes and design issues. *Issue Brief/National Health Policy Forum*, (832), 1–27.

Milani, F. (2010). Public option and private profits: What do markets expect? *Applied Health Economics & Health Policy, 8*, 155–165.

Millenson, M. L. (2001). Moral hazard vs. real hazard: Quality of care post-Arrow. *Journal of Health Politics, Policy & Law, 26*(5), 1069–1079.

Miller, R. H., & Luft, H. S. (1995). Estimating health expenditure growth under managed competition. *JAMA, 273*, 656–662.

Newhouse, J. P. (2006). Reconsidering the moral hazard-risk avoidance tradeoff. *Journal of Health Economics, 25*(5), 1005–1014.

Nichols, L. M. (2010). Implementing insurance market reforms under the federal health reform law. *Health Affairs, 29*(6), 1152–1157.

Nyman, J. A. (1998). Theory of health insurance. *Journal of Health Administration Education, 16*(1), 41–66.

Nyman, J. A. (1999a). The economics of moral hazard revisited. *Journal of Health Economics, 18*(6), 811–824.

Nyman, J. A. (1999b). The value of health insurance. *Journal of Health Economics, 18*, 141–152.

Nyman, J. A. (2004). Is "moral hazard" inefficient? The policy implications of a new theory. *Health Affairs, 23*(5), 194–199.

Nyman, J. A. (2008). Health insurance theory: The case of the missing welfare gain. European *Journal of Health Economics, 9*(4), 369–380.

Nyman, J. A., & Maude-Griffin, R. (2001). The welfare economics of moral hazard. *International Journal of Health Care Finance & Economics, 1*(1), 23–42.

Ohn, J., McMahon, L., & Carter, T. (2006). Another look at the relationship between socioeconomic factors and the Black-White health benefit inequality. *Journal of Hospital Marketing & Public Relations, 17*(1), 109–117.

Owen, C. L. (2009). Consumer-driven health care: Answer to global competition or threat to social justice? *Social Work, 54*(4), 307–315.

Pauly, M. (1986). Taxation, health insurance, and market failure in the medical economy. *Journal of Economic Literature, 26*, 629–675.

Pauly, M. V. (1989). Competition in health insurance markets. *Law and Contemporary Problems, 51*, 237–271.

Pauly, M. V., & Blavin, F. E. (2008). Moral hazard in insurance, value-based cost sharing, and the benefits of blissful ignorance. *Journal of Health Economics, 27*(6), 1407–1417.

Pauly, M. V., & Herring, B. J. (2000). An efficient employer strategy for dealing with adverse selection multiple-plan offerings: An MSA example. *Journal of Health Economics, 19*, 513–528.

Pauly, M. V., & Herring, B. (2007). Risk pooling and regulation: Policy and reality in today's individual health insurance market. *Health Affairs, 26*(3), 770–779.

Pauly, M. V., & Lieberthal, R. D. (2008). How risky is individual health insurance? *Health Affairs, 27*(3), w242–w249.

Pauly, M. V., & Ramsey, S. D. (1999). Would you like suspenders to go with that belt? An analysis of optimal combinations of cost sharing and managed care. *Journal of Health Economics, 18*, 443–458.

Perreira, K. M. (2006). Crowd-in: The effect of private health insurance markets on the demand for Medicaid. *Health Services Research, 41*(5), 1762–1781.

Pitsenberger, W. H. (2008). Limited provider panels: Their promise and problems in an individual health insurance market. *Journal of Health & Life Sciences Law, 1*(4), 67, 69–94.

Pylypchuk, Y. (2010). Adverse selection and the effect of health insurance on utilization of prescribed medicine among patients with chronic conditions. *Advances in Health Economics & Health Services Research, 22*, 233–272.

Regopoulos, L., Christianson, J. B., Claxton, G., & Trude, S. (2006). Consumer-directed health insurance products: Local-market perspectives. *Health Affairs, 25*(3), 766–773.

Reschovsky, J. D., Hadley, J., & Nichols, L. (2007). Why do Hispanics have so little employer-sponsored health insurance? *Inquiry, 44*(3), 257–279.

Reschovsky, J. D., Strunk, B. C., & Ginsburg, P. (2006). Why employer-sponsored insurance coverage changed, 1997–2003. *Health Affairs, 25*(3), 774–782.

Resende, M., & Zeidan, R. (2010). Adverse selection in the health insurance market: Some empirical evidence. *European Journal of Health Economics, 11*(4), 413–418.

Robinson, J. C. (2006). The commercial health insurance industry in an era of eroding employer coverage. *Health Affairs, 25*(6), 1475–1486.

Schiff, A. H. (2009). Physician collective bargaining. *Clinical Orthopaedics & Related Research, 467*(11), 3017–3028.

Schneider, J. E., Li, P., Klepser, D. G., Peterson, N. A., Brown, T. T., & Scheffler, R. M. (2008). The effect of physician and health plan market concentration on prices in commercial health insurance markets. *International Journal of Health Care Finance & Economics, 8*(1), 13–26.

Schoen, C., Stremikis, K., Collins, S., & Davis, K. (2009). Progressive or regressive? A second look at the tax exemption for employer-sponsored health insurance premiums. *Issue Brief (Commonwealth Fund), 53*, 1–8.

Seiber, E. E., & Florence, C. S. (2010). SCHIP's impact on dependent coverage in the small-group health insurance market. *Health Services Research, 45*(1), 230–245.

Siebrasse, P. B. (2007). Stark laws and fair market value exceptions: An introduction. *Journal of Medical Practice Management, 23*(1), 57–59.

Sloan, F. A., & Norton, E. C. (1997). Adverse selection, bequests, crowding out, and private demand for insurance: Evidence from the long-term care insurance market. *Journal of Risk and Uncertainty, 15*, 201–219.

Steinorth, P. (2011). Impact of health savings accounts on precautionary savings, demand for health insurance and prevention effort. *Journal of Health Economics, 30*(2), 458–465.

Stone, D. (2008). Protect the sick: Health insurance reform in one easy lesson. *Journal of Law, Medicine & Ethics, 36*(4), 607, 652–659.

Taylor, A., & Wilensky, G. R. (1983). The effect of tax policies on expenditures for private health insurance. In J.A. Meyer (Ed.), *Market reforms in health care*. Washington, DC: American Enterprise Institute for Policy Research.

Thomas, K. (1994–1995). Are subsidies enough to encourage the uninsured to purchase health insurance? An analysis of underlying behavior. *Inquiry, 31*, 415–424.

Thornton, J. A., & Rice, J. L. (2008). Does extending health insurance coverage to the uninsured improve population health outcomes? *Applied Health Economics & Health Policy, 6*, 217–230.

Turner, L. (2010). "Medical tourism" and the global marketplace in health services: U.S. patients, international hospitals, and the search for affordable health care. *International Journal of Health Services, 40*(3), 443–467.

Vaithianathan, R. (2006). Health insurance and imperfect competition in the health care market. *Journal of Health Economics, 25*(6), 1193–1202.

van den Berg, B., Van Dommelen, P., Stam, P., Laske-Aldershof, T., Buchmueller, T., & Schut, F. T. (2008). Preferences and choices for care and health insurance. *Social Science & Medicine, 66*(12), 2448–2459.

van Kleef, R. C., van de Ven, W. P., & van Vliet, R. C. (2009). Shifted deductibles for high risks: More effective in reducing moral hazard than traditional deductibles. *Journal of Health Economics, 28*(1), 198–209.

Vera-Hernandez, M. (2003). Structural estimation of a principal-agent model: Moral hazard in medical insurance. *Rand Journal of Economics, 34*(4), 670–693.

Wagstaff, A. (2010). Social health insurance reexamined. *Health Economics, 19*(5), 503–517.

Yegian, J. M. (2006). Coordinated care in a "consumer-driven" health system. *Health Affairs, 25*(6), w531–w536.

Zweifel, P., & Breuer, M. (2006). The case for risk-based premiums in public health insurance. *Health Economics, Policy, & Law, 1*(Pt. 2), 171–188.

Economics of Disease Prevention and Health Promotion

Al-Khatib, S. M., Sanders, G. D., Bigger, J. T., Buxton, A. E., Califf, R. M., Carlson, M, ... Expert Panel participating in a Duke's Center for the Prevention of Sudden Cardiac Death conference. (2007). Preventing tomorrow's sudden cardiac death today: Part I: Current data on risk stratification for sudden cardiac death. *American Heart Journal, 153*(6), 941–950.

Alden, N. E., Bessey, P. Q., Rabbitts, A., Hyden, P. J., & Yurt, R. W. (2007). Tap water scalds among seniors and the elderly: Socio-economics and implications for prevention. *Burns, 33*(5), 666–669.

Armstrong, E. P. (2007). Economic benefits and costs associated with target vaccinations. *Journal of Managed Care Pharmacy, 13*(7 Suppl. B), S12–S15.

Asche, C., LaFleur, J., & Conner, C. (2011). A review of diabetes treatment adherence and the association with clinical and economic outcomes. *Clinical Therapeutics, 33*(1), 74–109.

Baillie, K. (2008). Health implications of transition from a planned to a free-market economy—An overview. *Obesity Reviews, 9*(Suppl. 1), 146–150.

Basu, S., Chapman, G. B., & Galvani, A. P. (2008). Integrating epidemiology, psychology, and economics to achieve HPV vaccination targets. *Proceedings of the National Academy of Sciences of the United States of America, 105*(48), 19018–19023.

Bliss, D. Z., Zehrer, C., Savik, K., Smith, G., & Hedblom, E. (2007). An economic evaluation of four skin damage prevention regimens in nursing home residents with incontinence: Economics of skin damage prevention. *Journal of Wound, Ostomy, & Continence Nursing, 34*(2), 143–52; discussion 152.

Chaloupka, F. J., Straif, K., Leon, M. E., & Working Group, International Agency for Research on Cancer. (2011). Effectiveness of tax and price policies in tobacco control. *Tobacco Control, 20*(3), 235–238

Chang, C. F., Waters, T. M., & Mirvis, D. M. (2004). The economics of prevention in a post-managed-care environment. *Applied Health Economics & Health Policy, 3*(2), 67–70.

Chow, I., Lemos, E. V., & Einarson, T. R. (2008). Management and prevention of diabetic foot ulcers and infections: A health economic review. *Pharmacoeconomics, 26*, 1019–1035.

Conrad, D. A., & Perry, L. (2009). Quality-based financial incentives in health care: Can we improve quality by paying for it? *Annual Review of Public Health, 30*, 357–371.

Cook, E., Marchaim, D., & Kaye, K. S. (2011). Building a successful infection prevention program: Key components, processes, and economics. *Infectious Disease Clinics of North America, 25*(1), 1–19.

Davis, J. C., Robertson, M. C., Comans, T., & Scuffham, P. A. (2011). Guidelines for conducting and reporting economic evaluation of fall prevention strategies. *Osteoporosis International, 22*(9), 2449–2459.

De Luca d'Alessandro, E., Bonacci, S., & Giraldi, G. (2011). Aging populations: The health and quality of life of the elderly. *Clinica Terapeutica, 162*(1), e13–e18.

Douen, A., Pageau, N., & Medic, S. (2007). Usefulness of cardiovascular investigations in stroke management: Clinical relevance and economic implications. *Stroke, 38*(6), 1956–1958.

Dunn, J. D. (2008). Managed care considerations. *American Journal of Managed Care, 14*(6, Suppl. 2), S227–S237.

Ellis, R. P., & Manning, W. G. (2007). Optimal health insurance for prevention and treatment. *Journal of Health Economics, 26*(6), 1128–1150.

Elsler, D., Treutlein, D., Rydlewska, I., Frusteri, L., Kruger, H., Veerman, T., … Taylor, T. N. (2010). A review of case studies evaluating economic incentives to promote occupational safety and health. *Scandinavian Journal of Work, Environment & Health, 36*(4), 289–298.

Feely, J., & Bennett, K. (2008). Epidemiology and economics of statin use. *Irish Medical Journal, 101*(6), 188–191.

Gortmaker, S. L., Swinburn, B. A., Levy, D., Carter, R., Mabry, P. L., Finegood, D. T., … Moodie, M. L. (2011). Changing the future of obesity: Science, policy, and action. *Lancet, 378*(9793), 838–347.

Herman, W. H. (2011). The economics of diabetes prevention. *Medical Clinics of North America, 95*(2), 373–384.

Hilbert, A., Ried, J., Schneider, D., Juttner, C., Sosna, M., Dabrock P., … Heberbrand, J. (2008). Primary prevention of childhood obesity: An interdisciplinary analysis. *Obesity Facts, 1*(1), 16–25.

Holmes, C. B., Atun, R., Avila, C., & Blandford, J. M. (2011). Expanding the generation and use of economic and financial data to improve HIV program planning and efficiency: A global perspective. *Journal of Acquired Immune Deficiency Syndromes: JAIDS, 57* (Suppl. 2), S104–S108.

Hunt, N. A., Liu, G. T., & Lavery, L. A. (2011). The economics of limb salvage in diabetes. *Plastic & Reconstructive Surgery, 127*(Suppl. 1), 289S–295S.

Jansman, F. G., Postma, M. J., & Brouwers, J. R. (2007). Cost considerations in the treatment of colorectal cancer. *Pharmacoeconomics, 25*(7), 537–562.

Johansson, P., & Tillgren, P. (2011). Financing intersectoral health promotion programmes: Some reasons why collaborators are collaborating as indicated by cost-effectiveness analyses. *Scandinavian Journal of Public Health, 39*(Suppl. 6), 26–32.

Jones, L., & Bakler, M. R. (1986). The application of health economics to health promotion. *Community Medicine, 8,* 224–229.

Kenkel, D. S. (1994). The demand for preventive medical care. *Applied Economics, 26,* 313–325.

Klinkmann, H., & Vienken, J. (2008). Health is wealth! Is wealth health? *Makedonska Akademija na Naukite i Umetnostite Oddelenie Za Bioloshki i Meditsinski Nauki Prilozi, 29*(2), 13–23.

Kong, M. H., Peterson, E. D., Fonarow, G. C., Sanders, G. D., Yancy, C. W., Russo, A. M., … Al-Khalib, S. M. (2010). Addressing disparities in sudden cardiac arrest care and the underutilization of effective therapies. *American Heart Journal, 160*(4), 605–618.

Lenoir-Wijnkoop, I., Dapoigny, M., Dubois, D., van Ganse, E., Gutierrez-Ibarluzea, I., Hutton, J., … Nuijten, M. J. (2011). Nutrition economics—Characterising the economic and health impact of nutrition. *British Journal of Nutrition, 105*(1), 157–166.

Lewis, S. (2010). Creating incentives to improve population health. *Preventing Chronic Disease, 7*(5), A93.

Lo, Y. T., Chang, Y. H., Lee, M. S., & Wahlqvist, M. L. (2009). Health and nutrition economics: Diet costs are associated with diet quality. *Asia Pacific Journal of Clinical Nutrition, 18*(4), 598–604.

Malagelada, J. R. (2011). Diseases of the digestive tract: Is prevention possible and feasible? *Digestive Diseases, 29*(2), 255–263.

Mihalopoulos, C., Vos, T., Pirkis, J., & Carter, R. (2011). The economic analysis of prevention in mental health programs. *Annual Review of Clinical Psychology, 7,* 169–201.

Murphy, J. G., Correia, C. J., & Barnett, N. P. (2007). Behavioral economic approaches to reduce college student drinking. *Addictive Behaviors, 32*(11), 2573–2585.

Pelletier, K. R., Herman, P. M., Metz, R. D., & Nelson, C. F. (2010). Health and medical economics applied to integrative medicine. *Explore: The Journal of Science & Healing, 6*(2), 86–99.

Perencevich, E. N., Stone, P. W., Wright, S. B., Carmeli, Y., Fisman, D. N., Cosgrove, S. E., & Society for Healthcare Epidemiology of America. (2007). Raising standards while watching the bottom line: Making a business case for infection control. *Infection Control & Hospital Epidemiology, 28*(10), 1121–1133.

Piziak, V., Morgan-Cox, M., Tubbs, J., & Rajab, M. H. (2010). Elevated body mass index in Texas Head Start children: A result of heredity and economics. *Southern Medical Journal, 103*(12), 1219–1222

Roy, K., Chen, Z. A., & Crawford, C. A. (2009). Economic perspective on strategic human capital management and planning for the Centers for Disease Control and Prevention. *Journal of Public Health Management & Practice, 15*(6 Suppl.), S79–S89.

Ruger, J. P., Emmons, K. M., Kearney, M. H., & Weinstein, M. C. (2009). Measuring the costs of outreach motivational interviewing for smoking cessation and relapse prevention among low-income pregnant women. *BMC Pregnancy & Childbirth, 9*, 46.

Russell, L. B. (1984). The economics of prevention. *Health Policy, 4*, 85–100.

Sadatsafavi, M., Marra, C., Li, D., & Illes, J. (2010). An ounce of prevention is worth a pound of cure: A cost-effectiveness analysis of incidentally detected aneurysms in functional MRI research. *Value in Health, 13*, 761–769.

Sanders, G. D., Al-Khatib, S. M., Berliner, E., Bigger, J. T., Buxton, A. E., Califf, R. M., ... Expert Panel participating in a Duke Center for the Prevention of Sudden Cardiac Death-sponsored conference. (2007). Preventing tomorrow's sudden cardiac death today: Part II: Translating sudden cardiac death risk assessment strategies into practice and policy. *American Heart Journal, 153*(6), 951–959.

Schackman, B. R. (2010). Implementation science for the prevention and treatment of HIV/AIDS. *Journal of Acquired Immune Deficiency Syndromes: JAIDS, 55*(Suppl. 1), S27–S31.

Scheffler, R. M., & Paringer, L. (1980). A review of the economic evidence on prevention. *Medical Care, 18*, 473–484.

Schwappach, D. L. (2007). The economic evaluation of prevention—Let's talk about values and the case of discounting. *International Journal of Public Health, 52*(6), 335–336.

Scurlock, C., Raikhelkar, J., Mechanick, J. I. (2011). The economics of glycemic control in the ICU in the United States. *Current Opinion in Clinical Nutrition & Metabolic Care, 14*(2), 209–212.

Shepard, R. J. (1987). The economics of prevention: A critique. *Health Policy, 7*, 49–56.

Sipahi, O. R. (2008). Economics of antibiotic resistance. *Expert Review of Antiinfective Therapy, 6*(4), 523–539.

Trueman, P., & Whitehead, S. J. (2010). The economics of pressure relieving surfaces: An illustrative case study of the impact of high-specification surfaces on hospital finances. *International Wound Journal, 7*(1), 48–54.

Ungar, W. J. (2007). Paediatric health economic evaluations: A world view. *Healthcare Quarterly, 10*(1), 134–40, 142–145; discussion 145–146.

Vaczy, E., Seaman, B., Peterson-Sweeney, K., & Hondorf, C. (2011). Passport to health: An innovative tool to enhance healthy lifestyle choices. *Journal of Pediatric Health Care, 25*(1), 31–37.

Yazdy, M. M., Honein, M. A., Rasmussen, S. A., & Frias, J. L. (2007). Priorities for future public health research in orofacial clefts. *Cleft Palate-Craniofacial Journal, 44*(4), 351–357.

Yu, J., Smith, K. J., & Brixner, D. I. (2010). Cost effectiveness of pharmacotherapy for the prevention of migraine: A Markov model application. *CNS Drugs, 24*, 695–712.

Chapter 11

The Labor Market

OBJECTIVES

1. Define the role of the market for labor and explain how this market is linked to health and health care.

2. Describe a model of the demand for labor.

3. Describe a model of labor supply.

4. Explain how health insurance benefits are related to the supply of labor.

5. Explain the factors that affect the determination of wages and total compensation.

6. Explain how a model of the labor market can be used to explain wage and employment figures for healthcare workers.

7. Describe how health status affects workers' compensation.

8. Explain how market power can affect labor market outcomes in the healthcare sector.

11.1 INTRODUCTION

The labor market is the institution by which workers and employers come together to engage in the production of output. As a result of their interactions, the amount of labor that is hired and its compensation are determined. There are a number of health-related issues related to this market. Employers hire and pay workers according to their productivity and in some instances, a healthy worker will be more productive than an unhealthy one. Productivity is a key determinant in the employer's demand for labor. A second set of issues is related to labor supply: a worker's health status may influence his or her decision to seek full-time employment, part-time employment, or no employment at all. A third issue is related to total compensation rather than just wages. In the United States, workers receive part of their compensation in the form of fringe benefits, including health insurance. The demand for health insurance is thus connected with the labor market. To understand how policies that influence the purchase of health insurance work, it is necessary to understand how labor markets work.

Another set of issues related to the labor market deal with the determination of wages and employment for healthcare workers. Physicians, nurses, technicians, and other professionals and workers perform under the vagaries of the healthcare labor market. Numerous issues have arisen in this market, including shortages of nurses and other health professionals, and rising wages for healthcare workers.

11.2 DEMAND FOR LABOR

11.2.1 Demand for Labor by the Individual Firm

In this section, an analysis of the demand for a specific resource by an individual provider is developed. The provider could be a healthcare-producing entity, such as a hospital, laboratory, or physician's office, or it could be a nonhealthcare producer. The focus will be on healthcare providers, but the analysis can be applied to any type of institution in which they are employed. The dependent variable of interest is the demand for labor input. The labor input can be expressed in time units, such as hours or days. The labor demand curve, or function, is defined as the quantity of labor units that a firm will demand at any given price or wage.

In economic terms, this demand is a derived demand. That is, the firm does not demand labor, or any other input, for itself. Rather, an input is demanded because of the revenue or output it can generate for the firm. In short, the value of an input is derived from the usefulness of the input in achieving some objective. In traditional economic analysis, this objective is profits. Although healthcare firms may indeed have other objectives than profits, the profit maximization hypothesis is a good one to start with in analyzing the demand for labor and other inputs.

To help with the analysis, the example of a commercial laboratory that provides blood tests will be used. The time frame for the analysis will be a single day. The firm's product (or output) is defined as the number of blood tests produced per day. The firm has a series of inputs, which include capital equipment, materials and supplies, fixed management time, and variable labor time. Indeed, labor units, in the form of lab technician time, are assumed to be the only variable input (although, in reality, reagents will vary with the number of blood tests performed).

- *Production function.* With inputs and outputs defined, the relationship between them (the production function) is hypothesized. In Table 11-1, a numerical example of the relationship for the range of variable inputs from one to seven lab technician days is presented. With one lab technician, the lab can produce 50 blood tests; with two lab technicians, it can produce 110 tests; and so on. This relationship at first exhibits increasing marginal productivity, followed by decreasing marginal productivity (the third technician produces 50 extra tests, the fourth produces 40, and so on). Marginal productivity is the additional output achieved with the employment of one additional unit of input. Marginal productivity usually initially increases because of the ability to use the fixed resources more efficiently. As more inputs are used to produce output, marginal productivity will begin to fall as inefficiencies occur from employing less effective units and from difficulty in coordinating activities.

- *Revenue derived from worker production.* The firm's valuation of technician time rests not on the number of lab tests per se but on the revenue derived from these lab tests. The assumption is that each lab test has a fixed price of $6. Therefore, for each extra lab test produced, the firm brings in $6 in extra revenue. The total revenue from all lab tests at each level of input is shown in the fourth column of Table 11-1 (one technician brings in $300 in revenues, two bring in $660, etc.). The fifth column shows the *marginal value product* (*MVP*) obtained when the firm adds successive technicians. The *MVP* is defined as the additional revenue obtained from hiring one more unit of input. As with marginal productivity, this variable at first increases but then decreases. (The first technician has an *MVP* of $300, the second has an *MVP* of $360, and the *MVP* of the third is down to $300). The *MVP* curve is shown in Figure 11-1.

- *Labor cost.* We assume that each lab technician earns $160 per week. Because each lab technician earns the same amount, the marginal cost of the input is $160.

- *Firm's objectives.* The firm is assumed to have a goal of profit maximization. Profits, as defined here, are equal to revenue minus cost. The point at which maximum profits are attained occurs when the revenue gained from adding an additional worker equals the additional cost.

Table 11-1 The Demand for Labor by a Commercial Laboratory

(1)	(2)	(3)	(4)	(5)	(6)
Number of Laboratory Technicians	Number of Laboratory Tests (Total Product)	Additional Tests per Technician (Marginal Product)	Total Revenue from All Units of Production (Price of Product × Number of Units)	Additional Revenue from Addition of One Laboratory Technician (Marginal Value Product)	Wage Rate
1	50	50	$300	$300	$160
2	110	60	660	360	160
3	160	50	960	300	160
4	200	40	1,200	240	160
5	230	30	1,380	180	160
6	250	20	1,500	120	160
7	260	10	1,560	60	160

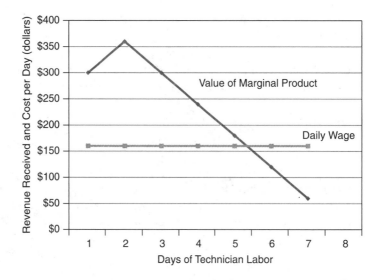

Figure 11-1 Demand Curve for Labor. The demand curve for labor is based on the additional revenue generated by each additional labor unit (days of technician labor), called the value of the marginal product (*VMP*). Provider profitability is determined by comparing the *VMP* with the price paid for labor.

The predictions of the model are as follows. On profitability grounds, the firm would hire the first worker, as the resulting marginal value product ($300) exceeds the marginal cost ($160). Indeed, the firm would continue to hire workers as long as it was profitable to do so. In this example, the firm would hire up to five workers for reasons of profitability. It would reduce its profits by hiring a sixth worker. Given the assumptions in the model, the firm's quantity of labor demanded equals five workers.

The demand curve was defined as the quantity of inputs a firm demands at a specific price. If the price of a unit of input changes, so will the quantity demanded. For example, a fall in the wage rate paid by the firm to $100 will increase the quantity of labor demanded to six units, and an increase in the wage rate will reduce the quantity of labor demanded. The quantity demanded will be traced out by the *MVP* curve, as this curve shows what the additional revenue will be for any given wage rate. Therefore, the *MVP* curve is the demand curve for the input.

The demand curve will shift outward if labor becomes more productive (yielding more output and revenue for given quantities of labor) or output prices increase. Labor can become more productive if the firm increases its degree of mechanization. For example, if the firm buys more capital equipment, each worker will be able to produce more. Also, if the price per lab test increases, then each worker will also yield more revenue (although not more output).

To extend the analysis, the effects of benefits as a form of compensation are introduced. Figure 11-2 shows a firm's demand curve for labor at alternative daily wage rates. For example, at a wage rate of $60, the firm will demand

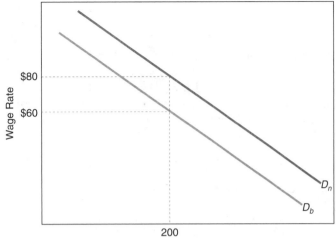

Figure 11-2 The Effect of Fringe Benefits on Demand for Labor. Curve D_n shows the demand for labor when the firm does not pay benefits. At a wage rate of $80 per day, the firm demands 200 labor days. In this case, the total wage is the same as total compensation. If health insurance benefits worth $20 per day are instituted, the demand curve relating the wage rate to the quantity of labor will fall by $20 at every quantity. This is because the firm, although still demanding 200 units at an average compensation cost of $80, is now providing each worker only $60 in wages as part of its $80 compensation package.

200 labor days. The demand curve for this rate (curve D_n) is based on the assumption that wages are the only form of compensation; that is, the firm does not offer fringe benefits such as health insurance.

Suppose, however, the firm agrees to provide $20 worth of fringe benefits per day. This adds $20 to the total labor compensation for each worker, but it does not add anything to the value of the output (the marginal value product). Therefore, the firm will still be willing to pay only $60 in total compensation for the 200th labor day—$40 in wages and $20 in fringe benefits. Thus, under the new benefits agreement, the firm would be willing to hire 200 workers at a wage rate of $40 rather than $60 ($40 in wages plus $20 in benefits is equivalent to $60 in wages with no benefits), and there is a new demand curve for labor. This curve, D_b, is the curve D_n shifted downward by exactly $20 at every quantity of labor. Any further increase in benefits would shift the demand curve down further. Furthermore, D_b, like the original demand curve, will shift in response to such factors as the price of output and the productivity of labor.

Now, taxes on corporate profits are introduced as a complicating factor. Assume that the firm pays a 10% profits tax. If an extra worker brings in $120 in revenues and costs the firm $100, then the before-tax profits will be $20 and the after-tax profits will be $18 [$20 × (1 − 0.10)]. If both wages and insurance premiums were deductible expenses, then it would not matter to the firm whether it paid out its compensation in the form of wages or insurance benefits. Under current tax law, insurance premiums are not taxed as employee income. Thus, this form of compensation is preferred by the employee because insurance purchased with pre-tax dollars "costs" the employee less than the same amount of coverage purchased with after-tax income. Assuming an individual desires health insurance coverage, then taking part of his/her wages in the form of health insurance instead of salary allows additional take home pay equal to the tax rate of the individual times the value of the insurance premium. This explains, in part, why benefits are so popular a form of compensation.

11.2.2 Market Demand for Labor

The market demand for labor or other inputs can be derived in the same way as other types of market demand. Assume the number of firms demanding labor in a certain market and the demand curve for each is known. The quantities demanded for labor at each wage rate can be added together to derive a market demand curve for labor. The supposition is retained that the price of the service or product is fixed. The market demand for labor (or other inputs) is thus a downward-sloping demand curve that shifts with changes in variables, such as the number of firms demanding labor and the productivity of each worker.

11.3 LABOR SUPPLY

11.3.1 Individual Labor Supply

The analysis of the supply of labor focuses on the quantity of labor individuals are willing to supply in order to earn income. The general framework used in this analysis is the consumer demand model. One main assumption of this model is that each consumer has a demand for income (usable to obtain goods and services) and for leisure time. The model examines how individuals alter their willingness to work in response to changes in labor compensation, such as wages. The end result of the analysis is a supply-of-labor curve relating the quantity of labor supplied to the wage rate.

The unit of observation in this model is the individual consumer (although some analysts have used the household as the observation unit because in many cases, data are collected at the household rather than the individual level), and the dependent variable is the number of hours an individual is willing to work. The assumptions in the analysis are as follows.

Imagine a utility-maximizing individual who has a utility function that encompasses two distinct goods: income (usable to purchase selected goods and services) and leisure time. As more is obtained of each good, the individual moves to higher levels of utility. It is also assumed that more is preferred to less, and so a higher utility level is preferred to a lower level.

The amounts of the two goods that will yield the same level of utility are shown in Table 11-2. If the individual has no income, he or she will be willing to take 60 hours in leisure. This combination of income and leisure will

Table 11-2 Income and Leisure Time Combinations at the Same Level of Utility

Income Per Week (Work Hours × Wage [$20/hour])	Leisure Hours Per Week (out of a total of 60 available hours)	Work Hours Per Week (Leisure + Work = 60 Hours)
$0	60	0
200	50	10
360	42	18
480	36	24
560	32	28
600	30	30

yield the same utility as $200 per week and 50 hours of leisure, $400 and 42 hours, and so on. Note that, whereas income increases in equal increments, leisure hours are reduced in successively smaller increments. This indicates a diminishing relative valuation placed on income. The individual will give up 10 hours of leisure to get the first $200 in income, but only 8 additional hours of leisure to get the next $200.

The individual has a total of 60 available hours per week. If 50 hours are spent on leisure, then 10 hours will be spent working. Finally, the individual can work for a wage of $20 per hour for up to 60 hours. Total income equals the product of wages and hours worked.

The conclusions of the model are as follows. The individual will increase work time hours from zero as long as the value of lost leisure is less than the wage rate. For example, at the point when the individual has full-time leisure, he or she is willing to give up 10 hours of leisure (work 10 more hours) for $200 in wages, a unit value of $20 per hour. However, once the individual has achieved this new point, he or she will be willing to give up only an additional 8 hours of leisure for an extra $200 in income. This implies a marginal value of leisure of $25 per hour at the new point. The individual places a lower value on the next $200 increase in income and would be willing to give up only 6 more hours of leisure, implying a marginal value of $33.33 per hour of leisure. Thus, the individual must be compensated at increasingly higher wage rates to induce him or her to give up more leisure (i.e., to work more).

Assume a wage rate of $30 an hour. The individual is faced with a choice of whether and how much to work. The individual will work at least 10 hours because the marginal value of the first 10 hours of work is $20. The individual would also choose to work the next 8 hours because the value of leisure time is less than the wage. Beyond that, the value of lost leisure is greater than the wage rate. Therefore, the individual will choose to work 18 hours. If the wage rate increases, say, to $40, then the individual would be willing to give up 6 more hours of leisure, and work for a total of 24 hours per week.

The positive relationship between wages and labor time measures what is called the *substitution effect of income for leisure*. The substitution effect of a wage increase is the increased incentive to work because work has a relative higher reward than leisure. Figure 11-3 shows how the quantity of labor changes as

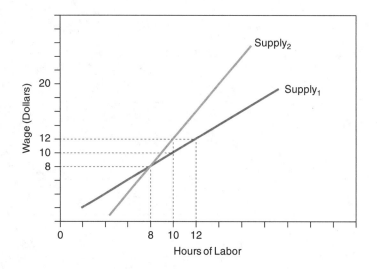

Figure 11-3   Alternative Labor Supply Curves. Curve Supply₁ shows a positive relationship between the wage rate and labor hours. Curve Supply₂ is a curve with a similar direction, but a steeper slope, which means that an increase in the wage rate from \$8 to \$10 will induce a smaller increase in the number of hours supplied.

the wage rate increases (curve Supply₁). There is also an income effect, which may offset the substitution effect. The income effect of a wage increase is the increase in purchasing power, enabling the worker to afford more leisure. As the wage rate increases, the total income that the individual can receive will increase, and the individual can purchase more goods and services; the individual will want to spend more leisure time consuming goods and services and hence will want to work less. It is possible that this income effect can more than offset the substitution effect, resulting in a backward-bending labor portion of the supply curve, especially at higher wage rates and income levels. However, statistical studies have shown that this is not a common event.

Supply curves for labor can have varying slopes. If an individual does not have a strong willingness to work more as wages increase, then the curve will be steeply sloped (Supply₂ in Figure 11-3). An individual more willing to work for small increases will have a curve like Supply₁. In Figure 11-3, an increase in wages from \$10 to \$12 will, depending on the labor supply curve, increase the labor supply to 10 hours (Supply₂) or 12 hours (Supply₁).

11.3.2 Health Insurance Benefits and Labor Supply

The most common way of financing health insurance in the United States is through the payment of health insurance premiums for individuals in the workplace. Health insurance coverage is a component of total worker compensation, which consists of wages plus fringe benefits. From the viewpoint of the individual worker, the amount of total compensation is what influences labor supply. However, economists have modeled labor supply decisions using wage rates as the base price. That tradition will be followed here.

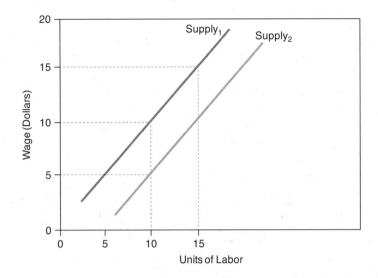

Figure 11-4 Labor Supply Curves with and without a Benefits Package. Curve Supply₁ shows the relationship between the wage rate and units (hours) of labor supplied when there are no benefits. The assumption is made that workers place a $1 value on each dollar of benefits. A $5 benefits package is introduced, and curve Supply₂ indicates the new quantity supplied at each wage rate. The reason why the curve shifts is as follows. The $5 wage rate now represents $10 in compensation and will induce the same amount of labor as will a $10 wage rate with no benefits. This is true for all wage rates. If, however, $1 in benefits is worth less to the worker than $1 in wages, the shift in the curve will be less.

In Figure 11-4, we present two labor supply curves, one for the case in which fringe benefits exist and one for the case in which there are none. Begin the analysis by focusing on the situation without fringe benefits. Curve Supply₁ relates the quantity of labor supplied to money wages. At a wage of $10, a total of 10 units of labor are supplied; at a wage of $15, a total of 15 units of labor are supplied; and so on.

Now, introduce fringe benefits worth $5 per worker (an amount independent of hours worked). Assume each worker places a value of $5 on these benefits. It is certainly possible of course for a worker to place a value lower than $5 on these benefits, and indeed fringe benefits may be worth very little to some workers. Under the current assumption, however, the value to the worker of compensation is $10 when the wage is $5; when the wage is $10, it is $15; and so on. Put another way, the curve that relates the wage rate to the quantity of labor supplied will shift downward and to the right (Supply₂). At a wage of $5 (plus $5 worth of fringe benefits), the supply of labor will be the same as it would be at a wage of $10 without fringe benefits. An additional $5 increase in benefits, wages held constant, will further shift the supply curve downward and to the right. (Of course, if the workers place a lower value on these benefits than their face value, the shift will be less than $5.)

11.3.3 Market Supply of Labor

The market labor supply is composed of the sum of labor supply curves of all the individuals in the market. As with the demand curve, the labor supply curve of the market comprises the summed quantity for each individual at each wage rate. An increase in the number of individuals in the market will cause the supply curve to shift to the right.

11.4 THE COMPETITIVE LABOR MARKET

11.4.1 Assumptions

This labor market analysis will focus on the market for lab technicians. To develop a competitive labor market model, assumptions must be made about market supply and demand factors, and how they interact. The basic model is shown graphically in Figure 11-5. The original market demand curve is shown as curve D_1. At a market wage of $20 per day, the firms in the market demand 20,000 days of lab technician services. At lower wages, the quantity of days demanded increases. The market supply curve is upward sloping, as hypothesized; this curve is shown as S_1 in Figure 11-5. At a market wage of $17.50, a total of 17,500 days of lab technician labor will be supplied in the market. If the wage increases to $20, then 20,000 days will be supplied. In the competitive model, an equilibrium condition is assumed; that is, the quantity supplied is equal to the quantity demanded.

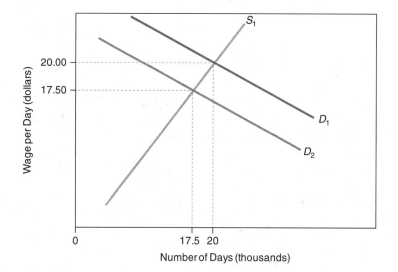

Figure 11-5 Labor Market Demand and Supply. The demand for labor is shown as curve D_1, and the supply curve is shown as curve S_1. Equilibrium occurs at a wage rate of $20 per day and a quantity of 20,000 labor days. If fringe benefits worth $5 a day are introduced, the demand curve shifts down uniformly by $5 (to D_2). The new equilibrium will be at a quantity of 17,500 days and a wage rate of $17.50.

11.4.2 Predictions

11.4.2.1 Supply, Demand, and Wage Rate

The first prediction of the model is that there will be a single equilibrium wage set at $20. Bargaining among demanders and suppliers of labor will result in this single equilibrium price at the equilibrium quantity of 20,000 labor days. Additionally, the equilibrium quantity and price will change with any changes in the related factors. With regard to shifts in demand, increases in the price of the product or the number of firms in the market will result in increased wage rates and increased labor days. Increases in the supply of labor will result in lower wages and higher quantities of labor. This model can be of help in analyzing the effect of using health insurance benefits as a form of compensation. Assume that the labs pay a $5 health insurance premium per labor day for each worker. The effect of this is to shift the demand curve uniformly down by $5, to curve D_2. Assume that there is no effect on supply. The prediction, in this case, is that the wage rate will fall to $17.50 and the quantity of labor employed will be reduced to 17,500 days. In this case, the finance method does reduce the quantity of employment.

11.4.2.2 Health and Labor Market Outcomes

Economists have recognized the role of health in labor market outcomes. The topic that has received the most attention has been the impact of health on the supply of labor. Good health will increase the likelihood that a worker will be employed and that a worker who is employed will work longer hours (e.g., will accept full-time rather than part-time employment). In terms of the competitive labor market model, poor health will shift the labor supply curve to the left. At any given wage rate, the quantity of labor supplied will be reduced when health status is decreased. Looking at the workings of the entire market, a reduction (leftward shift) in the supply of labor will reduce the overall amount of employment and increase the wage rate of those who continue to participate in the market.

Much of the evidence of the effect of health status on earnings has come from the developing countries (Duraisamy & Sathiyavan, 1998; Jack, 1999). A number of such studies have shown that improved health status, or factors that are associated with health status, such as nutrition and the body mass index, have a positive effect on wages. This finding is as expected, because, in many developing countries, there is a very low general level of health.

However, the same trends have been noted in developed countries as well. Using a national sample survey of residents in the United States, Kahn (1998) studied the comparative impact of labor market performance of persons with and without diabetes. He found that 64% of males who had diabetes and were between the ages of 50 and 60 were employed; the comparative figure for males without diabetes was 82%. The corresponding statistics for women were 40% and 60%, respectively. Thus, persons with diabetes are 18 to 20 percentage points (or 28 to 50%) less likely to be employed than persons without diabetes. Kahn's statistics indicate that there is a considerable effect of diabetes on labor market behavior, especially with regard to whether persons are employed.

Beck, Crain, Solberg, Unutzer, Glasgow, Maciosek,& Whitebird (2011) investigated the relationship between the severity of the symptoms of depression and productivity. They found for every one point increase on the Patient Health Questionnaire 9-item screen (PHQ-9), there was a corresponding 1.65% additional average loss in productivity. In addition, these authors found that a loss in productivity from individuals with symptoms of depression occurred in both full-time and part-time employment, and with self-reported poor or excellent health. This loss in productivity decreases the marginal value of the worker, possibly indicating it would be beneficial for employers to invest in treatment for these individuals.

11.4.2.3 Occupational Risk and Labor Market Outcomes

Injury and mortality rates vary considerably among occupations and industries. In 2010, there were 4,547 work-related fatalities in the United States, a rate of 3.5 per 100,000 full-time equivalent workers. The occupation with the largest number was construction (751), followed by transportation (631 deaths). On the basis of relative risks, workers in construction had a fatality rate of 9.5 deaths per 100,000 workers. By comparison, workers in education and health services had a fatality rate of 0.9 per 100,000, roughly one-tenth that of the construction workers (U. S. Bureau of Labor Statistics, 2010a). In 2010, there were 12 million nonfatal injuries and illnesses, or 118 per 10,000 equivalent full-time workers. Rates varied among occupations for illnesses and injuries as well. For example, there were 309.2 injuries per 10,000 workers in the protective services occupations and 10.8 injuries per 10,000 computer and mathematical occupations (U. S. Bureau of Labor Statistics, 2010b).

If workers correctly perceive differences among risks in different occupations, then according to utility-maximizing principles, they will prefer low-risk to high-risk occupations (all else held constant). Indeed, starting with a very low risk occupation (e.g., education and health services, in which there are 0.9 deaths per 100,000 workers), workers will demand risk premiums in order to induce them to accept occupations with higher risks (Viscusi, 1993). There are widespread differences in wages among occupations. The factors that influence these differences include both demand variables (worker productivity, occupational characteristics, price of the final product) and supply variables (worker age, education, and skill level). The on-the-job risk of mortality is one of many factors that influences the wage rate for any occupation. If adjustments could be made for all factors affecting supply and demand *other than risk*, then the interoccupational differences in wages would just compensate for differences in risk.

Once measures of that component of interoccupational wage differentials that reflects differences in occupational risks of mortality have been developed, these measures can be extrapolated to obtain an estimate of the value of a statistical life. For example, assume that there are two occupations with varying risks, but that all other factors are the same. Assume that a 50-year-old male has a life expectancy of 65 in the absence of a fatal work-related injury. The individual has a choice of two occupations: construction or education.

Construction workers experience 9.5 deaths per 100,000 workers, whereas educators experience only 0.9 deaths. The difference is 8.6 deaths per 100,000 workers (0.00086). The adjusted wage differential (net of other factors) is $400 annually. A projection can be made of the monetary value for the remainder of the person's lifetime. Ignoring the discounting factor (i.e., the discount rate is 0%), then the wage difference between the two occupations is $6,000 (15 years at $400 per year). The value of a statistical life can then be calculated as $69.767 million ($6,000 ÷ 0.00086). If more precision is desired, this estimate should be qualified so it can be made more realistic: future years' wages would be discounted, and many characteristics that are difficult to measure would have to be accounted for, such as the pleasantness of the work environment. Having made these adjustments, the estimate would be a better approximation of the valuation of risk that workers actually accept in the marketplace.

Indeed, a considerable number of studies have been conducted to measure the value of life using labor market differentials (Hirth, Chernew, Miller, Fendrick, & Weissert, 2000). These results show a very wide variation in the value of life. For a 40-year-old male, estimates ranged from $923,000 to over $19 million. Such differences are hard to reconcile, and they have created confusion on the part of policy makers. Nevertheless, the importance of the topic for policy-making purposes, including in the healthcare area, ensures that a great deal of additional work will be done in this area.

11.5 MARKET POWER IN LABOR MARKETS

11.5.1 Buyer's Market Power

In the past, there have been periods of time when widespread nursing shortages were reported by hospitals. A shortage is a situation in which, at the given wage rate, the quantity of labor demanded exceeds the quantity supplied. Economists have tried to explain shortages by means of economic models. The model of a hospital's buying power in the market for nurses can be used for this purpose. Assume that there is a single buyer of nursing services, a hospital in a small city. For this single buyer, an economic model is presented to predict pricing and output decisions.

- *Supplier costs.* With respect to the supply side of the market, assume there are a number of nurses available to be hired by the hospital (their supply curve is drawn in Figure 11-6). At a wage of $200 weekly, two nurses will supply their services; if the wage is increased to $300, three nurses will supply their services; and so on. With respect to the demand side of the market, the successive marginal value that the single hospital places on nurses is also shown in Figure 11-6.

- *Revenues.* Assume (1) that additional nurses allow the hospital to treat more patients, but the marginal productivity of these extra nurses diminishes; and (2) that the price received for each extra patient by the hospital is constant. The hospital's value curve has been derived from the estimated additional revenue that the hospital expects the additional nurses will generate. The marginal revenue (equal to the price

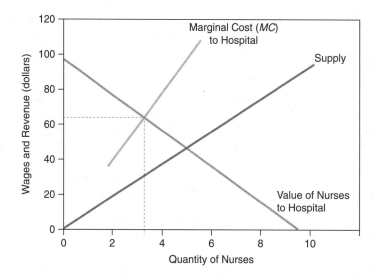

Figure 11-6   Equilibrium Wage and Number of Nurses Hired in Monopsonistic Market. The monopsonistic (single-buyer) firm's marginal cost (*MC*) for hiring additional nurses is derived from the schedule of nurses in the market. The value of an additional nurse is based on the amount of output that the hospital can produce with nurses (productivity) and the price of the output (the amount of revenue brought in by hiring an additional nurse). The profit-maximizing hospital will continue to hire nurses up to the point where the marginal cost equals the additional revenue from hiring another nurse.

of output times the marginal output yielded by an extra nursing unit) is $90 for the first nurse, $80 for the second, $70 for the third, and so on. Note that the total value to the hospital of three nurses is $240 ($90 + $80 + $70).

- *Behavioral assumption.* Finally, we will assume that the hospital wishes to maximize profits.

The implications of this model are that the profit-maximizing hospital will hire additional nurses as long as the marginal cost of doing so is less than the additional revenue. But the *MC* of nurses to the hospital is not the nurses' supply curve, *S*. Because *S* is sloped up, each successive nurse wants an extra dollar of pay. Assuming that the hospital must pay all nurses the same wage, by hiring the second nurse, it must pay a higher wage to the first as well. As a result, the *MC* curve is more steeply sloped than the supply curve (see Figure 11-6). For example, the *MC* of the second nurse is $30, but that of the third nurse is $50 (the difference between the total cost of 3 nurses at $90 and the total cost of 2 nurses at $40). The profit-maximizing hospital will hire three nurses (between 3 and 4 in Figure 11-6), for then the hospital's added revenue will equal its *MC* for hiring nurses. At such a level of hiring, it will pay a wage of $30 because that is the wage at which three nurses will supply their services.

In a monopsonistic (single-buyer) market, fewer nurses would be hired than in a competitive market. In a competitive market, competitive forces would drive the wage up to the level at which supply equals demand; more nurses would be hired, and wages would be higher. However, a monopsonistic buyer can prevent more nurses from being hired thus maintaining its profits. At the same time as it depresses wages, it creates a restriction in supply.

11.5.2 Unions as Monopoly Sellers of Labor

Feldman and Scheffler (1982) stated that in the early 1980s, unions increased nurses' wages by about 8%. A more recent study (Hirsch & Schumacher, 1995) questioned this finding. In 1999, nurses earned $20.86 per hour, compared to $21.53 for librarians and $27.86 for high school teachers (U.S. Department of Labor, 1999), despite the fact that there was a considerable degree of unionism among nurses. In this section, we present the theoretical argument that unions increase wages.

A union is an organized group of workers that allows individual workers to act as a cohesive unit when bargaining with employers. In terms of economic analysis, unions allow sellers of labor (in this case nurses) to wield monopoly power, raising their wages relative to those of nonunion workers. The monopoly model applied to the labor market is used to predict the impact of a union on wage levels. In Figure 11-7, a model of the labor market for nurses is presented, with hospitals as the buyers. Assume that there are several hospitals in the market but only one unit (a union) supplying them labor. The price

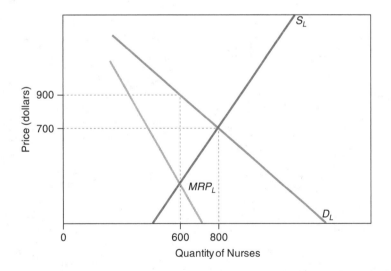

Figure 11-7 Monopolistic Seller of Labor. The marginal revenue product curve (MRP_L) is derived from the seller's demand for Labor (D_L). The seller will select the profit maximizing position at 600 nurses, where MRP_L equals S_L (supply of labor curve).

(wage) is measured along the vertical axis, and the quantity of nurses who are hired monthly is shown along the horizontal axis. The monthly demand for nurses is presented as curve D_L. The marginal revenue (MR) curve is derived from the demand curve. It shows the addition to total wage income of union members associated with expanded employment.

The marginal cost curve for nurses is shown as curve S_L. As the quantity of nursing time provided increases, the wage that nurses are willing to accept increases as well.

Assume that the union will maximize its "surplus," defined as the total compensation received by the workers minus any costs. Profits are defined in terms of the entire group of labor suppliers, who are behaving in unison as a labor union.

The union will bargain for a wage at that quantity of labor at which the members' wage income is maximized. The profit-maximizing position is where the marginal revenue equals marginal cost; that is, at the intersection of MR and S_L. In Figure 11-7, the profit-maximizing wage is $900 a month. The union would bargain for that wage and supply 600 nurses. In contrast, the wage in a competitive market would be $700 a month, and 800 nurses would be supplied at that price. The prediction of the model then is that unions increase wages and restrict employment.

As stated previously, the question as to whether the union has raised nursing wages is an open one. Other models have been developed that incorporate both hospital and union market power. Under such conditions, the wage would be determined by the relative degree of market power of both bargaining entities, and the same conclusions would not necessarily hold.

EXERCISES

1. The Midwest Clinic is a profit-maximizing organization. It has the capacity to hire up to five nursing hours. The production function for the clinic, in terms of clinic visits, is shown in the accompanying table.

Number of Nursing Hours	Number of Clinic Visits
1	12
2	22
3	30
4	36
5	40

Midwest charges a fee of $10 for each clinic visit. It pays nurses $50 an hour. What is the quantity of labor demanded by Midwest?

What will be the profit-maximizing quantity of labor demanded if the company adds $15 to the wage of each worker to pay for health insurance premiums?

2. What happens to the market supply function of public health nursing labor if:
   a. Wages increase in hospitals.
   b. Licensing requirements are made stricter for public health nurses.
   c. Nursing schools close down.
   d. There is a minimum wage imposed on nurses.
   e. The public image of public health nursing is improved.

3. What happens to the demand curve for labor of a clinic if each of the following occurs:
   a. The wage falls.
   b. The clinic purchases equipment that increases worker productivity.
   c. The price of clinic visits increases.
   d. The clinic hires more workers.
   e. The clinic hires better trained workers who are more productive.
   f. The clinic nurses provide care that is of a higher quality but takes more nursing time.

4. Explain the relationship between the wage rate and the quantity of labor supplied.

5. How does the introduction of health insurance as a benefit influence the supply curve for labor?

6. Assume a competitive model of the market for laboratory technicians in an environment of profit-maximizing laboratories. How will each of the following affect the wage rate for laboratory technicians:
   a. New equipment that increases the productivity of technicians is introduced.
   b. The local university increases the size of the graduating class of technicians.
   c. Technicians take more time in conducting tests in order to be more thorough.
   d. The government issues a generous retirement scheme for technicians over 60.
   e. The government licenses laboratories, restricting their numbers.
   f. Workers bargain for an increase in health insurance benefits; the laboratories provide insurance instead of wages.

7. Using the competitive labor market model, derive a prediction of the impact of poor health on employee wages.

8. The following is a labor supply function:

Wage Per Hour	Quantity of Nurse Supplied
$20	1
40	2
60	3
80	4
100	5
120	6

Nurses are used by the clinic to provide clinic visits. Each visit brings in $20 in revenue for the clinic. The relationship between nursing units and clinic visits is as follows:

Quantity of Nurses	Total Clinic Visits
1	5
2	9
3	12
4	14
5	15

The provider is assumed to maximize profits. Determine the provider's equilibrium wage and how many nursing units it will hire. The provider is a monopsonist, which means it is the sole purchaser of labor in the market.

BIBLIOGRAPHY

Labor Markets for Healthcare Workers

Abdrbo, A. A., Hudak, C. A., Anthony, M. K., & Douglas, S. L. (2011). Information systems use, benefits, and satisfaction among Ohio RNs. *CIN: Computers, Informatics, Nursing, 29*(1), 59–65.

Albreht, T. (2011). Health workforce in times of financial crisis. *European Journal of Public Health, 21*(1), 1.

Augustine, S., Lawrence, R. H., Raghavendra, P., & Watts, B. (2010). Benefits and costs of pay for performance as perceived by residents: A qualitative study. *Academic Medicine, 85*(12), 1888–1896.

Bacon, D. (2010). Results of the 2010 AORN Salary and Compensation Survey. *AORN Journal, 92*(6), 614–630.

Carlson, J. (2010). Keeping pay in check. Growing complexity of operating hospitals, systems adds to argument for compensating not-for-profit governing boards, but don't expect a big push soon. *Modern Healthcare, 40*(40), 26, 28.

Curran, C. R., & Totten, M. K. (2010). Board oversight of executive performance and compensation. *Nursing Economics, 28*(5), 343–345, 355.

Darbar, M., Emans, S. J., Harris, Z. L., Brown, N. J., Scott, T. A., & Cooper, W. O. (2011). Part-time physician faculty in a pediatrics department: A study of equity in compensation and academic advancement. *Academic Medicine, 86*(8), 968–973.

Dean, E. (2011). Staff discontent rises as inflation continues to devalue salaries. *Nursing Standard, 26*(3), 12–13.

Demaria, A. N. (2011). The primary care cardiologist. *Journal of the American College of Cardiology, 58*(8), 881–882.

Feldman, A. (2010). Protecting your employee resource and your practice. *New York State Dental Journal, 76*(6), 15–17.

Ford, J. (2011). A changing landscape. The job outlook for NPs & PAs. *Advance for NPs & PAs, 2*(1), 22–24.

Gewin, V. (2010). The spread of postdoc unions. *Nature, 467*(7316), 739–741.

Goodman, T. R., Forman, H. P., Stein, S., Bronen, R., & Brink, J. A. (2010). An "a la carte" academic radiology compensation plan: Something for everyone. *Journal of the American College of Radiology, 7*(11), 885–890.

Holtman, A. G., & Idson, T. L. (1993). Wage determination of registered nurses in proprietary and nonprofit nursing homes. *Journal of Human Resources, 28,* 55–79.

Kalist, D. E., Molinari, N. A., & Spurr, S. J. (2011). Cooperation and conflict between very similar occupations: The case of anesthesia. *Health Economics, Policy, & Law, 6*(2), 237–264.

Kheterpal, S., Tremper, K. K., Shanks, A., & Morris, M. (2011). Workforce and finances of the United States anesthesiology training programs: 2009–2010. *Anesthesia & Analgesia, 112*(6), 1480–1486.

Kocher, R., & Sahni, N. R. (2011). Hospitals' race to employ physicians—The logic behind a money-losing proposition. *New England Journal of Medicine, 364*(19), 1790–1793.

Kramer, J., & Santerre, R. E. (2010). Not-for-profit hospital CEO performance and pay: Some evidence from Connecticut. *Inquiry, 47*(3), 242–251.

Krueger, K. J., & Halperin, E. C. (2010). Perspective: Paying physicians to be on call: A challenge for academic medicine. *Academic Medicine, 85*(12), 1840–1844.

Lindsay, C. M. (1976). More real returns to medical education. *Journal of Human Resources, 11,* 127–129.

Mullenbach, K. F. (2010). Senior nursing students' perspectives on the recruitment and retention of medical-surgical nurses. *MEDSURG Nursing, 19*(6), 341–344.

Nakata, Y., & Miyazaki, S. (2011). Nurses' pay in Japan: Market forces vs. institutional constraints. *Journal of Clinical Nursing, 20,* 4–11.

Palmeri, M., Pipas, C., Wadsworth, E., & Zubkoff, M. (2010). Economic impact of a primary care career: A harsh reality for medical students and the nation. *Academic Medicine, 85*(11), 1692–1697.

Richardson, I., Slifkin, R., Randolph, R., & Holmes, G. M. (2010). A rural-urban comparison of allied health professionals' average hourly wage. *Journal of Allied Health, 39*(3), e91–e96.

Robeznieks, A. (2011). Par for doc pay? Annual compensation survey shows who gained the most and who lost ground. *Modern Healthcare, 41*(29), 22.

Saether, E. M. (2004). Nurses' labour supply with an endogenous choice of care level and shift type: A nested discrete choice model with nonlinear income. *Applied Health Economics & Health Policy, 3*(4), 273–280.

Salkever, D. (1975). Hospital wage inflation. *Quarterly Review of Economics and Business, 15,* 33–84.

Schumacher, E. J. (2011). Foreign-born nurses in the US labor market. *Health Economics, 20,* 362–378.

Schwartz, M. D., Durning, S., Linzer, M., & Hauer, K. E. (2011). Changes in medical students' views of internal medicine careers from 1990 to 2007. *Archives of Internal Medicine, 171*(8), 744–749.

Shah, T. (2011). Hospital CMO pay up. But their peers didn't fare as well. *Modern Healthcare, 41*(2), 34.

Shepherd, A. J., & Majchrzak, S. (2010). Employment of female and male graduates of US veterinary medical colleges, 2010. *Journal of the American Veterinary Medical Association, 237*(8), 922–925.

Simoens, S., & Giuffrida, A. (2004). The impact of physician payment methods on raising the efficiency of the healthcare system: An international comparison. *Applied Health Economics & Health Policy, 3*(1), 39–46.

Simons, A. B. (2009). What's a practice worth? *Journal of Medical Practice Management, 25*(3), 160–165.

Sloan, F.A. (1976). Real returns to medical education. *Journal of Human Resources, 11,* 118–126.

Smith, P. (2011). Workforce. Pay freeze for jobs—Deal or no deal? *Health Service Journal, 121*(6245), 26–27.

Snow, T. (2011a). Trust denies pay rise to staff with more than ten days off sick. *Nursing Standard, 25*(35), 5.

Snow, T. (2011b). Unfair wage deal could fuel tension between nursing staff and HCAs. *Nursing Standard, 25*(30), 14–15.

Szabo, J. (2010). With physician employment on the rise, new compensation models emerge. *Hospitals & Health Networks, 84*(12), 10.

Temple, A., Dobbs, D., & Andel, R. (2011). Exploring correlates of turnover among nursing assistants in the National Nursing Home Survey. *Journal of Nursing Administration, 41*(7/8 Suppl.), S34–S42.

Thornton, J. (1998). The labor supply effects of self-employed solo practice physicians. *Applied Economics, 30,* 85–94.

Timmons, J. C., Hall, A. C., Fesko, S. L., & Migliore, A. (2011). Retaining the older workforce: Social policy considerations for the universally designed workplace. *Journal of Aging & Social Policy, 23*(2), 119–140.

Tinsley, R. (2010). The 12-step way to reduce practice expenses: Part 1: Staffing efficiencies. *Family Practice Management, 17*(2), 38–43.

Tracy, E. E., Wiler, J. L., Holschen, J. C., Patel, S. S., & Ligda, K. O. (2010). Topics to ponder: Part-time practice and pay parity. *Gender Medicine, 7*(4), 350–356.

U. S. Department of Labor. (1999a). *National Compensation Survey: Occupational wages in the United States, 1998.* Washington, DC: Bureau of Labor Statistics.

Weinstein, A. R., Reidy, K., Norwood, V. F., & Mahan, J. D. (2010). Factors influencing pediatric nephrology trainee entry into the workforce. *Clinical Journal of the American Society of Nephrology: CJASN, 5*(10), 1770–1774.

Weissmann, G. (2011). Up the down pay scale: Teachers vs. football coaches. *FASEB Journal, 25*(5), 1433–1437.

Welch, J. L., Wiehe, S. E., Palmer-Smith, V., & Dankoski, M. E. (2011). Flexibility in faculty work-life policies at medical schools in the Big Ten conference. *Journal of Women's Health, 20*(5), 725–732.

Welton, J. M. (2011). Hospital nursing workforce costs, wages, occupational mix, and resource utilization. *Journal of Nursing Administration, 41,* 309–314.

Wilkins, K., & Shields, M. (2011). Employer-provided support services and job dissatisfaction in Canadian registered nurses. *Journal of Nursing Administration, 41*(7/8 Suppl.), S45–S53.

Williams, D. (2011). Nurses to fight changes to pay. *Nursing Times, 107*(19/20), 2–3.

Williams, T. E., Jr., Satiani, B., Thomas, A., & Ellison, E. C. (2009). The impending shortage and the estimated cost of training the future surgical workforce. *Annals of Surgery, 250*(4), 590–597.

Wright, D. B. (2010). Time is money: Opportunity cost and physicians' provision of charity care 1996–2005. *Health Services Research, 45,* 1670–1692.

Zarchy, M., Kinnunen, T., Chang, B. M., & Wright, R. F. (2011). Increasing predoctoral dental students' motivations to specialize in prosthodontics. *Journal of Dental Education, 75*(9), 1236–1243.

Health Insurance and Labor Markets

Abelsen, B. (2011). Pay scheme preferences and health policy objectives. *Health Economics, Policy, & Law, 6*(2), 157–173.

Barusch, A. S. (2011). Deficit commission targets social security: Privatization revisited? *Journal of Gerontological Social Work, 54*(1), 1–5.

Cutler, D. M., & Madrian, B. C. (1998). Labor market responses to rising health insurance costs: Evidence on hours worked. *Rand Journal of Economics, 29*(3), 509–530.

Flynn, P., Wade, M., & Holahan, J. (1997). State health reform: Effects on labor markets and economic activity. *Journal of Policy Analysis & Management, 16*(2), 219–236.

Garrett, B., & Chernew, M. (2008). Health insurance and labor markets: Concepts, open questions, and data needs. *Inquiry, 45*(1), 30–57.

Gerdtham, U. G., & Ruhm, C. J. (2006). Deaths rise in good economic times: Evidence from the OECD. *Economics & Human Biology, 4*(3), 298–316.

Gruber, J., & Madrian, B. C. (1997). Employment separation and health insurance coverage. *Journal of Public Economics, 66*, 349–382.

Kreuger, A. B., & Reinhardt, U. E. (1994). Economics of employer versus individual mandates. *Health Affairs, 13*, 34–54.

Marquis, M. S., & Long, S. H. (2001). Employer health insurance and local labor market conditions. *International Journal of Health Care Finance & Economics, 1*(3/4), 273–292.

Montagne, C. (2002). Bargaining health benefits in the workplace: An inside view. *Milbank Quarterly, 80*(3), 547–567.

Rhine, S. L., & Ng, Y. C. (1998). The effect of employment status on private health insurance coverage: 1977 and 1987. *Health Economics, 7*, 63–80.

Rogowski, J., & Karoly, K. (2000). Health insurance and retirement behavior. *Journal of Health Economics, 19*, 529–539.

Tompa, E., Trevithick, S., & McLeod, C. (2007). Systematic review of the prevention incentives of insurance and regulatory mechanisms for occupational health and safety. *Scandinavian Journal of Work, Environment & Health, 33*(2), 85–95.

Market Power in Labor Markets

Anderson, C., & Sensmeier, J. (2011). Nursing informatics scope of practice expands, salaries increase. *CIN: Computers, Informatics, Nursing, 29*(5), 319–320.

Bauml, B. (2011). Value for your profession. Does payroll outsourcing make sense for your practice? *Texas Dental Journal, 128*(2), 226–228.

Blakemore, S. (2010). Nurses face productivity drive despite projected budget rise. *Nursing Management (Harrow), 17*(8), 6–7.

Blesch, G. (2010). Time is money: Lawsuits hit hospitals for improper pay calculation. *Modern Healthcare, 40*(47), 32.

Brown, D. (2010). On local pay negotiations. Beware raiders of the lost cause. *Health Service Journal, 120*(6232), 16–17.

Carlson, J. (2009). A cut in pay. Many healthcare execs seeing smaller raises, flat salaries or even decreases in compensation, according to our annual survey. *Modern Healthcare, 39*(31), 26–30.

Carlson, J. (2011a). Feeling the squeeze. Healthcare execs see smaller raises overall, but some still net strong increases while others lose ground. *Modern Healthcare, 41*(33), 20, 22, 24–26, passim.

Carlson, J. (2011b). Pay loses its perk. *Modern Healthcare, 41*(20), 26–30.

Clamp, P. J., & Carswell, A. J. (2010). Comparative trends in ENT junior doctor pay. *Clinical Otolaryngology, 35*(4), 345–346.

Dean, E. (2010). Health unions prepare for battle to defend nurses' pension rights. *Nursing Standard, 25*(6), 5.

Feldman, R., & Scheffler, R. (1982). The union impact of hospital wages and fringe benefits. *Industrial and Labor Relations Review, 35*, 196–206.

Galloro, V. (2011). Strong performance. Healthcare executives reaped big rewards in 2010, with returning hospital CEOs seeing a 58.2% gain in compensation. *Modern Healthcare, 41*(33), 1, 6–7, 16.

Halley, M. D., & Reiser, W. S. (2011). Physician compensation: 5 mistakes, 1 solution. *Healthcare Financial Management, 65*(7), 82–86.

Hirsch, B. T., & Schumacher, E. J. (1995). Monopsony power and relative wages in the labor market for nurses. *Journal of Health Economics, 14,* 443–476.

Kendall-Raynor, P. (2011a). Employers threaten job cuts after unions stand firm on pay. *Nursing Standard, 25*(20), 5.

Kendall-Raynor, P. (2011b). Healthcare staff asked to work unpaid shifts in bid to save cash. *Nursing Standard, 25*(40), 5.

Kendall-Raynor, P. (2011c). Unions prepare for difficult decision over increment freeze. *Nursing Standard, 25*(18), 12–14.

Leigh, J. P., Tancredi, D., Jerant, A., & Kravitz, R. L. (2010). Physician wages across specialties: Informing the physician reimbursement debate. *Archives of Internal Medicine, 170*(19), 1728–1734.

Link, C. R., & Landon, J. H. (1975). Monopsony and union power in the market for nurses. *Southern Economic Journal, 14,* 649–659.

Lo Sasso, A. T., Richards, M. R., Chou, C. F., & Gerber, S. E. (2011). The $16,819 pay gap for newly trained physicians: The unexplained trend of men earning more than women. *Health Affairs, 30*(2), 193–201.

Mallidou, A. A., Cummings, G. G., Estabrooks, C. A., & Giovannetti, P. B. (2011). Nurse specialty subcultures and patient outcomes in acute care hospitals: A multiple-group structural equation modeling. *International Journal of Nursing Studies, 48*(1), 81–93.

Messersmith, J. G., Guthrie, J. P., Ji, Y. Y., & Lee, J. Y. (2011). Executive turnover: The influence of dispersion and other pay system characteristics. *Journal of Applied Psychology, 96*(3), 457–469.

Mooneyham, J. W., Goss, T., Burwell, L., Kostmayer, J., & Humphrey S. (2011). Employment incentives for new grads. *Nursing Management, 42*(3), 39–44.

Osinski, M. (2011). Here comes the sun: New policies will bring better times ahead for the nephrology specialty. *Nephrology News & Issues, 25*(3), 34–37.

Phillips, T. (2011). Exploitation in payments to research subjects. *Bioethics, 25,* 209–219.

Richards, D. (2011). Unionised workplaces make the difference. *Australian Nursing Journal, 18*(11), 21.

Roehr, B. (2011). New male doctors earned 17% more than female doctors in US in 2008. *BMJ, 342,* d798.

Schumacher, E. J. (1997). Relative wages and the returns to education in the labor market for registered nurses. *Research in Labor Economics, 16,* 149–176.

Schumacher, E. J., & Hirsch, B. T. (1997). Compensating differentials and unmeasured ability in the labor market for nurses: Why do hospitals pay more? *Industrial and Labor Relations Review, 50,* 557–579.

Spetz, J., Ash, M., Konstantinidis, C., & Herrera, C. (2011). The effect of unions on the distribution of wages of hospital-employed registered nurses in the United States. *Journal of Clinical Nursing, 20,* 60–67.

Yett, D. (1970). The chronic "shortage" of nurses. In H. Klarman (Ed.), *Empirical studies in health economics.* Baltimore, MD: Johns Hopkins University Press.

Effects of Health Status on Labor Markets

Bartel, A., & Taubman, P. (1979). Health and labor market success: The role of various diseases. *Review of Economics and Statistics, 61,* 1–8.

Beck, A., Crain, A. L., Solberg, L. I., Unutzer, J., Glasgow, R. E., Maciosek, M. V., and Whitebird, R. (2011). Severity of depression and magnitude of productivity loss. *Annals of Family Medicine, 9*(4), 305–11.

Berndt, E R., Finkelstein, S. N., Greenbert, P. E., Howland, R. H., Rush, A. J., Russell, J., & Keller, M. B.. (1998). Workplace performance effects from chronic depression and its treatment. *Journal of Health Economics, 17,* 511–535.

Bhattacharya, J., & Sood, N. (2011). Who pays for obesity? *Journal of Economic Perspectives, 25*(1), 139–158.

Boot, C. R., Koppes, L. L., van den Bossche, S. N., Anema, J. R., & van der Beek, A. J. (2011). Relation between perceived health and sick leave in employees with a chronic illness. *Journal of Occupational Rehabilitation, 21,* 211–219.

Bound, J. (1989). The health and earnings of rejected disability applicants. *American Economic Review, 79,* 482–503.

Duraisamy, P., & Sathiyavan, D. (1998). Impact of health status on wages and labour supply of men and women. *Indian Journal of Labour Economics, 41,* 67–84.

Ettner, S. L., Crain, A. L., Solberg, L. I., Unutzer, J., Glasgow, R. E., Maciosek, M. V., & Whitebird, R. (1997). The impact of psychiatric disorders on labor market outcomes. *Industrial and Labor Relations Review, 51,* 64–81.

Fenn, P.T., & Vlachonikolis, I. G. (1986). Male labor force participation following illness or injury. *Economics, 53,* 379–391.

Hamilton, B. H., & Hamilton, V. H. (1997). Down and out: Estimating the relationship between mental health and unemployment. *Health Economics, 6,* 397–406.

Jack, W. (1999). *Principles of health economics for developing countries.* Washington, DC: World Bank.

Judge, T. A., & Cable, D. M. (2011). When it comes to pay, do the thin win? The effect of weight on pay for men and women. *Journal of Applied Psychology, 96*(1), 95–112.

Kahn, M. E. (1998). Health and labor market performance: The case of diabetes. *Journal of Labor Economics, 16,* 878–899.

Karoly, L., & Rogowski, J. (1994). The effect of access to post-retirement health insurance and the decision to retire early. *Industrial and Labor Relations Review, 48,* 103–123.

Luft, H. (1975). The impact of poor health on earnings. *Review of Economics and Statistics, 57,* 43–57.

Sun, S. X., Dibonaventura, M., Purayidathil, F. W., Wagner, J. S., Dabbous, O., & Mody, R. (2011). Impact of chronic constipation on health-related quality of life, work productivity, and healthcare resource use: An analysis of the National Health and Wellness Survey. *Digestive Diseases & Sciences, 56*(9), 2688–2695.

Waenerlund, A. K., Virtanen, P., & Hammarstrom, A. (2011). Is temporary employment related to health status? Analysis of the Northern Swedish Cohort. *Scandinavian Journal of Public Health, 39*(5), 533–539.

Human Capital

Burns, H., Auvergne, L., Haynes-Maslow, L. E., Liles, E. A., Jr., Perrin, E. M., & Steiner, M. J. (2011). A qualitative analysis of career transitions made by internal medicine-pediatrics residency training graduates. *North Carolina Medical Journal, 72*(3), 191–195.

Durlak, J. A., Weissberg, R. P., Dymnicki, A. B., Taylor, R. D., & Schellinger, K. B. (2011). The impact of enhancing students' social and emotional learning: A meta-analysis of school-based universal interventions. *Child Development, 82,* 405–432.

Frogner, B. K. (2010). The missing technology: An international comparison of human capital investment in healthcare. *Applied Health Economics & Health Policy, 8,* 361–371.

Podsakoff, N. P., Whiting, S. W., Podsakoff, P. M., & Blume, B. D. (2009). Individual- and organizational-level consequences of organizational citizenship behaviors: A meta-analysis. *Journal of Applied Psychology, 94*(1), 122–141.

Rizzo, J. A., Abbott, T. A., & Pashko, S. (1996). Labour productivity effects of prescribed medicines for chronically ill workers. *Health Economics, 5,* 249–266.

Rochlin, J. M., & Simon, H. K. (2011). Does fellowship pay: What is the long-term financial impact of subspecialty training in pediatrics? *Pediatrics, 127*(2), 254–260.

Schultz, T. P. (1997). Assessing the productive benefits of nutrition and health: An integrated human capital approach. *Journal of Econometrics, 77,* 141–158.

Thomas, D., & Strauss, J. (1997). Health and wages: Evidence on men and women in urban Brazil. *Journal of Econometrics, 77,* 159–185.

Wada, R., & Tekin, E. (2010). Body composition and wages. *Economics & Human Biology, 8*(2), 242–254.

Wright, T. A., & Bonett, D. G. (2002). The moderating effects of employee tenure on the relation between organizational commitment and job performance: A meta-analysis. *Journal of Applied Psychology, 87*(6), 1183–1190.

Effects of Compensation Practices on Health

Damman, M., Henkens, K., & Kalmijn, M. (2011). The impact of midlife educational, work, health, and family experiences on men's early retirement. *Journals of Gerontology Series B-Psychological Sciences & Social Sciences, 66*(5), 617–627.

Dierick-van Daele, A. T., Steuten, L. M., Romeijn, A., Derckx, E. W., & Vrijhoef, H. J. (2011). Is it economically viable to employ the nurse practitioner in general practice? *Journal of Clinical Nursing, 20,* 518–529.

Finkelstein, J., Lifton, J., & Capone, C. (2011). Redesigning physician compensation and improving ED performance. *Healthcare Financial Management, 65*(6), 114–117.

Flodgren, G., Eccles, M. P., Shepperd, S., Scott, A., Parmelli, E., & Beyer, F. R. (2011). An overview of reviews evaluating the effectiveness of financial incentives in changing healthcare professional behaviours and patient outcomes. *Cochrane Database of Systematic Reviews,* (7), CD009255.

Gainsbury, S. (2010). Foundations seek to halt automatic pay rises. *Health Service Journal, 120*(6225), 4–5.

Gans, D. N. (2011). Unequal pay for unequal work. *MGMA Connexion/Medical Group Management Association, 11*(4), 17–18.

Good, E., & Bishop, P. (2011). Willing to walk: A creative strategy to minimize stress related to floating. *Journal of Nursing Administration, 41*(5), 231–234.

Happell, B., & Palmer, C. (2010). The Mental Health Nurse Incentive Program: The benefits from a client perspective. *Issues in Mental Health Nursing, 31*(10), 646–653.

Helmchen, L.A., & Lo Sasso, A. T. (2010). How sensitive is physician performance to alternative compensation schedules? Evidence from a large network of primary care clinics. *Health Economics, 19*(11), 1300–1317.

Hill, S.C. (2011). Individual insurance and access to care. *Inquiry, 48*(2), 155–168.

Jaskiewicz, W., Tulenko, K., Rockers, P., Wurts, L., & Mgomella, G. (2010). Retaining hospital workers: A rapid methodology to determine incentive packages. *World Hospitals & Health Services, 46*(3), 8–11.

Lindquist, L.A., Jain, N., Tam, K., Martin, G. J., & Baker, D. W. (2011). Inadequate health literacy among paid caregivers of seniors. *Journal of General Internal Medicine, 26*(5), 474–479.

Liong, A. S., & Liong, S. U. (2010). Financial and economic considerations for emergency response providers. *Critical Care Nursing Clinics of North America, 22*(4), 437–444.

McGovern, P., Dowd, B., Gierdingen, D., Moscovice, I., Kochevar, L., & Lohman, W. (1997). Time off work and the postpartum health of employed women. *Medical Care, 35,* 507–521.

Morgan, C. L., & Beerstecher, H. J. (2011). Satisfaction, demand, and opening hours in primary care: An observational study. *British Journal of General Practice, 61*(589), e498–e507.

Occupational Risk and Labor Market Outcomes

Berger, M. C., Blomquist, G. C., Kenkel, D., & Tolley, G. S. (1987). Valuing changes in health risks: A comparison of alternative measures. *Southern Economic Journal, 53,* 867–984.

Blazeviciene, A., & Novelskaite, A. (2010). New and old professional groups in health care: Formal re-definitions of the nursing profession and the internal qualities of professionals. *Medicina (Kaunas, Lithuania), 46*(Suppl. 1), 71–78.

Blomquist, G. (1979). Value of life saving: Implications of life saving. *Journal of Political Economy, 87*, 540–558.

Blomquist, G. (1981). The value of human life: An empirical perspective. *Economic Inquiry, 19*, 157–164.

Christian, M. S., Bradley, J. C., Wallace, J. C., & Burke, M. J. (2009). Workplace safety: A meta-analysis of the roles of person and situation factors. *Journal of Applied Psychology, 94*(5), 1103–1127.

Dalal, R. S. (2005). A meta-analysis of the relationship between organizational citizenship behavior and counterproductive work behavior. *Journal of Applied Psychology, 90*(6), 1241–1255.

Dillingham, A. E. (1985). The influence of risk variable definition on value-of-life estimates. *Economic Inquiry, 24*, 277–294.

Evans, M. (2011). Saving it for later. Healthy hospitals turn to layoffs to bend own cost curve. *Modern Healthcare, 41*(26), 1, 6–7.

Fisher, A., Fisher, A., Chestnut, L. G., & Violette, D. M. (1989). The value of reducing risks of death: A note on new evidence. *Journal of Policy Analysis and Management, 8*, 88–100.

Hirth, R. A., Chernew, M. E., Miller, E., Fendrick, A. M., & Weissert, W. G. (2000). Willingness to pay for a quality-adjusted life year. *Medical Decision Making, 20*, 332–342.

Kaplan, K. (2010). Academia: The changing face of tenure. *Nature, 468*(7320), 123–125.

Ker, K., Edwards, P. J., Felix, L. M., Blackhall, K., & Roberts, I. (2010). Caffeine for the prevention of injuries and errors in shift workers. *Cochrane Database of Systematic Reviews,* (5), CD008508.

Linnerooth, J. (1979). The value of human life: A review of the models. *Economic Inquiry, 17*, 52–74.

Maxson-Cooper, P. A. (2011). Empowering nurses through an innovative scheduling model. *Nursing Clinics of North America, 46*(1), 59–65.

Mintz, M. (2011). Something for everyone. New practice models for primary care physicians offer revenue and lifestyle advantages. *Medical Economics, 88*(10), 41–42, 44–45.

Mobley, K., & Turcotte, C. (2010). Structuring competitive physician compensation models. *Healthcare Financial Management, 64*(12), 76–82.

Mohle, B. (2010). Should a better life include more risk for workers? *Queensland Nurse, 29*(6), 5.

Reid, K. R., Attlesey-Pries, J. M., Syverson, R. C., Uthke, L. D., Wottreng, D. M., & Muehlenbein, M. J. (2011). Sustaining a successful RN compensation model through transparency and communication. *Journal of Nursing Administration, 41*(2), 58–63.

Robinson, J. C. (1986). Hazard pay in unsafe jobs. *Milbank Quarterly, 64*, 650–677.

Rosen, S. (1981). Valuing health risk. *American Economic Review, 71*, 241–245.

Schuring, M., Mackenbach, J., Voorham, T., & Burdorf, A. (2011). The effect of re-employment on perceived health. *Journal of Epidemiology & Community Health, 65*(7), 639–644.

Scott-Marshall, H., & Tompa, E. (2011). The health consequences of precarious employment experiences. *Work, 38*(4), 369–682.

Soberg, H. L., Roise, O., Bautz-Holter, E., & Finset, A. (2011). Returning to work after severe multiple injuries: Multidimensional functioning and the trajectory from injury to work at 5 years. *Journal of Trauma-Injury Infection & Critical Care, 71*(2), 425–434.

Sturman, M. C., Cheramie, R. A., & Cashen, L. H. (2005). The impact of job complexity and performance measurement on the temporal consistency, stability, and test-retest reliability of employee job performance ratings. *Journal of Applied Psychology, 90*(2), 269–283.

Thaler, R., & Rosen, S. (1975). The value of saving a life: Evidence from the labor market. In N. E. Terleckyj (Ed.), *Household production and consumption*. New York, NY: National Bureau of Economic Research.

U. S. Bureau of Labor Statistics. (2010a). *Census of fatal occupational injuries (CFOI)—Current and revised data*. Retrieved from http://www.bls.gov/iif/oshcfoi1.htm

U. S. Bureau of Labor Statistics. (2010b). *Occupational injuries and illnesses by selected characteristics*. Retrieved from http://www.bls.gov/news.release/osh2.toc.htm

U. S. Department of Labor. (1999). *Workplace injuries and illnesses in 1998*. Washington, DC: Bureau of Labor Statistics.

U. S. Department of Labor. (2000). *National census of fatal occupational injuries, 1999.* Washington, DC: Bureau of Labor Statistics.

Virtanen, P., Janlert, U., & Hammarstrom, A. (2011). Exposure to nonpermanent employment and health: Analysis of the associations with 12 health indicators. *Journal of Occupational & Environmental Medicine, 53*(6), 653–657.

Viscusi, W. K. (1978a). Wealth effects and earnings premiums for job hazards. *Review of Economics and Statistics, 60,* 408–416.

Viscusi, W. K. (1978b). Labor market valuations of life and limb. *Public Policy, 26,* 360–386.

Viscusi, W. K. (1993). The value of risks to life and health. *Journal of Economic Literature, 31,* 1912–1946.

Wadsworth, E. J., Chaplin, K. S., & Smith, A. P. (2010). The work environment, stress and well-being. *Occupational Medicine (Oxford), 60*(8), 635–639.

PART III: Evaluative Economics

Economic Evaluation of Health Services

12.1 INTRODUCTION

Economic evaluation analysis involves the quantification of changes in health resource use and outcomes due to the introduction of new interventions. Policy makers are increasingly turning to these analyses in order to acquire information for making decisions about alternatives in health care. Managers of drug formularies, especially publicly funded ones, resort to economic evaluations in order to determine which drugs to pay for under the insurance plan. Government policy makers use health technology assessments, which are based largely on economic evaluations, to shed light on the economic implications of new interventions.

Economic evaluations are used to inform decisions when there is a concern that a market is not yielding the right allocation of resources. The studies attempt to replace poor information or provide missing information on outcomes and their valuations, and on the costs of interventions. The direct measure of these concepts can provide important insights as to how resources should be allocated.

In this chapter, the methods that are used in economic evaluation studies are introduced. First, an overview of the subject, indicating the questions that are posed and the tools that have been developed to answer them, is presented. Following this, the guidelines for a sound economic evaluation and the key components of three major types of economic evaluation studies—cost-effectiveness (including incremental cost-effectiveness ratios), cost-utility, and benefit-cost studies—are presented.

12.2 THE PURPOSES OF ECONOMIC EVALUATION

There are several distinct reasons to perform economic evaluation studies. First, alternative courses of action that are substitute solutions for the same conditions can be compared. For example, two drugs for the treatment of migraine headaches might be compared, or the use of drugs versus surgery for treating blocked arteries might be compared. Recent studies have shown that the complications of diabetes can be treated effectively with intensive glucose control, which includes frequent monitoring of glucose levels and frequent clinic visits. The alternative intervention is the more conventional treatment, which includes careful diet and exercise, but less careful monitoring and less frequent insulin doses (Diabetes Control and Complications Trial Research Group, 1995, 1996). An economic evaluation study would allow us to compare the benefits and costs of the two treatments. Second, the question of whether a treatment is worthwhile can be investigated. For example, we might ask the question of whether diabetes should be treated at all can be examined. Note that there is an important difference between this and the first purpose. In a study of alternatives, the changes in health that occur as a result of the use of additional resources would be examined, but whether the changes were worth the cost would not be considered. In the second kind of study, that exact question would in fact be asked.

12.3 STEPS IN ECONOMIC ANALYSIS

Regardless of which economic analysis method is employed, the same basic steps are employed; the major differences are in the magnitude and complexity of the events being evaluated. The first step in any analysis is to define the problem clearly and explicitly. The way the problem is defined establishes the boundaries of the viable alternatives—the more broadly the problem is defined, the more alternatives are available for solving the problem. The second step is to explicitly state the degree to which the objectives are to be met; these objectives are quantifiable outcomes associated with the problem being addressed. For example, the problem is identified as rising costs, and the objective is to keep rising costs below 20% of GDP in the United States.

The third step in any economic analysis is to identify alternatives or options available for achieving the objective or addressing the problem identified.

In identifying the alternatives, it is often useful to graph the chronological ordering of the possible sequence of events. The graphing assists in formulating the mathematical model and in identifying the probabilities associated with each decision or outcome in the analysis. In graphing the alternatives a decision tree can be used in addressing linear style problems, while Markov models are more applicable if the events being analyzed occur repeatedly or over a long period of time.

Step four involves identifying the benefits or outcomes to be achieved. These benefits can be either direct or indirect. Regardless of the type of benefit, they need to be able to be quantified or measured. To compare benefits across alternatives, they need to be measured in comparable units. Although the comparable unit is often monetary, that is not required for any of the approaches; the only thing that is required is that the benefits can be measured and compared with common units. Step five involves identifying and quantifying all expected resources to be expended or consumed. These costs can also be direct and indirect and need to be measured and valued in common units. The requirement for common units of measurement enables various alternatives to be compared for decision making.

Step six involves the identification of the perspective from which the analysis is being viewed; the question identified to be answered should determine the perspective to be taken because the benefits and costs may be different for each type of entity. Identifying the perspective enables decisions to be made with the best information possible.

In addition to the perspective, it is important to identify the time frame of the alternatives being assessed. Unless all costs and benefits occur in the same period of time, then it becomes necessary to perform discounting—step seven. Because the value of money is greater in the present than it is in the future, the preference is to receive money as soon as possible, requiring future benefits and costs to be discounted. Although there is little disagreement regarding the need for discounting, the discount rate to be applied is much more controversial. There is not a single discount rate appropriate for all situations. In general, the discount rate applied should reflect the best estimate of the risk involved in the situations.

The eighth step involves analyzing the uncertainties associated with the events; this involves performing sensitivity analysis on the key variables to determine the importance of the variables to the results of the analysis. A range of values should be applied to each variable employing the "what if . . . " scenario. If the variation in the value of the key variable is substantial, then the variable will need close scrutiny in the decision-making process.

Step nine involves comparing the benefits and costs of the alternatives. The results of this comparison can provide important information regarding relative impact of the alternatives. This doesn't imply that the results of the comparison should be the only input into the decision-making process, but rather the analysis can be an important input into the decision-making process. Once the comparative results have been derived, it becomes important to discuss the results with others to check the validity of the assumptions made and to consider the ethical issues surrounding the decision. The final step involves monitoring and reevaluating conditions after the decision has been made. This reassessment can be used to assist in decisions to modify the size or focus of the program implemented, depending on changes that have occurred in the environment.

An economic evaluation doesn't provide all the answers, but it does provide explicit consideration of the goals and objectives to be achieved, the perspective taken, the alternatives considered, and the values assigned to costs, benefits, and risks. This explicit consideration should improve the decision-making process.

12.4 SELECTING THE RIGHT TYPE OF ANALYSIS

Once the purpose of the evaluation is clear, the appropriate type of study can be selected. There are five different types of comparative studies in economic evaluation analysis: cost-effectiveness analysis, cost-utility analysis, cost-minimization analysis, cost-consequence analysis, and benefit-cost analysis (Drummond, O'Brien, Stoddart, & Torrance, 1997). In cost-effectiveness analysis, the difference in costs is compared to the difference in outcomes (in which the outcomes are of a single type, such as years of life following treatment). The formula for cost-effectiveness analysis is

$$(c_2 - c_1) / (q_2 - q_1)$$

in which 1 and 2 refer to alternative interventions (e.g., conventional versus intensive treatment for diabetes), c is the cost per person, and q is the outcome. Cost-effectiveness analysis is used when there are alternative ways of attaining a single type of outcome, such as life years or quality of life. The outcomes do not have to be the same amount, simply a comparable type of outcome. Associated with cost-effectiveness analysis is cost-consequences analysis. In this type of analysis, multiple types of outcome are possible, such as time to death and quality of life, but the outcomes are not aggregated into a single scale (Bakker, Hidding, van der Linden, & van Doorslaer, 1994). Cost-consequence analysis is similar in purpose to cost-effectiveness analysis and so the two methods are grouped together.

Another form of cost-effectiveness is incremental cost-effectiveness ratio (ICER). This method of evaluation assesses the difference between cost and effectiveness of two different events or interventions. The formula for ICER is

$$ICER = (Cost_{new} - Cost_{old}) / (Effect_{new} - Effect_{old})$$

In health care, this method is useful when a new medical treatment is being considered to replace an existing treatment. In making the comparisons, a number of outcomes are possible. For example, the new treatment may be less expensive than the old treatment, and it may also be more effective. In this case, then the new treatment dominates and should be adopted. In another case, for example, the new treatment may cost less than the old treatment, but it may also be less effective. In this case, neither treatment is dominant, so the decision involves determining if the decrease in health outcomes is worth the savings in cost. Another case, for example, occurs when the new treatment costs more, but it is also more effective. Again, in this case, neither treatment is dominant; the question to be answered is whether the gain in health outcome is worth the increase in costs. Finally, for example, the new treatment may be more costly and less effective than the old treatment. In this case, the old treatment is dominant and should not be replaced with the new treatment.

The ICER method is also relevant when a new medical treatment is developed when no treatment previously existed. In this case, the formula is simply

$$\text{ICER} = (\text{Cost}_{new} / \text{Effect}_{new})$$

The focus here is now on determining if the results are worth the costs incurred in its production. Although the ratio does not provide an absolute answer, it does provide valuable information for decision making. A shortcoming of this method, however, is that there is no consensus as to what the threshold point is when the new treatment is not considered to be worth the additional cost of its production. Historically, medical interventions have been evaluated in terms of improving health or extending life, with very little attention given to costs. What is the maximum cost per additional year of life saved that should be viewed favorable—$50,000? $75,000?

In cost-utility analysis, differences in the "utility" of interventions is compared with differences in cost. The cost-utility formula is

$$(c_2 - c_1) / (u_2 - u_1)$$

in which the outcome *(u)* is an index of consumer health status (consumer health status is a composite measure encompassing more than one component of health).

In certain circumstances, cost-minimization analysis can be used as a special form of cost-effectiveness or cost-utility analysis. When the outcomes are the same for all of the interventions being studied, then the interventions can be evaluated just by looking at costs. A cost-minimization analysis would then be used. In benefit-cost analysis, the health indices are typically replaced with dollar measures of benefits. The assessment is the difference between benefits and costs, all of which are usually expressed in monetary terms. Although benefits are usually expressed in monetary terms, this is not necessary. Monetary values are typically used because they are a common measure across multiple types of projects. However, all that is necessary is that the benefits be measured by a common unit. The formula for the benefit-cost analysis of an intervention is

$$\text{NB} = b - c \text{ or Ratio} = b/c$$

in which NB is the net benefit, *b* stands for the value of the benefits from the intervention, and *c* is the additional cost of the intervention. There is of course an implicit alternative, in that the resources could be used in another way, reflecting the opportunity costs of the activity.

The net benefit approach *(b − c)* compares projects on the basis of the excess of benefits over costs; total costs are subtracted from total benefits to determine the greatest value of net benefit. In this approach, the project with the greatest net benefit is selected. Although the results provide information on the absolute value of net benefits, they ignore the relative magnitude of the projects. For example, a net benefit of $1,000 could reflect the difference of total costs of $100 and the total benefits of $1,100, or it could reflect total costs of $100,000 and total benefits of $101,000.

The benefit-cost ratio approach (b/c) compares projects on the basis of the average benefit per unit cost; in this approach, the project with the greatest ratio of benefits to costs is selected. The results of this approach can be impacted by the classification of an event as a cost or a benefit. For example, if a project reduces hospitalization utilization, the reduction in utilization can be viewed as an increase in benefits, thereby increasing the numerator, or as a decrease in costs, thereby decreasing the denominator. Where it is classified will impact the value of the ratio. For example, if the original project had costs of $5,000 and benefits of $10,000, then the ratio is 2:1 ($10,000/$5,000). Now, assume hospitalization is reduced, decreasing expenditures by $1,000. If the reduction is viewed as an increase in benefits, the ratio is now 2.2:1 ($11,000 /$5,000). However, if the reduction is viewed as a decrease in costs, then the ratio is now 2.5:1 ($10,000/$4,000). It is very important therefore to state explicitly the assumptions made in the analysis because it will impact the outcomes.

There is an appropriate type of analysis for each study objective. If analysts want to compare outcomes and costs for alternative interventions using a single outcome measure (or unweighted multiple outcomes), then they will use cost-effectiveness analysis. If they want to compare costs and outcomes when there is more than one component of outcome, and these are combined into a single index whose weights are a reflection of someone's valuations, then they would use cost-utility analysis. Finally, if they are asking whether the intervention should be adopted (i.e., whether is it worthwhile), then they would use benefit-cost analysis.

12.5 GUIDELINES FOR CONDUCTING A COST-EFFECTIVENESS ANALYSIS

In the past several years, a number of publications have appeared that provide guidance on what steps to take in conducting an economic evaluation analysis in the healthcare field (Canadian Coordinating Office for Health Technology Assessment, 1997; Cookson, Drummond, & Weatherly, 2009; Drummond, O'Brien, Stoddart, & Torrance, 1997; Gold, McCoy, & Siegel, 1996; Menon, Schubert, & Torrance, 1996; Nixon Stoykova, Glanville, Christie, Drummond, & Kleijnen, 2000; Sorenson, Tarricone, Siebert, & Drummond, 2011). In this section, an outline of the elements of cost-effectiveness and cost-utility analyses in the light of what these guidelines recommend is presented. The exposition will be conducted using an example of comparing an intensive treatment of diabetes and the conventional treatment. First, an example is briefly presented, then the use of the guidelines to conduct economic evaluation analyses is presented.

The example is based on several pivotal clinical trials for diabetes control (Diabetes Control and Complications Trial Research Group, 1995, 1996) in which newly diagnosed diabetes patients were randomized to one of two interventions. In the first intervention, called conventional care, the individual tests his or her glucose level daily, takes one or two insulin injections daily, and visits a clinic every three months. In the second intervention, intensive or tight control, the individual tests his or her glucose four times daily, visits a health team often, follows a special diet, exercises regularly, and takes insulin at least four times daily.

Information on deaths and alternative outcomes for the patients in each group are shown in Table 12-1. Alternative outcomes are presented in terms of quality of life, willingness to pay, and quality-adjusted life years (QALYs). The annual cost per person is $10,000 for individuals with tight glucose control and $3,000 for individuals with conventional control. The details of costs are shown in Table 12-2. These include physician visits, inpatient hospitalization, self-care (including the cost of insulin), and adverse events not treated on an inpatient basis. Most of the difference in cost between interventions is due to the self-care category. Using this example, the various economic evaluation studies that can be conducted are outlined.

Table 12-1   Outcome Measures for Alternative Interventions in Diabetes Control

	Year 1	Year 2	Year 3
Tight insulin control			
Survivors	997	997	990
Deaths	3	3	4
Life years	998.5	995.5	992.0
Quality of life per person	0.9	0.9	0.9
Quality-adjusted life years	898.65	895.50	892.80
Willingness to pay for an additional QALY	$80,000	$80,000	$80,000
Annual cost per person	$10,000	$10,000	$10,000
Annual cost for 1,000 persons	$10,000,000	$10,000,000	$10,000,000
Conventional care			
Survivors	995	990	984
Deaths	5	5	6
Life years	997.5	992.5	987.0
Quality of life per person	0.8	0.8	0.7
Quality-adjusted life years	798.0	794.0	690.9
Willingness to pay for an additional QALY	$80,000	$80,000	$80,000
Annual cost per person	$3,000	$3,000	$3,000
Annual cost for 1,000 persons	$3,000,000	$3,000,000	$3,000,000

Table 12-2   Annual Cost Per Person of Alternative Interventions for Diabetes Control

Category	Calculation Details	Cost per Person
Conventional care		
Inpatient hospital care	0.10 probability of hospitalization × $5,000 per hospitalization	$500
Outpatient visits	1 annual examination × $500 plus 3 visits × $100	$800
Self-care expenses	Monitoring supplies, insulin, and supplies for administering insulin	$1,400
Cost of adverse effects	1 visit to an emergency room per year	$300
Total costs		$3,000
Intensive therapy program		
Inpatient hospital care	0.02 probability of hospitalization × $5,000 per hospitalization	$100
Outpatient visits	1 annual examination × $500 plus 11 visits × $100	$1,600
Self-care expenses	Monitoring supplies, insulin, and supplies for administering insulin	$8,270
Cost of adverse effects	1 visit to an emergency room per year at $300 per visit	$30
Total costs		$10,000

12.5.1 Perspective

Perspective means the viewpoint taken by the investigator. Broadly, there are two types of perspective, private and societal. The private viewpoint is that of any single or group of providers, patients, or payers. If the individuals of interest are patients, the intent is to understand how the intervention impacts these people. If the payer's viewpoint is taken, the concern is with how much of the payer's own resources are used. The societal perspective is the perspective of all persons. It is an "all resources" perspective, in that it focuses on all resources used by all persons who are involved in the care—providers, patients, and caregivers. In our diabetes example, the assumption is an "all healthcare resources" perspective, except that it excludes the nonhealthcare resource losses (e.g., lost work time) incurred by unpaid caregivers and patients. Most guidelines recommend taking the broadest societal perspective; however, the choice of perspective is a value judgment, and there are uses for studies that take each perspective.

12.5.2 Time Horizons

The time horizon is the period over which costs and outcomes are measured. Most guidelines recommend that the analyses incorporate a long enough timeline to take into account all resources and outcome effects, including downstream events. Sometimes, downstream events are hard to identify. For example, if a patient is treated in a neonatal intensive care unit, he or she might experience effects years after the treatment. These events are rarely captured in study databases, and so the investigators must develop a hypothetical model to project such events. In this example, a time horizon of three years is assumed.

12.5.3 Outcomes

Outcome measures fall into two major categories, as shown in Table 12-3. These will be termed *clinical* and *holistic*. Clinical outcome measures include complete, partial, or no response in relation to cancer tumors, blood pressure, and cholesterol level. Clinical outcome measures are usually used in clinical trials because they provide objective evidence of illness.

Clinical outcome measures do not indicate how patients regard their own conditions. A condition with very little objective evidence, such as dyspepsia, may still be of enormous importance to the patient because it produces discomfort.

Clinical outcome measures do not provide information on patients' perceptions of their own conditions. As patient and consumer empowerment has

Table 12-3   Measures Used in Economic Studies

Clinical measures (examples)
Hypertension: Blood pressure measurement
Diabetes: Hemoglobin A1c control
Diabetes: Low density Lipoprotein (LDL) management and control
Diabetes: Diabetic retinopathy examination
Tobacco use assessment
Adult weight screening and follow-up
Influenza immunization for patients 50 years old or older
Childhood immunization status
Holistic measures
Measures based on mortality
Survival time
Time of survival (life years)
Health-related quality of life measures
Disease-specific indicators
General health indicators
Preference-based measures

increased, there has been a growing interest in developing outcome measures that reflect patients' perceptions. These are termed *holistic measures,* in large part because the concept of a holistic measure is so broad, as is the set of the phenomena the concept is designed to characterize. As seen in Table 12-3, measures based on mortality are included in the holistic category. In fact, they would fit into either category. In any case, mortality-related measures are very commonly used because they are easy to obtain and because mortality is of such importance. Mortality measures include the occurrence of death, as well as survival time (called *life years*).

The indicator of time until death illustrates the role that the time dimension plays in outcome analysis. Individuals experience different health states through time, and so the benefits and hardships they experience as a result of these health states should include a time dimension. The time-inclusive counterpart of mortality is the number of years of survival. In this example, out of 1,000 persons with diabetes who undertook the tight insulin control intervention, there were 997 survivors at the end of the first year, 994 at the end of the second, and 992 at the end of three years (see Table 12-1). One key outcome would be total deaths within three years, which is 10 for the tight insulin control intervention and 16 for the conventional care intervention. If the time dimension is added and life years as the outcome measure is used, then in the first year, there are 998.5 life years in the tight insulin control arm (the three individuals who died are assumed to live one-half year each). The total life years for the tight control intervention equal 2,986 over the three-year period, and the total life years for the conventional care arm equal 2,977.

Life tables have been developed that show, for each age of the population, the probability that a person of that age will not survive until his/her next birthday. From this, it is possible to calculate the probability of surviving any particular year of age, and the remaining life expectancy of people at different ages can also be calculated. For example, in 2009, life expectancy for females at age 65 in the United States was 20.0 years, while for males it was only 17.3 years.

Health-related quality-of-life years may differ from each other because the quality of life that individuals experience can vary considerably. In order to capture the variation in quality of life, a large number of health-related quality-of-life indexes have been developed. Some of the indexes are specific to a particular disease, some are objectively determined indexes oriented toward health status in general, and some are based on consumers' own preferences. A disease-specific index contains items that are relevant to the particular disease, whether it be asthma, cancer, or breast cancer. Objective health status indexes contain items that are relevant to all or many conditions. Both types of indexes will contain a number of questions about aspects of health status. For example, a person might be asked about his or her mobility. The questionnaire might provide five or six levels of mobility (none, ability to sit up in bed, etc.), and the individual marks the level appropriate to his or her condition. The responses determine the index score, although in some quality-of-life indexes, there are scores for the separate components. Guidelines on economic evaluations recommend the inclusion of health-related quality-of-life indexes.

Health-related quality-of-life indexes are usually confined to a patient's health status at a given point in time. Extrapolations can be made to cover intervals between responses. However, if patients die during the measurement interval, then the indexes generally do not incorporate this factor into the assessment. Death must be taken into account as a separate indicator. By the same token, mortality measures do not take the quality of life into account. Additionally, none of the measures that have been discussed take into account the consumer's own valuations or preferences for each health state. In order to address these concerns, several different research groups have developed preference-based, or utility, measures of health outcome (see Table 12-4). These preference-based measures are each based on a set of health dimensions. In the 15-D (15 dimensions of health) measure (Sintonen, 1981b), each of the 15 health dimensions has five categories, and there is a description for each category. For example, the five descriptions for the Vitality dimension are as follows:

1. I feel healthy and energetic.
2. I feel slightly weary, tired, or feeble.
3. I feel moderately weary, tired, or feeble.
4. I feel weary, tired, or feeble, almost exhausted.
5. I feel extremely weary, tired, or feeble, totally exhausted.

Table 12-4 Health Dimensions in the 15-D Health-Related Quality of Life Index

Dimension	Importance Weight
Breathing	0.075
Mental functioning	0.044
Speech	0.065
Vision	0.075
Mobility	0.046
Usual activities	0.057
Vitality	0.074
Hearing	0.104
Eating	0.040
Eliminating	0.033
Sleeping	0.090
Distress	0.079
Discomfort/symptoms	0.072
Sexual activity	0.084
Depression	0.062
Total	1.000

Source: Adapted from H. Sintonen. The 15D Instrument of Health-related Quality of Life: Properties and Applications, *Annals of Medicine*, Vol. 33, pp. 328–335, © 2001.

A score for each category was elicited from a sample of interviewees, each of whom placed his or her own valuation on the category.

A second level of weights, sometimes called *importance weights*, was assigned by a sample group to each of the 15 dimensions (see Table 12-4). All of the importance weights add up to a value of 1.00. As a result, the highest possible score on the 15-D measure is 1.00, which is achieved if a respondent scores at the highest level in each of the categories. Some investigators, both in the 15-D and other preference systems, have assigned a value of 0 to death. This is a very convenient assumption because it allows investigators to score on a single scale those interventions that have both death and changes in quality of life as outcomes. Within the context of such systems, the magnitude of QALYs can be calculated, which is an extremely convenient outcome measure. In this example, in each of the three years, a QALY value of 0.9 has been assigned to the persons who practice tight insulin control. Each surviving person would experience a total of 2.7 QALYs over the three years.

There are some deaths in this diabetes example, and the QALY valuation for a deceased persons is zero (deaths are assumed to occur at midpoint in the year). The assignment of a value of zero to death, while convenient, is controversial. When investigators develop weights for alternative health conditions, they usually ask members of a representative group to provide their own values. If patients who have experienced a specific health state are asked for their evaluations, they can provide a value that is based on an understanding of the condition. However, most weights have been developed from surveys of the general population, many of whom have not experienced the health states. In these instances, the valuations are thus projections of what the respondents think they might experience in a given state. The assignment of a value of zero to death is clearly an instance of projection. Individuals who have been surveyed have not experienced the condition, and so its valuation has little basis. Indeed, in all quality-of-life valuation surveys, the investigators did not even ask respondents about what they thought they might experience in death. They made their own extrapolations.

An additional issue in preference-based indicators is whose valuations to include in the measure of outcome. Investigators have alternatively focused on the values of providers (physicians and nurses), the general population, and specific patient groups. In addition, a number of economists have used introspection (inserting valuations of what they think is reasonable), along with sensitivity analyses. At present, there is no agreement as to whose values to incorporate into the weights. The patients are the only ones who have actually experienced many of the conditions, but the results of decisions often fall on payers of insurance premiums (employees or employers) or taxpayers.

12.5.4 Efficacy and Effectiveness

When there are two or more interventions, each of which will achieve a given purpose, there must be a method to determine the *differences* in outcomes among these interventions. One method is to use experimental techniques, such as randomized controlled trials. Properly set up, these techniques create carefully specified protocols for selected groups of patients, who are randomized to alternative interventions so that the selection of one intervention or another is beyond the control of the investigators. The investigators can then be sure that the two (or more) groups contain comparable patients. In a randomized controlled trial or other clinical setting, the differences in outcomes between interventions yield a measure called *efficacy*. This term refers only to differences between interventions under experimental or controlled clinical conditions. Efficacy measures do not always translate into everyday practice. Randomized controlled trials usually follow very tight protocols and monitor patients closely. If the trial is not done in a hospital (and most are not), the trial staff must devote considerable resources to monitoring patient adherence to protocols. In many instances, the treatments have unpleasant side effects, and clinical staff try to ensure that the trial protocols are maintained by the patients (e.g., that they take medicines at the prescribed intervals). No such monitoring is possible for practitioners in everyday circumstances. As a result, efficacy measures obtained from clinical trials or clinical settings are not always good indicators of how an intervention will work in actual practice.

The concept of effectiveness is related to differences in outcomes between interventions under nonexperimental, or everyday, conditions. Effectiveness must be determined from data collected from routine operations. Billing data, collected by insurers, often provide information that can be used to determine effectiveness. However, administrative or billing data usually do not contain information about quality of life and often does not contain enough clinical information to allow researchers to determine if indeed the patients within each comparison group are truly identical (which they would be in a clinical trial). Thus, unlike in randomized or clinical setting trials, investigators using statistical studies are less sure that the populations that they are comparing are the same. Despite these problems in determining effectiveness, it is this measure of difference, not that of efficacy, that is sought in a cost-effectiveness model. This is because the cost-effectiveness model is used to inform policy or management decisions, both of which are carried out under actual conditions.

In this diabetes example, it is assumed that the measures of outcomes are similar to those that would be obtained in actual practice conditions. Effectiveness, then, is measured by the difference in outcomes between interventions. There are several different effectiveness measures in this example. One is the number of lives saved during a given time frame. By the end of year three, there were 992 survivors in the tight insulin control arm and 984 in the conventional care arm. The difference, 8 lives, is the effectiveness measure. If all life years in each intervention are summed, then the effectiveness in terms of life years is 9 (2,986 − 2,977). In terms of QALYs, the effectiveness measure is 404.05 years (2,686.95 − 2,282.9). It should be noted that we have counted a QALY occurring in any year as having the same value as QALYs occurring in other years. Some analysts propose that a discount factor be applied to the benefits that occur in future years. That issue will be discussed next.

12.5.5 Costs

Economic costs are equivalent to the combined value of *resources* used in an intervention. Economic costs should be distinguished from transfer payments, which are unrelated to resources. Transfer payments include taxes, unemployment insurance payments, social security payments, and so on. From the point of view of the payer, such payments would appear as costs; from the viewpoint of recipients, they would appear as revenues. However, they are not payments for resource use and production and so are not indicators of how the economy's resources are being used.

Economic costs are subdivided into direct and lost productivity (also called indirect) costs. Direct costs are equivalent to the combined value of goods and services for which payment is received. They can be paid for by insurers, governments, or consumers (out of pocket). To be direct costs, the services must have embodied a resource, and they must have been purchased. Indirect, or lost productivity, costs are the costs of those services that included resources but were not purchased. If a patient travels to a clinic or sits idly in a waiting room, he or she may be losing valuable productive time and income. In effect, the patient's time, which is a resource, is not being purchased; payment has been foregone. The value of time lost will never be objectively observed, but it is real, and an economic value should be imputed to the resource.

Economic evaluation studies call for different perspectives. An insurer is interested mainly in what it pays out, for resources and any other sickness benefits. A patient is interested only in what he or she pays out of pocket and in any time lost from work. The patient will also be interested in sickness-related transfer payments, as these will reduce his or her sickness costs. The broadest perspective, called the societal perspective, is the viewpoint of all social resources. It excludes transfer payments because these are viewed as nonproductive payments. The relationship between the perspective of a study and the cost measures that are included in it is shown in Table 12-5. As can be seen, all resources are included in the societal perspective. In any other perspective, the costs suffered by just certain groups will be the sole focus of attention. Economic evaluation guidelines generally propose that the broadest viewpoint be taken. However, economic evaluation studies are often initiated by special interest groups, such as government drug benefit companies and hospitals. These groups are only secondarily concerned with the societal perspective, however commendable it may be.

The costs that are identified should be the marginal costs of the interventions. These costs are equivalent to the combined value of all

Table 12-5   Costs Included in Economic Evaluation Studies

Perspective of Study	Direct Costs	Indirect Costs	Transfer Payments
Payer	✓		✓
Provider	✓*		✓
Patient and caregiver	✓**	✓	✓†
Societal	✓	✓	

*Includes only payer portion
**Includes only out-of-pocket expenses
†Includes sickness benefit payments received by patients

additional resources used to deliver the intervention. In this diabetes example, the hypothetical marginal cost of two interventions are presented (see Table 12-2). Each cost estimate was divided into four components: inpatient hospitalization from complications of diabetes, routine outpatient visits, self-care, and adverse events that typically lead to emergency room treatment. Hospital costs are the expected costs of hospitalization, and they are based on the probability of being hospitalized and the cost of a hospitalization. Outpatient costs consist of the physician fees for routine visits. Adverse events costs are the emergency room costs that might result from complications that do not lead to hospitalization or that precede hospitalization. The costs of self-care include the costs of monitoring glucose levels, insulin, and medical supplies. Many of these costs will be out-of-pocket costs incurred by the patient. The value of lost productivity is excluded in this analysis, which therefore falls somewhat short of taking a full societal viewpoint.

As seen in Table 12-2, intensive insulin therapy costs $10,000 per person per year, whereas conventional therapy costs $3,000. The annual difference between the two interventions ($7,000) is primarily due to the costs of self-care, which total $8,270 for the intensive treatment and $1,400 for conventional care.

12.5.6 Discounting Future Costs and Benefits

Individuals place a higher value on present utilities than future ones. The discount rate is an expression of the preferences of present over future benefits. All future period costs should therefore be discounted to make them equivalent to costs in the present time. Assume a 5% discount rate. The discounted costs of the first year for conventional care (assuming, as is traditional, that the costs occur at the end of the year) are $2,857 ($3,000/1.05). For the second year, these costs are $2,722 ($3,000/[1.05]^2), and for the third year they are $2,592. The present value for all three years is the sum of these values, $8,171. The discounted costs for all three years of intensive treatment is $27,230, and the difference in the present value of costs between the two interventions (i.e., $c_2 - c_1$) is $19,059.

There is a controversy over the question of whether to also discount nonmonetary benefits. Investigators who wrote on the issue in the 1970s (Weinstein & Stason, 1977) stated that benefits and costs should be placed on the same plane and should both be discounted. More recently, some investigators (Parsonage & Neuberger, 1992) have claimed that, if we discount the benefits from health promotion activities, many of which are not experienced until years after the intervention, the present value will be reduced significantly. For example, the present value of $1,000 received in 20 years at a discount rate of 5% is only $396. Yet a gap of 20 years between health promotion activities and health benefits is not unusual. In light of these findings, a debate has occurred over whether to discount health benefits because doing so places many health promotion activities on very shaky grounds. The investigators contend that a social time preference discount rate may be less than a private one. In recognition of this, guidelines now recommend conducting a sensitivity analysis that includes a zero (no discount) rate for benefits.

12.5.7 Cost-Effectiveness Ratios

In this diabetes example, a series of cost-effectiveness ratios can be calculated. Three such ratios are calculated: cost per life saved, cost per life year saved, and cost per quality-adjusted life year saved. Table 12-6 summarizes the costs and outcomes for two groups of 1,000 persons with diabetes. The net discounted costs for 1,000 persons under intensive treatment are $27,230,000 and for persons under conventional care they are $8,166,000. The net difference in costs ($c_2 - c_1$) is therefore $19,064,000. The difference in deaths equals four, and so the cost per life saved is $4,766,000 ($19,064,000/4). Similarly, the cost per life year saved is $1,121,412, and the cost per QALY is $47,182.

The interpretation of these ratios is as follows. With regard to the QALY outcomes, an additional $47,182 in costs will yield an additional quality-adjusted life year. The ratio by itself does not tell us whether it would be worth it to spend the extra resources, and thus it does not provide all the information that is needed to choose one type of intervention over the other. It merely says what, in physical terms, will be obtained for the money.

12.5.8 Sensitivity Analysis

Most evaluations, even those that are based on randomized clinical trials, will be developed using assumed values for some variables. In this analysis, QALY information may have been obtained from different sources than the information for lives saved; for example, the QALY data may have been extrapolated from another study. If the valuation of QALYs for the two populations was uncertain, they could be subjected to a sensitivity analysis to see what would be the effect of making different assumptions. If the results changed appreciably, especially if they resulted in different conclusions, then much less confidence could be placed on the analysis (Briggs, Sculpher, & Buxton., 1994).

Assume that the QALY value for the intensive treatment was 0.85 rather than 0.90 for each of the three years. Then the outcome would be 2,537 life years for the three-year period. The value of $q_2 - q_1$ would be 255 QALYs rather than 404, and the cost-effectiveness ratio, if all else remained the same, would be $74,761 per life year saved. This is considerably more than the original ratio; however, whether it would change the recommendation depends on whether the cost-effectiveness ratio exceeded some assumed threshold. Some standards

Table 12-6   Summary Data for Alternative Cost-Effectiveness Ratios

Program	Net Discounted Costs for 1,000 Persons	Deaths	Life Years	Quality-Adjusted Life Years
Intensive Care	27,230,000	6	2,986	2,686.95
Conventional Care	8,166,000	10	2,969	2,282.90
Difference	19,064,000	4	17	404.05

would need to be set to determine what was an acceptable cost-effectiveness ratio. In the following section, the setting of standards is discussed.

12.5.9 Interpreting the Results

The cost-effectiveness ratio takes on additional meaning if it can be compared to some standard. The development of a standard will require some value judgments to be made about what is an acceptable improvement in cost per QALY. Several investigators (Laupacis, Feeny, Detsky, & Tugwell, 1992) have developed a conceptual tool to help interpret such findings. In Figure 12-1, the cost-effectiveness results are presented in graphic form, reflecting an illustration of an ICER evaluation. The two axes represent increases (or decreases) in QALYs and increases (or decreases) in cost. The original coordinates are the levels of cost and the QALY outcome for one of the interventions, say, c_1 and q_1. Let c_1 be $8,166,000 per 1,000 persons and q_1 be 2,282.9 QALYs, which is the value for conventional diabetes care in this example.

Based on the coordinates in Figure 12-1, there are four quadrants, labeled A, B, C, and D. The origin is c_1 and q_1. Relative to these points, c_2 will be the same, greater, or less than c_1; and q_2 will be the same, greater, or less than q_1. At any point in quadrant A, the intensive treatment intervention will cost less and produce more QALYs than the conventional intervention. On both cost and outcome grounds, the intensive intervention is preferred to the conventional one;

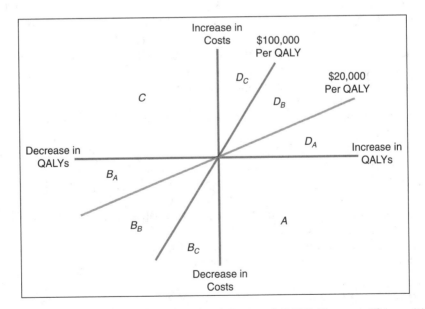

Figure 12-1 Alternative Combinations of Cost and QALY Changes. The position of each point represents a cost-effectiveness ratio. The position of the point will provide a standard that can be interpreted as dominant (quadrants A and C), strong evidence (quadrants D_A and B_A), moderate evidence (quadrants B_B and D_B), and weak evidence (quadrants D_C and B_C).

it is termed *dominant*. On policy grounds, the intensive intervention should be adopted. The same type of reasoning holds for any rate that falls into quadrant C; only in this case, the conventional alternative is dominant.

If, relative to c_1 and q_1, the points c_2 and q_2 fall into quadrant D, then intervention 2 (intensive treatment) costs more *and* yields more QALYs. To derive a policy conclusion, a value judgment must be used to set a standard. One group of researchers (Laupacis, Feeny, Detsky, & Tugwell, 1992) proposed the following set of value judgments:

- If intervention 2, relative to intervention 1, results in a cost-effectiveness ratio that is less than $20,000 per year, then there is *strong* evidence supporting the adoption of intervention 2.

- If intervention 2, relative to intervention 1, results in a cost-effectiveness ratio that is between $20,000 and $100,000 per year, then there is *moderate* evidence supporting the adoption of intervention 2.

- If intervention 2, relative to intervention 1, results in a cost-effectiveness ratio that is greater than $100,000 per year, then there is *weak* evidence supporting the adoption of intervention 2.

These guidelines are presented graphically in Figure 12-1. The line indicating a cost-effectiveness ratio of $20,000 per QALY separates area D_A from the rest of the quadrant D. The line indicating a cost-effectiveness ratio of $100,000 per QALY separates D_C from the remainder of quadrant D. Thus, quadrant D is now divided into three areas related to the values stated. If the cost-effectiveness ratio falls into the area of D_A (cost-effectiveness ratio below $20,000 per QALY), then this provides strong evidence supporting its adoption. If it falls into area D_B (i.e., it is between $20,000 and $100,000), then there is moderate evidence. And if it falls into area D_C (i.e., it exceeds $100,000), then weak evidence for adoption is provided. Similar reasoning holds for ratios that fall into quadrant B.

Analyses such as these make more explicit the value judgments that are related to policy analyses. In this example, the standards were somewhat loosely based on average annual salaries. A low-income person earns about $20,000, and so if the cost per QALY is below that, then the authors conclude that adoption would be warranted. However, these values are by no means universally accepted. Other investigators have chosen the standard of $50,000 to delineate whether an intervention should be recommended (Hirth, Chernew, Miller, Fendrick, & Weissert, 2000). A number of investigators have recommended the development and use of community surveys on what the general public is willing to pay for a QALY (Olsen & Donaldson, 1998).

12.6 BENEFIT–COST ANALYSIS

Cost-effectiveness analysis and cost-utility analysis provide information about the differences in outcomes in relation to differences in costs. As already stated, they do not provide information on whether the differences in outcomes are worth the differences in cost. To determine whether they are, one must either inject one's own (or somebody else's) valuations of the outcomes or else seek monetary valuations of the outcomes.

12.6.1 Valuation of Outcomes

Among the outcomes for health care are improved health, an ability to work or engage in leisure activities, and desired characteristics of the services themselves, such as convenience. Investigators have placed valuations on all of these.

12.6.2 Human Capital

One method of outcome valuation, called the *human capital approach,* focuses on lost work and lost leisure time. According to this approach, individuals' lost time from work (or leisure) is valued at the opportunity cost of time. This cost can be either the value of lost wages or the amount one must pay someone else to do the replacement work. For example, if a woman has heavy bleeding and loses five days from work, one can place a value on this time by estimating the per diem wage (e.g., $80 per day) and multiplying this wage by the length of time. An alternative way of measuring human capital losses would be through measuring the replacement costs for lost time. If a homemaker was sick for five days and could not engage in housework, then one could estimate the loss by determining the cost of hiring someone else to do the work.

The human capital method, once very popular, has fallen out of favor with economists for several reasons. First, studies in the Netherlands have questioned whether this method commonly overestimates productivity losses (Koopmanschap, Rutten, van Ineveld, & van Roijen, 1995). According to their friction-cost analyses, companies may replace individuals who are off the job with others; these replacement workers may have been previously unemployed or underemployed. The value of lost production would then be less than stated by the human capital method. Of course, the ease or difficulty of finding replacement workers would depend on overall economic conditions, such as the prevailing unemployment rate.

Second, if a person is sick, he or she loses work time and perhaps income, but there are other benefits lost as well. Individuals may still work, but at a lower capacity. Or if they are off work, they may simultaneously lose other benefits usually associated with good health. The lost wage from absence from work therefore may not be an understatement of the value of the losses to the individuals after all. For this reason, investigators have sought other means of measuring the value of lost work time.

Third, human capital incorporates a value system that places emphasis on those who are employed. Retirees and unemployed persons are valued at a very low rate, if at all. Yet a large portion of our health resources go to treat those who are not working, including persons who are retired. The human capital approach therefore would not serve as a good method of evaluating lost benefits from interventions that led to improved health but maybe not increased work time. Nevertheless, the human capital approach is still widely used, especially in cost-of-illness studies. Proponents of national economic policies espouse the goal of increasing total productivity and per-worker productivity. Improved health can often lead to the achievement of these goals. This may be why the human capital approach has not completely faded away.

12.6.3 Risk Preference

A second method for evaluating lost benefits is the "risk preference" approach, which is based on actual market data rather than inferred values, and so it reflects personal preferences. The widest use of this method has been in the labor market. The economic hypothesis states that individuals will demand a risk premium in order to accept more risky occupations. If the health risks in various occupations, as well as the wages paid in these occupations, can be quantified, then, after we adjust for other variables that might also affect wages (e.g., experience, training, and gender), the wage differential should be related to the risk differential. Put otherwise, the adjusted wage differential measures the extra amount of money that workers demand in return for working in an occupation with a higher risk of injury or death. This measure can be used to evaluate the probability of poor health or death. Somewhat indirectly, a value per QALY can be inferred from this information. If there is a 10% difference in risk of mortality between two occupations, and the annual pay differential is $5,000, then a value of $50,000 for the loss of a life ($5,000/0.10) can be inferred. In this way, some of the benefits from an increased probability of improved health can be estimated, namely, those associated with longevity. Many other health-related benefits cannot be dealt with through the use of this concept.

12.6.4 Contingent Valuation

A third method of measuring benefits is termed *contingent valuation*, in which individuals are asked what they would hypothetically pay if they could achieve the benefits that result from specific interventions. For example, if a person who undergoes kidney dialysis daily could, with no adverse effects, receive dialysis only twice a week, then he or she would benefit enormously. An interviewer could question this person about how much he or she valued (in monetary terms) such an occurrence. The stated value could be construed as the individual's willingness to pay for the improved kidney treatments.

In a contingent valuation study, the responses depend on what the respondents are asked. Much study has gone into this subject. Briefly, here are some guidelines for achieving a valid valuation:

- The effects of the intervention should be clearly stated and understood by the respondent.

- The questionnaire should stress that there are other goods and services competing for the respondent's money.

- The respondent should be told that he or she would have to reduce spending on other things.

- Generally, the respondent should be told that the additional spending would be in the form of higher taxes or product prices.

- The interview should include follow-up questions in order to determine the reasons for the respondent's valuations.

12.6.5 Techniques of Valuation

These valuation techniques described have been used by investigators in a number of different contexts. One group of investigators surveyed studies in which respondents expressed a willingness to pay in return for specific reductions in risk that would result in expected increases in QALYs. Using the estimates of these studies, the authors calculated a value of life (Hirth, Chernew, Miller, Fendrick, & Weissert, 2000). They estimated the age of persons in each study, the expected life years remaining, the QALYs per life year, and thus the number of QALYs. With this information, the investigators could estimate a cost per QALY for each study reviewed. The values arrived at differed widely and seemed to depend on the research approach. According to the human capital approach, the value for cost per QALY was $24,777. Using revealed preference studies, the authors estimated a value of $93,000. And using the contingent valuation approach, they estimated a value of $161,000. Given the large variation among methods, the authors concluded that the goal of determining a cost per QALY was elusive.

In theory, the value of a QALY is most important, as it provides a key to answering a central question in economic evaluation. However, the cost per QALY in practice seems to depend on the context of the analysis and on the method used to obtain information. The values arrived at using the method that is closest to revealed preferences—risk preference—cannot be easily linked to specific health states. As well, there are considerable differences in the results of the various studies. The contingent valuation method suffers from the difficulty of applying it to specific interventions and the difficulty of achieving comparability. This method also elicits hypothetical responses from individuals; faced with actual situations, people may value services differently. It would seem that the contingent valuation method is better suited to answering hypothetical questions about health-related programs than questions about the values placed on specific interventions. Often, respondents would require detailed knowledge about the interventions, and their information needs might tax the interviewing process. A great deal of detail about the results of specific interventions can be obtained from health-related quality-of-life indicators, including preference-based indicators. Willingness-to-pay measures cannot provide such detail. In sum, the best instrument to use depends on the purpose of the investigation.

12.6.6 Benefit–Cost Ratio

Benefit–cost analysis answers the question, Are the costs worth the benefits? Looking at a specific intervention, then this question implies that there is an alternative intervention, even if it amounts to "not conducting the intervention." The main point is that there are alternative uses of the resources involved. In a benefit-cost analysis, the alternative should be explicitly considered.

Ignoring discounting, the benefit-cost equation is expressed as

$$NB = b - c \text{ or Ratio} = b/c$$

in which b refers to the benefits resulting from the intervention and c to the additional costs.

Returning to the diabetes example, assume that at the current level of treating diabetes (i.e., using the conventional method), the cost per person is as before (i.e., the discounted, three-year value for c is $19,064 per person). This is the additional cost of tight insulin control, assuming that the conventional method would have been used in the absence of tight insulin control. The difference in QALYs per person is 0.404. If the willingness to pay for one additional QALY is $60,000, then the value of b is $24,240 (0.404 × $60,000). Thus, the net benefits are greater than zero. Because this measure incorporates the worth of a QALY, it provides an answer to the basic question, Is it worth it? In the absence of other considerations, a net present value in excess of zero would yield a recommendation to adopt the intervention.

The contingent valuation calculated will almost certainly be derived from studies that elicit answers under hypothetical conditions. The populations who are surveyed may not be representative of all relevant persons. Therefore, like all other measures, the willingness-to-pay measure must be interpreted with care.

EXERCISES

1. A health economist was asked to compare outcomes and costs of two diabetes therapies that affected both the severity of the disease and the survival rate. What evaluation concept should he use?

2. A health economist was asked to compare outcomes and costs for two prophylactic medicines that reduced deaths during surgical operations. The interventions did not influence quality of life. What concept should she use?

3. A health economist was asked whether a new drug that reduced mortality should be used. What concept should she use?

4. Patients who were hospitalized for asthma were placed on a new drug. The drug resulted in an extra day of hospitalization (the length of stay went from 6 to 7 days), which cost $800. There were no other differences in the treatment. The drug cost $300 for the dose. As well, it took an hour of nursing time (wage = $20 per hour) and $10 in supplies to administer it. The mortality rate was 10 deaths per 100 with the drug and 12 deaths per 100 without it. What is the cost-effectiveness ratio for using the drug?

5. In a population of 1,000 persons at the beginning of the year, 40 die during the year. How many life years were there during the year?

6. In one year, 30 persons per 1,000 die of asthma. A new drug reduces that number to 20 per 1,000. How is outcome defined, and what is the "effectiveness" of the drug?

7. In one year, 60 people per 100 die from complications of diabetes. A new drug will reduce that number to 40 per 100 *if*

everyone takes the drug, according to a recently conducted clinical trial. However, 25% of those who take the drug will discontinue it, even though this means that their death rate will be the same as the rate for those who don't take the drug. What is the efficacy and effectiveness of the drug?

8. In an asthma center, the nurse took two quality-of-life measurements using the 15-D questionnaire. The scores (on a scale of 1 to 5) for the first and the second are presented in the next table. The first measurement was taken when the patient entered the clinic, and the second was taken one week later, after the patient received asthma medicine. What is the effectiveness, in quality-adjusted life years, of the asthma medicine?

Health Dimension	Score at First Visit	Score at Second Visit
Breathing	2	3
Mental functioning	2	2
Speech	2	3
Vision	2	2
Mobility	2	2
Usual activities	2	2
Vitality	2	4
Hearing	2	2
Eating	2	3
Eliminating	2	3
Sleeping	2	3
Distress	2	2
Discomfort	2	3
Sexual Activity	4	5
Depression	2	2

9. A patient with asthma will live for six months if she does not take her medicine. The quality of life of that patient will be 0.8. If she takes asthma medicine, her quality of life will increase to 0.9 and her length of survival will be seven months. What is the effectiveness of the medicine?

10. Two interventions were each applied to 1,000 persons. Given the resulting data (contained in the table shown here), determine a cost-effectiveness ratio. The discount rate is 5%. Is this a high ratio?

	Year 1	Year 2
Intervention A		
Survivors	980	960
Quality of life	0.9	0.9
Cost per person	$30,000	$6,000
Intervention B		
Survivors	970	970
Quality of Life	0.85	0.85
Cost per person	$20,000	$4,000

BIBLIOGRAPHY

Benefit–Cost and Cost-Effectiveness Analysis: General

Bakker, C., Hidding, A., van der Linden, S., & van Doorslaer, E. (1994). Cost effectiveness of group physical therapy compared to individualized therapy for ankylosing spondylitis. *Journal of Rheumatology, 21,* 264–268.

Briggs, A., Sculpher, M., & Buxton, M. (1994). Uncertainty in the economic evaluation of health care technologies: The role of sensitivity analysis. *Health Economics, 3,* 95–104.

Canadian Coordinating Office for Health Technology Assessment. (1997). *Guidelines for economic evaluation of pharmaceuticals: Canada.* Ottawa: Canadian Coordinating Office for Health Technology Assessment.

Claxton, K., Sculpher, M., & Drummond, M. (2002). A rational framework for decision making by the National Institute For Clinical Excellence (NICE). *Lancet, 360*(9334), 711–715.

Cochrane, A. (1972). *Effectiveness and efficiency.* New York, NY: Oxford University Press.

Craig, B. M., & Busschbach, J. J. (2011). Toward a more universal approach in health valuation. *Health Economics, 20,* 864–875.

Culyer, A. J. (1985). The scope and limits of health economics. *Okonomie des gesundheitswesens (New ed.) 159,* 31–54.

Doubilet, P. (1986). Use and misuse of the term "cost effective" in medicine. *New England Journal of Medicine, 314,* 253–256.

Drummond, M., Griffin, A., & Tarricone, R. (2009). Economic evaluation for devices and drugs— Same or different? *Value in Health, 12*(4), 402–404.

Drummond, M., Manca, A., & Sculpher, M. (2005). Increasing the generalizability of economic evaluations: Recommendations for the design, analysis, and reporting of studies. *International Journal of Technology Assessment in Health Care, 21*(2), 165–171.

Drummond, M., Mason, A., & Towse, A. (2006). The desirability and feasibility of economic studies of drugs post-launch. *European Journal of Health Economics, 7*(1), 5–6.

Drummond, M., & Sculpher, M. (2005). Common methodological flaws in economic evaluations. *Medical Care, 43*(7 Suppl.), 5–14.

Drummond, M. F. (2003). The use of health economic information by reimbursement authorities. *Rheumatology, 42*(Suppl. 3), iii60–iii63.

Drummond, M. F., Aguiar-Ibanez, R., & Nixon, J. (2006). Economic evaluation. *Singapore Medical Journal, 47*(6), 456–461; quiz 462.

Drummond, M. F., & Davies, L. (1991). Economic analysis alongside clinical trials. *International Journal of Technology Assessment in Health Care, 7,* 561–573.

Drummond, M. F., Schwartz, J. S., Jonsson, B., Luce, B. R., Neumann, P. J., Siebert, U., & Sullivan, S. D. (2008). Key principles for the improved conduct of health technology assessments for resource allocation decisions. *International Journal of Technology Assessment in Health Care, 24*(3), 244–258; discussion 362–368.

Drummond, M. F., & Sculpher, M. J. (2006). Better analysis for better decisions: Facing up to the challenges. *Pharmacoeconomics, 24*(11), 1039–1042.

Drummond, M. F., Wilson, D. A., Kanavos, P., Ubel, P., & Rovira, J. (2007). Assessing the economic challenges posed by orphan drugs. *International Journal of Technology Assessment in Health Care, 23*(1), 36–42.

Drummond, M. F., Stoddart, G. L. & Torrance, G. W. (1987). *Methods for the economic evaluation of health care programmes.* Toronto, Canada: Oxford University Press.

Drummond, M. F., O'Brien, B. J., Stoddart, G. L., & Torrance, G. W. (1997). *Methods for the economic evaluation of health care programmes* (2nd ed.). Oxford, England: Oxford University Press.

Gold, M. R., McCoy, K., I., & Siegel, J. E. (1996). *Cost-effectiveness in health and medicine.* New York, NY: Oxford University Press.

Greenberg, D., Rosen, A. B., Wacht, O., Palmer, J., & Neumann, P. J. (2010). A bibliometric review of cost-effectiveness analyses in the economic and medical literature: 1976–2006. *Medical Decision Making, 30*(3), 320–327.

Haddix, A. C., Teutsch, S. M., Shaffer, P. A., & Dunet, D. O. (1996). *Prevention effectiveness: A guide to decision analysis and economic evaluation.* New York, NY: Oxford University Press.

Hatzriandrou, E. I., Koplan, J. P., Weinstein, M. C., Caspersen, C. J., & Warner, K. E. (1988). A cost-effectiveness analysis of exercise as health promotion. *American Journal of Public Health, 78,* 1417–1421.

Hellinger, F. J. (1980). Cost-benefit analysis of health care: Past applications and future prospects. *Inquiry, 17,* 204–215.

Hirth, R. A., Chernew, M. E., Miller, E., Fendrick, A. M., & Weissert, W. G. (2000). Willingness to pay for a quality-adjusted life year: In search of a standard. *Medical Decision Making, 20,* 332–342.

Laupacis, A., Feeny, D., Detsky, A. S., & Tugwell, P. X. (1992). How attractive does a new technology have to be to warrant adoption and utilization? Tentative guidelines for using clinical and economic evaluations. *Canadian Medical Association Journal, 146,* 473–481.

Luce, B. R., & Elixhauser, A. (1990). *Standards for the socioeconomic evaluation of health care services.* Berlin, Germany: Springer Verlag.

Marshall, D. A., Douglas, P. R., Drummond, M. F., Torrance, G. W., Macleod, S., Manti, O, Cheruvu, L., & Corvari, R. (2008). Guidelines for conducting pharmaceutical budget impact analyses for submission to public drug plans in Canada. *Pharmacoeconomics, 26*(6), 477–495.

Menon, D., Schubert, F., & Torrance, G. W. (1996). Canada's new guidelines for the economic evaluation of pharmaceuticals. *Medical Care, 34,* DS77–DS86.

Parsonage, M., & Neuberger, H. (1992). Discounting and health benefits. *Health Economics, 1,* 71–79.

Sculpher, M. J., Claxton, K., Drummond, M., & McCabe, C. (2006). Whither trial-based economic evaluation for health care decision making? *Health Economics, 15*(7), 677–687.

Sculpher, M., Drummond, M., & O'Brien, B. (2001). Effectiveness, efficiency, and NICE. *BMJ, 322*(7292), 943–944.

Sculpher, M. J., Pang, F. S., Manca, A., Drummond, M. F., Golder, S., Urdahl, H., Davies, L. M., & Eastwood, A. (2004). Generalisability in economic evaluation studies in healthcare: A review and case studies. *Health Technology Assessment (Winchester, England), 8*(49), iii–iv, 1–192.

Simes, R. J., & Glasziou, P. P. (1992). Meta analysis and quality of evidence in the economic evaluation of drug trials. *Pharmacoeconomics, 1,* 282–292.

Stoddart, G. L., & Drummond, M. F. (1984). How to read clinical journals. VII: To understand an economic evaluation. Parts A and B. *Canadian Medical Association Journal, 130,* 1428–1433, 1542–1549.

Suarez-Almazor, M. E., & Drummond, M. (2003). Regulatory issues and economic efficiency. *Journal of Rheumatology, 68* (Suppl.), 5–7.

Taylor, R. S., Drummond, M. F., Salkeld, G., & Sullivan, S. D. (2004). Inclusion of cost effectiveness in licensing requirements of new drugs: The fourth hurdle. *BMJ, 329*(7472), 972–975.

Thurston, S. J., Craig, D., Wilson, P., & Drummond, M. F. (2008). Increasing decision-makers' access to economic evaluations: Alternative methods of communicating the information. *International Journal of Technology Assessment in Health Care, 24*(2), 151–157.

Warner, K. E. (1982). *Cost-benefit and cost-effectiveness analysis in health care.* Ann Arbor, MI: Health Administration Press.

Warner, K. E., & Hutton, R. C. (1980). Cost-benefit and cost-effectiveness analysis in health care. *Medical Care, 18,* 1069–1084.

Weatherly, H., Drummond, M., Claxton, K., Cookson, R., Ferguson, B., Godfrey, C., ..., & Sowden, A. (2009). Methods for assessing the cost-effectiveness of public health interventions: Key challenges and recommendations. *Health Policy, 93*(2/3), 85–92.

Weinstein, M. C., & Stason, W. B. (1977). Foundations of cost-effectiveness analysis for health and medical practices. *New England Journal of Medicine, 296,* 716–721.

White, D. B., Katz, M. H., Luce, J. M., & Lo, B. (2009). Who should receive life support during a public health emergency? Using ethical principles to improve allocation decisions. *Annals of Internal Medicine, 150*(2), 132–138.

Williams, A. (1974a). The cost benefit approach. *British Medical Bulletin, 20,* 252–256.

Williams, A. (1974b). Measuring the effectiveness of health care systems. *British Journal of Preventive and Social Medicine, 28,* 196–202.

Diabetes-Related Studies

Axente, L., Sinescu, C., & Bazacliu, G. (2011). Heart failure prognostic model. *Journal of Medicine & Life, 4*(2), 210–225.

Christensen, T. E., Gundgaard, J., & Pilgaard, T. (2011). Healthcare costs of fast-acting insulin analogues versus short-acting human insulin for Danish patients with type 2 diabetes on a basal-bolus regimen. *Journal of Medical Economics, 14*(4), 477–485.

Diabetes Control and Complications Trial Research Group (DCCT). (1995). Resource utilization and costs of care in the Diabetes Control and Complications Trial. *Diabetes Care, 18,* 1468–1478.

Diabetes Control and Complications Trial Research Group (DCCT). (1996). Lifetime benefits and costs of intensive therapy as practiced in the Diabetes Control and Complications Trial. *JAMA, 276,* 1409–1415.

Freund, T., Peters-Klimm, F., Rochon, J., Mahler, C., Gensichen, J., Erler, A., ..., & Szecsenyi, J. (2011). Primary care practice-based care management for chronically ill patients (PraCMan): Study protocol for a cluster randomized controlled trial [ISRCTN56104508]. *Trials [Electronic Resource], 12,* 163.

Gebel, E. (2011). A matter of the sexes: The differences between men and women with diabetes. *Diabetes Forecast, 64*(10), 46–49.

Gray, A., Raikou, M., McGuire, A., Fenn, P., Stevens, R., Cull, C., ..., & Turner, R. . (2000). Cost effectiveness of an intensive blood glucose control policy in patients with type 2 diabetes: Economic analysis alongside randomized controlled trial (UKPDS 41). *British Medical Journal, 320,* 1373–1378.

Holscher, C. (2011). Diabetes as a risk factor for Alzheimer's disease: Insulin signalling impairment in the brain as an alternative model of Alzheimer's disease. *Biochemical Society Transactions, 39*(4), 891–897.

Lazar, H. L., McDonnell, M. M., Chipkin, S., Fitzgerald, C., Bliss, C., & Cabral, H. (2011). Effects of aggressive versus moderate glycemic control on clinical outcomes in diabetic coronary artery bypass graft patients. *Annals of Surgery, 254*(3), 458–463; discussion 463–464.

Le, T. K., Curtis, B., Kahle-Wrobleski, K., Johnston, J., Haldane, D., & Melfi. C. (2011). Treatment patterns and resource use among patients with comorbid diabetes mellitus and major depressive disorder. *Journal of Medical Economics, 14*(4), 440–447.

Putnam, W., Lawson, B., Buhariwalla, F., Goodfellow, M., Goodine, R. A., Hall, J., ..., & Godwin, M. S. l. (2011). Hypertension and type 2 diabetes: What family physicians can do to improve control of blood pressure—An observational study. *BMC Family Practice, 12,* 86.

Selea, A, Sumarac-Dumanovic, M., Pesic, M., Suluburic, D., Stamenkovic-Pejkovic, D., Cvijovic, G., & Micic, D. (2011). The effects of education with printed material on glycemic control in patients with diabetes type 2 treated with different therapeutic regimens. *Vojnosanitetski Pregled, 68*(8), 676–683.

Suh, D. C., Lee, D. H., McGuire, M., & Kim, C. M. (2011). Impact of rosiglitazone therapy on the lipid profile, glycemic control, and medication costs among type 2 diabetes patients. *Current Medical Research & Opinion, 27*(8), 1623–1633.

UK Prospective Diabetes Study Group. (1998). Intensive blood-glucose with sulphonylureas or insulin compared with conventional treatment and risk of complications in patients with type 2 diabetes (UKPDS33). *Lancet, 352,* 857–853.

Versnel, N., Welschen, L. M., Baan, C. A., Nijpels, G., & Schellevis, F. G. (2011). The effectiveness of case management for comorbid diabetes type 2 patients; The CasCo study. Design of a randomized controlled trial. *BMC Family Practice, 12,* 68.

Volpe, M., Cosentino, F., Tocci, G., Palano, F., & Paneni, F. (2011). Antihypertensive therapy in diabetes: The legacy effect and RAAS blockade. *Current Hypertension Reports, 13*(4), 318–324.

Wang, W., Balamurugan, A., Biddle, J., & Rollins, K. M. (2011). Diabetic neuropathy status and the concerns in underserved rural communities: Challenges and opportunities for diabetes educators. *Diabetes Educator, 37*(4), 536–548.

Webb, J. B., Applegate, K. L., & Grant, J. P. (2011). A comparative analysis of type 2 diabetes and binge eating disorder in a bariatric sample. *Eating Behaviors, 12*(3), 175–181.

Health-Related Quality of Life and QALYs

Airoldi, M., & Morton, A. (2009). Adjusting life for quality or disability: Stylistic difference or substantial dispute? *Health Economics, 18*(11), 1237–1247.

Ara, R., & Brazier, J. E. (2010). Populating an economic model with health state utility values: Moving toward better practice. *Value in Health, 13*(5), 509–518.

Attema, A. E., & Brouwer, W. B. (2010a). On the (not so) constant proportional trade-off in TTO. *Quality of Life Research, 19*(4), 489–497.

Attema, A. E., & Brouwer, W. B. (2010b). The value of correcting values: Influence and importance of correcting TTO scores for time preference. *Value in Health, 13,* 879–884.

Baker, R., Bateman, I., Donaldson, C., Jones-Lee, M., Lancsar, E., Loomes, G., ..., & SVQ Research Team. (2010). Weighting and valuing quality-adjusted life-years using stated preference methods: Preliminary results from the Social Value of a QALY Project. *Health Technology Assessment (Winchester, England), 14*(27), 1–162.

Bakker, C., Hidding, A., van der Linden, S., & van Doorslaer, E. (1994). Cost effectiveness of group physical therapy compared to individualized therapy for ankylosing spondylitis. *Journal of Rheumatology, 21,* 264–268.

Bobinac, A., Van Exel, N. J., Rutten, F. F., & Brouwer, W. B. (2010). Willingness to pay for a quality-adjusted life-year: The individual perspective. *Value in Health, 13,* 1046–1055.

Donaldson, C., Baker, R., Mason, H., Jones-Lee, M., Lancsar, E., Wildman, J., ..., & Smith, R. (2011). The social value of a QALY: Raising the bar or barring the raise? *BMC Health Services Research, 11,* 8.

Drummond, M. (2001). Introducing economic and quality of life measurements into clinical studies. *Annals of Medicine, 33*(5), 344–349.

Drummond, M., Brixner, D., Gold, M., Kind, P., McGuire, A., & Nord, E. (2009). Toward a consensus on the QALY. *Value in Health, 12*(Suppl. 1), S31–S35.

Erickson, P. (1966). Modeling health-related quality of life: The bridge between psychometric and utility-based measures. *Journal of the National Cancer Institute, Monograph 20,* 17–20.

Eskelinen, E., Rasanen, P., Alback, A., Lepantalo, M., Eskelinen, A., Peltonen, M., & Roine, R. P. (2009). Effectiveness of superficial venous surgery in terms of quality-adjusted life years and costs. *Scandinavian Journal of Surgery: SJS, 98*(4), 229–233.

Fukuhara, S., Ikegami, N., Torrance, G. W., Nishimura, S., Drummond, M., & Schubert, F. (2002). The development and use of quality-of-life measures to evaluate health outcomes in Japan. *Pharmacoeconomics, 20*(Suppl. 2), 17–23.

Gandjour, A., & Gafni, A. (2010). The additive utility assumption of the QALY model revisited. *Journal of Health Economics, 29*(2), 325–328; author reply 329–331.

Garau, M., Shah, K. K., Mason, A. R., Wang, Q., Towse, A., & Drummond, M. F. (2011). Using QALYs in cancer: A review of the methodological limitations. *Pharmacoeconomics, 29,* 673–685.

Grosse, S. D., Prosser, L. A., Asakawa, K., & Feeny, D. (2010). QALY weights for neurosensory impairments in pediatric economic evaluations: Case studies and a critique. *Expert Review of Pharmacoeconomics & Outcomes Research, 10*(3), 293–308.

Gudex, C., & Kind, P. (n.d.). *The QALY toolkit.* York, England: Center for Health Economics.

Hauber, A. B. (2009). Healthy-years equivalent: Wounded but not yet dead. *Expert Review of Pharmacoeconomics & Outcomes Research, 9*(3), 265–269.

Jelsma, J., De Weerdt, W., & De Cock, P. (2002). Disability adjusted life years (DALYs) and rehabilitation. *Disability & Rehabilitation, 24*(7), 378–382.

Kirkdale, R., Krell, J., Brown, C. O., Tuthill, M., & Waxman, J. (2010). The cost of a QALY. *QJM, 103*(9), 715–720.

Lipscomb, J., Drummond, M., Fryback, D., Gold, M., & Revicki, D. (2009). Retaining, and enhancing, the QALY. *Value in Health, 12*(Suppl. 1), S18–S26.

Neumann, P. J., & Greenberg, D. (2009). Is the United States ready for QALYs? *Health Affairs, 28*(5), 1366–1371.

Nord, E., Enge, A. U., & Gundersen, V. (2010). QALYs: Is the value of treatment proportional to the size of the health gain? *Health Economics, 19*(5), 596–607.

Normand, C. (2009). Measuring outcomes in palliative care: Limitations of QALYs and the road to PalYs. *Journal of Pain & Symptom Management, 38*(1), 27–31.

Nyman J. A. (2011). Measurement of QALYS and the welfare implications of survivor consumption and leisure forgone. *Health Economics, 20,* 56–67.

Oliver, A. (2003). Putting the quality into quality-adjusted life years. *Journal of Public Health Medicine, 25*(1), 8–12.

Shiroiwa, T., Sung, Y. K., Fukuda, T., Lang, H. C., Bae, S. C., & Tsutani, K. (2010). International survey on willingness-to-pay (WTP) for one additional QALY gained: What is the threshold of cost effectiveness? *Health Economics, 19*(4), 422–437.

Sintonen, H. (1981a). An approach to measuring and valuing health states. *Social Science and Medicine, 15C,* 55–65.

Sintonen, H. (1981b). *The 15-D measure of health related quality of life.* West Heidelberg, Australia: National Centre for Health Program Evaluation.

Smith, M. D., Drummond, M., & Brixner, D. (2009). Moving the QALY forward: Rationale for change. *Value in Health, 12*(Suppl. 1), S1–S4.

Torrance, G. W., & Feeny, D. (1989). Utilities and quality adjusted life years. *International Journal of Technology Assessment in Health Care, 5,* 559–575.

Ungar, W. J. (2011). Challenges in health state valuation in paediatric economic evaluation: Are QALYs contraindicated? *Pharmacoeconomics, 29,* 641–652.

Weyler, E. J., & Gandjour, A. (2011). Empirical validation of patient versus population preferences in calculating QALYs. *Health Services Research, 46,* 1562–1574.

Williams, A. (1985). Economics of coronary bypass grafting. *British Medical Journal, 291,* 326– 329.

Value of Health and Life

Beach, M. C., Asch, D. A., Jepson, C., Hershey, J. C., Mohr, T., McMorrow, S., & Ubel, P. A. (2003). Public response to cost-quality tradeoffs in clinical decisions. *Medical Decision Making, 23*(5), 369–378.

Blomquist, G. (1981). The value of human life: An empirical perspective. *Economic Inquiry, 19*, 157–164.

Churchill, L. R. (2011). Rationing, rightness, and distinctively human goods. *American Journal of Bioethics, 11*(7), 15–16.

Cook, J., Drummond, M., & Heyse, J. F. (2004). Economic endpoints in clinical trials. *Statistical Methods in Medical Research, 13*(2), 157–176.

Currie, G. R., Donaldson, C., O'Brien, B. J., Stoddart, G. L., Torrance, G. W., & Drummond, M. F. (2002). Willingness to pay for what? A note on alternative definitions of health care program benefits for contingent valuation studies. *Medical Decision Making, 22*(6), 493–497.

Donaldson, C. (1999). Valuing the benefits of publicly-provided health care: Does "ability to pay" preclude the use of "willingness to pay"? *Social Science and Medicine, 49*, 551–563.

Drummond, M. (2003). Prioritizing investments in health: Can we assess potential value for money? *Journal of Rheumatology, 68*(Suppl.), 19–20.

Dunlop, W. (2002). Revisiting the fair innings argument. *New Zealand Bioethics Journal, 3*(2), 22–26.

Fisher, A., Chestnut, L. G., & Violette, D. M l. (1989). The value of reducing risks of death. *Journal of Policy Analysis and Management, 8*, 88–100.

Friedman, A. W. (2011). Rationing and social value judgments. *American Journal of Bioethics, 11*(7), 28–29.

Gandjour, A. (2009). Ethical criteria for allocating health-care resources. *Lancet, 373*(9673), 1425; author reply 1425–1426.

Greenberg, D., & Neumann, P. J. (2011). Does adjusting for health-related quality of life matter in economic evaluations of cancer-related interventions? *Expert Review of Pharmacoeconomics & Outcomes Research, 11*(1), 113–119.

Harris, J. (2005). The age-indifference principle and equality. *Cambridge Quarterly of Healthcare Ethics, 14*(1), 93–99.

Hawkins, N., Epstein, D., Drummond, M., Wilby, J., Kainth, A., Chadwick, D., & Sculpher, M. (2005). Assessing the cost-effectiveness of new pharmaceuticals in epilepsy in adults: The results of a probabilistic decision model. *Medical Decision Making, 25*(5), 493–510.

Hay, J. W., Smeeding, J., Carroll, N. V., Drummond, M., Garrison, L. P., Mansley, E. C., ..., & Shi, L. (2010). Good research practices for measuring drug costs in cost effectiveness analyses: Issues and recommendations: The ISPOR Drug Cost Task Force report—Part I. *Value in Health, 13*(1), 3–7.

Jacobs, P., & Fassbender, K. (1998). The measurement of indirect costs in the health economics evaluation literature. *International Journal of Technology Assessment in Health Care, 14*, 799–808.

Johanneson, M., Jonsson, B. & Borqquist, L. l. (1991). Willingness to pay for antihypertensive therapy: Results of a Swedish pilot study. *Journal of Health Economics, 10*, 461–474.

Johanneson, M., Johansson, P. O., Kristrom, B., & Gerdtham, U. G. (1993). Willingness to pay for antihypertensive therapy: Further results. *Journal of Health Economics, 12*, 95–108.

Jones, V. F., Wheeler, F., & Aldrich, T. (2004). Which life? *Journal of the Kentucky Medical Association, 102*(6), 263–266.

Klein, D. A. (2011). Evaluating social value: On the intersection of mortality and economics in the distribution of publicly funded medical care. *American Journal of Bioethics, 11*(7), 18–20.

Koopmanschap, M. A., Rutten, F. F., van Ineveld, B. M., & van Roijen, L. (1995). The friction cost method for measuring indirect cost of disease. *Journal of Health Economics, 14*, 171–189.

Landefeld, J. S., & Seskin, E. P. (1982). The economic value of life: Linking theory to practice. *American Journal of Public Health, 72*, 555–566.

Li, M., Vietri, J., Galvani, A. P., & Chapman, G. B. (2010). How do people value life? *Psychological Science, 21*(2), 163–167.

Lieu, T. A., Ray, G. T., Ortega-Sanchez, I. R., Kleinman, K., Rusinak, D., & Prosser L.A. (2009). Willingness to pay for a QALY based on community member and patient preferences for temporary health states associated with herpes zoster. *Pharmacoeconomics, 27,* 1005–1016.

Lippert-Rasmussen, K., & Lauridsen, S. (2010). Justice and the allocation of healthcare resources: Should indirect, non-health effects count? *Medicine, Health Care & Philosophy, 13*(3), 237–246.

Mason, A., Weatherly, H., Spilsbury, K., Golder, S., Arksey, H., Adamson, J., & Drummond, M. (2007). The effectiveness and cost-effectiveness of respite for caregivers of frail older people. *Journal of the American Geriatrics Society, 55*(2), 290–299.

Mooney, G. (1977). *The valuation of human life.* New York, NY: Macmillan.

Muller, A., & Reutzel, T. J. (1984). Willingness to pay for a reduction in fatality risk. *American Journal of Public Health, 74,* 808–812.

Nord, E. (2005). Concerns for the worse off: Fair innings versus severity. *Social Science & Medicine, 60*(2), 257–263.

O'Brien, B., & Viramontes, J. L. (1994). Willingness to pay: A valid and reliable measure of health state preference? *Medical Decision Making, 14,* 289–297.

Olsen, J. A., & Donaldson, C. (1998). Helicopters, hearts, and hips: Using willingness to pay to set priorities for public sector programmes. *Social Science and Medicine, 46,* 1–12.

Pinto-Prades, J. L., Loomes, G., & Brey R. (2009). Trying to estimate a monetary value for the QALY. *Journal of Health Economics, 28*(3), 553–562.

Rice, D. P., & Hodgson, T. A. (1982). The value of human life revisited. *American Journal of Public Health, 72,* 536–538.

Schelling, T. C. (1968). The life you save may be your own. In S. B. Chase (Ed.), *Problems in public expenditure analysis.* Washington, DC: Brookings Institution.

Shogren, J. F., Shin, S. Y., Hayes, D. J., & Kliebenstein, J. B. (1994). Resolving differences in willingness to pay and willingness to accept. *American Economic Review, 84,* 255–270.

Thaler, R., & Rosen, S. (1975). The value of saving a life. In M. E. Terleckyj (Ed.), *Household production and consumption.* New York, NY: National Bureau of Economic Research.

Thompson, M. S. (1986). Willingness to pay and accept risks to cure chronic disease. *American Journal of Public Health, 76,* 392–397.

Ubel, P. A., Richardson, J., & Baron, J. (2002). Exploring the role of order effects in person trade-off elicitations. *Health Policy, 61*(2), 189–199.

Viscusi, W. K. (1978). Labor market valuations of life and limb. *Public Policy, 26,* 359–385.

Viscusi, W. K. (1993). The value of risks of life and health. *Journal of Economic Literature, 31,* 1912–1946.

Zeckhauser, R. (1975). Procedures for valuing lives. *Public Policy, 23,* 419–464.

Zhao, F. L., Yue, M., Yang, H., Wang, T., Wu, J. H., & Li, S. C. (2011). Willingness to pay per quality-adjusted life year: Is one threshold enough for decision-making?: Results from a study in patients with chronic prostatitis. *Medical Care, 49*(3), 267–272.

Specific Cost-Benefit and Cost-Effectiveness Analyses

Berwick, D. M., & Komaroff, A. L. (1982). Cost effectiveness of lead screening. *New England Journal of Medicine, 306,* 1392–1398.

Bloom, B. S., & Jacobs, J. (1985). Cost effects of restricting cost-effective therapy. *Medical Care, 23,* 872–880.

Cookson, R., Drummond, M., & Weatherly, H. (2009). Explicit incorporation of equity considerations into economic evaluation of public health interventions. *Health Economics, Policy, & Law, 4*(Pt. 2), 231–245.

Cowie, M. R., Marshall, D., Drummond, M., Ferko, N., Maschio, M., Ekman, M., ..., & Boriani, G. (2009). Lifetime cost-effectiveness of prophylactic implantation of a cardioverter defibrillator in patients with reduced left ventricular systolic function: Results of Markov modelling in a European population. *Europace, 11*(6), 716–726.

Coyle, D., Welch, V., Shea, B., Gabriel, S., Drummond, M., & Tugwell, P. (2001). Issues of consensus and debate for economic evaluation in rheumatology. *Journal of Rheumatology, 28*(3), 642–647.

Doherty, N., & Hicks, B. C. (1975). The use of cost-effectiveness analysis in geriatric day care. *Gerontologist, 15,* 412–417.

Drummond, M., Chevat, C., & Lothgren, M. (2007). Do we fully understand the economic value of vaccines? *Vaccine, 25*(32), 5945–5957.

Drummond, M., Weatherly, H., & Ferguson, B. (2008). Economic evaluation of health interventions. *BMJ, 337,* a1204.

Drummond, M. F. (2000). Health economic models: A question of balance—Summary of an open discussion on the pharmacoeconomic evaluation of non-steroidal anti-inflammatory drugs. *Rheumatology, 39*(Suppl. 2), 29–32.

Drummond, M. F. (2005). Economic evaluation of treatment strategies in gastroenterology. *American Journal of Gastroenterology, 100*(10), 2143–2145.

Elixhauser, A. (1989). The cost effectiveness of preventive care for diabetes mellitus. *Diabetes Spectrum, 2,* 349–353.

Evans, R. G., & Robinson, G. C. (1980). Surgical day care: Measurements of the economic payoff. *Canadian Medical Association Journal, 123,* 873–880.

Evans, R. G., & Robinson, G. C. (1983). An economic study of cost savings on a care-by-parent ward. *Medical Care, 21,* 768–782.

Franco, E. L., & Drummond, M. F. (2008). Cost-effectiveness analysis: An essential tool to inform public health policy in cervical cancer prevention. *Vaccine, 26*(Suppl. 5), F1–F2.

Hammond, J. (1979). Home health care cost effectiveness: An overview of the literature. *Public Health Reports, 94,* 305–311.

Lave, L. B. (1980). Economic evaluation of public health programs. *Annual Review of Public Health, 1,* 255–276.

Osnes-Ringen, H., Kvamme, M. K., Kristiansen, I. S., Thingstad, M., Henriksen, J. E., Kvien, T. K., & Daqfinrud, H. (2011). Cost-effectiveness analyses of elective orthopaedic surgical procedures in patients with inflammatory arthropathies. *Scandinavian Journal of Rheumatology, 40*(2), 108–115.

Peyasantiwong, S., Loutfy, M. R., Laporte, A., & Coyte, P. C. (2010). An economic evaluation of treatments for HIV-associated facial lipoatrophy: A cost-utility analysis. *Current HIV Research, 8*(5), 386–395.

Russell, L. B. (1986). *Is prevention better than cure?* Washington, DC: Brookings Institution.

Scheffler, R. M., & Paringer, L. (1980). A review of the economic evaluation of prevention. *Medical Care, 18,* 473–484.

Weinstein, M. C. (1983). Cost-effectiveness priorities for cancer prevention. *Science, 221,* 17–23.

Weisbrod, B. A. (1971). Costs and benefits of medical research. *Journal of Political Economy, 79,* 527–544.

Weisbrod, B. A., Test, M. A., & Stein, L. I. (1980). Alternative to mental hospital treatment. *Archives of General Surgery, 37,* 400–405.

Economic Evaluation and Technology Assessment

Davies, L., Drummond, M., & Papanikolaou, P. (2000). Prioritizing investments in health technology assessment. Can we assess potential value for money? *International Journal of Technology Assessment in Health Care, 16*(1), 73–91.

Detsky, A. S. (1985). Using economic analysis to determine the resource consequences of choices made in planning clinical trials. *Journal of Chronic Diseases, 38,* 753–765.

Drummond, M., & Banta, D. (2009). Health technology assessment in the United Kingdom. *International Journal of Technology Assessment in Health Care, 25*(Suppl. 1), 178–181.

Drummond, M., & Sorenson, C. (2009). Nasty or nice? A perspective on the use of health technology assessment in the United Kingdom. *Value in Health, 12*(Suppl. 2), S8–S13.

Drummond, M., & Weatherly, H. (2000). Implementing the findings of health technology assessments. If the CAT got out of the bag, can the TAIL wag the dog? *International Journal of Technology Assessment in Health Care, 16*(1), 1–12.

Drummond, M. F., & Stoddart, G. L. (1984). Economic analysis and clinical trials. *Controlled Clinical Trials, 5,* 115–128.

Hansen, D., Golbeck, A. L., Noblitt, V., Pinsonneault, J., & Christner, J. (2011). Cost factors in implementing telemonitoring programs in rural home health agencies. *Home Healthcare Nurse, 29*(6), 375–382.

Marshall, N. W., Monnin, P., Bosmans, H., Bochud, F. O., & Verdun, F. R. (2011). Image quality assessment in digital mammography: Part I. Technical characterization of the systems. *Physics in Medicine & Biology, 56*(14), 4201–4220.

Nielsen, C. P., Funch, T. M., & Kristensen, F. B. (2011). Health technology assessment: Research trends and future priorities in Europe. *Journal of Health Services & Research Policy, 16*(Suppl. 2), 6–15.

Nixon, J., Stoykova, B., Glanville, J., Christie, J., Drummond, M., & Kleijnen J. (2000). The U.K. NHS economic evaluation database. Economic issues in evaluations of health technology. International Journal of Technology Assessment in Health Care, 16(3), 731–42.

Patel, C. M., Sahdev, A., & Reznek, R. H. (2011). CT, MRI and PET imaging in peritoneal malignancy. *Cancer Imaging, 11,* 123–139.

Scott, S. H., & Dukelow, S. P. (2011). Potential of robots as next-generation technology for clinical assessment of neurological disorders and upper-limb therapy. *Journal of Rehabilitation Research & Development, 48*(4), 335–353.

Slaughter, M. S., Pederson, B., Graham, J. D., Sobieski, M. A., & Koenig, S. C. (2011). Evaluation of new Forcefield technology: Reducing platelet adhesion and cell coverage of pyrolytic carbon surfaces. *Journal of Thoracic & Cardiovascular Surgery, 142*(4), 921–925.

Sorenson, C., Tarricone, R., Siebert, M., & Drummond, M. (2011). Applying health economics for policy decision making: do devices differ from drugs?. Europace, 13 Suppl 2, ii54-8.

Steinman, M. A., Handler, S. M., Gurwitz, J. H., Schiff, G. D., & Covinsky, K. E. (2011). Beyond the prescription: Medication monitoring and adverse drug events in older adults. *Journal of the American Geriatrics Society, 59,* 1513–1520.

Stevens, A., Chalkidou, K., & Littlejohns, P. (2011). The NHS: Assessing new technologies, NICE and value for money. *Clinical Medicine, 11*(3), 247–250.

Tan, S. S., & Sarker, S. K. (2011). Simulation in surgery: A review. *Scottish Medical Journal, 56*(2), 104–109.

Trosman, J. R., Van Bebber, S. L., & Phillips, K. A. (2011). Health technology assessment and private payers's coverage of personalized medicine. *American Journal of Managed Care, 17*(Suppl. 5), SP53–SP60.

Weinstein, M. C. (1981). Economic assessments of medical practices and technologies. *Medical Decision Making, 1,* 309–330.

Williams, M. C., Reid, J. H., McKillop, G., Weir, N. W., van Beek, E. J., Uren, N. G., & Newby, D. E. (2011). Cardiac and coronary CT comprehensive imaging approach in the assessment of coronary heart disease. *Heart, 97*(15), 1198–1205.

Chapter 13

Value Judgments and Economic Evaluation

OBJECTIVES

1. Describe the type of question that evaluative economics is intended to answer.

2. Describe what a value judgment is and how it can be used in evaluative economics.

3. Using assumed valuations by individuals for services and costs, identify an efficient level of output in any market.

4. Compare alternative delivery arrangements in terms of their efficiency.

5. Describe how a market for health insurance can be efficient when there is less than complete insurance coverage.

6. Describe the extra-welfarist approach to identifying optimal economic arrangements.

7. Define the concept of equity.

8. Identify several alternative measures of equity and explain how these can be applied to evaluate alternative modes of finance and care delivery.

13.1 INTRODUCTION

In this chapter, the level of inquiry is not focused on the actual allocation of resources devoted to medical care, which is interested in explaining only the various allocations that might occur in different circumstances and not with whether any particular allocation is "good" or "acceptable" or "equitable," to mention only a few of the terms that might be used to label an allocation. In this chapter, the task of evaluating alternative possible allocations of resources is introduced. This task will lead to such questions as whether totally free care can be judged "better" than the provision of medical care in a simple market or whether and in what sense a regulated system is preferable to an unregulated one. Many of these questions, it should be pointed out, are policy issues. Indeed, evaluative analysis forms the cornerstone of policy analysis because the ultimate goal of policy is to bring about improvements in the use of resources.

Before undertaking evaluative analysis, the ground rules for conducting an evaluation must be established. That is the mission of this chapter. In Section 13.2, the importance of having a recognizable and unvarying standard for gauging alternative allocations is discussed. The values that individual persons place on specific services can be used as the basis of a social evaluation. One procedure for building a social evaluation is discussed in Section 13.3. The standard that results from this procedure, which is used frequently by economists, is referred to as an *efficiency criterion*. Such a yardstick takes individuals' starting situations as given and therefore bypasses questions relating to equity and need as determined by clinical criteria. The application of efficiency criteria to evaluate the performance of the health insurance market is discussed in Section 13.4, and policy goals emanating from this efficiency analysis are presented in Section 13.5. The relevance of the efficiency criteria as the sole benchmark of resource allocation has been questioned by many observers. An alternative approach, called *extra-welfarism*, is presented in Section 13.6. Finally, alternative measures of equity are considered in Section 13.7.

13.2 VALUES AND STANDARDS IN ECONOMIC EVALUATION

Suppose there is a situation in which A has a curable cancer but is receiving no medical care, and B is healthy but is spending $8,000 on surgical services for a facial lift. Would this be an acceptable allocation of medical resources? Many would say it is unfair, but scarcely anybody would take the trouble to set forth the basic standard being used to judge the situation. Suppose instead that it was necessary heart surgery B was receiving. Would this change one's evaluation of the situation? Would a different standard be used to gauge its fairness?

In this example, the resources are being allocated differently in the two situations. However, unless there is a standard that did not itself vary from situation to situation, it is really not possible to compare the two situations. That is, without an independent scale of fairness or acceptability, there would not be a measure capable of assessing alternative allocations. This section presents a classification of available systems of standards, focusing on the bases on which standards may be formed.

For the purposes of economic evaluation, there are two ways of deriving a system of values and then developing a ranking of alternative uses of resources. In the first method, called *delegatory* or *top-down*, a value system is imposed on the members of society. For example, it might be imposed by a higher being, such as a deity; by an interpreter of the ultimate word, such as Moses or Mohammed; or by a dictator, who settles on some value system based on his or her values. Alternatively, someone can assume the mantle of spokesperson for society, proclaiming "society wants a decent standard of health for all," or some such alleged "truth." Despite the nod toward democracy, any would-be ethical authority who chooses to speak for society without a mandate based on the views of individuals within the society is really imposing his or her own views on society.

The second method for deriving a system of values is called *participatory* or *bottom-up*. In this method, the views of all members of the community play a role. One assumption underlying this method is that *everyone's* values must be taken into account in ranking alternative ways of using resources. Another assumption is that each individual is the best judge of his or her own welfare.

Now attention is turned to the value systems themselves, which vary tremendously, ranging from the very specific to the very vague. They can take the form of specific laws handed down by a deity, or can be formulated in terms of such general concepts as *fairness*, *liberty*, and *equality*.

The field of health services analysis contains many examples of writers proposing value systems based on their own view of what seems desirable. For instance, some have posited a "right" to health or health care. One commentator used the principle of *agape* to derive this right (Outka, 1974), whereas another appealed to a "strong sense in the population" that this right exists (Mechanic, 1976).

Even assuming a single value system could be identified, the problem of translating the chosen value system into a gauge or ranking scheme to assess alternative ways of using resources would still need to be established. This translation step can be controversial itself. Because any value system will be somewhat vague, different ranking schemes with very different implications can be derived from it. The next problem encountered would then be the problem of which ranking scheme to choose. For example, the goal of "equality" can be interpreted in many ways—as equality of *health status* or equality of *medical care utilization*. If it is decided that it entails equal use of medical care for equal health status, then individuals who have poor health would receive more care than individuals who are basically healthy. This may seem plausible, but how is the decision reached on how much more care people with poor health should get? Also, if the medical care given to those in poor health is not effective, should they still receive it?

The last step, after having decided on a ranking scheme, is to apply it to actual or proposed states of resource use (e.g., distributions of health care or levels of health) to determine their desirability from a policy standpoint. It should be stressed that value systems imposed from earlier are not necessarily evil. The source of such a system may be a highly respected and beloved authority, and the system may contain laudatory ideals and translate into ranking schemes that seem reasonable and compassionate. Nevertheless, an imposed scheme is not built up from the values of the members of the society and therefore retains some degree of nonrepresentativeness.

In Sections 13.3 and 13.4, a participatory system of evaluation is developed. This system, well known in economic circles as the *Paretean system* (named after the famous 19th-century sociologist Vilfredo Pareto), allows arrival at an optimum position through examining changes that could be made in resource allocations if started from an initial position. This optimum holds only with reference to the initial starting point (i.e., the initial endowments each member of society possesses). The starting point is not judged, which may or may not be fair, a consideration discussed in Section 13.5.

13.3 EFFICIENT OUTPUT LEVELS

13.3.1 Individual Valuations of Goods and Services or Activities

If individuals' own valuations are accepted as the best indicators of their own welfare, then it must be determined, at least in principle, what these valuations might be. Because this analysis is concerned with specific goods and services, the task is simplified somewhat. The need is only to determine individuals' valuations with respect to those goods and services being considered.

Economists have developed a hypothesis regarding an individual's valuation of units of a specific good or service. The hypothesis, which is based on this demand analysis, is that the more of any good or service the individual has, the less successive units of the good or service will be worth to him or her (as compared with other goods and services). The analysis can be recast using money as the basic unit of value. To do this, it must be assumed that money itself is of constant value. That is, if an individual gives up $2, that $2 will always represent the same loss to the individual, however much income he or she has. This assumption will hold, at least partially, if the outlay for the good or service in question is a reasonably small portion of the individual's total budget.

If an individual has an income of $20,000, spending $200 or $300 on a good or service is unlikely to cause the valuation of each dollar to change for the individual. However, as the amount that must be given up to obtain a good or service becomes very large relative to income, the utility of, or the subjective valuation placed on, the marginal dollar will change. The assumption is being made in this section that it does not. It should be noted that this is a different assumption than often made regarding health insurance demand.

Given the assumption that money income has a constant value for individuals for all relevant ranges of expenditures, the individual valuations of successive units of a good or service in terms of money can be specified. It must be stressed that these valuations are the individuals' own evaluations of specific units of the good or service, and they qualify on participatory grounds for inclusion into the overall participatory social evaluation.

13.3.2 Values in a Selfish Market

To simplify the analysis, it is assumed initially that there are two individuals in the market, A and B. Each has a specific schedule of valuations for his or her own consumption of medical care. These valuations are referred to as *marginal valuations* (MVs). A marginal valuation is defined as the extra amount of money an individual would be willing to pay for an additional unit of a good or service. Thus, an MV is a measure of what an extra unit of the good or service is worth to the individual in money terms.

In the initial analysis, both A and B derive satisfaction, or value, from their own consumption of medical services, and theirs is the only satisfaction that anyone in society gets from their consumption. A places a marginal value of $160 on his first unit consumed, $140 on his second, and so on, as seen in columns 1 and 2 in Table 13-1. Note that the marginal values placed by each individual on successive units of medical care consumed diminish; all other factors, such as health status, income, and wealth, are held constant (i.e., the initial values of these variables are held constant). For purposes of social evaluation, then, this is a measure of the social worth of A's consumption of medical care (because no one else values this care other than A himself).

The assumed relation between marginal value and quantity consumed can be presented geometrically. In Figure 13-1, the curve MV_a represents A's marginal valuation of successive units of medical care. It is assumed, for ease of geometric exposition, that the units of medical care can be made very small, so that the MV curve becomes smooth. A's valuation of his own consumption is referred to as the *private* (or *internal*) valuation of his consumption. On the assumption that no one else cares about A's consumption, his private valuation is the same as the social valuation (the total value placed on A's consumption by all of society).

Similarly, the private valuations of B is presented in Table 13-1, and geometrically as MV_b in Figure 13-1. For whatever reason (she is poorer, more healthy, or less well educated), B places a lower value on each unit of health care than does A.

Indeed, her first unit has an MV of $50, her second has an MV of $40, and so on. These valuations might seem low, but because B is the ultimate judge of her own welfare, these valuations cannot be questioned, they are simply part of the data.

Table 13-1 Values and Costs of Medical Care

(1)	(2)	(3)	(4)	(5)	(6)	(7)
Quantity Consumed by A (Q_a)	A's Marginal Valuation (MV_a)	Quantity Consumed by B (Q_b)	B's Marginal Valuation (MV_b)	Quantity Consumed by A and B	Social Marginal Value of Consumption	Marginal Cost of Output at Consumption Level $Q_a + Q_b$
1	$160	0	$0	1	$160	$70
2	140	0	0	2	140	70
3	120	0	0	3	120	70
4	100	1	100	5	100	70
5	80	2	80	7	80	70
6	60	3	60	9	60	70
7	40	4	40	11	40	70
8	20	5	20	13	20	70
9	0	6	0	15	0	70

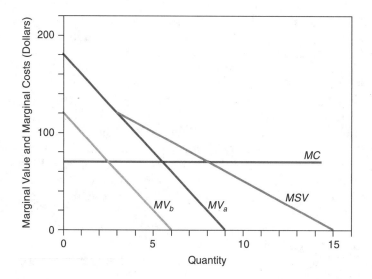

Figure 13-1   Representation of Efficient Output Level. Individuals A and B have private marginal valuations for medical care (MV_a and MV_b, respectively). Using these, the marginal social value (MSV) curve is calculated, which relates aggregate quantity to each individual's valuation. MC is the marginal social cost of medical care. The efficient level of output is that quantity at which MSV equals the MC.

According to the assumption, A and B are the only members of society who participate in the medical care market. The marginal social valuations of medical care coincide with the marginal private valuations. Column 5 of Table 13-1 lists the aggregated quantities that correspond to each level of MV. For example, at an aggregate quantity of five units of medical care (four used by A and one by B), each consumer's marginal value will be $100. If seven units were consumed (five by A and two by B), each individual's MV would be $80. It has now been hypothesized how much each additional unit of medical care is worth to each participant. Furthermore, an aggregate-level relationship has been derived between the quantity of medical care and the marginal value to each individual, if he or she was consuming at the level of consumption indicated by the MV curve (Figure 13-1). This aggregate curve, called the MSV (marginal social value) curve, shows the value to each member of the market if all individuals are consuming at the levels indicated by the curve. Because B does not have an MV above $120, for values above $120, the MSV curve coincides with A's MV curve.

An implicit assumption of this analysis is that consumer valuations are expressed in terms of a good or service, medical care. But medical care may not be valued for its own sake (except perhaps by a hypochondriac); it is usually *health* that is valued. In fact, each consumer's MV is made up of two components: an MV for health (termed H) and the marginal productivity of an additional unit of medical care (M) in producing health ($\Delta H/\Delta M$). Thus, the valuation of medical care is derivative, stemming from the two components.

Next, the cost of producing medical care must be determined. The initial assumption here is that each level of output is being produced at the minimum cost. This assumption is sometimes referred to as the *technical efficiency* assumption. It implies that, given production conditions and input prices, the lowest cost combination of inputs is used at any output level. In column 7 of Table 13-1 and in Figure 13-1, the minimum marginal cost at which providers can produce medical care is shown. It is assumed that this minimum marginal cost remains constant at $70 per unit as output increases. Note that the *MC* is the additional cost per unit of care; each extra unit costs $70 to produce.

One interpretation of *MC* is that it is the amount of money that must be paid to the inputs to hire them away from the next-highest valued use. If medical care was not produced, something else of value to consumers would be. It can be assumed then that the *MC* is the amount that would have to be paid to the resources to induce them not to produce that something else. This approach enables being able to put a value on unpaid resources that otherwise would appear to be "valueless" or "free." Thus, the *MC* is marginally above (and approximates) the value that someone else would have placed on these resources in an alternative use. Viewing the *MC* in this way means that it is essentially the opportunity cost of the resources used (the value that users of other goods and services would have placed on them).

13.3.3 The Socially Optimum Quantity of Medical Care

The next step in this analysis involves the definition and identification of desirable or optimum resource allocations. Because this method of evaluation is participatory, allocations of resources that would be considered better than alternatives by all members of the community need to be identified. As will be seen presently, it is possible using a participatory method to rank some allocations as superior to others, although every conceivable situation cannot be compared. The criterion here is this: the resources must be used in a way that maximizes social value. That is, if the resources are distributed in such a way that consumers are willing to pay the most for them, then output will be at the "right," or economically efficient, level.

Using the valuations of A and B and the *MC* of medical care, the market will be at a socially optimal (or economically efficient) level of output if the *MV*s of A and B equal the *MC* (i.e., $MV_a = MV_b = MC$). If output is at a level at which the *MV*s are greater than *MC*, say, at an aggregate quantity of 3 in Table 13-1, then an expansion of output to 5 (an increase of 1 for A and B each) would have an *MC* per unit of output of $70 but would yield $100 extra in value to A and B each. Similarly, if the *MC* is greater than the *MSV*, this indicates that resources are worth more elsewhere, and so output should fall. In Figure 13-1, the optimal level of medical care is 7 units. Given the assumptions stated earlier, this is how much medical care should be produced. This measure of efficiency—the distribution of output based on utility—is called *allocative efficiency*.

In reality, in a medical care market, too much or too little (as well as just enough) medical care could be produced. Too much could be produced if the government had a policy of financing medical care and giving it away for free.

At a zero price, demand will be at 15 units (when the *MV*s are zero); the *MC* of additional units will be well above this if the government is willing to ensure that all that is demanded is provided. The financing of the program could be through taxes. However, by meeting all demands, the government is clearly providing too much.

On the other hand, the market may provide too little. If medical care was in the hands of a monopolist, the monopolist would set a price well above a point at which *MV* = *MC*. If the price was $110, then three units in total would be demanded (all by A). Here, the market would be producing too little care.

In addition, the optimum level of resource use could result in little or even no use of medical care by some individuals. The height of the *MV* curve, which is in effect a demand curve, will depend on health status, wealth, income, and so on. Poor people (e.g., B) may have low *MV*s. Indeed, if the *MC* was higher than in our example, a socially optimal quantity of output would be perfectly consistent with no consumption of medical care by B. (This is true even though B may have poor health.) It might be argued that this is unfair, and indeed, depending on the definition of fairness, it might well be. It should be recognized however that the root cause of the inequitable distribution of medical care is the inequitable distribution of wealth. A higher income for B would mean higher demand and *MV* curves for medical care. Of course, as far as the notion of economic efficiency is concerned, initial wealth and income levels for each individual are given. A redistribution of income or wealth among individuals might seem fair to many observers, but it would not be evaluated within the bounds of the present notion of economic efficiency.

13.3.4 Optimal Output with Altruism

To preserve the present notion of economic efficiency and to extend it to cover some distributional issues, an analysis has been developed to allow for the concern of some individuals for the low medical care consumption levels of others. Here, the previous example is extended to allow for A's external demand for B's consumption of medical care. From A's viewpoint, it may well be that B has a level of consumption of medical care that is too low. If this is the case, some representation must be found of the value to A of B's medical care consumption. It is likely, of course, that A's concern for B's medical care consumption is not unlimited. A is concerned, but only up to a point, for A has other private and public concerns as well. In fact, as seen in Section 13.4.3, A's valuation of B's medical care consumption can be treated as any other good or service; the more B consumes, the less the marginal value to A of an additional unit. In Table 13-2, A's MV for B's consumption is $60 for the first unit, $40 for the second, and so on. In Figure 13-2, this external *MV* curve is shown as MV_a^b.

It may seem strange that A's altruistic concern for B's welfare can be translated into mercenary terms and be given a monetary measure. The ability to do this rests on the assumption that goods and services are scarce, and A must make some choices at the margin. Even if A decided to give all his money away and use none of it for his family or own personal use, there would still be hard decisions to make. Should the money be donated to the Cancer Society or Heart Association? Should the money go toward the preservation of New-foundland seals or bald eagles? Depending on their tastes, even the most altru-istic of people must make choices regarding scarcity and our analysis is merely a formalization of this fact. Of course, most people will engage in private consumption as well as altruistic consumption; their values can be presented by marginal valuation curves for both types of activities. The benefits to be

Table 13-2 Private and Social Values of B's Consumption of Medical Care

(1)	(2)	(3)	(4)
Quantity Consumed by B	Marginal Value to B of Own Consumption (MV_b)	Marginal Value to A of B's Consumption (MV_a)	Marginal Social Value of B's Consumption $(MV_b + MV_a)$
1	100	60	160
2	80	40	120
3	60	20	80
4	40	0	40
5	20	0	20

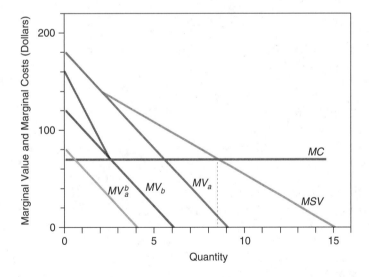

Figure 13-2 Representation of Efficient Output Level. Individuals A and B have private marginal valuations for medical care (MV_a and MV_b, respectively); in addition, individual A places an external value on B's consumption. The marginal social value of B's consumption is the sum of the values placed on B's consumption by both A and B. The MSV of all medical care also reflects this externality. The MC is the marginal social cost of medical care. The efficient level of output is where $MSV = MC$ (at approximately eight units).

obtained from others' consumption will be termed *external benefits,* and the values that people place on these benefits will be termed *external values.*

It is now possible to arrive at a measure of the value that society places on B's medical care. This value can be called a *social value,* and it is made up of all individuals' private and external values for the specific good or service. Thus, the marginal social value for B's consumption of medical care can be obtained by adding up the values both individuals place on each successive unit of medical care that B might consume. In Table 13-2, society has a marginal valuation of $160 for the first unit of B's medical care (equal to the sum of MV_b and MV_a^a), $120 for the second, and so on. These valuations are shown in Figure 13-2 as MSV_b^b, which is the vertical sum of MV_b and MV_a^b. *Vertical sum* means that each unit of B's consumption has a value to society (A and B) greater than the value placed on it by B alone. Because of this "public" dimension, all values placed on each unit of B's consumption are summed. Because each member's valuation of the commodity is measured along the vertical, or cost, axis, the summation of all members' valuations of this good or service is therefore a vertical sum.

The marginal valuation curve facing the market for medical care for A and B is *MSV,* which shows the quantity for all individuals at alternative *MSVs* for each individual. This curve is much like the *MSV* curve in Figure 13-1, except it incorporates A's valuation of B's consumption along with the private *MVs.*

The socially optimum level of output is similarly interpreted; the output is optimal at the quantity in which the *MSV* for all individuals equals the *MC.* In Figure 13-2, the optimum level of output is eight units of medical care. This optimum quantity incorporates each individual's private valuations, as well as any external valuations for the poor, the needy, the sick, and so on. The optimum quantity that incorporates the external concerns of A is greater than the optimum quantity if only selfish concerns exist (see Figure 13-1). However, these outcomes are the results of the data, and it may well be that B's optimal consumption is still at a low level.

The results of the extended analysis are consistent with some kind of transfer of funds from A to B for the purposes of increasing B's consumption of medical care. However, the analysis does not say what kind of transfer should take place. It may be voluntary (e.g., charitable donations given by A directly to B or to some providing agency) or tax based (e.g., taxes levied on A might be used to reimburse providers). Although, if taxation is used to raise funds, this analysis implies that it is voluntarily accepted by A. In either case, the optimal solution allows for some transfer, but it should be stressed that a transfer can be too much or too little. The government can over- or underprovide, based on A's criteria. All that this analysis shows is that *some* transfer is consistent with economic efficiency.

13.3.5 Alternative Delivery Arrangements

Now that an ideal or efficient output level has been identified, alternative delivery arrangements can be examined to see how they compare with the ideal. That is, it becomes possible to determine whether expected output under the alternatives is too little, just enough, or too much.

13.3.5.1 "Free" and Unlimited Care

First, assume that B is given all the medical care for free that she can consume. As column three of Table 13-1 indicates, she would choose to consume six units of output. The social optimum is eight units for A and B, and the *MC* at this quantity is $70. Optimally, B should consume three (i.e., when $MSV_b = MC$). For every unit B consumes beyond three, the value of B's consumption is less than the cost to society (everyone). Because someone must bear the burden of this care, and because *MC* exceeds *MSV* for all units beyond three, there is a net social loss for these units. B gains handsomely (i.e., her private benefits exceed her private costs), but overall, this type of arrangement may lead to a great deal of medical care being consumed with very little value attached to it.

13.3.5.2 Competitive Market, No Philanthropy

Another arrangement is now considered, that of a competitive market with no philanthropy or government programs. Equilibrium in a competitive market will occur when marginal private cost equals price. In the example here, A will consume the right amount for himself, but B will not. B's consumption will be less than the socially efficient amount because all society would have been willing to pay more for the first four units of B's consumption than the marginal cost. The competitive market does not provide a mechanism to express A's external demand for B's care. A freely operating competitive market with no philanthropy will yield less than the optimal level of output when externalities would have justified a larger output. As for a monopolistic market, the output of such a market will be less than the output of a competitive market, which means it will be even further below the optimal amount.

13.3.5.3 Competitive Market with Philanthropy

It has been contended that even with philanthropy, a competitive market will not produce the optimal amount of output. To understand why, consider a situation in which there are many donors of medical care, each of whom places a value on the consumption of medical care by the needy. In this case, some social arrangement must be found for ensuring that the values of these donors will be expressed in the market. If each of these potential donors offers to give what the output is worth to him or her, the social value will equal the sum of the private values. However, if each donor feels that the others will also give, he or she might give less, hoping to get a "free ride," that is, gain the benefit of the others' donations while giving less. It is in the interests of each private donor to initially offer less than the value he or she places on the output in the hope that someone else will pay the tab. If everyone behaves in this way, the total amount given in philanthropy will be less than the socially optimal amount. Analysts who accept the efficiency criterion frequently justify compulsory government programs on the basis that they make everyone pay what the programs are worth. Of course, it is difficult to decide how much a program would be worth to each taxpayer because the individual still has an incentive to understate the value of the program to him- or herself.

Even accepting this justification for government programs, it must still be discovered whether there exists an arrangement that will lead to the correct amount of medical care being utilized. As can be seen in Figure 13-2, if B was offered subsidized medical care, the efficient amount of medical care would be utilized. In this case, a charge of $60 per unit of medical care to B would lead to B's consumption of the optimal quantity—three units. The rest of society must now pick up the remainder of the tab. Because the total cost to all members of society of medical care consumed by B is $210, and because B will pay $180 of this, some arrangements must be made to collect the remaining $30 from the rest of society. This can be done in the form of taxes. Various arrangements are discussed in the next paragraphs.

It can be concluded from this analysis that some form of cost-sharing arrangement can lead to the provision of an optimal or efficient amount of the product. However, other arrangements can also be efficient. One is to have needy individuals pay nothing and to impose some other form of rationing. In practice, this type of arrangement requires that the rationing system used must produce the efficient outcome, and such systems are difficult to design and operate. This analysis can also be extended to a case in which the needy individuals have different levels of income. If their demands differ because of these income levels, a system of variable subsidies tailored to income levels could be designed to have each member consume the right level of output (Pauly, 1972).

What is critical in translating the preceding analysis into a policy prescription is a clear conception of what the external demands might be in actuality. Assuming that external demands for the medical care of some groups do exist and are significant, it is essential that it be exactly determined for what services these external demands are. If they are for good health, for example, then the external demanders (the A's in our analysis) may demand preventive care for consumption by the potential recipients of aid (the B's), however the demands may be much more specific than that. The demanders might show concern only for individuals who have catastrophic illnesses requiring large financial outlays. In this case, they will not want to pay for the medical care of needy individuals who have sore throats, ingrown toenails, or acne. Very little is known about the nature of medical care externalities (external demands). From an efficiency point of view however, it is necessary to know what the external demanders are concerned about before we design a delivery system that will incorporate these externalities.

Assuming that the nature of the external demands have been identified, then the preceding analysis can be used to answer the questions as long as the goal of efficiency is kept in mind. Once the demands have been pinpointed, the types of health care that might improve the situation, and the potential recipients, can be identified. The consumer's portion of cost sharing should be designed to ensure that there is no overuse, which is defined as any quantity beyond which marginal social benefits are less than marginal social costs. The reimbursement mechanism chosen should lead to the least-cost output.

13.4 OPTIMAL HEALTH INSURANCE

The provision of health insurance requires resources and incurs costs. In the same way that there is an optimal quantity of medical care, there is an optimal degree of insurance coverage. It is assumed that all individuals are the same in all respects except one—the amount they must pay to obtain insurance.

Let us assume that there are 900 individuals (the number is not important) who are members of a large group, and 100 individuals who are members of a small group. All individuals have an initial level of wealth of $2,000. There is a probability of 10% (0.10) that each individual will get sick (i.e., 10% of each group will get sick). For those individuals who do get sick, the medical costs are $400 per patient. The utility function for each member (all have the same tastes) is as shown in Table 13-3. Utility is assumed to reflect consumer welfare. Although total utility increases with increased wealth, it does so at a decreasing rate—diminishing marginal utility of wealth. This utility function

Table 13-3   Relationship Between Wealth and Utility.

Wealth	Total Utility	Marginal Utility
$1,600	57.0	4.2
1,620	61.2	4.0
1,640	65.2	3.8
1,660	69.0	3.6
1,680	72.6	3.4
1,700	76.0	3.2
1,720	79.0	3.0
1,740	81.8	2.8
1,760	84.4	2.6
1,780	86.8	2.4
1,800	89.0	2.2
1,820	91.0	2.0
1,840	92.8	1.8
1,860	94.4	1.6
1,880	95.8	1.4
1,900	97.0	1.2
1,920	98.0	1.0
1,940	98.8	0.8
1,960	99.4	0.6
1,980	99.8	0.4
2,000	100.0	0.2

can be interpreted as a measure of "consumer welfare." With regard to the supply side of the market, it is assumed that there is one insurer that provides insurance at cost. The loading cost to the insurer of a large group policy is $60, whereas the cost for a small group policy is $120. The objective is to maximize the overall utility of all members without detracting from that of any single member. This is the Paretean criterion.

The framework used focuses on consumer welfare (utility). In general, it is assumed that consumer welfare is maximized by shifting the risk onto the insurer whenever the expected utility with insurance is greater than the utility in the absence of insurance. The postinsurance utility is the net of the economic cost of accepting the risk. Therefore, utility (welfare) is maximized whenever the risk is appropriately shifted.

In this analysis, there are two groups of individuals. Each individual faces an expected loss of $40 (i.e., 10% of $400), and each can obtain insurance at a cost that includes the expected loss ($40) plus the appropriate loading cost. For members of the large group, the full premium, including the loading charge, is $100. For members of the smaller group, the premium is $160. For members of the large group, there is a utility, or welfare, gain by shifting the risk: at a cost of $100, the utility will be 97.0 units, which exceeds the expected utility of not insuring, which is 95.8 units. There is a social gain from shifting the risk. The same is not true for the members of the smaller group. Because the cost of insurance for them is $160, they would be better off to remain uninsured. This would be true even if the cost of insurance for the smaller group was subsidized (i.e., if someone else paid part or all of the premiums). This is because the criterion of social efficiency rather than individual efficiency is being used. When it is recognized that there is a *social* cost of insuring, then it must also be recognized that there is an *optimal* degree of insurance coverage. This optimal degree may be zero if the arrangements for providing insurance are too costly.

It must also be acknowledged that consumers may vary in many respects, including the following: risk of illness, income or wealth level, degree of risk aversion, and circumstances affecting the cost of illness. As each varies, the utility gain from shifting the risk of incurring medical expenses will also change. For example, individuals with a high risk of illness will gain more in terms of utility from shifting their risk than individuals with a low risk of illness. Thus, a situation in which individuals who are less healthy have greater insurance coverage could be an optimal situation. That is, variations in insurance coverage among individuals can be economically efficient.

There is a confounding factor in this analysis: moral hazard. There can be a net welfare gain resulting from the shifting of risk. Once the risk is shifted, the out-of-pocket price of medical care to the consumer falls. If there is any elasticity of demand for medical care, then moral hazard will come into play and the quantity demanded of health care will increase. If the out-of-pocket price of medical care is low enough, the individual might consume care up to the point at which $MC > MV$. There is a net welfare loss in the medical care market that occurs when the individual is ill. There are, then, two welfare effects of insurance: the welfare gain from shifting the risk and the welfare loss from consuming beyond the optimal point when the individual is ill. True optimality requires that both effects together be considered (Gianfrancesco, 1978). Usually, investigators focus on the insurance market (Gianfrancesco, 1983; Pauly, 1990) or the medical care market (Pauly, 1972) in isolation from one another.

13.5 EXTRA-WELFARISM

The framework used until now has included a number of value judgments and principles. A key principle is that each person is the best judge of his or her own welfare. Welfare, in this framework, depends exclusively on the utility of goods and services as valued by the individuals. If there is any "public" component of goods and services, it is introduced through external demand, which is the value some people place on other people's consumption. Beyond this, there is no justification for publicly provided health care that can be derived from the Paretean welfare framework.

The Paretean framework has come under criticism in recent years on the grounds that it does not include all that people value in life (Culyer, 1990; Rice, 1992). There are other sources of personal well-being besides goods and services. Many of these other sources of well-being are embodied in the characteristics of people rather than the characteristics of the goods and services that people consume. People value mobility, absence from pain, and absence from distress, and they value these for other people as well. Although it is true that there are goods and services (including medical care) that are linked to these more ultimate sources of well-being, there is no automatic link between them. Consequently, a social evaluation based on goods and services consumed, and nothing else, appears much too narrow.

"Health" is often viewed as a composite of characteristics of people, such as mobility, absence of distress, and so forth. A number of economists have asserted that health is important, and not only because we want it for ourselves. They regard health as one of several entities that "society" recognizes should be made available to everyone (Culyer, 1993), regardless of willingness to pay. This position has often appeared in the healthcare literature (Fein, 1972; Outka, 1974). If health really is a socially recognized good, then health *services* cannot be evaluated strictly in terms of their market value. In particular, the distribution of health services must be evaluated on a social basis.

The researchers who hold this position largely avoid the question of who the judge of welfare will be, a question directly addressed in the Paretean framework. They merely assert that some decision maker, chosen (or elected) by society, should be responsible for conducting the evaluation. Thus, in this extra-welfarist viewpoint, it is no longer clear who the judge of welfare is. Indeed, extra-welfarism is consistent with the use of any social judge other than the consumers; the approach merely posits that there are some entities whose social value is determined outside of the consumers themselves. The role of economists is to act as advisors for the distributive organization and uncover the implications of incorporating efficiency and other objectives into the economic analysis. It should be pointed out that people's direct evaluations of their health services can be included in the extra-welfarist economic calculus, as can other (nondirect) evaluations of their health care.

The extra-welfarist position is concerned with how health is distributed among all members of society. Whoever the judge of well-being becomes (the government, a community league, etc.), value judgments must still be made in order to decide how to distribute health services and health. One way to operationalize the extra-welfarist approach (i.e., turn it into an evaluative tool) is to provisionally accept the principle that health care should be distributed according to "need." If need is defined as the ability to benefit from health services (Culyer, 1995), then the "decision maker" is faced with the question of how to allocate health services so as to enhance or preserve different individuals' health status. Even if this approach evades the issue (or at least leaves the issue open) of who is to decide on the distribution, it helps make explicit the wide array of distributions that are possible (using the principle of need and other principles as well).

Figure 13-3 is a graph that shows the health of two individuals, A and B, measured along the two axes (Wagstaff, 1991). The following (nonvalue-laden) assumptions are made: individual A has a self-assessed health status of h_1 and individual B has a self-assessed health status of h_2. The health status of both can be improved, but there is a limit. Curve H shows the maximum amount of health that can be produced with the resources available for health care (assumed to be fixed for society as a whole). More health can be produced

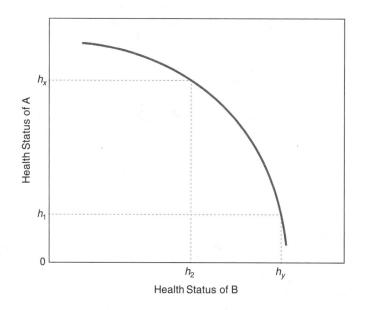

Figure 13-3 Potential Health Status of Two Indivudals. The health status of A and the health status of B are currently at h_1 and h_2. Through expending more resources, their health status can move up to h_x and h_y, respectively. However, since the available resources are finite, the limit of improvement for both individuals combined is shown by curve H.

for A, but only at the expense of resources and health for B. With available resources, A's health can be increased up to h_x (with no change in B's health) and B's health can be increased up to h_y (with no change in A's health). The exact shape of the H curve will depend on how effective the additional resources are in improving each individual's health. If very little extra can be done to improve B's health, then the curve will be steeply sloped. Our curve shows that more can be done for both.

Mentioned previously was the principle that health resources should be distributed according to need. There are a number of different ways to express "need."

- *Equal health status.* One value judgment is to allocate resources so that everyone ends up with an equal level of health. If this principle is used, then more resources must be provided to A to ensure that, in the end, both A and B are equally healthy. Equal health implies that each person is on a 45° line from the origin.

- *Maximizing total health regardless of its distribution.* In order to implement this criterion, the trade-off in health status between the two persons must be known. If the health transformation curve, H, favors person A, then resources will be more productive in improving A's health status rather than B's. An optimal point will occur on the H curve above the 45° line. The characteristic of the optimal point will be where the additional health per dollar of expenditure will be the same for the two people.

- *Equalizing additional health per dollar.* This criterion is most like the Paretean optimum. According to this criterion, the initial starting point (h_1, h_2) is accepted and allocation of additional resources occurs so that the total health gain is as large as possible. The optimum point will at a position northeast of the initial position on the transformation curve, H.

The usefulness of the extra-welfarist approach is that it allows us to go further in exploring resource allocation than the Paretean or welfarist position, and if society places special importance on characteristics such as health, then alternative distributions of healthcare resources need extremely careful evaluation.

13.6 CONCEPTS OF EQUITY

Distributional equity is important in analyzing both access to and consumption of medical care (e.g., differences in utilization among groups) and its financing (e.g., differences in payments), and so it is essential to have measures of equity. We focus here on three types of distributional equity: intergenerational equity, vertical equity, and horizontal equity (Long & Smeeding, 1984).

Intergenerational equity, in a financial context, concerns the distribution of payments among different generations. For example, if the population is divided into retirees (who are generally 65 or older and eligible for Medicare benefits), those of working age (say, those 18 to 64), and others, then the classification scheme could be regarded as dividing the population along generational lines. Because the Medicare hospital insurance program is financed largely through the flow of payroll taxes into the Hospital Insurance Trust Fund, these taxes will be borne largely by individuals in the working-age group. In other words, the working-age generation is largely financing the care of the generation of retirees. The equity implications of this kind of tax are very different than those of the tax used to expand the Medicare program's benefits in 1988. This latter was a 15% tax on the taxable income of the retirees, and it proved to be so unpopular that the program expansion was repealed by Congress. This last type of tax involves a minimal intergenerational transfer of funds.

Current employment-based private health insurance provides another example of intergenerational transfer. All employees pay a similar health insurance premium, which is based on the average utilization pattern for all workers. According to insurance principles, if workers were rated separately by age group, younger workers would have a lower premium than older workers because their utilization is less. The financing method of charging everyone in the plan the same rate (community rating) is, in effect, intergenerationally inequitable.

The second type of equity, vertical equity, concerns the economic burden experienced by different income groups. For example, imagine there are three income groups: those who make under $40,000, those who make from $40,000 to $80,000, and those who make over $80,000. A tax is progressive if members of a higher income group pay a larger portion of their income in tax than those with a lower income; it is neutral if the portion is the same for all groups; and it is regressive if members of a lower income group pay a higher portion of their income in tax than those with a higher income.

An example of vertical inequity would be a flat tax charged to all individuals regardless of their income level. A fixed premium for Medicare enrollees is such a tax. Lower income groups pay the same rate as higher income groups do, and this premium amounts to a higher portion of their income.

Horizontal equity concerns the degree to which equals are taxed equally. An example of a horizontally inequitable tax is a tax on specific goods and services such as alcohol, tobacco products, and hospital care. Consumption, or sales, taxes on the former two products fall on groups who use these products more heavily. Such taxes have been a popular means of financing health insurance programs for indigents. Even though these taxes are horizontally inequitable, it has been argued that because these individuals are likely to be less healthy and use the healthcare system more, they should pay higher taxes. That is, if not just taxes but rather the net of healthcare services minus taxes paid are considered, then horizontal *inequity* is not present. Another type of tax that has been recommended as a way to pay for medical care for indigents is a tax on hospital admissions. Such a tax will also be inequitable, although to a large extent it will be less visible because it will be passed on to the third parties who reimburse the providers. (Of course, the insurers in turn will pass the tax on by charging higher health insurance premiums.)

13.7 GOALS OF HEALTH POLICY

There are a number of different ways that the goals of health policy can be articulated. At one level, one can articulate a set of environmental conditions that will allow for a smoother operating policy. For example, many feel that if consumers are given a range of health plans to select from, and the freedom to choose among those plans, then social goals will be advanced. At a lower, operational level, there are goals that deal with operating performance, such as efficiency, equity, and public financial constraints. Finally, social goals can be articulated in terms of the health outcomes of a group of individuals. In order for the policy goal to be operational, policies will still have to specify how each person's health status is to be included (e.g., whether everyone is counted the same). In addition, the policy makers should take into account the economic aspects of the policy goals. There are insufficient resources to allow everyone to maximize their health status, therefore goals have to be set that allow one to rank social measures of health status resulting from different policies.

One might combine policy goals from the different categories. For example, a policy maker might deem equity of resource use to be important. However, once individuals have equal resources available to them (e.g., through spending vouchers), the policy maker might value freedom of choice to allow individuals to select those types of care that they feel would best suit them. As another example, a policy maker might value a population's health status highly but also want to ensure technical efficiency is achieved. The policy maker would select policies that would forward both objectives. Each of the goals is discussed briefly in the following section.

13.7.1 Environmental Conditions

A market is an institution in which free choice is exercised by the participants who are in pursuit of their own well-being. A social goal that falls under this category is allowing persons the freedom to seek care from whatever health plan they want to join. It might also be suggested that anyone who wants to provide health services may do so. Generally, choice in healthcare markets is not extended to anyone who wants to be a provider. This is a reflection of other policy goals, such as the protection of quality, being sought.

13.7.2 Efficiency

In order to achieve economic efficiency, (1) demand must be at an appropriate level, neither too restrictive (e.g., because of monopolistic prices) nor too low (such that there be an excessive demand); and (2) providers must produce an adequate supply of services, (3) at an appropriate quality level, and (4) at a low cost of production.

13.7.2.1 Demand Barriers

Demand barriers are impediments to the reception of care. Within the context of the present model, price is the prime impediment. Additional care demanded can be encouraged by lowering the direct price through the purchase of insurance, public programs, or charity. To the degree that additional medical care utilization is thought to be desirable, the extent of financial demand barriers can be measured by the availability of insurance or the direct price faced by individuals.

However, money price is not the only factor related to demand barriers. Waiting costs and travel costs can also obstruct access of care. If medical care consumption is to be encouraged, these costs must be addressed, either through subsidies, relocating facilities to lower travel time and expenses, or expanding facilities and increasing operating hours to decrease waiting time. However, it should be remembered that, from an efficiency standpoint, demand can be too great as well as insufficient.

13.7.2.2 Adequacy of Supply

Adequacy of supply refers to the availability of sufficient resources to provide care at the efficient level (given the level of quality). Adequacy of supply depends on the incentive (payment) system developed, the level of payment, and the adequacy of funds.

13.7.2.3 Technical Efficiency

Technical efficiency is a measure of the cost of producing a given level and quality of output. Technical efficiency is usually expressed in terms of money costs, but care must be taken when comparing costs among facilities to be sure that all other factors (e.g., quality, input prices, and case mix) have been taken into consideration.

13.7.2.4 Quality of Care

On the assumption that quality is not free, it costs more to achieve a higher quality of care. Therefore, like any other characteristic of output, quality can come in too great or too little a quantity. Quality of care is an often-cited policy goal in health care. Regulation and licensing of professionals are often enacted in the name of the protection of quality of care.

13.7.3 Equity

Equity is a very broad concept. Two aspects of equity are considered here: equity of utilization and equity of finance.

13.7.3.1 Equity of Utilization

A service can be provided efficiently, and yet some individuals who could benefit from more of it simply cannot pay for it. Society or policy makers can set utilization goals above those provided in a market situation. In this case, the direct price or other barriers to care must be removed. Thus, some efficiency may be lost in order to attain a higher degree of equity.

13.7.3.2 Equity of Finance

Equity of finance can refer to direct out-of-pocket prices as well as taxation and premiums, factors that may not directly affect utilization. Healthcare premiums may be deemed too low, in which case some individuals would be viewed as not paying a fair portion of the cost of medical care. Equity of finance would call for an increase in these premiums.

13.7.4 Public Financial Constraints

Strictly speaking, the government budget does not fall within the scope of this model. Of course, a transfer of funds from A to B is consistent with a tax on A by a government body and subsequent expenditures on medical care for B. But the model says nothing about the size of the tax, the expenditure, or the difference (the contribution to the deficit). In recent years, however, the budget deficit and public spending have come under a great deal of scrutiny, and cutbacks in government programs have been widespread. Typically, the rationale for cutting a program's expenditures is not lack of worthiness of the program but the program's contribution to the overall budget deficit. To the extent that cutbacks can be achieved merely through increases in technical efficiency, true savings are provided to society, and there are gains in social efficiency. However, cutbacks may also result in reduced supply. This is not necessarily bad if output was greater than the socially optimum level originally. However, if the initial output was at the socially optimum level or below it, cutbacks will lead to reductions in social efficiency because the value of the output that is lost is greater than the savings resulting from the cutbacks.

13.7.5 Health Status of the Population

In recent years, many investigators have focused on population-based measures of health status as a goal of policy. Many of the other goals can be viewed as leading to better health, and so these investigators focus on direct measures of health as a policy objective. Of course, the costs of achieving various levels of health status must be considered as well. Thus, the system is confronted with the constrained objective of maximizing population health subject to resource constraints. Additionally, focusing on this goal does not do away with equity considerations. Once there are more than one individual whose health is measured, the problem of how to add up the health status of all the individuals is encountered. These problems have been discussed in this chapter, and they need to be addressed in any policy consideration.

EXERCISES

1. Distinguish between Paretean and delegatory value systems in terms of who determines the preferences.
2. In a world of completely selfish individuals, if we could measure each person's marginal value for his or her own medical care, what conditions must be met in order for the healthcare market to be at an optimal level of output?
3. What do we mean by the socially optimal level of medical care?

4. In a society with two persons, if one is altruistic and values the other's use of medical care, how will this influence the socially optimal quantity of medical care that is produced.

5. According to the Paretean criterion, if medical care is given away free and in unlimited quantities, will this yield a socially optimal outcome?

6. What is a consumption externality for medical care?

7. Will a freely competitive market without philanthropy yield a socially optimal output when there are consumption externalities?

8. What conditions must be met in order for there to be an optimal degree of insurance coverage?

9. If individuals are fully insured for all healthcare services, will this necessarily result in a socially optimal amount of insurance coverage?

10. List five goals of health policy.

11. What is the extra-welfarist approach to defining an optimal amount of output and how does it compare with the Paretean approach?

12. Given the following *MV* information, what is the optimal allocation of care according to the Paretean criteria, when the marginal cost of care is constant at $200.

Person A		Person B	
Quantity of care consumed	Marginal value (MV)	Quantity of care consumed	Marginal value (MV)
1	$200	1	$150
2	180	2	120
3	162	3	92
4	146	4	66
5	134	5	42
6	122	6	20
7	112	7	0
8	104	8	0
9	99	9	0

BIBLIOGRAPHY

Efficiency Criteria

Arrow, K. J. (1963). Uncertainty and the welfare economics of medical care. *American Economic Review, 53,* 941–973.

Arrow, K. J. (2004). Uncertainty and the welfare economics of medical care. 1963. *Bulletin of the World Health Organization, 82*(2), 141–149.

Baker, D. W., Sudano, J. J., Albert, J. M., Borawski, E. A., & Dor., A. (2002). Loss of health insurance and the risk for a decline in self-reported health and physical functioning. *Medical Care, 40*(11), 1126–1131.

Buchanan, J. M. (1965). *The inconsistency of the National Health Service.* London, England: Institute of Economic Affairs.

Butler, J. R. G. (1992). Welfare economics and cost-utility analysis. In P. Zweifel & H. E. Frech, III (Eds.), *Health economics worldwide.* Amsterdam, The Netherlands: Kluwer Academic.

Chernew, M. E. (2005). Achieving value in healthcare. *American Journal of Managed Care, 11*(3), 138–139.

Chernew, M., & Fendrick, A. M. (2008). Value and increased cost sharing in the American health care system. *Health Services Research, 43*(2), 451–457.

Claxton, K., Paulden, M., Gravelle, H., Brouwer W., & Culyer, A. J. (2011). Discounting and decision making in the economic evaluation of health-care technologies. *Health Economics, 20,* 2–15.

Culyer, A. J. (1971). The nature of the commodity "health care" and its efficient allocation. *Oxford Economic Papers, 23,* 189–211.

Culyer, A. J. (1977). On the relative efficiency of the National Health Service. *Kyklos, 25,* 266–287.

Culyer, A. J. (2001). Economics and ethics in health care. *Journal of Medical Ethics, 27*(4), 217–222.

Dineen, C. (2011). Finding the right way to ration. *American Journal of Bioethics, 11*(7), 26–28.

Dor, A., & Watson, H. (1998). Welfare consequences of alternative insurance contracts in the mixed for-profit/nonprofit hospital market. *Southern Economic Journal, 64,* 698–712.

Dowd, B., & Feldman, R. (2002). Having it all: National benefit equity and local payment parity in Medicare. *Health Affairs, 21*(3), 208–214.

Evans, R. G. (1997). Going for the gold. *Journal of Health Politics, Policy and Law, 22,* 427–465.

Feldman, R., & Dowd, B. (1993). What does the demand curve for medical care measure? *Journal of Health Economics, 12,* 193–200.

Fendrick, A. M., & Chernew, M. E. (2007). "Fiscally responsible, clinically sensitive" cost sharing: Contain costs while preserving quality. *American Journal of Managed Care, 13*(6, Pt. 2), 325–327.

Fendrick, A. M., & Chernew, M. E. (2009). Value based insurance design: Maintaining a focus on health in an era of cost containment. *American Journal of Managed Care, 15*(6), 338–343.

Frick, K. D., & Chernew, M. E. (2009). Beneficial moral hazard and the theory of the second best. *Inquiry, 46*(2), 229–240.

Paris, J. J. (2011). Rationing: A "decent minimum" or a "consumer driven" health care system? *American Journal of Bioethics, 11*(7), 16–18.

Parsi, K. (2010). Toward a more just health care system. *Annals of Health Law, 19*(1, Spec. no.), 53–56.

Pauly, M. V. (1968). The economics of moral hazard. *American Economic Review, 58,* 531–537.

Pauly, M.V. (1972). *Medical care at public expense.* New York, NY: Praeger.

Pauly, M.V. (2004). Medicare drug coverage and moral hazard. *Health Affairs, 23*(1), 113–122.

Pauly, M. V., & Blavin, F. E. (2008). Moral hazard in insurance, value-based cost sharing, and the benefits of blissful ignorance. *Journal of Health Economics, 27*(6), 1407–1417.

Peele, P. B. (1993). Evaluating welfare losses in the health care market. *Journal of Health Economics, 12,* 205–208.

Rice, T. (1993a). Demand curves, economists and desert islands. *Journal of Health Economics, 12,* 201–204.

Rice, T. (1993b). A model is only as good as its assumptions. *Journal of Health Economics, 12,* 209–211.

Rice, T. (1997). Can markets give us the health system we want? *Journal of Health Politics, Policy and Law, 22,* 383–426.

Scanlon, D. P., Swaminathan, S., Lee, W., & Chernew, M. (2008). Does competition improve health care quality? *Health Services Research, 43*(6), 1931–1951.

Schneiderman, L. J. (2011). Rationing just medical care. *American Journal of Bioethics, 11*(7), 7–14.

Thorne, E. D. (1998a). When private parts are made public goods. *Yale Journal on Regulation, 15,* 149–175.

Thorne, E. D. (1998b). The shortage of market-inalienable human organs: Consideration of non-market failures. *American Journal of Economics and Sociology, 57,* 247–260.

Weisbrod, B. A. (1964). Collective consumption services of individual consumption goods. *Quarterly Journal of Economics, 78,* 471–477.

Optimal Health Insurance

Abraham, J. M., & Feldman, R. (2010). Taking up or turning down: New estimates of household demand for employer-sponsored health insurance. *Inquiry, 47*(1), 17–32.

Antos, J., Bertko, J., Chernew, M., Cutler, D., de Brantes, F., Goldman, D., ..., & Shortell, S. (2010). Bending the curve through health reform implementation. *American Journal of Managed Care, 16*(11), 804–812.

Arrow, K. J., & Levin, S. A. (2009). Intergenerational resource transfers with random offspring numbers. *Proceedings of the National Academy of Sciences of the United States of America, 106*(33), 13702–13706.

Atherly, A., Dowd, B. E., & Feldman, R. (2004). The effect of benefits, premiums, and health risk on health plan choice in the Medicare program. *Health Services Research, 39*(4, Pt. 1), 847–864.

Blomquist, A., & Johansson, P.-O. (1997). Economic efficiency and mixed public/private insurance. *Journal of Public Economics, 66,* 505–516.

Chernew, M., Cutler, D. M., & Keenan, P. S. (2005). Increasing health insurance costs and the decline in insurance coverage. *Health Services Research, 40*(4), 1021–1039.

Chernew, M. E., Juster, I. A., Shah, M., Wegh, A., Rosenberg, S., Rosen, A. B., ..., & Fendrick, A. M. (2010). Evidence that value-based insurance can be effective. *Health Affairs, 29*(3), 530–536.

Chernew, M. E., Rosen, A. B., & Fendrick, A. M. (2007). Value-based insurance design. *Health Affairs, 26*(2), w195–w203.

Chernew, M., Frick, K., & McLaughlin, C. G. (1997). Worker demand for health insurance in the non-group market: A note on the calculation of welfare loss. *Journal of Health Economics, 16,* 375–380.

Chu, W. H. (1997). Health insurance and the welfare of health care consumers. *Journal of Public Economics, 64,* 125–133.

Cleeton, D. (1989). The medical uninsured: A case of market failure? *Public Finance Quarterly, 17,* 55–83.

Desmond, K. A., Rice, T., & Fox, P. D. (2006). Does greater Medicare HMO enrollment cause adverse selection into Medigap? *Health Economics, Policy, & Law, 1*(Pt. 1), 3–21.

Dowd, B. E., Coulam, R. F., Feldman, R., & Pizer, S. D. (2005). Fee-for-service Medicare in a competitive market environment. *Health Care Financing Review, 27*(2), 113–126.

Fendrick, A. M., & Chernew, M. E. (2006). Value-based insurance design: Aligning incentives to bridge the divide between quality improvement and cost containment. *American Journal of Managed Care, 12* (Spec. no.), SP5–SP10.

Fendrick, A. M., & Chernew, M. E. (2007). "Fiscally responsible, clinically sensitive" cost sharing: Contain costs while preserving quality. *American Journal of Managed Care, 13*(6, Pt. 2), 325–327.

Gianfrancesco, F. D. (1978). Insurance and medical care expenditure: An analysis of the optimal relationship. *Eastern Economics Journal, 4,* 225–234.

Gianfrancesco, F. D. (1983). A proposal for improving the efficiency of medical insurance. *Journal of Health Economics, 2,* 175–184.

Hanoch, Y., & Rice, T. (2006). Can limiting choice increase social welfare? The elderly and health insurance. *Milbank Quarterly, 84*(1), 37–73.

Hirth, R. A., Baughman, R. A., Chernew, M. E., & Shelton, E. C. (2006). Worker preferences, sorting and aggregate patterns of health insurance coverage. *International Journal of Health Care Finance & Economics, 6*(4), 259–277.

Jack, W., & Sheiner, L. (1997). Welfare: Improving health expenditure subsidies. *American Economic Review, 87,* 206–221.

Patel, V., & Pauly, M. V. (2002). Guaranteed renewability and the problem of risk variation in individual health insurance markets. *Health Affairs,* (Suppl. Web Exclusives), W280–W289.

Pauly, M.V. (1990). The rational nonpurchase of long-term-care insurance. *Journal of Political Economy, 98,* 153–168.

Pauly, M.V. (2004). Means-testing in Medicare. *Health Affairs,* (Suppl. Web Exclusives), W4-546–W4-557.

Pauly, M. V., & Herring, B. (2007). Risk pooling and regulation: Policy and reality in today's individual health insurance market. *Health Affairs, 26*(3), 770–779.

Rice, T., Lavarreda, S. A., Ponce, N. A., & Brown, E. R. (2005). The impact of private and public health insurance on medication use for adults with chronic diseases. *Medical Care Research & Review, 62*(2), 231–249.

Scanlon, D. P., Chernew, M., Swaminathan, S., & Lee, W. (2006). Competition in health insurance markets: Limitations of current measures for policy analysis. *Medical Care Research & Review, 63*(6 Suppl.), 37S–55S.

Selden, T. M. (1997). More on the economic efficiency of mixed public/private insurance. *Journal of Public Economics, 66,* 517–523.

Vladeck, B. C., & Rice, T. (2009). Market failure and the failure of discourse: Facing up to the power of sellers. *Health Affairs, 28*(5), 1305–1315.

Extra-Welfarism

Brouwer, W. B., Culyer, A. J., van Exel, N. J., & Rutten, F. F. (2008). Welfarism vs. extra-welfarism. *Journal of Health Economics, 27*(2), 325–338.

Chernew, M. E., Baicker, K., & Hsu, J. (2010). The specter of financial armageddon—Health care and federal debt in the United States. *New England Journal of Medicine, 362*(13), 1166–1168.

Chernew, M., Gibson, T. B., & Fendrick, A. M. (2010). Trends in patient cost sharing for clinical services used as quality indicators. *Journal of General Internal Medicine, 25*(3), 243–248.

Culyer, A. J. (1989). The normative economics of health care finance and provision. *Oxford Review of Economic Policy, 5,* 34–58.

Culyer, A. J. (1990). Commodities, characteristics of commodities, characteristics of people, utilities, and the quality of life. In S. Baldwin, C. Godfrey, & C. Propper . (Eds.), *Quality of life: Perspectives and problems.* London, England: Routledge.

Culyer, A. J. (1991). Conflicts between equity concepts and efficiency in health: A diagrammatic approach. *Osaka Economic Papers, 40,* 141–154.

Culyer, A. J. (1993). Health, health expenditures, and equity. In E. van Doorslaer, F. Rutten, & A. Wagstaff . (Eds.), *Equity in the finance and delivery of health care: An international perspective.* Oxford, England: Oxford University Press.

Culyer, A. J. (1995). *Equality of what in health policy? Conflicts between the contenders.* Discussion paper 142. York, England: University of York, Center for Health Economics.

Cummings, J. R., Lavarreda, S. A., Rice, T., & Brown, E. R. (2009). The effects of varying periods of uninsurance on children's access to health care. *Pediatrics, 123*(3), e411–e418.

Cummings, J. R., Lavarreda, S. A., Rice, T., & Brown, E. R. (2010). Perspective and desire in comparative effectiveness research: The relative unimportance of mere preferences, the central importance of context. *Pharmacoeconomics, 28,* 889–897.

Fein, R. (2010). Values in health policy and health services research. *Health Services Research, 45*(3), 851–870.

Fendrick, A. M., Chernew, M. E., & Levi, G. W. (2009). Value-based insurance design: Embracing value over cost alone. *American Journal of Managed Care, 15*(10 Suppl.), S277–S283.

Fendrick, A. M., Smith, D. G., & Chernew, M. E. (2010). Applying value-based insurance design to low-value health services. *Health Affairs, 29*(11), 2017–2021.

Kolstad, J. T., & Chernew, M. E. (2009). Quality and consumer decision making in the market for health insurance and health care services. *Medical Care Research & Review, 66*(1 Suppl.), 28S–52S.

Pauly, M. V. (1994). Reply to Roberta Labelle, Greg Stoddart, and Thomas Rice. *Journal of Health Economics, 13,* 495–496.

Pauly, M. V., Mitchell, O. S., & Zeng, Y. (2007). Death spiral or euthanasia? The demise of generous group health insurance coverage. *Inquiry, 44*(4), 412–427.

Rice, T. (1992). An alternative framework for evaluating welfare losses in the health care market. *Journal of Health Economics, 11,* 85–92.

Rice, T., & Desmond, K. A. (2004). The distributional consequences of a Medicare premium support proposal. *Journal of Health Politics, Policy & Law, 29*(6), 1187–1226.

Wagstaff, A. (1991). QALYs and the equity-efficiency trade-off. *Journal of Health Economics, 10,* 21–41.

Equity and Other Social Goals

Anderson, G. M., Bronskill, S. E., Mustard, C. A., Culyer, A., Alter, D. A., & Manuel, D. G. (2005). Both clinical epidemiology and population health perspectives can define the role of health care in reducing health disparities. *Journal of Clinical Epidemiology, 58*(8), 757–762.

Arrow, K. J., Bensoussan, A., Feng, Q., & Sethi, S. P. (2007). Optimal savings and the value of population. *Proceedings of the National Academy of Sciences of the United States of America, 104*(47), 18421–18426.

Beauchamp, D. E. (1976). Public health as social justice. *Inquiry, 13,* 3–14.

Blake, P. R., & McAuliffe, K. (2011). "I had so much it didn't seem fair": Eight-year-olds reject two forms of inequity. *Cognition, 120*(2), 215–224.

Bundorf, M. K., & Pauly, M. V. (2006). Is health insurance affordable for the uninsured? *Journal of Health Economics, 25*(4), 650–673.

Carter, B. (2010). Adult guardianship: Human rights or social justice? *Journal of Law & Medicine, 18*(1), 143–155.

Churchill, L. R. (2011). Rationing, rightness, and distinctively human goods. *American Journal of Bioethics, 11*(7), 15–16.

Cozzolino, P. J. (2011). Trust, cooperation, and equality: A psychological analysis of the formation of social capital. *British Journal of Social Psychology, 50,* 302–320.

Culyer, A. J. (2001). Equity—Some theory and its policy implications. *Journal of Medical Ethics, 27*(4), 275–283.

Culyer, A. J. (2006). The bogus conflict between efficiency and vertical equity. *Health Economics, 15*(11), 1155–1158.

Culyer, A. J. (2007). Equity of what in healthcare? Why the traditional answers don't help policy—And what to do in the future. *Healthcarepapers, 8*(Spec no.), 12–26.

Daniels, N. (1982). Equity of access to health care. *Milbank Quarterly, 60,* 51–81.

Dor, A., Sudano, J., & Baker, D. W. (2006). The effect of private insurance on the health of older, working age adults: Evidence from the health and retirement study. *Health Services Research, 41*(3, Pt. 1), 759–787.

Faden, R., & Powers, M. (2011). A social justice framework for health and science policy. *Cambridge Quarterly of Healthcare Ethics, 20,* 596–604.

Fein, R. (1972). On achieving access and equity in health care. In J. B. McKinlay (Ed.), *Economic aspects of health care.* New York, NY: Watson.

Fein, R. (2003). Universal health insurance—Let the debate resume. *JAMA, 290*(6), 818–820.

Fleck, L. M. (2011). Just caring: Health care rationing, terminal illness, and the medically least well off. *Journal of Law, Medicine & Ethics, 39,* 156–171.

Friedman, A. W. (2011). Rationing and social value judgments. *American Journal of Bioethics, 11*(7), 28–29.

Friedman, L. M. (1971). The idea of right as a social and legal concept. *Journal of Social Issues, 27,* 189–198.

Gilmer T., Kronick, R., & Rice, T. (2005). Children welcome, adults need not apply: Changes in public program enrollment across states and over time. *Medical Care Research & Review, 62*(1), 56–78.

Goldfarb, R., Havrylyshyn, O., & Mangum, S. (1984). Can remittances compensate for manpower outflows. *Journal of Development Economics, 15*, 1–17.

Hammell, H. (2011). Is the right to health a necessary precondition for gender equality? *Review of Law & Social Change, 35*(1), 131–193.

Hemenway, D. (1982). The optimal location of doctors. *New England Journal of Medicine, 306*, 397–401.

Keenan, P. S., Cutler, D. M., & Chernew, M. (2006). The "graying" of group health insurance. *Health Affairs, 25*(6), 1497–1506.

Klein, D. A. (2011). Evaluating social value: On the intersection of mortality and economics in the distribution of publicly funded medical care. *American Journal of Bioethics, 11*(7), 18–20.

Koroukian, S. M., Xu, F., Dor, A., & Cooper, G. S. (2006). Colorectal cancer screening in the elderly population: Disparities by dual Medicare-Medicaid enrollment status. *Health Services Research, 41*(6), 2136–2154.

LaVeist, T. A., Gaskin, D., & Richard, P. (2011). Estimating the economic burden of racial health inequalities in the United States. *International Journal of Health Services, 41*(2), 231–238.

Lewis, C. F., Fein, R., & Mechanic, D. (1976). *A right to health.* New York, NY: Wiley-Interscience.

Long, S. H., & Smeeding, T. M. (1984). Alternative Medicare financing sources. *Milbank Quarterly, 62*, 325–348.

Manderscheid, R. (2011). Reflecting on social justice. *Behavioral Healthcare, 31*(5), 38.

McGee, S. J. (2011). To friend or not to friend: Is that the question for healthcare? *American Journal of Bioethics, 11*(8), 2–5.

Mechanic, D. (1976). Rationing health care. *Hastings Center Report, 9*(1), 34–37.

Mitchell, B. M., & Phelps, C. E. (1976). National health insurance: Some costs and effects of mandated employee coverage. *Journal of Political Economy, 84*, 553–571.

Outka, G. (1974). Social justice and equal access to health care. *Journal of Religious Ethics, 2*, 11–32.

Pagan, J. A., & Pauly, M. V. (2006). Community-level uninsurance and the unmet medical needs of insured and uninsured adults. *Health Services Research, 41*(3, Pt. 1), 788–803.

Schwartz, W. B., & Joskow, P. L. (1978). Medical efficacy versus economic efficiency: A conflict in values. *New England Journal of Medicine, 299*, 1462–1464.

Shroufi, A., Chowdhury, R., Aston, L. M., Pashayan, N., & Franco, O. H. (2011). Measuring health: A practical challenge with a philosophical solution? *Maturitas, 68*(3), 210–216.

Simm, K. (2011). The concepts of common good and public interest: From Plato to biobanking. *Cambridge Quarterly of Healthcare Ethics, 20*, 554–562.

Stoddart, G. L., & Labelle, R. J. (1985). *Privatization in the Canadian health care system.* Ottawa, Ontario: Health and Welfare Department, Government of Canada.

Strand, R. (2011). Health ideologies, objectivism, and the common good: On the rights of dissidents. *Cambridge Quarterly of Healthcare Ethics, 20*, 605–611.

Sudgen, R., & Williams, A. (1978). *The principles of practical cost-benefit analysis.* Oxford, England: Oxford University Press.

Sutrop, M. (2011). Changing ethical frameworks: From individual rights to the common good? *Cambridge Quarterly of Healthcare Ethics, 20*, 533–545.

Szende, A., & Culyer, A. J. (2006). The inequity of informal payments for health care: The case of Hungary. *Health Policy, 75*(3), 262–271.

Taylor, E. F., Chernew, M., & McLaughlin, C. (2006). Do determinants of medicare supplemental coverage choice vary by income. *Journal of Health & Social Policy, 22*(1), 1–18.

Thurow, L. C. (1985). Medicine versus economics. *New England Journal of Medicine, 313*, 611–614.

Ubel, P. A., Hirth, R. A., Chernew, M. E., & Fendrick, A. M. (2003). What is the price of life and why doesn't it increase at the rate of inflation? *Archives of Internal Medicine, 163*(14), 1637–1641.

van Doorslaer, E., Wagstaff, A., Bleichroft, H., Catonge, S., Gerdtham, U. G., Gerlin, M., …, & Winkelhake, O. (1997). Income-related inequalities in health: Some international comparisons. *Journal of Health Economics, 16*, 93–112.

Whipple, D. (1974). Health care as a right. *Inquiry, 11*, 65–68.

Financing Health Care

14.1 INTRODUCTION

There are three major methods of financing healthcare services—out-of-pocket payments by the consumers, insurance premiums, and taxation—and within each category there are a number of different financing techniques. For example, out-of-pocket payments include deductibles, copayments, coinsurance, and full consumer payments. Insurance premiums can be paid directly by the consumer or paid by the employer or by the government. And taxes can be levied on income or on specific products or services. Further, the different financing methods can interact: insurance premiums can be excluded from taxation (as is the case in the United States) or can be taxed.

Each method will impact differently on groups with different characteristics, such as income level or family size. Determining how the burden of each financing method will fall is not a straightforward matter. The burden of insurance premiums that are paid out of pocket by consumers will fall on the consumers directly, but income taxes can influence this burden, and when insurance is obtained through the workplace (as is usually the case in the United States), the burden of payment is not clear-cut. Furthermore, different kinds of taxes will have the same impact on groups with varying income levels. Economic analysis is a very useful tool for sorting out the effects of these varying finance methods. The first part of this chapter examines how explanatory economics can be used to analyze the burden of the various financing methods. How these various methods can be assessed in terms of specific criteria or policy objectives are also discussed.

Different financing methods also have significantly different costs. In the case of private insurance, there are the costs of marketing, rating alternative consuming groups, paying providers, and monitoring utilization. In the case of government finance, there are the costs of collecting taxes and administering public programs. A debate has been occurring in the United States in recent years over whether healthcare coverage for the population should be financed primarily through private markets (with appropriate subsidies) or public financing. This chapter illustrates how economic analysis can be used to compare these options.

14.2 INSURANCE TERMINOLOGY

A brief discussion of basic insurance concepts is presented before analyzing the financing of health care because these various concepts also have implications for financing health care and the burden of healthcare costs. These various features have implications for the various methods of financing health care.

Consumers may pay various amounts toward a medical bill. Many insurance packages require the consumer to pay a *deductible* before insurance pays anything. This deductible is a flat, or fixed, amount that must be paid by the consumer before the insurance company begins to pay all or part of the remaining amount. For example, an insurance package may require the beneficiary to pay the first $500 of medical expenses for each year before the insurance pays anything. Deductibles have an impact on the administrative costs of the insurance company by eliminating the processing of claims for small amounts and therefore the transaction costs associated with the settling of claims. The higher the deductible, the fewer the claims that will need to be processed. However, the use of deductibles, especially high deductibles, may be a deterrent for some beneficiaries accessing needed medical care. In addition, the deductible creates a greater burden on lower income individuals than on higher income individuals because the deductible represents a larger percentage of total income for the lower income beneficiary.

Another common feature of insurance is the use of a *copayment*, which requires the beneficiary to pay a fixed amount each time a service is used. For example, an insurance package may require the beneficiary to pay $10 each time a visit is made to a primary care physician, $20 each time a visit is made to a specialist, and $50 for each visit to an emergency room. A copayment places similar burdens on lower income individuals as deductibles because they represent a larger portion of income. A copayment would not have the same impact on administrative costs as deductibles because they would not necessarily reduce the number of claims filed.

Coinsurance requires the beneficiary to pay a specified percentage of the price of the medical service, and the insurance company pays the balance.

For example, an insurance package may require the individual to pay 20% of the price after the deductible and the insurance company will pay 80%. Assuming that the price of the medical encounter was $1,000, if the beneficiary had a $500 deductible and 20% coinsurance rate, then the beneficiary would have to pay $600 and the insurance company would pay $400 ($1000 − $500 − [$500 × 0.8]) = $400. A coinsurance feature lowers the price of the covered medical care by the percentage the insurance company pays; in this case, it lowers the price by 80% after the deductible. A coinsurance feature reduces the price of the service, but still provides an incentive to be a cost-conscious consumer, because the consumer pays a percenage of whatever the price is. The actual impact will depend on the price elasticity of demand of the consumer—the more price elastic, the greater the impact on demand.

Many insurance plans included a "stop-loss" feature, which sets an upper limit on the amount the consumer will have to pay. This reduces the risk of a serious medical condition resulting in a catastrophic loss. For example, an insurance package may contain the provision that once out-of-pocket expenditures reach a specified amount (e.g., $5,000), then the insurance company will pay all remaining medical expenses associated with covered services. Although stop-loss features apply to beneficiaries, insurance companies seek protection by setting maximums and limits. For example, the insurance package may specify a *maximum* annual amount it will cover, such as $100,000 of medical care or 30 days of hospital care. The policy may also contain lifetime *limits* that the insurance company will pay for medical expenses incurred by an individual, such as a limit of $2 million for covered services by the individual. These maximums and limits are not reached by most individuals, but raise the fear that medical bankruptcy is a possibility, even for individuals with good health insurance coverage.

The two basic methods of establishing insurance premiums are *community rating* and *experience rating*. Under the community rating method, all enrollees in the plan are charged the same premium, although even it is usually separated into single coverage and family coverage. Under this method, high users of medical services in the community are subsidized by low users. If the low users determine that the premiums are too high for the benefits received, they may simply drop coverage and become uninsured. Also, redistributing resources from low users to high users may actually transfer income from low-income individuals to high-income individuals because income level is not considered in establishing the premium.

Experience rating relies upon the characteristics of groups of individuals or upon the prior experiences of those groups in establishing the premium to be charged. As a result, different groups are charged different rates depending upon their expected use of medical services. Under this method, low-risk, low-user groups are charged a lower premium for the package of covered services. Under the experience rating method, the *medical loss ratio*, benefits paid out/premium is close to 1.0, with only a small loading fee charged. A loading fee is the amount above the pure premium (amount of medical claims paid) that the insurance company charges to cover marketing expenses, administration, claims processing, reserves, and profits.

14.3 FINANCING MEANS AND BURDENS IN THE UNITED STATES

Currently in the United States, a variety of financing mechanisms are used in health care. These mechanisms and the amounts raised through each are shown in Table 14-1. As can be seen, a total of $2.5936 trillion was spent on health care in 2010. Of this amount, $299.7 billion (about 11.6%) was financed by out-of-pocket payments by consumers. In comparison, in 1965, consumers financed about 43.5% of expenditures out of pocket.

A total of $848.7 billion (33%) was financed through private health insurance in 2010, compared to 24% in 1965. The percentage of the under-65 population covered by private health insurance has been declining since 2001, decreasing to 64% in 2010. The majority of the population with private health insurance receive coverage through employment-based insurance (55.3% of the under-65 population, or 86.4% of the privately insured population), with 13.6% of the privately insured purchasing individual policies (DeNavas-Wait, Proctor, & Smith, 2011). As illustrated in Table 14-2, for individuals with employer-based coverage, employers financed 83% of the $5,429 of premiums for single coverage employees in 2011 and 72.6% of the $15,073 for family coverage. Between 1999 and 2011, both the premiums for insurance coverage and the percentage of premiums paid by the employee increased. As a result, the employee's cost for single coverage increased from $318 to $921, and the employee's cost for family coverage increased from $1,543 to $4,129 during that period.

As shown by the data presented in Table 14-2 with regard to health insurance provided through the workplace, the majority of the premiums are paid for by employers, with a smaller amount being paid for directly by employees. However, this does not mean that the employers bear the burden of the majority of the health insurance expenses. For one thing, premiums paid for by employers are workplace benefits that are not subject to income tax. Therefore, there is a sizable public subsidy given to employees who obtain their insurance in this way; their taxes will be lower than if they paid for their premiums directly. In addition, there is considerable evidence that when all the wage effects are taken into account, the employees do indeed bear a major share of these premium costs through lower direct wages, even if the picture at first glance does not show it that way.

The third form of finance that is used is public finance, or taxation. In 2010, over $1.35 trillion (52.1%) of total financing for health care involved taxation, compared to 31% in 1965. Most of this 2010 amount went to pay for the federal Medicare program, which covers individuals 65 and over and those totally and permanently disabled, and the joint federal-state Medicaid program, which is primarily for certain categories of lower income groups. These programs are largely, but not entirely, financed by taxation. With regard to taxation, the major federal tax that pays for the hospital portion (Part A) of Medicare is a payroll tax of 2.9% of all wages, paid equally (1.45 %) by employers and employees. As of January 2013, individuals filing jointly will pay an additional 0.9% on income greater than $250,000 and single individuals will pay the additional 0.9% on incomes over $200,000. The employers tax rate will not increase from 1.45%. In addition, there is a Medicare "premium"

Table 14-1 Sources of Funds for National Health Expenditures, 1965 and 2010 (Millions of Dollars)

Source of Funds	1965 ($)	1965 (%)	2010 ($)	2010 (%)
Private funds				
Out-of-pocket	$18,262.2	43.5	$299,694.6	11.6
Private health insurance	10,000.1	23.8	848,701.2	32.7
Other private	693.9	1.7	93,996.5	3.6
Total private funds	*$28,956.2*	69.0	*$1,242,392.3*	47.9
Public funds				
Medicare	0	0.0	524,551	20.2
Medicaid				
Federal	0	0.0	269,504.5	10.4
State & Local	0	0.0	131,913.2	5.1
CHIP				
Federal	0	0.0	8,147.2	0.3
State & Local	0	0.0	3,520.6	0.1
Department of Defense	831.3	2.0	38,438.7	1.5
Veterans Affairs	1,119.5	2.7	46,016.5	1.8
Indian Health Services	0	0.0	3,578.8	0.1
Workers Compensation	869.5	2.1	37,248.3	1.4
General Assistance	121.7	0.3	6,965.9	0.3
Maternal/Child Health				
Federal	80	0.2	584.9	0.0
State & Local	164	0.4	2,221.8	0.1
Vocational Rehabilitation				
Federal	26.8	0.1	418.8	0.0
State & Local	14.6	0.0	117.9	0.0
SAMHSA	0	0.0	3,385.1	0.1
Other Federal Programs	830.7	2.0	7,324	0.3
Other State & Local	3,389.4	8.1	31,285.7	1.2
School Health	168.2	0.4	4,494.9	0.2
Public Health Activity				
Federal	213.8	0.5	15,482	0.6
State & Local	407	1.0	67,007.4	2.6
Research	1,521	3.6	49,267	1.9
Structures and Programs	3,243.6	7.7	99,777.5	3.8
Total Public Funds	*$13,001.2*	31.0	*$1,351,251.7*	52.1
TOTAL HEALTH $	*$41,957.3*	100.0	*$2,593,644.0*	100.0

Source: Data from Centers for Medicare & Medicaid Services. "National Health Expenditures by Type of Service and Source of Funds, CY 1960-2010." Accessed April 11, 2012 from http://www.cms.gov/NationalHealthExpendData/02_NationalHealthAccountsHistorical.asp#TopOfPage.

Table 14-2 Average Annual Premiums and Average Annual Worker Premium Contributions Paid by Covered Worker for Single and Family Coverage, 1999–2011

Year	Single Coverage	Single Paid by Worker	% Paid by Worker	Family Coverage	Family Paid by Worker	% Paid by Worker
1999	$2,196	$318	14.5	$5,791	$1,543	26.6
2000	2,471	334	13.5	6,438	1,619	25.1
2001	2,689	355	13.2	7,061	1,787	25.3
2002	3,083	466	15.1	8,003	2,137	26.7
2003	3,383	508	15.0	9,068	2,412	26.6
2004	3,695	558	15.1	9,950	2,661	26.7
2005	4,024	610	15.2	10,880	2,713	24.9
2006	4,242	627	14.8	11,480	2,973	25.9
2007	4,479	694	15.5	12,106	3,281	27.1
2008	4,704	721	15.3	12,680	3,354	26.5
2009	4,824	779	16.1	13,375	3,515	26.3
2010	5,049	899	17.8	13,770	3,997	29.0
2011	5,429	921	17.0	15,073	4,129	27.4

Source: Data from "Employer Health Benefits 2011 Annual Survey—Report," (#8225). The Henry J. Kaiser Family Foundation, September 2011.

paid by enrolled beneficiaries for medical care (physician services) and health maintenance organization (Part B) coverage, which was $99.90 per month in 2012. Most of the remainder of the federal portion was raised through general taxation, the largest portion from direct income taxation. Of the $1.35 trillion spent by governments on health care, $204.8 billion was raised through state government taxation. Most of state taxation is in the form of direct income and indirect sales taxes.

Table 14-1 provides an indication of from where the money is coming, but it cannot be used directly to assess the "burden" of medical care financing (defined as the reduction in real income due to payments and taxes). The complexity of the situation and the prominent role played by each of the financing methods calls for a much more detailed analysis. Each financing method imposes different burdens on different groups. The pattern of these burdens will be discussed after examining the positive economics of the burdens.

14.4 ECONOMIC ANALYSIS OF ALTERNATIVE PAYMENT SOURCES

This section presents economic analyses of alternative payment methods. The focus of the analyses is the economic impact of the payment methods on the resource owners (primarily employees and owners of companies).

Insurance premiums (in particular, the impact of employer-paid premiums, taxation, and mandated benefits) and taxation (the impact of payroll and sales taxes) will be examined.

A primary question relates to the economic incidence of a tax, that is, who ends up bearing the economic burden. The group that bears the burden of the tax may be different from the group from which it is originally collected. For example, a government tax on cigarettes may be collected from tobacco retailers. However, to the extent that prices of tobacco products are higher because of the tax, the incidence is on the smokers, who bear the burden of the higher price.

14.4.1 Private Health Insurance

14.4.1.1 Insurance Premiums

Insurance can be obtained through the workplace or by individual purchase. Insurance obtained in the workplace can be paid for directly by the employees (through payroll deductions), by the employers, or by a combination of employees and employers. There is no controversy over the incidence of premiums paid by employees or by individuals; the purchasers bear the cost of their insurance purchases.

The economic incidence of employer-paid premiums is more complicated. The cost of insurance benefit packages are viewed by employers as an expense, much like wages are. An employer has a demand curve for labor and will regard the costs of various forms of compensation as monetarily equivalent. If the marginal employee is worth (has a marginal value of) $100 to the employer, then the employer will be willing to pay up to $100 in compensation, whether in the form of wages or fringe benefits (Kreuger & Reinhardt, 1994). If benefits are increased, then the employer will reduce monetary wages. Thus, the economic burden of all health insurance benefits will fall on the employee, either directly (out of pocket) or indirectly (through a lower wage).

14.4.1.2 Taxation and Insurance Premiums

Health insurance benefits paid by the employer are exempt from personal income and the social security taxes of the employee. This reduces the cost to the employee of employer-paid health insurance and increases the quantity demanded for health insurance. However, it cannot be assumed that once a subsidy is put into place, the quantity demanded and supplied will remain the same. To see why, consider the analysis of a tax subsidy provided here.

In Figure 14-1, the initial demand curve for health insurance (with no tax subsidies) is D_1. According to this curve, when the premium rate is $1000, a total of 75 individuals will be willing to shift their risks to insurers. Now introduce a 50% subsidy. This will in effect lower the out-of-pocket price for insurance at every premium rate. Thus, at a premium rate of $1,000, the out-of-pocket price to the consumer is $500, and at this price, 100 individuals will be willing to shift their risks. The market demand curve will then be D_2.

According to the supply curve for insurance (S in Figure 14-1), insurers will be willing to accept 92 risks at a price of $1,350. Generally, a higher supplier price will be required to induce the insurers to accept more risks.

Initially, assume that there is no tax subsidy. Then 75 risks will be shifted (or individuals insured) at a premium rate of $1,000. This is the equilibrium price and quantity. Using this position as a base point, a subsidy on premiums of 50% will now be introduced. That is, the individuals are in a 50% income tax bracket and are allowed to deduct insurance premiums before calculating income taxes. A preliminary analysis of the effects of the subsidy might be as follows. The premium price would remain the same ($1,000), but half would be paid ($500) out of pocket by the consumer and half would fall on taxpayers (because the individual would get $500 back from the public purse). This analysis might be applied to 75 insurance policies in order to determine the "shifting" effect. However, a sounder economic analysis would result from supposing that the new quantity on which the subsidy will be based will be neither the old quantity nor the quantity demanded at a premium of $1,000. In order to determine the likely effects of the subsidy, an economic analysis of the type presented in Figure 14-1 must be conducted.

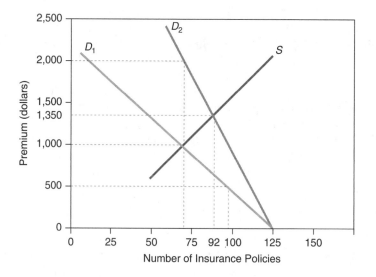

Figure 14-1   The Effect of a Subsidy on the Quantity of Health Insurance. The demand curve for insurance without any tax subsidy is shown in the above diagram as D_1. This curve shows that, at an unsubsidized premium rate of $1000, 75 individuals will demand insurance. Now, introduce a 50-percent subsidy (e.g., at a premium rate of $1000, the individual will pay $500). The market demand curve will shift to D_2. The supply curve for insurance is also shown. At a market price of $1000 the insurance industry is willing to supply 75 policies (accept 75 risks). Without a subsidy, 75 individuals will shift risks to the insurers. With a 50-percent subsidy, the out-of-pocket premium price would initially drop to $500. There would be a large excess demand at this price, but the industry would not be willing to accept 100 risks at $1000. The price would be increased until a new equilibrium is reached—at $1350 (and 92 policies sold risks shifted).

As shown in the figure, the subsidy raises quantity demanded at each price, and so more individuals will seek to shift risks at the premium rate of $1,000. However, suppliers (insurers) will require higher premiums in order to accept more risks. The premium rate will rise, and fewer risks will be shifted than were originally indicated by demand conditions alone. In our example, the final premium rate will be $1,350, and at this price, 92 risks will be shifted.

The cost of the premium will be borne half by the consumer and half by the taxpayer. However, the amount of subsidy will be based on the new price of $1,350. And the quantity of risks shifted will be the new equilibrium quantity. The final equilibrium (and the burden of the subsidy) will depend on the elasticities of demand and supply. In the extreme, if the supply curve were upward sloping, indicating no change in risks shifted, then the analysis would indicate that the premium would rise by the full amount of the subsidy. The taxpayers would pay a subsidy of $1,000 based on a new premium of $2,000, with 75 risks still being shifted. It is more likely the supply curve is horizontal, indicating an unlimited supply of risks accepted at a price of $1,000. Then the consumer would get a full $500 subsidy paid for by the taxpayers; in this case, 100 risks would be shifted.

Our analysis does not take into account subsequent effects of the increased insurance coverage on the medical care market. Nevertheless, even this simple analysis indicates that the demand-and-supply analysis should be considered when determining the full effects of a tax subsidy on premiums.

14.4.1.3 Mandated Benefits

Mandated insurance benefits are government-required coverage benefits that individuals privately purchase or employers must provide. Mandated benefits can have a considerable impact on labor markets depending on how they are viewed by consumers, and this impact will in turn affect the incidence of benefits.

An economic analysis of mandated benefits using a labor market analysis, such as that presented in Figure 14-2, will be considered. In the initial situation, there are no mandated benefits. The demand for labor is shown as D_1, and the supply of labor is shown as $S_{v=0}$. Equilibrium wages are at $80, and equilibrium employment is at 300 workers.

Now mandated insurance benefits that cost $20 per worker are introduced. In terms of total compensation, the employer's demand curve for labor will remain the same; however, when expressed in terms of the wage rate, the demand curve will shift down by $20, because $20 is added to the wages for each worker to calculate total compensation. In terms of wages, the new demand curve for labor is D_2.

It would be tempting to say that the employees will bear the entire burden of the mandated benefits and take a $20 reduction in wages, in which case employment would remain the same. Such will be the case only if the workers fully value the benefits (see curve $S_{v=b}$); the new price in this instance would be $60.

If the workers do not value the benefits at all, there will be a reduction in wages (but by less than $20) to $70 (or some such amount, depending on the elasticity of labor supply) and also a reduction in employment. The burden

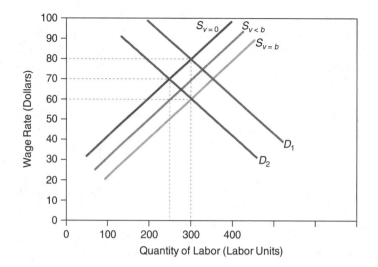

Figure 14-2 The Effect of Mandated Insurance Coverage on Labor Markets. The demand for labor when the employer does not provide any benefits is shown as D_1. For example, at a wage rate of $80, 300 workers (the labor units) will be demanded. Now, introduce mandated benefits of $20 per worker. The employer will still value each worker's productivity the same, but at each quantity of labor, the total compensation that must be paid by the employer is $20 above the wage rate. Therefore, the demand curve is shifted down by $20 at each quantity of labor (D_2). Three alternative supply curves for labor are posited. The first supply curve ($S_{v=0}$) is for the situation where the mandated benefits have no value to the workers. Each employee's supply curve for labor, in terms of the wage rate, remains the same after the benefits are mandated. The second supply curve ($S_{v=b}$) is for the situation where the workers value benefits and wages equally. The supply curve relating wages to the quantity of labor supplied shifts down by the full amount of the mandated benefits ($20 in this case). The third supply curve ($S_{v<b}$) is for the intermediate situation, where the workers place some value on the benefits, but less than the $20 that they cost the employer. Initially, without the mandated benefits, the market equilibrium is at a wage of $80 and a quantity of 300 workers employed. When mandated benefits are instituted, the new equilibrium position will depend on the value placed on the benefits by the workers. With full valuation, the new equilibrium will occur where wages fall by $20, but there will be no change in employment. However, if the benefits are not valued at all, then wages will fall (to $70 in this case) and employment will be reduced. If some value (less than $20) is placed on the benefits by the workers, there will be an intermediate result.

---

of the mandate will then fall, to some degree, on the workers who lose their jobs. If benefits are only partially valued ($S_{v<b}$), the net result will be somewhere in between.

In an extreme case, such as a vertical supply curve, there will be no employment effect, but a full wage effect. In fact, several studies have shown that this result is approximated in reality (Kreuger & Reinhardt, 1994), and so the workers bear the full burden of the mandate. In sum then, mandated benefits may have similar effects to those that might be posited without a more formal economic analysis; but this is the case only because the supply curve of labor is in reality close to vertical (zero elasticity) in the relevant ranges.

14.4.2 Taxation

Much health care (52.1%) is publicly funded, and much of the funding comes through taxation. However configured, taxes can be regarded as reductions in income or wealth without any attached benefits. Although it is true that benefits may come as a result of the use of funds, under taxation, these benefits are not directly linked to the taxes. Only full-scale economic analyses using heroic assumptions can link the benefits resulting from the spending of taxes to the costs of the taxes themselves.

Taxation can be direct or indirect. Direct taxes are those that are directly levied on income. They cannot therefore be shifted (i.e., the burden cannot be made to fall on someone other than the taxpayer). Indirect taxes on goods and services can be shifted (in essence, avoided) to some degree. Economic analysis is useful in determining the economic impact and burden of taxation. In the next section, the burden of two types of taxes commonly used to finance health care—payroll taxes and sales taxes—will be analyzed.

14.4.2.1 Payroll Taxes

A payroll tax is levied on wages. Medicare uses a payroll (social security) tax of 1.45% of total payroll (payable by both the employer and employee for a total of 2.9%) to finance the hospital portion of Medicare. The burden of an employee-paid payroll tax is quite clear: it is paid by the worker. However, because it lowers take-home wages, some workers may decide not to supply labor. Employment will therefore fall. The burden is thus equally shared among workers. The economic effects resulting from the imposition of a payroll tax that is paid by employers is less clear and deserves closer attention.

In Figure 14-3, the analysis of the effect of a payroll tax on labor and wages is introduced. Initially, there is a competitive labor market with a given supply of labor (S) and a given demand for labor (D_1). The output measure is labor hours, and, in this market, equilibrium occurs with a wage rate of $40 per unit and a quantity of 300 labor hours. Note that a very steep supply curve for labor has been drawn. This indicates that workers will not change their work habits very much when wages increase or decrease. A vertical curve would indicate that they would not change their habits at all. Now an employer-paid payroll tax of 100% of wages is introduced.

If the employers are in a competitive industry, they cannot raise the price of their output, and so their demand-for-labor curve cannot be increased through higher prices. Therefore, the employers would have to either absorb the tax themselves or lower wages. At first blush, the inclination might be to say that wages would stay at $40, taxes of $40 would be paid, and employment would remain the same. This is a very unlikely outcome given the forces behind the employment for labor. Figure 14-3 presents an economic analysis of what will happen. The effect of this tax is to shift down the demand-for-labor curve, which is based on the marginal revenue of the product that labor produces. At a wage of $20, each employer must pay a tax of $20 (which is 100% of the wage). Each worker costs twice as much to the firm. Therefore, whereas the employers formerly demanded 300 labor hours when the wage was $40, they will now demand 300 hours of labor at a wage of $20. Note also

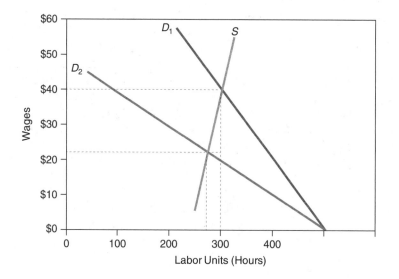

Figure 14-3 The Effect of Imposing an Employer-Paid Payroll Tax. Initially, the demand for labor without a payroll tax is shown in terms of wages. With the given supply curve for labor, equilibrium occurs with a wage of $40 and a quantity of employment of 300 work hours. The effect of a payroll tax of 100 percent of wages is to shift the demand curve in terms of wages down by 50 percent. For example, at a wage rate of $20, the employers pay a tax of $20, for a total payout of $40, and, thus, the demand with the tax is the same as it would be if the wage was 100 percent higher, but there was no tax. The new equilibrium will be determined by the intersection of supply and demand for labor. In this case, the supply curve is almost vertical. There will be very little reduction in employment, and an almost 50 percent reduction in wages.

that because the tax is expressed as a percentage of wages, the new demand-for-labor curve (in terms of wages) is a fixed percentage lower than the old one. The higher the wage, the greater the discrepancy between the old and new curves.

With the employers' demand-for-labor curve (in terms of wages) shifting downward, employees will receive lower wages. The equilibrium volume of labor and the corresponding wage rate are just under 300 hours and just over $22. This means that the quantity of labor will hardly have changed, but the wage rate will have fallen by almost the full amount of the tax. The workers have not substituted away from working and have borne almost the entire burden of the tax through a reduction in their wage rate. In this case, the supply-of-labor curve is almost vertical, and workers would rather accept lower wages than lose employment. Other situations are possible. For example, if workers were very sensitive to their wage rates, and the supply-of-labor curve was close to horizontal, the labor supply would fall when wages fell. In this instance, the workers would avoid the tax entirely by refusing to work at lower wages. At the new wage, the tax would have been shifted to the employers, who also would hire fewer workers.

The effect of the payroll tax then will be to reduce employment and wages. How much of the tax will be borne by the workers (through a decrease in wages) will depend on how much they are willing to adjust their wages and their work—information summarized by the supply-of-labor curve.

14.4.2.2 Sales Taxes

A very similar analysis applies to sales taxes. A sales tax is levied on a product or service. Most states use sales taxes as a major source of revenue. Sales taxes can be general (on all items), modified general (on most items except, for example, food and children's clothes), or specific (on gasoline, alcohol, tobacco products, health insurance premiums, etc.). In the case of tobacco and alcohol, these taxes may affect consumer behavior with regard to drinking and smoking and thus health status (and healthcare demand). Certainly this was the rationale for a large tobacco tax that the state of Maine imposed in order to pay for more publicly funded healthcare benefits in the 1980s.

In order to analyze the effects of sales taxes, the example of a sales tax on prescription drugs will be used. The initial situation, without the sales tax, is shown in Figure 14-4. There is a demand for the drugs, as is shown by the

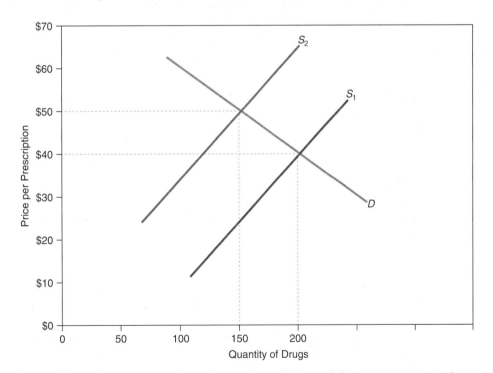

Figure 14-4 Effect of a Sales Tax. The supply and demand for prescriptions are shown above. Equilibrium without the sales tax is where the price is $40 and the quantity of prescriptions is 200 (where S_1 and D intersect). If a sales tax of $20 per prescription is imposed, to be paid by suppliers, the suppliers' costs will increase by exactly $20, as will the supply curve (S_2). The new equilibrium will take into account the demand elasticity. In the above case, the price will increase by $10 and the quantity sold will be reduced by 150 prescriptions. The consumer will, in effect, have shifted some of the tax onto the suppliers by reducing their demands.

demand curve (D). This is the demand of the consumers of the drugs. And there is also a curve for the supply without the sales tax (S_1). In a competitive market, equilibrium will occur at a price of $400 and a quantity of 200 prescriptions filled (at the intersection of D and S_1).

Now impose a sales tax of $20 on each prescription, to be paid by the pharmacists. Initially, it might be imagined that the pharmacists will simply raise the price of each prescription to $60 and collect the tax on each of the 200 prescriptions. But this would occur only if the demand curve for prescriptions was vertical and consumers would demand their prescriptions at any price. This is not a realistic scenario in the case of drugs or most other goods and services. There is an elasticity of demand for drugs, as indicated by the downward-sloping demand curve.

The tax will cause the prices charged by the pharmacists to increase (if they pay the tax), and they might at first charge $60 for each prescription (although they would receive $40, as before). But there is a limit to what consumers will pay. In this case, some consumers will refuse to fill their prescriptions, thus avoiding the tax entirely. A new equilibrium will be set at $50, and only 150 prescriptions will be filled. The pharmacists will receive only $30 for each prescription and will supply fewer (150 at the net-of-tax price of $30).

The market will have shifted part of the tax onto the pharmacists, who now pay one-half of it by receiving a lower price. The consumers end up paying $10 of the prescription tax by reducing the quantity they demand. The burden of the sales tax will thus be shared. It should be pointed out that there are other possible outcomes, depending on the slopes of the supply and demand curves. However, it is not likely that all of the tax will be borne by the consumers. As pointed out earlier, sales taxes on a variety of products related to health are very common. Many states impose a tax on health insurance premiums. Such a tax will have an effect on the number of individuals who shift their risks to an insurer, and it can be analyzed using the sales tax model.

14.5 THE IMPLICATIONS OF ALTERNATIVE TYPES OF HEALTHCARE FINANCING

In this section, attention is turned to the implications of alternative types of healthcare financing. The term *implications* does not have a precise meaning. The term is used to denote the pattern of distribution of burdens of various financing methods (Due, 1957). The focus will be on one key characteristic of individuals—their level of income—and four different types of financing: insurance premiums, income taxes, sales taxes, and payroll taxes. Although highly simplified, the analysis is intended to provide a basic understanding of the major issues.

In evaluating the implications of taxes, the focus is on the regressiveness of the tax. A tax is considered to be regressive if it has a larger relative impact on the income of low-income individuals than on the incomes of higher income individuals. A tax is considered to be progressive if it has a larger relative impact on the incomes of high-income individuals than on low-income individuals. A tax is considered to be neutral if it has the same relative impact on all income cohorts. The impact is viewed as a relative burden on the various income cohorts.

Assume that there are four income groups, each with 100 families (see Table 14-3). Each family in the lowest income group has earnings of $20,000; in the next-lowest group, of $40,000; in the next group, of $60,000; and in the highest income group, of $80,000.

Each family incurs healthcare expenditures of $5,000. There are no differences in healthcare usage by income level. However, all expenditures are financed, and the out-of-pocket cost is zero. Total medical expenses for all groups is $2 million.

Each family's total consumption of commodities, including food but not medical care, is given in column 5 of Table 14-3. The lowest income group spends all it earns on goods and services, the next group spends 90%, the third group spends 80%, and the highest income group spends 70%. The members of a group save what they do not spend. If they have to pay for medical care, they will reduce other expenditures but will not reduce their savings. If they do pay for medical care itself, it will be through the purchase of insurance.

The financing problem is how to pay for the $2 million in medical care expenses. There are four options: insurance premiums, a sales tax, a payroll tax, and an income tax. The task is to determine the incidence of each type of financing on the different income groups. The conclusions reached are summarized in Figure 14-5.

Premiums. Each family bears the same risk of health expenses, and so it would seem reasonable to charge every family the same premium rate (use a community rating). There are 400 families, and $2 million in healthcare funds must be raised. Therefore, each family will pay a premium of $5,000.

The burden of the financing method on each family is the premium divided by family income. This would be 25% for the lowest income families, 12.5% for the families earning $40,000, a total of 8.3% for the families earning $60,000, and 6.25% for the highest income families. The incidence of premiums is such that the burden decreases steadily as income increases.

Table 14-3   Income and Expenditures for Four Income Groups

Income Group	Earnings Per Family	Number of Families	Total Income	Total Consumption Expenditures	Healthcare Expenditures Per Family	Total Health-care Expenditures
A	$20,000	100	$2,000,000	$2,000,000	$5,000	$500,000
B	40,000	100	4,000,000	3,600,000	5,000	500,000
C	60,000	100	6,000,000	4,800,000	5,000	500,000
D	80,000	100	8,000,000	5,600,000	5,000	500,000
Total		400	20,000,000	16,000,000		2,000,000

Payroll Taxes. In the case of a payroll tax, a fixed percentage of wages is charged, but there is usually a cap above which income is not taxed. In this case, assume that this cap is $60,000. This means that all wages up to $60,000 are taxed. The members of the highest income group (those earning $80,000) will pay taxes on only the first $60,000 of their wages. Total taxable wages are $18 million for all families. In order to raise the required $2 million, a tax rate of 11.1% must be levied on all wages up to $60,000.

The burden of the tax will be the same for the three groups whose members have incomes at or below $60,000. However, the highest income group pays only $6,660 in payroll taxes per family, for an effective tax rate of 8.325%. As shown in Figure 14-5, the burden of the payroll tax is the same for the three lowest groups but falls somewhat for the highest income group.

Sales Taxes. Sales taxes can be imposed on any of a variety of consumption expenditures. Assume here that sales taxes are imposed on all consumption expenditures except medical care expenditures. Total consumption expenditures for all families equal $16 million. In order to raise the required $2 million in funds, the overall sales tax rate must be 12.5% ($2 million/16 million). The lowest income group pays $250,000 on its $2 million in expenditures; the next group pays $450,000; the next group, $600,000; and the highest income group pays $700,000.

Income Taxation. The burden of the income tax will depend on the actual tax rates, and these are subject to policy decisions by Congress. Assume here that the tax rates are such that the highest income class pays roughly four times the rate of the lowest group. This is very roughly the ratio in the United States today. Specifically, assume that given an average overall rate, the lowest

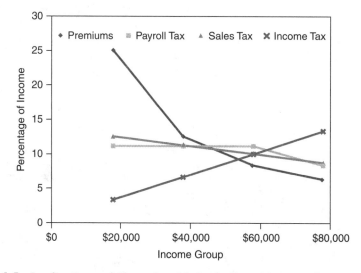

Figure 14-5 Implications of Financing Methods. Premiums are the most regressive source of financing, income tax is the most progressive, and sales and payroll taxes fall in between.

group will pay 40% of this rate (i.e., 0.4), the second group will pay 80% of the rate, the third highest group will pay 120% of the rate, and the highest group will pay 160% of the rate. Let x stand for the overall tax rate. The overall rate can be determined by solving for x in this equation:

$$0.4(\$2 \text{ million})x + 0.8(\$4 \text{ million})x + 1.2(\$6 \text{ million})x + 1.6(\$8 \text{ million})x = \$2 \text{ million}$$

The $2 million is the amount to be collected by the income tax. If the equation is solved for x, the average overall rate is found to be 8.33%. Based on the ratios determined by "policy," the four groups pay 3.33%, 6.64%, 9.99%, and 13.33% of income in income taxes, respectively.

The overall incidence of the funding methods can be compared. Premiums are the most "regressive" and income taxes are the most "progressive." The other two methods fall in between (under the assumptions here, they are mildly regressive).

Omitted from this analysis are out-of-pocket expenditures. The use of this type of financing will result in lower overall usage (because of the downward-sloping demand curve for medical care). Thus, if families had to pay out of pocket for health care, total expenditures would likely fall below $2 million. The overall burden would depend on the response of each income group.

The assessment of financing options will depend on the policy goals. Much of the focus in evaluating types of financing is on considerations of equity. However, efficiency issues need to be addressed as well.

14.6 THE ADMINISTRATIVE COST OF ALTERNATIVE TYPES OF HEALTHCARE FINANCING

There has been a lively debate in recent years about administrative costs associated with the healthcare financing system in the United States. Much of the debate has been focused on the costs associated with the marketing of health insurance and hospital services; the monitoring of utilization and the regulating of payment by insurers; the billing of third parties by providers; and the collecting of deductibles, coinsurance, and copayments from patients by providers. Because of the complexity of the U.S. system of healthcare finance, more resources are devoted to these functions than in other healthcare systems, such as those of Canada and the United Kingdom. A study conducted using 1987 data estimated that between $96 billion and $120 billion were spent on administration in the United States, out of a total spent of $488 billion for all healthcare-related services (Woolhandler & Himmelstein, 1991). This study primarily added up the money costs of these functions.

Pozen and Cutler (2010) found that the largest difference in spending between the United States and Canada was in administrative costs, with 44% more administrative staff in the United States than in Canada. When all administrative costs were included, they found administrative costs accounted for 39% of the difference between the United States and Canada. Other authors (Blanchfield, Heffernan, Osgood, Sheehan, & Meyer, 2010; Davis, Schoen, Schoenbaum, Doty, Holmgren, Kriss, & Shea, 2007; Luxembourg Income Study, 2011) have also found that the United States has many more administrative staff than do other countries. Cutler and Ly (2011) provide an excellent overview of comparative administrative findings.

This debate has served to highlight the fact that a healthcare financing system requires resources and that different systems have different costs. The Canadian system, for example, has lower administrative costs than does the U.S. system. However, the amount of administrative costs is not the only factor that needs to be taken into account when choosing a national healthcare "system." Morra. Nicholson, Levinson, Gans, Hammons, & Casalino (2011) found that physicians in the United States spend almost four times as much interacting with payers as do physicians in Canada.

Marketing functions serve to inform potential customers about the characteristics of various health plans. Consumers can better select among health plans if they have more information. Regulation and payment functions serve to help ensure that the care provided is of a high quality and results in good outcomes. Although these functions are not always completely effective, nevertheless, when we evaluate a financing system, we must look at the benefits of the various financing practices in addition to their costs.

EXERCISES

1. What proportion of total health expenses are made by out-of-pocket, government, and health insurance sources of finance?
2. An employee is worth $100 a week to her employer. The worker demands $20 in health insurance benefits, to be paid by the employer. What would the employer be willing to pay in terms of wages?
3. What is the effect on the market for health insurance of a government tax subsidy on health insurance premiums?
4. What will be the effect of mandated health insurance benefits on the market for labor if the workers do not place any value on these benefits? If they fully value the benefits?
5. What is a payroll tax? How will the imposition of a payroll tax affect the wage rate and the quantity of labor employed?
6. How will the imposition of a sales tax on a commodity affect the price and quantity sold of that commodity? Will the consumer usually bear the entire burden of the tax?
7. How do each of the following methods of financing the healthcare system impact on persons according to their income group?
   a. Income tax
   b. Sales tax
   c. Payroll tax
   d. Insurance premiums

BIBLIOGRAPHY

The Burden of Insurance

Abraham, J. M., & Feldman, R. (2010). Taking up or turning down: New estimates of household demand for employer-sponsored health insurance. *Inquiry, 47*(1), 17–32.

Baicker, K., & Goldman, D. (2011). Patient cost-sharing and healthcare spending growth. *Journal of Economic Perspectives, 25*(2), 47–68.

Banthin, J. S., & Bernard, D. M. (2006). Changes in financial burdens for health care: National estimates for the population younger than 65 years, 1996 to 2003. *JAMA, 296*(22), 2712–2719.

Berman, H., Lerner, A., Madden, P., Van Horn, L., & McPherson, B. (2011). Nonprofit health care market concentration and the public interest. *Inquiry, 48*(2), 102–108.

Bernard, D. M., Banthin, J. S., & Encinosa, W. E. (2006). Health care expenditure burdens among adults with diabetes in 2001. *Medical Care, 44*(3), 210–215.

Bhattacharya, J., & Bundorf, M. K. (2009). The incidence of the healthcare costs of obesity. *Journal of Health Economics, 28*(3), 649–658.

Bhattacharya, J., & Sood, N. (2011). Who pays for obesity? *Journal of Economic Perspectives, 25*(1), 139–158.

Book, E. L. (2005). Health insurance trends are contributing to growing health care inequality. *Health Affairs,* (Suppl. Web Exclusives), W5-577–W5-579.

Chernew, M., Cutler, D. M., & Keenan, P. S. (2005). Increasing health insurance costs and the decline in insurance coverage. *Health Services Research, 40*(4), 1021–1039.

Claxton, G., DiJulio, B., Whitmore, H., Pickreign, J., McHugh, M., Finder, B., & Osei-Anto, A. (2009). Job-based health insurance: Costs climb at a moderate pace. *Health Affairs, 28*(6), w1002–w1012.

Claxton, G., Gabel, J., Gil, I., Pickreign, J., Whitmore, H., Finder, B., & Osei-Anto, A. (2006). Health benefits in 2006: Premium increases moderate, enrollment in consumer-directed health plans remains modest. *Health Affairs, 25*(6), w476–w485.

Coffee, M. (2011). Insurance. Employers continue to shift health care costs onto workers. *Hospitals & Health Networks, 85*(10), 22.

Collins, S. R. (2007). Employer-based health insurance: Past, present, and future. *Healthcare Financial Management, 61*(12), 34–37.

Cutler, D. M. (1995). The cost and financing of health care. *American Economic Review, 85*(Suppl.), 32–37.

DeNavas-Wait, C., Proctor, B. D., & Smith, J. C. (2011). *Income, poverty, and health insurance coverage in the United States: 2010.* Washington DC: U.S. Government Printing Office. Retrieved from http://www.census.gov/prod/2011pubs/p60-239.pdf

Doty, M., Rustgi, S. D., Schoen, C., & Collins S. R. (2009). Maintaining health insurance during a recession: Likely COBRA eligibility: An updated analysis using the Commonwealth Fund 2007 Biennial Health Insurance Survey. *Issue Brief (Commonwealth Fund), 49*, 1–12.

Ellis, R. P., & Albert Ma, C. T. (2011). Health insurance, cost expectations, and adverse job turnover. *Health Economics, 20*, 27–44.

Gabel, J., Claxton, G., Gil, I., Pickreign, J., Whitmore, H., Finder, B., ..., & Rowland, D. (2005). Health benefits in 2005: Premium increases slow down, coverage continues to erode. *Health Affairs, 24*(5), 1273–1280.

Gabel, J., Pickreign, J., McDevitt, R., Whitmore, H., Gandolfo, L., Lore, R., & Wilson, K. (2007). Trends in the golden state: Small-group premiums rise sharply while actuarial values for individual coverage plummet. *Health Affairs, 26*(4), w488–w499.

Galbraith, A. A., Wong, S. T., Kim, S. E., & Newacheck, P. W. (2005). Out-of-pocket financial burden for low-income families with children: Socioeconomic disparities and effects of insurance. *Health Services Research, 40*(6, Pt. 1), 1722–1736.

Gruber, J., & Krueger, A. B. (1991). The incidence of mandated employer-provided insurance: Lessons from workers' compensation insurance. In D. Bradford (Ed.), *Tax policy and the economy*. Cambridge, MA: National Bureau of Economic Research.

Himmelstein, D. U., Thorne, D., Warren, E., & Woolhandler, S. (2009). Medical bankruptcy in the United States, 2007: Results of a national study. *American Journal of Medicine, 122*(8), 741–746.

Himmelstein, D. U., Thorne, D., & Woolhandler, S. (2011). Medical bankruptcy in Massachusetts: Has health reform made a difference? *American Journal of Medicine, 124*(3), 224–228.

Himmelstein, D. U., Warren, E., Thorne, D., & Woolhandler, S. (2005). Illness and injury as contributors to bankruptcy. *Health Affairs*, (Suppl. Web Exclusives), W5-63–W5-73.

Heim, B. T., & Lurie, I. Z. (2009). Do increased premium subsidies affect how much health insurance is purchased? Evidence from the self-employed. *Journal of Health Economics, 28*(6), 1197–1210.

Keenan, P. S., Cutler, D. M., & Chernew, M. (2006). The "graying" of group health insurance. *Health Affairs, 25*(6), 1497–1506.

Kreuger, A., & Reinhardt, U. E. (1994). Economics of employer versus individual mandates. *Health Affairs, 13*, 34–54.

Leonard, J., & Rosenbaum, S. (2011). Health insurance exchanges: Implications for public health policy and practice. *Public Health Reports, 126*(4), 597–600.

Linehan, K. (2010). Keeping health insurance after a job loss: COBRA continuation coverage and subsidies. *Issue Brief/National Health Policy Forum*, (837), 1–9.

Marquis, M. S., Buntin, M. B., Kapur, K., & Yegian, J. M. (2005). Using contingent choice methods to assess consumer preferences about health plan design. *Applied Health Economics & Health Policy, 4*(2), 77–86.

Mitchell, B. M., & Phelps, C. E. (1976). National health insurance: Some costs and effects of mandated employee coverage. *Journal of Political Economy, 84*, 553–571.

Monheit, A. C. (2008). Using health insurance premiums to change health behaviors. *Inquiry, 45*(3), 252–255.

Monheit, A. C., & Vistnes, J. P. (2005). The demand for dependent health insurance: How important is the cost of family coverage? *Journal of Health Economics, 24*(6), 1108–1131.

November, E. A., Cohen, G. R., Ginsburg, P. B., & Quinn, B. C. (2009). Individual insurance: Health insurers try to tap potential market growth. *Research Briefs*, (14), 1–8.

Patchias, E. M., & Waxman, J. (2007). Women and health coverage: The affordability gap. *Issue Brief (Commonwealth Fund), 25*, 1–12.

Pauly, M. V., & Herring, B. (2007). Risk pooling and regulation: Policy and reality in today's individual health insurance market. *Health Affairs, 26*(3), 770–779.

Pauly, M. V., Mitchell, O. S., & Zeng, Y. (2007). Death spiral or euthanasia? The demise of generous group health insurance coverage. *Inquiry, 44*(4), 412–427.

Polsky, D., Stein, R., Nicholson, S., & Bundorf, M. K. (2005). Employer health insurance offerings and employee enrollment decisions. *Health Services Research, 40*(5, Pt. 1), 1259–1278.

Shen, Y. C., & Long, S. K. (2006). What's driving the downward trend in employer-sponsored health insurance? *Health Services Research, 41*(6), 2074–2096.

Summers, L. H. (1989). Some simple economics of mandated benefits. *American Economic Review, 79*, 177–183.

Whitmore, H., Gabel, J. R., Pickreign, J., & McDevitt, R. (2011). The individual insurance market before reform: Low premiums and low benefits. *Medical Care Research & Review, 68*(5), 594–606.

Wilensky, G. R., & Taylor, A. K. (1982). Tax expenditures and health insurance: Limiting employer-paid premiums. *Public Health Reports, 97*, 438–444.

Woolhandler, S., & Himmelstein, D. U. (2007a). Consumer-directed healthcare: Except for the healthy and wealthy it's unwise. *Journal of General Internal Medicine, 22*(6), 879–881.

Woolhandler, S., & Himmelstein, D. U. (2007b). Double catastrophe: Injury-related bankruptcies. *Medical Care, 45*(8), 699–701.

The Burden of Taxation

Aaron, H. J. (1992). Equity in the finance and delivery of health care. *Journal of Health Economics, 11*(4), 467–471.

Aaron, H. J. (1994. Tax issues in health care reform. *National Tax Journal, 47,* 407–416.

Akazili, J., & Mooney, G. (2011). Social health insurance: To each according to his needs; From each according to his means—But what might that mean? *International Journal of Health Services, 41*(4), 679–690.

Brandon, W. P. (1982). Health-related tax subsidies. *New England Journal of Medicine, 302,* 947– 950.

Browning, E. K., & Johnson, W. R. (1980). Taxation and the cost of national health insurance. In M. V. Pauly (Ed.), *National health insurance.* Washington, DC: American Enterprise Institute.

Burman, L. E., & Williams, R. (1994). Tax caps on employment-based health insurance. *National Tax Journal, 47,* 529.

Christanson, J. B., Tu, H. T., & Samuel, D. R. (2011). Employer-sponsored health insurance: Down but not out. *Issue Brief/Center for Studying Health System Change,* (137), 1–5.

Doty, M. M., Collins, S. R., Nicholson, J. L., & Rustgi, S. D. (2009). Failure to protect: Why the individual insurance market is not a viable option for most U.S. families: Findings from the Commonwealth Fund Biennial Health Insurance Survey, 2007. *Issue Brief (Commonwealth Fund), 62,* 1–16.

Dror, D. M., Radermacher, R., Khadilkar, S. B., Schout, P., Hay, F. X., Singh, A., & Koren, R. (2009). Microinsurance: Innovations in low-cost health insurance. *Health Affairs, 28*(6), 1788–1798.

Due, J. F. (1957). *Sales taxation.* London, England: Routledge and Kegan Paul.

Feldstein, M., Friedman, B., & Luft, H. (1972). Distributional aspects of national health insurance benefits and finance. *National Tax Journal, 25,* 497–510.

Gabel, J., Pickreign, J., McDevitt, R., & Briggs, T. (2010). Taxing Cadillac health plans may produce Chevy results. *Health Affairs, 29*(1), 174–181.

Graves, J. A., Curtis, R., & Gruber, J. (2011). Balancing coverage affordability and continuity under a basic health program option. *New England Journal of Medicine, 365*(24), e44.

Gruber, J., & Hanratty, M. (1995). The labor-market effects of introducing national health insurance: Evidence from Canada. *Journal of Business and Economic Statistics, 13,* 163–173.

Gruber, J., & Washington, E. (2005). Subsidies to employee health insurance premiums and the health insurance market. *Journal of Health Economics, 24*(2), 253–276.

Hall, M. A. (2011). Risk adjustment under the Affordable Care Act: A guide for federal and state regulators. *Issue Brief (Commonwealth Fund), 7,* 1–12.

Hall, M. A., & Monahan, A. B. (2010). Paying for individual health insurance through tax-sheltered cafeteria plans. *Inquiry, 47*(3), 252–261.

Himmelstein, D. U., & Woolhandler, S. (2008). Privatization in a publicly funded health care system: The U.S. experience. *International Journal of Health Services, 38*(3), 407–419.

Himmelstein, D. U., & Woolhandler, S. (2009). The regressivity of taxing employer-paid health insurance. *New England Journal of Medicine, 361*(10), e101.

Lahey, J. N. (2012). The efficiency of a group-specific mandated benefit revisited: The effect of infertility mandates. *Journal of Policy Analysis & Management, 31*(1), 63–92.

Marquis, M. S., & Buchanan, J. L. (1994). How will changes in health insurance tax policy and employer health plan contributions affect access to health care and health care costs? *JAMA, 271,* 939–944.

Mitchell, J. B., Haber, S. G., & Hoover, S. (2005). Premium subsidy programs: Who enrolls, and how do they fare? *Health Affairs, 24*(5), 1344–1355.

Richman, B. D. (2007). Insurance expansions: Do they hurt those they are designed to help? *Health Affairs, 26*(5), 1345–1357.

Royalty, A. B., & Hagens, J. (2005). The effect of premiums on the decision to participate in health insurance and other fringe benefits offered by the employer: Evidence from a real-world experiment. *Journal of Health Economics, 24*(1), 95–112.

Schoen, C., Fryer, A. K., Collins, S. R., & Radley, D. C. (2011). Realizing health reform's potential: State trends in premiums and deductibles, 2003–2010: The need for action to address rising costs. *Issue Brief (Commonwealth Fund), (26)*, 1–38.

Schoen, C., Stremikis, K., Collins, S., & Davis, K. (2009). Progressive or regressive? A second look at the tax exemption for employer-sponsored health insurance premiums. *Issue Brief (Commonwealth Fund), 53*, 1–8.

Sommers, B. D. (2005). Who really pays for health insurance? The incidence of employer-provided health insurance with sticky nominal wages. *International Journal of Health Care Finance & Economics, 5*(1), 89–118.

Administrative Costs

Aaron, H. J. (2003). The costs of health care administration in the United States and Canada—Questionable answers to a questionable question. *New England Journal of Medicine, 349*(8), 801–803.

Aaron, H. J. (2006). A message to friends of social insurance: Wake up! *Health Affairs, 25*(3), w135–w137.

Aaron, H. J. (2007). Budget crisis, entitlement crisis, health care financing problem—Which is it? *Health Affairs, 26*(6), 1622–1633.

Aaron, H. J. (2009). Why paying for health care reform is difficult and essential—Numbers and rules. *New England Journal of Medicine, 361*(10), 937–939.

Aaron, H. J. (2011). The central question for health policy in deficit reduction. *New England Journal of Medicine, 365*(18), 1655–1657.

Aaron, H. J., & Bosworth, B. P. (1996). The budget meets the Boomers. *Brookings Review, 14*(4), 10–13.

Aaron, H. J., & Butler, S. M. (2008). A federalist approach to health reform: The worst way, except for all the others. *Health Affairs, 27*(3), 725–735.

Aaron, H. J., & Ginsburg, P. B. (2009). Is health spending excessive? If so, what can we do about it? *Health Affairs, 28*(5), 1260–1275.

Aaron, H. J., & O'Neill, P. H. (2007). The worst system of health care reform—except for all the others: A federalist approach to health care reform. *Journal of Policy Analysis & Management, 26*(1), 178–187.

Aaron, H. J., & Reischauer, R. D. (1998). "Rethinking Medicare reform" needs rethinking. *Health Affairs, 17*(1), 69–71.

Blanchfield, B. B., Heffernan, J. L., Osgood, B., Sheehan, R. R., & Meyer, G. S. (2010). Savings billions of dollars—and physicians' time—by streamlining billing practices. *Health Affairs, 29*(6), 1248–1254.

Chandra, C., Kumar, S., & Ghildayal, N. S. (2011). Hospital cost structure in the USA: What's behind the costs? A business case. *International Journal of Health Care Quality Assurance, 24*(4), 314–328.

Cutler, D. M., & Ly, D. P. (2011). The (paper) work of medicine: Understanding international medical costs. *Journal of Economic Perspectives, 25*(2), 3–25.

Davis, K., Schoen, C., Schoenbaum, S. C., Doty, M. M., Holmgren, A. L., Kriss, J. L., & Shea, K. K. (2007). Mirror, mirror on the wall: An international update on the comparative performance of American health care. *The Commonwealth Fund*. Retrieved from http://www.commonwealthfund. org/Publications/Fund-Reports/2007/May/Mirror--Mirror-on-the-Wall--An-International-Update-on-the-Comparative-Performance-of-American-Healt.aspx

Dorn, S. (2007). Administrative costs for advance payment of health coverage tax credits: An initial analysis. *Issue Brief (Commonwealth Fund), 24*, 1–12.

Ellis, R. P., & Albert Ma, C. T. (2011). Health insurance, cost expectations, and adverse job turnover. *Health Economics, 20*, 27–44.

Epstein, A. M., Aaron, H. J., Baicker, K., Hacker, J. S., & Pauly, M. V. (2009). Health care reform in perspective. *New England Journal of Medicine, 361*(16), e30.

Fairman, K. A., & Curtiss, F. R. (2011). How do seniors respond to 100% cost-sharing for prescription drugs? Quality of the evidence underlying opinions about the Medicare Part D coverage gap. *Journal of Managed Care Pharmacy, 17*(5), 382–392.

Goodman, R. (2011). Variation of fee-for-service specialist direct care work effort with patient overall illness burden. *Health Services Management Research, 24,* 130–141.

Hall, M. A., Hager, C. L., & Orentlicher, D. (2011). Using payroll deduction to shelter individual health insurance from income tax. *Health Services Research, 46,* 348–364.

Himmelstein, D. U., & Woolhandler, S. (1986). Cost without benefit: Administrative waste in U.S. health care. *New England Journal of Medicine, 314,* 441–445.

Himmelstein, D.U., Lewontin, J. P., & Woolhandler, S. (1996). Who administers? Who cares? Medical administrative and clinical employment in the United States and Canada. *American Journal of Public Health 69,* 172–178.

Himmelstein, D. U., Woolhandler, S., & Wolfe, S. M. (2004). Administrative waste in the U.S. health care system in 2003: The cost to the nation, the states, and the District of Columbia, with state-specific estimates of potential savings. *International Journal of Health Services, 34*(1), 79–86.

Hirose, K., Shore, A. D., Wick, E. C., Weiner, J. P., & Makary, M. A. (2011). Pay for obesity? Pay-for-performance metrics neglect increased complication rates and cost for obese patients. *Journal of Gastrointestinal Surgery, 15*(7), 1128–1135.

Johnson, C. E., Lemak, C. H., Hall, A. G., Harman, J. S., Zhang, J., & Duncan, R. P. (2010). Outsourcing administrative functions: Service organization demonstrations and Florida Medicaid PCCM program costs. *Journal of Health Care Finance, 37*(1), 1–12.

Luxembourg Income Study (LIS). (2011). *Database.* Retrieved from http://www.lisproject.org/techdoc.htm

Mar, P. L., Yu, R. A., & Yu, J. C. (2011). Division or department: A microeconomic analysis. *Plastic & Reconstructive Surgery, 127*(6), 2487–2495.

Morra, D., Nicholson, S., Levinson, W., Gans, D. N., Hammons, T., & Casalino, L. P. (2011). US physician practices versus Canadians: Spending nearly four times as much money interacting with payers. *Health Affairs, 30*(8), 1443–1450.

Newhouse, R. P. (2010). Do we know how much the evidence-based intervention cost? *Journal of Nursing Administration, 40*(7/8), 296–299.

Pozen, A., & Cutler, D. M. (2010). Medical spending differences in the United States and Canada: The role of prices, procedures, and administrative expenses. *Inquiry, 47*(2), 124–134.

Rooney, D., Pugh, C., Auyang, E., Hungness, E., & Darosa, D. (2010). Administrative considerations when implementing ACS/APDS skills curriculum. *Surgery, 147*(5), 614–621.

Smith, C., Wood, S., & Beauvais, B. (2011). Thinking lean: Implementing DMAIC methods to improve efficiency within a cystic fibrosis clinic. *Journal for Healthcare Quality, 33,* 37–46.

Smith, M. W., Chow, A., Kimerling, R. (2010). Estimating lost revenue from a free-care mandate in the U.S. Department of Veterans Affairs. *Psychiatric Services, 61*(11), 1150–1152.

Stock, G. N., & McDermott, C. (2011). Operational and contextual drivers of hospital costs. *Journal of Health Organization & Management, 25*(2), 142–158.

Stremikis, K., Schoen, C., & Fryer, A. K. (2011). A call for change: The 2011 Commonwealth Fund Survey of public views of the U.S. health system. *Issue Brief (Commonwealth Fund), 6,* 1–23.

Wong, B. J., Cifaldi, M. A., Roy, S., Skonieczny, D. C., & Stavrakas, S. (2011). Analysis of drug and administrative costs allowed by U.S. private and public third-party payers for 3 intravenous biologic agents for rheumatoid arthritis. *Journal of Managed Care Pharmacy, 17*(4), 313–320.

Woolhandler, S., Campbell, T., & Himmelstein, D. U. (2004). Health care administration in the United States and Canada: Micromanagement, macro costs. *International Journal of Health Services, 34*(1), 65–78.

Woolhandler, S., & Himmelstein, D. U. (1991). The deteriorating administrative efficiency of the U.S. healthcare system. *New England Journal of Medicine, 324,* 1253–1258.

Woolhandler, S., & Himmelstein, D. U. (2004). The high costs of for-profit care. *CMAJ Canadian Medical Association Journal, 170*(12), 1814–1815.

Woolhandler, S., & Himmelstein, D. U. (2007). Competition in a publicly funded healthcare system. *BMJ, 335*(7630), 1126–1129.

Zimmerman, C. (2011). Compared to Canadians, U.S. physicians spend nearly four times as much money interacting with payers. *Findings Brief: Health Care Financing & Organization, 14*(8), 1–3.

Chapter 15

Public Health Insurance

15.1 INTRODUCTION

In this chapter, an economic framework is used to analyze selected aspects of public health insurance coverage in the United States. Health insurance is a key element of the healthcare system, and public policies related to insurance influence the functioning of the healthcare market. In this chapter, it is shown how the economic framework can be used to analyze policy choices, discuss policy goals in relation to the economic framework, and assess policy choices in terms of the social objectives.

In Section 15.2, an overview of public health insurance in the United States is presented, focusing on Medicare and Medicaid, the two major national public health insurance plans. In Section 15.3, the issue of health insurance coverage is discussed. In Section 15.4, some information on trends in public health insurance is presented. In Section 15.5, the social goals of Medicare are discussed. In Section 15.6, some of the solutions proposed in recent years are described and how each solution contributes to or obstructs the achievement of specific health policy goals is explained. Section 15.7 considers alternatives to Medicaid.

15.2 PUBLIC HEALTH INSURANCE

Public health insurance in the United States for nonmilitary populations involves two key programs aimed at target populations. These are the Medicare and Medicaid programs. Some states also have additional public health insurance programs. Often these additional programs will be tied in some way to Medicaid, but in some circumstances they are not. In this chapter, the focus is on Medicare and Medicaid.

15.2.1 Medicare

15.2.1.1 Who Is Covered

Medicare is a national health insurance program for a subset of the U.S. population. Medicare was established in 1965 under Title XVIII of the Social Security Act and began coverage of beneficiaries on January 1, 1966. Originally, Medicare covered individuals 65 years of age or older, regardless of income or medical history, as long as they or their spouse contributed to Social Security for 10 years (40 quarters), Railroad Retirement, or federal retirement programs. In 1972, Medicare was expanded to cover individuals under 65 with permanent disabilities or who had end-stage renal disease (ESRD). Medicare was again expanded in 2001 to cover individuals with amyotrophic lateral sclerosis (ALS, or Lou Gehrig's disease).

In 2010, Medicare covered about 47 million people (39 million 65 and older and 8 million disabled), or about 15% of the total population (Annual Report of the Boards of Trustees, 2011). Between 1966 and 2000, the population covered by Medicare doubled and is projected to double again to about 80 million by 2030. The population served is also diverse. For example, in 2010, about 56% of the beneficiaries were female, 78% were non-Hispanic White, and 70% were between the ages of 65 and 84. As the characteristics of the population change over time, the diversity of the covered population will become more racially and ethnically diverse. About 30% of beneficiaries reported only fair to poor health in 2010, with disproportionate representation in the nonelderly, Black, Hispanic, and lower-income populations. Also, about 90% of noninstitutionalized Medicare beneficiaries have one or more chronic illnesses, with 46% with three or more chronic conditions.

15.2.1.2 What Is Covered?

Medicare consists of four parts: Part A, Hospital Insurance; Part B, Supplemental Medical Insurance; Part C, for Medicare Advantage; and Part D for Prescription Drugs. Each of these will be discussed in more detail in the following paragraphs.

Part A, Hospital Insurance (HI), covers inpatient hospital services, limited skilled-nursing facility services for rehabilitation, home health care, and hospice services. Most individuals are automatically eligible for Part A coverage if they are a U.S. citizen or permanent resident, if they or their spouse are eligible for Social Security payments, have made payroll tax contributions for 40 quarters (10 years), and are age 65 or older. These individuals are eligible regardless of income or asset level or any preexisting medical condition. Individuals under age 65 qualify for Medicare Part A if they have received Social Security Disability Income (SSDI) payments for at least 24 months and they do not have to have made payroll tax contributions for 40 quarters. In addition, people with end-stage renal disease or Lou Gehrig's disease are eligible for Medicare as soon as they begin receiving SSDI payments. Individuals who are eligible for Part A do not pay a premium; individuals age 65 and older not eligible (e.g., have not contributed for 40 quarters) can enroll in Part A by paying a monthly premium. Part A beneficiaries are responsible for a deductible before Medicare begins to pay; in 2010, the Part A deductible was $1,100 for each episode or "spell of illness" for an in-hosptial stay. In addition, beneficiaries generally pay a coinsurance amount for extended hospital stays (days 61–90) or skilled-nursing facility stays (days 21–100). In 2010, the cost per day of extended hospital stay was $275, and for extended nursing facility stay it was $137.50 per day.

Part B, Supplementary Medical Insurance (SMI), assists beneficiaries paying for physician services, outpatient services, home health services, preventive services, ambulance services, clinical laboratory services, durable medical equipment, kidney supply and services, outpatient mental health services, and diagnostic tests. In addition, it covers an annual comprehensive wellness visit and personalized prevention plan. Unlike Part A, however, Part B is voluntary and beneficiaries are required to pay a premium for the program ($110.50 per month in 2010). For about 95% of beneficiaries, the rate of increase in the premium is limited to the cost-of-living increase in Social Security benefits. Also, the premium paid is related to income; single individuals with an income greater than $85,000 or couples with an income greater than $170,000 in 2010 pay a higher premium, ranging from $154.70 to $353.60 per month. In 2010, only about 5% of beneficiaries paid the income-related Part B premium. Part B benefits are also subject to annual deductibles ($155 in 2010) and a 20% coinsurance rate, although the preventative services are exempt from the coinsurance and deductible. Over 90% of eligible beneficiaries enroll in Part B.

Part C, Medicare Advantage, is an alternative to the traditional Medicare Plan and allows individuals to enroll in a private plan, such as a health maintenance organization (HMO), preferred provider organization (PPO), or a private fee-for-service plan. These plans receive payments from Medicare for covered services, and beneficiaries are eligible for all benefits covered under Parts A, B, and D. Typically, enrollees pay the monthly Part B premium and often pay an additional premium directly to their plan (in 2010, the unweighted average premium was $56 per month, but varied from $40 for HMOs to $74 for private fee-for-service plans). Most beneficiaries have limited out-of-pocket costs under Part C, but cost-sharing requirements vary widely across plans. Participants in Part C are heavily concentrated in only six states.

Part D, Outpatient Prescription Drug Benefit, is a recent addition to Medicare, implemented in 2006. Private plans contract with Medicare to provide coverage to voluntarily enrolled beneficiaries. Beneficiaries enrolled in the plan typically pay a monthly premium, and individuals with modest income and assets are eligible for assistance. Beginning in 2011, the health reform law establishes a new Part D premium program similar to the Part B program and gradually phases in coverage of the Part D coverage gap (the donut hole) by 2020. In 2010, the standard benefit required had a $310 deductible and a 25% coinsurance rate, up to an initial coverage limit of $2,830 in total drug costs. Beneficiaries then pay 100% of drug costs until they have spent $4,550 out-of-pocket for prescriptions. Then, beneficiaries begin paying 5% of the drug cost or a copayment ($2.50 for generic, $6.30 for brand name) per prescription for the remainder of the year.

15.2.1.3 Financing Medicare

The primary sources of Medicare funding are general revenues (40%), payroll tax revenues (38%), and premiums (12%) paid by beneficiaries. In addition, taxation of Social Security benefits, payments from states, and interest also help fund the other 10% of Medicare.

Part A, the Hospital Insurance Trust Fund, receives funding through a dedicated tax levied against earnings. This tax (2.9%) is paid equally by employers and employees (1.45% each), with self-employed individuals paying both parts. Beginning in 2013, the health reform law increases the tax for higher-income individuals (greater than $200,000 per individual and greater than $250,000 per couple) to 2.35% from 1.45%. This tax is levied against earnings (salary and wages), not total income.

Part B, the Supplementary Medical Insurance Trust Fund, is financed in part from general revenues and in part by premiums paid by beneficiaries voluntarily enrolled in the program. Premiums are automatically set to cover 25% of the costs of Part B, and general revenues cover 75%. Higher-income individuals pay a larger share, ranging from 35 to 80%.

Part C, the Medicare Advantage program, is not separately funded. It provides benefits under Parts A, B, and D and so receives its funding through these sources.

Part D, the Prescription Drug program, receives funding from general revenues, premiums from beneficiaries, and state payments for dual eligibles. The monthly premiums from beneficiaries are established to cover 25.5% of the costs of the standard plan and Medicare funds the other 74.5%. As under Part B, higher-income individuals pay a larger share of the coverage and receive a smaller subsidy from Medicare.

Financing the Medicare program continues to face a number of challenges. These challenges include rising healthcare costs, a population that continues to age, and a declining ratio of workers contributing to the system to beneficiaries enrolled in the program. Efforts to control the costs of Medicare remain a federal priority because it accounts for about 15% of the total federal budget (Potetz, Cubanski, & Neuman, 2011).

15.2.1.4 Paying Providers

Except for Medicare Advantage (Part C) managed care arrangements, Medicare pays providers on a fee-for-service basis, with bundling of services occurring under the hospital prospective payment system with MS-DRGs. Physician fees include an aggregation of elements under the RBRVS system, and home health is paid a bundled, capitated amount.

Medicare financed about 20% of total personal healthcare expenditures in 2010, with its share varying by the type of service. For example, Medicare was expected to fund about 40% of the total spending on home health care, but only about 20% of nursing home care. The most rapidly growing service funded by Medicare is prescription drugs, in which Medicare financed about 24% of national drug spending in 2010, compared to only 3% in 2005, the year prior to implementation of Part D. Hospitals received about 29% of their funding from Medicare in 2010.

15.2.1.5 Supplemental Insurance Coverage

Because of the risk of substantial out-of-pocket costs to Medicare beneficiaries, about 90% of beneficiaries have supplemental coverage to Medicare. This supplemental coverage takes several forms, but the goal is to assist the beneficiaries in covering the relatively high cost-sharing expenses of Medicare and also to cover benefits that Medicare does not cover currently. While traditionally the primary source of supplemental coverage was employer-sponsored benefits, large employers offering retiree health benefits have declined substantially due to rising costs and the economic environment. However, the number of beneficiaries enrolled in Medicare Advantage plans has been increasing, and the additional coverage offered by these plans has helped to cushion some of these changes.

Another source of supplemental coverage comes from state Medicaid programs, which provide some assistance to low-income Medicare beneficiaries who also have modest assets. The Medicaid programs often pay the Part B and Part D premiums for these eligible beneficiaries to ensure they have coverage under these voluntary programs. Medicaid may also pay premiums for individuals who don't qualify for subsidized enrollment but are eligible to pay premiums to join the program. More about these "dual-eligible" beneficiaries will be provided in the Medicaid section.

Medicare beneficiaries also have the ability to purchase supplemental private insurance plans, usually called Medigap plans. These Medigap policies help cover the cost-sharing requirements of Medicare and to fill in the gaps in the benefits. These policies are designed to cover the deductibles, coinsurance, and copayments associated with Medicare-covered services. While these plans reduce financial burdens to the beneficiaries, they do reduce the typical incentives associated with having beneficiaries retain some financial responsibility, impacting the price consciousness of consumers. In general, these Medigap policies must conform to 1 of 10 standard benefit packages. Each of these packages offers coverage of a different set of benefits from which the beneficiaries can select. The monthly premium charged varies by the benefits covered, the insurer, the age of the beneficiary, and the place of residence.

Some beneficiaries enroll in multiple supplementary plans to provide more complete coverage of medical expenses. Even with all these supplemental policies, many Medicare beneficiaries still experience substantial out-of-pocket expenses. For example, Medicare beneficiaries currently spend over 16% of their income out-of-pocket for health care, and that percentage has been increasing with economic conditions and changes in premiums and services covered. As out-of-pocket costs increase, Medicare beneficiaries face additional challenges to maintaining daily necessities. As cost-sharing increases, more Medicare beneficiaries may have to choose between basic necessities and health care, with the results being adversely impacted health.

15.2.2 Medicaid

15.2.2.1 Who Is Covered?

Medicaid is another public insurance program. Medicaid was established in 1965 as part of the "Great Society" program under Title XIX of the Social Security Act; it was implemented as of July 1, 1966. Medicaid was established as an entitlement program to provide financial assistance for healthcare services and long-term care services for certain low-income individuals and families who were receiving cash assistance (welfare recipients). However, since its beginning, it has been expanded to increase eligibility to cover additional individuals living below or near the poverty level. Today, Medicaid covers both working and jobless families, individuals with a variety of physical and mental conditions, and elderly individuals. The role of Medicaid is slated to expand substantially under health reform.

Unlike Medicare, which is a federally operated program under guidelines established by the Social Security Administration and administered through the Centers for Medicare and Medicaid Services (CMS), Medicaid is a state-federal partnership program. Medicaid participation by states is voluntary, and it is financed jointly by federal and state governments, with the federal government "matching" dollars expended by the states. The federal match rate (Federal Medical Assistance Percentage, or FMAP) to the states varies and is based on state per capita income relative to the national average. FMAP is at least 50% (meaning that for every dollar the state spends on Medicaid, the federal government will provide another dollar for Medicaid services) and reaches as high as 73%. The higher the FMAP, the greater the percentage of total Medicaid costs that are financed by the federal government. In 2009, the American Recovery and Reinvestment Act temporarily increased the FMAP, and for 2010, the FMAP ranged from 5 to 85%. This increased the federal share of total Medicaid spending in 2010 from 57 to 66%, enabling states to cover additional individuals due to the economic conditions. Because most private insurance is obtained through place of employment, when individuals lose employment, they also usually lose insurance coverage. The expansion in Medicaid during this period was designed to provide financial assistance to individuals until they became reemployed and began receiving insurance coverage again (Holahan & Chen, 2011).

Under the partnership, Medicaid is administered by the states under broad federal guidelines and oversight by CMS. The broad federal guidelines enable states to exercise considerable variation in the design of their programs. While state participation in Medicaid is voluntary, currently all states participate. The federal government defines minimum requirements that states must meet, but the states have broad authority to establish eligibility criteria, benefits covered, provider payments, delivery systems, and a number of other conditions for their program. As a result, the percentage of the population covered across states varies widely.

In addition, states may request a waiver from the federal government, enabling them to design and operate their program outside the federal guidelines. A typical reason for requesting a waiver is to adopt a new model of coverage and delivery system for their low-income population. The waiver capability and the inherent flexibility of the Medicaid program have enabled states to adapt and evolve to meet the needs of their populations better. States can adjust more quickly to changing economic conditions or medical conditions (such as the HIV/AIDS pandemic) to coordinate and manage the health of their populations. The flexibility also means that there is substantial diversity in who is covered across the states.

In general terms, not only must an individual qualify based on financial criteria, but the individual must also belong to a group designated as "categorically" eligible for coverage. The federal government mandates that pregnant women and children under six with family incomes less than 133% of the federal poverty level (FPL) be covered. In addition, children age six to eighteen with family income below 100% of the FPL must be covered, as must parents below states' 1996 welfare eligibility levels. Most elderly populations and individuals with disabilities and on SSI must also be covered. States do, however, have flexibility in determining what counts as income for the program, with most states including assets in the measure. In addition to the minimum mandatory groups, states have the option of expanding coverage to additional groups. These optional groups covered typically extend the upper income levels for covered groups.

Medicaid is an entitlement program. Once a state has established the eligibility criteria for its Medicaid program, then all individuals in the state meeting the criteria have a federal right to Medicaid coverage; the individuals are entitled to coverage, and enrollment cannot be limited by the state, nor can waiting lists be applied. One federal criterion is that individuals must be American citizens or specific categories of lawfully residing immigrants who have resided in the United States for five years.

Medicaid is currently core to the financing structure of the U.S. healthcare system and is expected to expand substantially under health reform. Currently, more children are covered under Medicaid than any other source. Also, the majority of adults who are covered under Medicaid are in working families, holding low-paying jobs without access to employer-based health insurance. Many nonelderly individuals with disabilities unable to obtain coverage in the private market or for whom the coverage available does not meet all their needs, rely on Medicaid. Medicaid also covers pregnant women, with about 40% of all births occurring to Medicaid mothers.

Another group of Medicaid enrollees are the low income individuals on Medicare, the "dual-eligible" individuals. The dual-eligible populations are poorer than the other Medicare populations and also tend to have poorer health. About one in six Medicare beneficiaries are also enrolled in Medicaid, which assists enrollees in paying their premiums for Part B and D, cover the cost-sharing obligations of Medicare, and cover services not covered under Medicare, especially custodial long-term care in nursing facilities. Because of poorer health and services needed, these individuals place greater financial strain on the Medicaid program than the typical Medicaid recipient.

In 1997, the State's Children's Health Insurance Program (S-CHIP) was created under Title XXI of the Social Security Act. S-CHIP allowed states substantial flexibility in the expansion of insurance coverage of children. This program is also a federal-state program and can either be included with the state's Medicaid program or established as an independent program or as a combination. The independent design allows states more flexibility and requires states to describe the characteristics of their program in a state health plan. If the state includes S-CHIP in their Medicaid program, then the same rules apply as to other recipients, although eligibility is extended to higher income individuals. As eligibility for coverage became more expansive, concerns were raised that the public insurance program would "crowd out" private insurance coverage. The concern was that the lower, subsidized premium of S-CHIP would cause parents to drop dependent children from their private insurance plan and enroll them in the public program.

Even with the expanded coverage under Medicaid, there are still groups, or categories, of individuals who are not eligible for Medicaid, regardless of income level. Low income is a necessary condition but not a sufficient condition for coverage. One group is the parents of children who are on Medicaid because the income requirements are more restrictive for adults than for children. Another group is adults without dependent children, who no matter how low their income is, unless they are pregnant or disabled, they do not qualify for Medicaid. Most states do not cover lawfully resident immigrants during their first five years in the United States. Federal law prohibits undocumented immigrants from being covered by Medicaid.

15.2.2.2 What Is Covered?

Medicaid covers a broad array of services, some of which are mandatory, while others are optional. Because of the rather diverse needs of the Medicaid population, not only are the typical benefits covered under private insurance provided, but Medicaid programs also typically cover dental, vision, transportation, translation services, and long-term care services and support. Table 15-1 provides a list of mandatory services as well as typical optional services covered. States employ a number of strategies to limit utilization of services, such as utilization review, prior authorization, restrictive definitions of medical necessity, and case management.

For children under 21, the mandatory coverage of Early and Periodic Screening, Diagnostic, and Treatment (EPSDT) benefit provides a very comprehensive set of services to correct or ameliorate acute and chronic physical and mental health conditions. The services covered under the EPSDT benefit are broader than most private insurance plans and are especially important for children with disabilities.

Also not widely provided under private insurance are the long-term services and support provided under Medicaid. Medicaid includes services provided in skilled and intermediate-level nursing homes, as well as such community-based services as home health, rehabilitation therapy, medical equipment, adult daycare, and respite care for caregivers, to enable individuals to live as independently as possible. Medicaid is the largest public payer of

Table 15-1 Services Covered by Medicaid Programs

Mandatory Services	Commonly Offered Optional Services
Inpatient hospital services	Prescription drugs
Outpatient hospital services	Clinic services
Early and periodic screening, diagnostic, and treatment (EPSDT) services for individuals under 21 years of age	Physical therapy
Nursing facility services	Occupational therapy
Home health services	Speech, hearing, and language disorder services
Physician services	Respiratory care services
Rural health clinic services	Other diagnostic, screening, preventive, and rehabilitative services
Federally qualified health center services	Podiatry services
Laboratory and X-ray services	Optometry services
Family planning services	Dental services
Certified pediatric and family nurse practitioner services	Dentures
Freestanding birth center services (when licenses or otherwise recognized by the state)	Prosthetics
Transportation to medical care	Eyeglasses
Tobacco cessation counseling for pregnant women	Chiropractic services
Tobacco cessation, http://www.governing.com/news/state/gov-Study-Medicaid-Anti-Smoking-Programs-Lead-to-Significant-Savings.html	Other practitioner services
	Private duty nursing services
	Personal care
	Hospice
	Case management
	Services for individuals age 65 or older in an Institution for Mental Disease (IMD)
	Services in an intermediate care facility for the mentally retarded
	State Plan home and community based services 1915(i)
	Self-directed personal assistance services 1915(i)
	Community First Choice Option 1915(k)
	Other services approved by the Secretary*

*This includes services furnished in a religious nonmedical healthcare institution, inpatient psychiatric services for individuals under age 21, emergency hospital services by a non-Medicare certified hospital, and critical access hospital (CAH).

Source: Data from Centers for Medicare & Medicaid Services (2012). Medicaid Benefits. Accessed February 3, 2012 from http://www.medicaid.gov/Medicaid-CHIP-Program-Information/By-Topics/Benefits/Medicaid-Benefits.html.

mental health care, and Medicaid also covers about two-thirds of all nursing home residents and about 40% of individuals with HIV.

15.2.2.3 Financing Medicaid

The federal-state partnership organizational structure of Medicaid results in financing also shared between the two. There is a statutory formula that dictates how the federal government matches the spending of each state. The federal match rate, FMAP, is based upon a state's per capita income relative to the national average—the lower a state's per capita income, the higher the rate paid by the federal government. There is not a limit on total Medicaid expenditures, but expenditures are limited by the ability of the state to generate its share of the expenses.

For most states, Medicaid is the largest source of federal revenue for the state, while it tends to be the second-largest sector of a state's budget, behind education. Because states must balance their budgets, generating revenue to support Medicaid can be difficult, especially in economic downturns, when state revenues decline while the enrollment in Medicaid increases. However, because increased Medicaid spending by the state results in an influx of federal dollars, it increases the multiplier effect of those dollars, as businesses and residents generate successive rounds of earnings and purchases. This influx of federal dollars into the state's economy provides an incentive for states to focus on health care and not reduce coverage of their populations, although states are forced to control costs to balance their budget.

15.2.3 Paying the Providers

15.2.3.1 Fee-for-Service

There are two generic types of healthcare financial coverage for providers under Medicare: fee-for-service and per capita (or capitation) payment. In the fee-for-service plan, the Medicare program sets prices for individual patient contacts or encounters. Medicare has developed systems for classifying services of providers for most types of care supplied; these systems now include inpatient hospitalization, outpatient care, home care, and skilled-nursing facility care. Any classification system can divide cases or patients into groups of patients or encounters; the patients within each group are assumed to use a similar amount of resources. Each group is assigned a *relative weight,* and a dollar value is assigned to a weighted unit. Medicare adjusts the monetary prices for a variety of factors, including whether the provider is in an urban or rural area, area wage and cost-of-living levels, and provider characteristics (e.g., teaching versus nonteaching units). The result is a complex array of prices.

Inpatient hospital care is funded by the Medicare Severity Diagnosis Related Group (MS-DRG) system. The original DRG system was implemented in 1983, with 467 DRGs, and the system was modified to incorporate the severity of cases within the DRGs in 2007, with over 700 groups. Each of the groups is assigned a basic payment rate, reflecting the average resources used to treat Medicare patients in that DRG. This payment rate is divided into two components: labor related and nonlabor related, with proportions based on the wage index. In 2012, if the wage index was greater than one, then the labor share accounted for 68.8% of the relative weight, or $3,584.30 per unit, and the non-labor share accounted for 31.2%, or $1,625.44 per unit. If the wage index was equal to or less than one, then the labor share was 62.0%, or $3,230.04 per unit, and the nonlabor share was 38.0%, or $1,979.70 per unit. These base rates are multiplied by the relative weight of the MS-DRG to obtain the amount the hospital will receive for a patient hospitalized with that diagnosis.

Hospitals may receive an add-on payment to the base payment if they treat a high percentage of low-income patients, known as the disproportionate share hospital (DSH) adjustment. If a hospital is an approved teaching hospital, then it receives an indirect medical education (IME) adjustment percentage add-on payment. This rate depends upon the ratio of residents-to-beds for operating costs and on the ratio of residents to average daily census for capital costs.

The final adjustment is made for unusually costly patients—the outlier adjustment. This adjustment is designed to protect hospitals from unusually expensive cases. The total payment hospitals receive for a patient in a MS-DRG then, reflects the base payment plus DSH adjustment, plus IME adjustment, plus outlier adjustment (see https://www.cms.gov/AcuteInpatientPPS/01_overview.asp#TopOfPage).

Medicare has also implemented a prospective payment system for post-acute home care. A classification system was developed that is based on the patient's diagnosis and on therapeutic needs (physical, speech-language pathology, and occupational) (Liu, Gage, Harvell, Stevenson, & Brennan, 1999). As with inpatient care, a weight is assigned to each group in the class, and a price per weighted unit is set. The Medicare home care payment system replaced a system by which home care providers billed for individual services. It thus represents a bundling of services, in comparison with the payment system prior to 1999, when the prospective payment system was introduced.

Unlike hospital and home care reimbursement, the payment for physicians under Medicare remains on an individual service basis. Physicians are paid by fee category, called *Current Procedural Terminology* (CPT). Each service is assigned a weight; currently, the weighting system is called the *Resource-Based Relative Value System* (RBRVS). The RBRVS contains separate component weights that reflect work performed, practice expenses, liability insurance, and regional cost variations. A dollar value is assigned by Medicare, which converts the resource-based weights to dollar payments. In 2012, this conversion figure was $24.6712. CMS has established 89 physician fee schedule (PFS) localities reflecting geographical cost variation to adjust the payment rates for physicians.

15.2.3.2 Managed Care

Until 1998, the overall level of payment for a risk (HMO) contract was 95% of the fee-for-service level of expenditures in any single county. Beginning in 1998, a blended rate, reflecting local and national costs, was set, subject to a minimum amount per enrollee. In 2000, a risk-adjustment model, called the *Principal Inpatient Diagnostic Cost Group* (PIP-DCG), was introduced. According to this risk-adjustment model, patients who had been hospitalized in the prior year for specific diagnoses were projected to have higher total costs and thus were entitled to a higher payment (see www.hcfa.gov/stats/ hmorates/45d1999/45d02.htm). This payment change was made to encourage HMOs to enroll persons with poorer health status and to encourage HMOs to operate in lower cost areas.

15.3 UNCOVERED CARE

Despite the existence of Medicare and Medicaid, many individuals either have no health insurance coverage at all or have large gaps in coverage. According to estimates by the U.S. Bureau of the Census, 16.3% of all individuals (about 49.9 million) had no insurance coverage in 2010 (DeNavas-Walt, Proctor, & Smith, 2011). A substantial number of this group were young and/ or healthy, but the group included many who were in fair or poor health and also 7.3 million children (DeNavas-Walt, Proctor, & Smith, 2010). Further, 28 million of the noncovered individuals were employed, which poses a problem because employment is the usual route through which health insurance is obtained. The percentage of people covered by private insurance has been decreasing since 2001.

It should be pointed out that *uninsured* is not the same thing as *unserved*. Many individuals with no insurance still receive medical care: they either pay the full price for this care or receive subsidized or charity care. What is likely, however, is that they receive less care than they would if they had insurance coverage.

In addition to those with no coverage, a substantial number of individuals have gaps in coverage. The Medicare deductibles and copayments can add up to a large amount, and individuals who are covered by Medicare but do not have additional private (Medigap) or Medicaid coverage can, if they become ill, incur substantial out-of-pocket costs, including individuals who need nursing home care. There is very little in the way of long-term care insurance coverage at present, and so individuals in nursing homes (especially intermediate-care facilities) will be required to pay for such care themselves, unless they "spend down" to the point at which both their income (less medical expenses) and their assets are below the state Medicaid limits.

Lack of coverage has also surfaced as a major policy issue in the area of inpatient hospital care. The burden of treating indigent patients has not fallen evenly on hospitals. Teaching hospitals, public hospitals, and hospitals that partially specialize in certain product lines (e.g., obstetrics) provide larger portions of charity care and have higher rates of bad debt (Mulstein, 1984).

15.4 SOME TRENDS IN PUBLIC HEALTH INSURANCE

In recent years, several public insurance trends have captured interest in the public policy arena. In this section, these trends are reviewed briefly.

15.4.1 Disbursements of the Hospital Insurance Trust Fund

Medicare's HI funding is tied to the growth of the portion of the Social Security tax that is earmarked for the Hospital Insurance Trust Fund. However, there is no automatic link between the growth of trust fund revenues and the growth of fund expenditures, which primarily go to reimburse hospitals (Iglehart, 1999; Wolkstein, 1984). The revenues are based on a percentage of payrolls and so cannot be increased by more than the increase in payrolls, unless the Social Security tax rate is increased or, as happened recently, the base on which the tax is levied is increased (i.e., employment and wages have increased). In the absence of such increases in tax revenues, large deficits in the fund had been experienced, and until very recently, increasingly large deficits had been predicted.

According to the 2011 Annual Report of the Board of Trustees of the Federal Hospital Insurance and Federal Supplementary Medical Insurance Trust Funds, expenditures from the HI trust fund exceeded revenues. In 2010, the deficit was $32.3 billion. Deficits in the trust fund are projected to continue in all future years, requiring redemption of trust fund assets to pay expenditures. It is estimated that trust fund assets will be depleted/exhausted in 2024.

15.4.2 Medicare's SMI Revenues and Expenditures

SMI funds come from two main sources: premiums paid directly by the enrollees (or by Medicaid for those qualifying for Medicaid coverage) for Part B and Part D revenue funds and from general revenue funds. Part B and Part D are maintained in separate accounts in the SMI. Originally, the premium rate for Part B was set so that premium revenues of the SMI trust fund were one-half of all revenues. From 1973, the growth of premiums was mandated to be no greater than the growth of Social Security cash benefits. As a result, since then, the premium share of total fund revenues in Part B has fallen to about 30%. The nature of financing for both Part B and Part D is similar, with premiums and the transfer from general revenues for each part established annually at a level sufficient to cover the following year's estimated expenditures. Accordingly, each account within SMI is automatically financially balanced each year.

Reimbursements from the fund grew by about 23% annually from 1966 to 1994 (Health Care Financing Administration, 1995). Because the number of enrollees grew by only about 2.2% during this period, most of this growth has been in expenditures per enrollee. As in the case of the Hospital Insurance Trust Fund, this growth in expenditures has been a major cause of concern. However, unlike Hospital Insurance Trust Fund outlays, Medical Insurance Trust Fund expenditures can be increased by government appropriations.

According to the Trustee's Report (2011), expenditures for Part B grew at an average annual rate of 6.9% over the past five years. Part B cost increases are projected to grow at an annual rate of 4.7% from 2011 to 2015, and if legislative changes to physician payment occur, the rate is projected to average 7.5% through 2015. A "hold harmless" provision does not allow Part B premium increases to cause a beneficiary's net Social Security benefits to decrease, limiting the amount of revenue generated for premiums.

The Medicare Part D program began in 2006. Expenditures in this account are projected to grow at an average annual rate of 9.7% from 2011 to 2020. Given the structure, revenues and expenditures will balance.

15.4.3 Out-of-Pocket Expenditures for Medicare Enrollees

Because of the Medicare premiums, deductibles, coinsurance, and copayments, Medicare enrollees incur considerable out-of-pocket expenses. Higher income Medicare enrollees often seek private insurance options to help cover the copayments, coinsurance, and deductibles, while many enrollees maintain health insurance through their former employers beyond retirement. About 90% of all Medicare enrollees maintain these types of Medigap coverage or receive assistance from Medicaid as a dual eligible enrollee. However, about 10% have no additional coverage beyond Medicare.

In 2009, Medicare households spent about 15% of their total budget on health-related expense, an amount that was about three times the amount of non-Medicare households. The largest share of their expenses (65.7%) went to pay for Part B and Part D premiums and premiums for supplemental insurance coverage. When health insurance premiums are excluded, Medicare beneficiaries spent, on average in 2009, about 5.1% of total household income on health care, compared to 2.1% of the non-Medicare population.

Healthcare spending as a percentage of household income increases with age of the beneficiaries; individuals 65–69 years of age spent 12.7% of their income, compared to 18.2% of those 80 years old or older. Because of disabilities, the under-65 cohort on Medicare spent 11.5% on average. The increased spending with age reflects poorer health status due to aging and the increased need for long-term care.

Individuals with income levels just above the poverty level incurred a greater financial burden for health than did individuals below the poverty level, partly because those below poverty often qualified for Medicaid, while those just above poverty did not. In 2009, Medicare households at less than 100% of the federal poverty level (FPL) spent 13.6% of their income on health care, compared to 16.4% for those with incomes between 100 and 199% of the FPL, and 12.9% for those with incomes of 400% or greater of the FPL. Medicare households below poverty with members also covered by Medicaid spent on average $493, compared to Medicare households below poverty not covered by Medicaid that had expenses of $3,323.

In summary, while Medicare provides substantial coverage for its beneficiaries, the population can still face the risk of high financial burdens. For example, out-of-pocket costs can be high because of premiums, deductibles, copayments, coinsurance, annual maximums, plan maximums, and noncovered services. While Medicare beneficiaries do not pay premiums for Part A hospital insurance if they have accumulated credits for 40 Social Security quarters, if they have only 30–39 quarters, they would be required to pay $248 per month for coverage in 2012, or $451 per month if they had fewer than 30 quarters. In addition, Medicare had a $1,156 deductible in 2012, plus after 60 days in the hospital, beneficiaries had to pay $289 per day for days 61–90 and $578 per day for days 91–150. After 150 days, there is no coverage by Medicare for hospital care.

For skilled-nursing facility care, beneficiaries had to pay $144.50 per day for days 21–100. The first 20 days are covered for rehabilitation purposes, and no coverage is provided after 100 days. Medicare payments for psychiatric hospitalization are the same as inpatient hospital care, except there is a maximum of 190 days of care over the lifetime of the beneficiary. Medicare pays 100% of home health care, except the beneficiary pays 20% of the Medicare-approved amount for medical equipment. For hospice care in 2012, prescriptions cost $5 and the beneficiary paid 5% per day of the Medicare-approved amount, up to a maximum of $1,156.

For Part B coverage, most individuals paid a $99.90 per month premium because of the limit tied to increases in Social Security benefits. For individuals not meeting this requirement, the premium was $115.40 per month. For Part B, there was a $140 deductible and a 20% coinsurance rate of the Medicare-approved amount for physician services (the amount could be more if the physician did not accept Medicare). In 2012, outpatient hospital care could incur a maximum of $1,156. Laboratory tests were completely covered, as were certain preventative care services. Noncovered preventative services had the same coinsurance rate as physician services. For medical equipment and supplies, Medicare pays 80% of the "approved charge," and the beneficiary may pay more than 20% if charges are above the Medicare-approved charge. For outpatient mental health services, the beneficiary pays 45% of the approved charge. Partial hospitalization for mental health services has the same coverage and expenses as inpatient hospital services.

The amount varies by plan for Part D coverage. However, no plan's deductible could exceed $320 in 2012. The coinsurance and/or copayment amounts vary by plan, with some plans having different levels, or tiers, for different types of drugs. The initial coverage limit was $2,930 in 2012, and the out-of-pocket threshold was $4,700. The donut hole (no coverage) was between $2,930 and $4,700. In 2012, beneficiaries receive a 50% discount on brand name drugs while in the donut hole and will pay a maximum of 86% on generic drugs.

Part C, Medicare Advantage plans, replace Part A and Part B insurance with combined coverage. Often additional benefits, including Part D, are provided by these private insurance plans. What is covered and costs vary by plan.

15.5 GOALS OF MEDICARE

In order to discover what the policy issues are with Medicare, the preceding facts need to be assessed in light of the social goals of Medicare. It was only recently that these goals were stated explicitly (Cutler, 2000; U.S. General Accounting Office, 1999). Among these stated goals were affordability, equity, adequacy, feasibility, and acceptance. The definitions of these concepts given here are those of the U.S. Government Accounting Office (GAO), which differ from the standard economic definitions. *Affordability* refers to the total costs incurred by the program. When stating this goal, the GAO is referring to the public component of the program and its burden on public spending. *Equity* refers to the burden of payments on specific groups. Individuals can be viewed as paying too much if they don't have sufficient coverage or if their premiums are too high. Individuals can also be paying too little for premiums and copayments; with low direct costs, they would be using too much care (from a strict efficiency viewpoint). *Adequacy* refers to the availability of care.

Feasibility refers to the ability of Medicare to actually implement changes in policy. *Acceptance* refers to the acceptability of the program to consumers, intermediaries, and providers.

These goals bear some resemblance to the following very general economic goals of health policy: economic efficiency (which has demand, technical efficiency, and adequacy-of-supply aspects), equity in utilization and equity in payment, quality of care, and public expenditure control. The economic goal of public expenditure control translates into the GAO goal of affordability. The economic goal of equity of payment translates into the GAO goal of equity. The economic goals of equity in utilization and adequacy of supply translates into the GAO goal of adequacy. The economic goals of quality of care and technical efficiency are not directly addressed in the GAO goals, although quality assurance activities are a very important component of Medicare activities (Medicare Payment Advisory Commission, 2000). The GAO goals of feasibility and acceptance are not directly addressed in the general economic goals.

In order to assess Medicare policies, Medicare performance must be evaluated in light of the policy goals. As seen in the previous section, the major issues include rising expenditures, hospital trust-fund deficits, and large out-of-pocket payments for some groups. These phenomena are related to the goals of affordability, equity of payment, and adequacy of supply. Most importantly, the goals may well conflict with each other (otherwise there would not be an economic problem). In the late 1990s, the Health Care Financing Administration (the agency that administered Medicare) and the Congress instituted a series of reforms designed to address the goal achievement balance under Medicare. The policy initiatives were Medicare Part C and the Balanced Budget Act of 1997. In the following section, an overview of the policies that are available to Medicare are provided.

15.6 POLICY ALTERNATIVES FOR MEDICARE

15.6.1 Economic Analysis and Alternative Solutions

Six basic types of policies can be identified that can be used to help achieve policy goals. The first set of policies deals with the setting of the broad outline of the program. For example, Medicare can change who is entitled to benefits or what benefits individuals receive. The second set of policies deals with health insurance premiums. Medicare can change Part B premiums, and it can change the out-of pocket price of supplementary private insurance premiums. As well, Medicare can arrange for supplementary coverage in other programs, such as Medicaid. The third set deals with the direct price of care. Medicaid can change the deductibles and copayments paid by enrollees and in the process, impact the demand for care (subject, of course, to the purchase of supplementary insurance). The fourth set deals with provider reimbursement. Medicare can change the basis of reimbursement. For example, home health care was formerly funded on the basis of individual services. Most recently, Medicare developed a home healthcare classification system that bundled individual services within diagnostic and needs-based groups. In addition to changing the definition of what output they will fund, Medicare can change the rate of payment. Fifth, Medicare can introduce competitive practices into its reimbursement mechanism. It can fund care on the basis of vouchers, encouraging individuals to shop around for their care. And sixth, Medicare can regulate the behavior of providers (i.e., make them provide care based on specific norms set by the program).

15.6.2 The Scope of the Program

Currently, Medicare's main line of business is to provide insurance coverage for persons 65 years of age and older. In 1997, Congress set up the Medicare Commission to make recommendations about policies that could affect the future of Medicare. One of the policies recommended by the two committee chairs was to increase the age of Medicare beneficiaries to 67. This proposal did not achieve policy status, but it is an obvious way of changing the number of beneficiaries in the system. One proposal intended to extend the Medicaid mandate was to provide prescription drug insurance coverage (Davis, Poisal, Chulis, Zarabozo, & Cooper., 1999; Soumerai & Ross-Degnan, 1999). Prescription drug coverage was implemented in 2006 with a wide variety of features, including additional premiums, copayments and deductibles, prescription limits, and so forth. Its inclusion added a new dimension to the program, and administrative costs increased considerably.

15.6.3 Insurance Premiums

Individuals and groups have proposed policies that would both increase and decrease health insurance premiums. Concern over the growth in first-dollar coverage has led some observers to propose a premium tax on Medigap policies. The introduction of such a tax would raise the price of Medigap coverage and reduce the amount of coverage purchased. The reduction in such coverage would lead to a reduction in the use of medical services in the short run.

There is a premium only for Part B and Part D Medicare. About one-quarter of Part B revenues come from this premium and the rest from general government revenues. The Balanced Budget Act of 1997, which overhauled Medicare's finances, did not substantially increase the premium; however, the premium is based on Social Security payments, and as such payments increase, so will the Part B premium. In 2000, the premium was $45.50 per month; by 2012, it increased to $ 99.90 (or $115.40 for those not under the Social Security cap). An increase in the premium influences the goal of equity in payment.

15.6.4 Copayments, Coinsurance, and Deductibles

Copayments, coinsurance, and deductibles serve to regulate demand for covered healthcare services and to reduce government revenues. Coinsurance is fixed as a percentage of medical charges, and it increases as charges rise. Copayments and deductibles are based on usage and are not always predictable. Individuals seek predictability by purchasing Medigap insurance coverage, which pays for the copayments and deductibles. The deductible in 2012 was $ 1,156 for Part A and $ 99.90 for Part B. There was also 20% coinsurance for Part B. These payments have increased annually, but they have not been a major part of Medicare's cost-cutting plans. Higher copayments, deductibles, and coinsurance reduce affordability.

15.6.5 Provider Payments

In 1983, Medicare began paying for inpatient hospitalization on a DRG basis, and expanded to MS-DRG in 2007. A price is applied to the MS-DRG weighted units to obtain a given price per weighted unit, which is what the hospitals receive. Every year, this price is increased by a given update factor in order to account for inflation and technological change. The update factor is supposed to cover changes in capital input prices, technology changes, and any real changes in the case-mix factor. The Balanced Budget Act of 1997 made changes to Medicare that were projected to result in $116 billion in savings between 1998 and 2002. Two-thirds of these savings were to come from limits in the update factors for inpatient care (Moon, Gage, & Evans., 1997). For the first year, there was a freeze on payment rates (Levit, Cowan, Lazenby, Sensenig, McDonnell, Stiller, Martin, & the Health Accounts Team., 2000).

The Medicare Part A payment strategy also included a switch from fee-for-service to prospective payment systems for home health care and outpatient care. Classification systems have been developed for home health care (Goldberg, Delargy, Schmitz, Moore, & Wrobel, 1999) and outpatient care (Health Care Financing Administration, 2000). Such systems are expected to increase control over spending in these areas by Medicare. They may also reduce availability.

15.6.6 Managed Care and Competition

In the original Medicare scheme for HMO coverage, the fees paid to HMOs were based on total medical care expenditures per beneficiary. Using the adjusted average per capita cost (AAPCC) method of rate setting, fees were set at 95% of the total medical costs for persons in the geographic area (usually the county). Included in the rate was the enrollee's Part B premium. The health plan decided on any benefit package in excess of the standard Medicare A and B coverage (e.g., whether to include drug coverage), additional premiums (if any), and copayments for medical visits. The basic rate was risk adjusted for age, gender, eligibility for Medicaid supplemental coverage, and whether the enrollee was institutionalized. Under the AAPCC formula, there were wide geographic variations in premium rates. In 1997, rates ranged from $250 per month to $760. There were also wide variations in managed care enrollments among states. Only 5% of the eligible population enrolled in risk contracts in Arizona in 1997; in California, the statistic was 27%. In addition, there was some evidence that Medicare risk plans enrolled persons who were lower users of health services (Brown, Clement, Hill, Retchin, & Bergeron, 1993); as a result, their costs were below the risk premiums set by Medicare, and the HMOs' profits were sometimes considerable.

Many observers have placed high hopes on managed care to achieve acceptable levels of health care for the covered population. The failure of Medicare to achieve a uniformly high degree of managed care coverage was attributed to the wide regional variations in the AAPCC rates and the inability of the risk-rating formula to account for high-cost enrollees. In 1998, Congress enacted a new Part C of Title XVIII of the Social Security Act, creating the Medicare + Choice program. The program had two new features. First, it created a blended national-regional rate for the managed care premium. In this rate, Medicare combined a national rate ($398 per month) with the county rates (the old AAPCC rates). There was to be a floor below which no county-specific rate would fall. This resulted in a severing of the link between fee-for-service costs and managed care rates (McClellan, 2000). Second, Congress instituted a new risk-adjustment variable, called the *Principal Inpatient Diagnostic Cost Group* (PIP-DCG). According to the PIP-DCG, a patient who is hospitalized in the previous year for a specific (serious) condition will fall into a higher risk category, and the HMO will receive a higher rate adjustment for this patient. The intent of these changes is to encourage HMOs to establish programs in areas that are now poorly served and to accept higher risk patients who have been hospitalized for serious conditions. Other features of the Medicare risk system remained. These include the variable benefits package, additional premiums tied to the benefits package, and consumer premiums and copayments.

Several criticisms have been aimed at the Medicare + Choice program (Aaron, 1999). One is that Medicare + Choice may still not appropriately adjust for risk. The nature of the enrollees of the Medicare program and the circumstances of enrollment make it easier for HMOs to select low-cost enrollees. Medicare enrollees select into the program as individuals rather than within groups, and HMOs can target low-cost individuals for membership much easier than they can target employees who join as a group. In addition, Medicare enrollees have a great variability in cost. In any society, most of the people with very high medical costs are older individuals, and in the United States, all of the older individuals are in the Medicare program. There are thus considerable benefits to be gained by HMOs from seeking out the lower cost individuals. It is thus particularly important for the Medicare program to have an adequate risk-adjustment mechanism.

A second criticism of the program is that Medicare + Choice offers a services and benefits package. Medicare pays for a basic core of services plus whatever additional services the HMO offers. These extra services are included in the HMO additional premium, if there is one. As a result, Medicare is not paying for a defined group of services, and enrollees may become confused as to what is in the Medicare package and what is extra.

In 2003, the Medicare Modernization Act was renamed Medicare + Choice Medicare Advantage (MA). The focus of MA became one of expanding access to private plans and providing additional benefits to private plan enrollees rather than cost control. The result is that Medicare pays more per enrollee in these plans than it does per enrollee in the traditional Medicare plan. In 2010, the health reform act caused another shift by beginning to reduce payments to MA plans in an effort to bring their costs back in line with the fee-for-service Medicare system. A bonus system was also introduced into the MA program in which bonuses would be paid according to quality ratings for the plan. In addition, by 2014, the plans would be required to maintain a medical loss ratio of at least 85%, limiting administrative expenses and profits to 15%.

In 2011, about 25% of Medicare beneficiaries were enrolled in Medicare Advantage plans. There is wide variation across states, with less than 1% enrolled in Alaska, and 44% in Minnesota. The penetration rate also varies by county, with urban counties enrolling 26%, compared to 15% in rural counties.

Medicare Advantage plans are paid a capitated amount to provide all Part A and Part B benefits. A separate amount is paid to cover Part D. The rate paid is established in a bidding process based on estimated costs per enrollee for covered services. All bids that meet the necessary condition are accepted. The bids are compared to a benchmark amount, and the benchmarks become the maximum amount Medicare will pay a plan in a given area. If the bid from a plan is higher than the benchmark, then enrollees pay the difference in the form of a monthly premium. If it is lower, the plan and Medicare split the difference. The plan's share is known as a rebate and must be used to offer supplemental benefits to enrollees. Medicare's payments to plans reflect the enrollees' risk profile. The 2010 health reform law reversed the methodology for paying plans and reduced the benchmarks. The amount of the rebate in the future will depend upon the quality rating of the plan.

In the coming years, there will be many reform proposals seeking to push Medicare toward becoming a competitive system. It is questionable whether such reforms would solve the problems associated with introducing managed care principles into the Medicare program. Medicare enrollees still join HMOs individually and have high and variable costs. The very significant incentive to select healthier cases will remain as long as the risk-adjustment tools do not permit the identification of high-risk individuals. As well, any attempt to regulate competitive practices will result in an extremely complex set of rules. However, the set of rules may not be any more complex than the set of current fee-for-service rules, in which a multitude of prices and adjustments have been introduced within a complicated regulatory framework. Further, the definition and regulation of the basic product characteristics will prove to be a daunting task. Medical care is a service with many aspects, and the among-patient and among-provider differences are very subtle.

A successful capitation program will better allow Medicare to achieve a greater degree of control over public expenditures. Competition should lead to a greater degree of efficiency in the market. The achievement of the other social goals may be more controversial. The ability of Medicare to ensure uniformly high-quality services is still open to question. And the availability of care may be hampered by the continual attempt by managed care plans to enroll low-cost patients. Nevertheless, any system must be judged by comparing it to other feasible systems. Currently, fee-for-service is the alternative to Medicare Advantage. Fee-for-service may perform better in terms of availability and quality of care, but it is lacking in regard to the goals of efficiency and expenditure control. In the end, the policy maker is faced with a trade-off, and the choice of system will depend on the degree of importance given to each of the social goals.

15.7 POLICY ALTERNATIVES FOR MEDICAID

Medicaid programs are run by the states and financed by them and the federal government. Individual states have a great deal of discretion in the policies they institute to govern the programs, which indeed exhibit substantial variability. Part of this variability is due to the fact that Medicaid serves several very different populations, including the poor aged, poor families with dependent children, and the blind and disabled.

Medicaid's problems are somewhat different from those of Medicare. To begin with, there are a large number of uninsured children in the United States who are eligible for coverage under the Accountable Care Act but who have not been enrolled for one reason or another. For example, there were 49.9 million persons without insurance coverage in 2010. In addition, there are many persons over 65 who have low incomes but no supplementary coverage and who are thus at risk for considerable out-of-pocket expenditures. In 2010, about 21% of the Medicaid population was over 65 years old and had joint Medicare-Medicaid coverage (DeNavas-Walt, Proctor, & Smith, 2011). Until 1990, the growth in total expenditures for Medicaid was moderate. However, beginning in 1990, following the expansion of the program to cover children and women whose incomes were above the poverty level but still low, the growth in expenditures was substantial, although in 1996 and 1997, expenditure growth leveled off. At its inception, the Medicaid program accounted for 2.9% of all national health expenditures. In 2010, state and federal outlays for Medicaid totaled $401.4 billion, accounting for 15.5% of the nation's health expenditures.

15.7.1 Scope of the Program

Until 1987, only low-income women (under age 65 and not blind or disabled) and their children who were receiving AFDC payments were eligible for Medicaid enrollment. The Medicaid program expanded eligibility in 1987 to include low-income women and children who were not on the AFDC program. At their discretion, states could offer coverage to families whose incomes reached 185% of the poverty level. This expansion of coverage led to a rapid increase in Medicaid enrollment and expenditures beginning in 1990 (Cutler & Gruber, 1996a, 1996b).

Medicaid's scope of coverage is very broad. It usually includes outpatient drugs and dental care. Because the breadth of coverage is wider than that for Medicare, Medicaid also enrolls low-income Medicare enrollees who do not have supplementary coverage.

Although the variety of services was not affected, the state of Oregon instituted a benefit limitation policy in 1994. It created a ranking of the costs and benefits of alternative medical procedures and proposed to pay for only those procedures whose benefit-cost ratios ranked above a certain cutoff point. Near the top of the list were treatments for disorders such as bone cancer and multiple sclerosis, which, it was claimed, yield substantial benefits per dollar of cure. Lower on the list were disorders whose treatments have a lower rate of return, including chronic ulcers and sleep disorders. Thus, the scope of the services was to be limited by type of treatment. This program was quite controversial and has generated a great deal of discussion.

15.7.2 Copayments

Generally, Medicaid does not charge recipients for their services. However, states can institute a copayment for some services. As of 2004, some 41 states had copayments for prescription drugs, usually ranging from $0.50 to $1.00 per prescription. In addition, some states have mandated limits on the quantity of drugs prescribed and the number of refills. After the enrollee reaches these limits, the drugs are no longer covered. There is evidence that these copayments affect the utilization of drugs, and there is limited evidence that health status is adversely affected (Stuart & Zacker, 1999).

15.7.3 Provider Payments

Medicaid programs are noted for the low levels of fees paid to providers (Gruber, 1997). Low fee levels discourage providers from serving Medicaid enrollees and thus reduce availability. This is a problem often noted when Medicaid is discussed.

15.7.4 Competitive Bidding by Suppliers

Competitive bidding, which has been implemented by the California and Arizona Medicaid programs, has the objective of providing cost-effective care for indigents. If the buyer has a considerable degree of market power, it can extract a lower price from competitive sellers, and if there is any room for cost reductions, either through increasing efficiency or lowering quality, the reductions will be incorporated into the providers' bids. However, the bidding process is a complex one and may not automatically lead to savings.

15.7.5 Managed Care

Many states are looking to managed care programs in order to consolidate their efforts at provision. In 1998, about 53% of the Medicaid population was enrolled in managed care plans, while by 2010, over 71% were enrolled in managed care. The proportion of persons who were enrolled in managed care varied by group.

Many older individuals receive long-term care coverage through Medicaid (as well as through their Medicare coverage). Long-term care utilization, for those who need it, is less controllable than other types of care (acute care), and long-term care is thus less amenable to HMO-type coverage. Older Medicaid long-term care patients would therefore tend not to be enrolled in a Medicaid managed care plan. Indeed, only 4.9% of Medicaid enrollees who are served by HMOs are age 65 or older. The majority of Medicaid HMO enrollees are children (51%) and parents (22%).

Under Medicaid, HMOs face the same issues as under Medicare. There is a wide variation in fee-setting practices and in fees among states (Holahan, 1999). In addition, as in the fee-for-service sector, managed care rates in general are quite low (Bruen & Holahan, 1999). As well, risk-adjustment factors have not been well developed, and so biased selection in membership may be a problem. In short, Medicaid has problems enrolling members and maintaining the provision of care for these individuals. This policy has the effect of reducing the availability of care for these populations.

15.8 PAY-FOR-PERFORMANCE INITIATIVES

A number of different pay-for-performance (P4P) models have been proposed and tried in recent years. The Centers for Medicare and Medicaid Services (CMS) have supported a number of demonstration projects to evaluate their effectiveness in improving quality and decreasing costs. The health reform law also calls for a number of additional demonstrations to incorporate value-based purchasing into the payment system.

Basically, P4P links the payment system to the accomplishment of predefined performance measures. These performance measures can contain either positive incentives or disincentives. An example of a positive incentive is to link the amount paid to the provider to the documented achievement of a certain level of preventive services performed (e.g., percentage of women in the practice over age 50 who have received mammography screenings in the last two years). The provider receives higher payment if his/her practice percentage is equal to or greater than the desired, predefined percentage. A disincentive establishes a penalty for the occurrence or nonoccurrence of certain events. For example, Medicare has established a policy that it will no longer pay providers for the increased costs associated with medical errors or hospital-acquired infections. Another area being carefully scrutinized currently is the rate of readmission to hospitals in less than 30 days, especially for the same diagnosis or for diagnoses related to the original admission.

An issue that needs to be carefully considered in the development of incentives and/or disincentives is the potential negative impacts on patients. Will a P4P incentive encourage adverse selection of patients that will assist the provider in reaching the desired goal? How will patients who have serious and complex conditions be treated in a P4P system when the patient interacts with multiple providers in multiple locations. Will a P4P system decrease access to care for the sickest, most vulnerable populations? In the complex, fragmented delivery system, can a P4P model be developed that can accurately and appropriately attribute responsibility for the outcome of care for complex patients?

Pay-for-performance models and demonstration projects have been undertaken and supported by CMS in an effort to transform itself from a passive payer for services delivered to its beneficiaries to an active, value-based purchaser of higher quality, affordable healthcare services. To become a value-based purchaser, CMS is attempting to establish incentives and disincentives designed to change the behavior of providers by linking effective resource utilization and clinical measures to a redesigned payment system, increasing joint clinical and financial accountability in the healthcare system.

When evaluating the transformation of the system to achieve value in the healthcare system, Christianson, Leatherman, & Sutherland (2007), provide a number of issues that require consideration and answers. First, is the goal of the incentive/disincentive to achieve improvement or attainment? If the goal is improvement, then rewarding change may maximize the potential improvements in quality, because the low-performing providers can improve the most. On the other hand, rewarding achievements would tend to focus and reward the providers who were delivering superior care.

The second issue revolves around deciding if the goal is to reward achievement of an absolute value or standard or to achieve a relative rating or percentage of a target. Establishing an absolute value to be achieved can be difficult and expensive to establish the correct benchmark and keep it up to date. It can also be expensive, if most providers surpass the threshold established. A relative rating (such as using quartiles), can be easier to calculate, but may not be very informative if there is very little variation among the providers; if the first quartile and the fourth quartile are clustered close together, then differentiating between them for payment is relatively worthless.

Third, how should risk adjustments or exemptions/exclusions be handled? Risk adjustments are typically undertaken to reflect differences in case mix or severity of patients in a panel or practice. Determining and appropriately measuring the risk and establishing a valid adjustment factor is difficult, or even not applicable to certain metrics (e.g., immunizations). On the other hand, if exemptions or exclusions for certain patients or providers are allowed based on predetermined/prespecified conditions or characteristics, then opportunities for gaming the system are increased.

Another issue encountered in applying P4P criteria to individual physicians is the small sample size of eligible patients or procedures. If a practice has very few patients, procedures, or conditions eligible to be scored in the metric, then a single outlier can significantly impact the results, making them uninformative. As a result, these providers can either be excluded from the P4P system, or multiple years of data combined to achieve larger numbers. A problem with using multiple years is that it may camouflage important changes over time.

When patients see multiple providers, it is especially difficult to obtain outcome measures that can be attributed to an individual provider. This ties into the next issue of obtaining physician engagement to improve care processes: if the physician doesn't see the relevancy to their own activities, it is hard to get him/her motivated to participate and change behavior.

P4P may also have unintended consequences. For example, the selection of the measurement criteria may lead to better documentation rather than an actual improvement in the outcome being measured. Physicians could also either move practices or select patients that are more likely to manage their own care, thereby reducing access to services for certain groups of patients. Providers could also focus on the areas that are included in the incentives and let other areas decline because they are not being measured. Coordination of care could also decrease for patients with multiple conditions, and administrative costs could increase, as additional time is needed to comply with the quality metrics, document care provided, or track rewards to individual providers in a group.

As this discussion indicates, implementing a value-based, pay-for-performance system is not without problems. However, careful evaluation of incentives/disincentives created will enable Medicare and other purchasers to become more prudent purchasers, not just payers.

EXERCISES

1. What populations are covered by Medicare?
2. What are the most important services covered by Medicare Parts A and B?
3. What are the major sources of funding for Medicare Parts A and B?
4. What populations are covered by Medicaid?
5. What services are covered by Medicaid?
6. What is the major source of funding for Medicaid?
7. What is Medigap and what purpose does it serve?
8. Can a Medicare enrollee join a managed care plan, and if so, what premiums does he or she pay?
9. What are the key characteristics of persons without health insurance in the United States?
10. Why can't the Medicare program increase Part A spending on hospital care by applying for funds out of general taxation revenues?
11. What are the goals of Medicare?
12. List five policies for Medicare and identify what goal(s) each addresses.
13. What are the most important problems faced by Medicaid and what policies might be used to help solve them?

BIBLIOGRAPHY

Medicare

2011 Annual Report of the Boards of Trustees of the Federal Hospital Insurance and Federal Supplementary Medical Insurance Trust Funds. https://www.cms.gov/Research-Statistics-Data-and-Systems/Statistics-Trends-and-Reports/ReportsTrustFunds/downloads/tr2011.pdf

Aaron, H. J. (1999). Medicare choice: Good, bad, it all depends. In A. J. Rettenmaier & T. R. Saving (Eds.), *Medicare reform: Issues and answers*. Chicago, IL: University of Chicago Press.

Aaron, H. J., & Reischauer, R. D. (1995). The Medicare reform debate: What is the next step? *Health Affairs, 14,*(4), 8–30.

American Association of Retired Persons. (1999). *Out-of-pocket spending on health care by Medicare beneficiaries age 65 and older: 1999 projections*. Washington, DC: American Association of Retired Persons.

American Medical Association. (2000). *Medicare RBRVS*. Chicago, IL: American Medical Association.

Baker, L. C. (1997). The effect of HMOs on fee-for-service health care expenditures: Evidence from Medicare. *Journal of Health Economics, 16,* 453–481.

Berenson, R., & Holahan, J. (1992). Sources of growth in Medicare physician expenditures. *JAMA, 267,* 687–691.

Biles B., Arnold, G., & Guterman, S. (2011). Medicare Advantage in the era of health reform: Progress in leveling the playing field. *Issue Brief (Commonwealth Fund), 5,* 1–14.

Birnbaum, M., & Patchias, E. M. (2010). Measuring coverage for seniors in Medicare Part A and estimating the cost of making it universal. *Journal of Health Politics, Policy & Law, 35*(1), 49–62.

Blustein, J. (2000). Drug coverage and drug purchases by Medicare beneficiaries with hypertension. *Health Affairs, 19,*(2), 219–230.

Briesacher, B. A., Ross-Degnan, D., Wagner, A. K., Fouayzi, H., Zhang, F., Gurwitz, J. H., & Soumerai, S. B. (2010). Out-of-pocket burden of health care spending and the adequacy of the Medicare Part D low-income subsidy. *Medical Care, 48*(6), 503–509.

Brown, R. S., Clement, D. G., Hill, J. W., Retchin, S. M., & Bergeron, J. W. (1993). Do health maintenance organizations work for Medicare? *Health Care Financing Review, 15*(1), 7–23.

Brunt, C. S., & Jensen, G. A. (2010). Medicare Part B reimbursement and the perceived quality of physician care. *International Journal of Health Care Finance & Economics, 10*(2), 149–170.

Congressional Budget Office. (1983). *Changing the structure of Medicare benefits.* Washington, DC: Congressional Budget Office.

Cutler, D. M. (1999). What does Medicare spending buy us? In A. J. Rettenmaier & T. R. Saving (Eds.), *Medicare reform: Issues and answers.* Chicago, IL: University of Chicago Press.

Cutler, D. M. (2000). Walking the tightrope on Medicare reform. *Journal of Economic Perspectives, 14,* 45–56.

Davis, K., & Rowland, D. (1984). Medicare financing reform: A new Medicare premium. *Milbank Quarterly, 62,* 300–316.

Davis, M., Poisal, J., Chulis, G., Zarabozo, C., & Cooper, B. (1999). Prescription drug coverage, utilization, and spending among Medicare beneficiaries. *Health Affairs, 18*(1), 231–243.

DeNavas-Walt, Proctor, & Smith, 2011.

Dunn, A. (2010). The value of coverage in the Medicare Advantage insurance market. *Journal of Health Economics, 29*(6), 839–855.

Elliott, M. N., Haviland, A. M., Orr, N., Hambarsoomian, K., & Cleary, P. D. (2011). How do the experiences of Medicare beneficiary subgroups differ between managed care and original Medicare? *Health Services Research, 46,* 1039–1058.

Ettner, S. L. (1995). The opportunity costs of elder care. *Journal of Human Resources, 31,* 189–205.

Ettner, S. L. (1997). Adverse selection and the purchase of Medigap insurance by the elderly. *Journal of Health Economics, 16,* 543–562.

Feder, J. (1995/1996). Some thoughts on the future of Medicare. *Inquiry, 32,* 376–378.

Friedman, B., & Jiang, H. J. (2010). Do Medicare Advantage enrollees tend to be admitted to hospitals with better or worse outcomes compared with fee-for-service enrollees? *International Journal of Health Care Finance & Economics, 10*(2), 171–185.

Fuchs, V. R. (2000). Medicare reform: The larger picture. *Journal of Economic Perspectives, 14,* 57–70.

Gillis, K. D., & Lee, D. W. (1997). Medicare, access, and physicians' willingness to accept new Medicare patients. *Quarterly Review of Economics and Finance, 37,* 579–603.

Ginsburg, P. B., & Moon, M. (1984). An introduction to the Medicare financing problem. *Milbank Quarterly, 62,* 167–182.

Gluck, M. A. 1999). *Medicare prescription drug benefit.* Medicare Brief no. 1. Washington, DC: National Academy of Social Insurance.

Gold, M. (2009). Medicare's private plans: A report card on Medicare Advantage. *Health Affairs, 28*(1), w41–w54.

Goldberg, H. B., Delargy, D., Schmitz, R. J., Moore, T., & Wrobel, M. (1999). *Case mix adjustment for a national home health prospective payment system: Second interim report.* Cambridge, MA: Abt Associates.

Goody, B., Friedman, M. A., & Sobaski, W. (1994). New directions for Medicare payment systems. *Health Care Financing Review, 16*(2), 1–11.

Hariri, S., Bozic, K. J., O'Connor, M. I., & Rubas, H. E. H. (2008). Medicare Part B: Physician participation options. *Journal of Bone & Joint Surgery—American Volume, 90*(10), 2282–2291.

Health Care Financing Administration. (1995). *Medicare and Medicaid statistical supplement.* Baltimore, MD: Health Care Financing Administration.

Health Care Financing Administration. (1998). *The profile of Medicare: Chart book 1998.* Baltimore, MD: Health Care Financing Administration.

Health Care Financing Administration. (2000, April 7). Medicare program prospective payment system for hospital outpatient services; Final rule. *Federal Register, 65*(68) 18433–18820.

Hernandez, J. S. (2008). The ABCs of Medicare Advantage. *Journal of Ahima, 79*(11), 82–84.

Hofstra, P., & Zupko, K. (2009). Medicare Part C: A basic primer and some practical advice about Medicare private fee-for-service plans. *Journal of Medical Practice Management, 24*(5), 297–299.

Hsiao, W. C., & Kelly, N. L. (1984). Medicare benefits: A reassessment. *Milbank Quarterly, 62,* 207–229.

Hsiao, W. C., Dunn, D. L., & Verrilli, D. K. (1993). Assessing the implementation of physician payment reform. *New England Journal of Medicine, 328,* 928–933.

Iglehart, J. K. (1999). The American health care system—Medicare. *New England Journal of Medicine, 340,* 327–332.

Kominski, G. F., & Long, S. H. (1997). Medicare's disproportionate share adjustment and the cost of low-income patients. *Journal of Health Economics, 16,* 177–190.

Lee, A. J., & Mitchell, J. B. (1994). Physician reaction to price changes: An episode-of-care analysis. *Health Care Financing Review, 16*(2), 65–83.

Levit, K., Cowan, C., Lazenby, H., Sensenig, A., McDonnell, P., Stiller, J., Martin, A., & the Health Accounts Team. (2000). Health spending in 1998: Signals of change. *Health Affairs, 19*(1), 124–132.

Liu, K., Gage, B., Harvell, J., Stevenson, D., & Brennan, N. (1999). *Medicare's post-acute care benefit.* Washington, DC: Urban Institute.

Long, S. H., & Smeeding, T. M. (1984). Alternative Medicare financing sources. *Milbank Quarterly, 62,* 325–348.

Luft, H. S. (1984). On the use of vouchers for Medicare. *Milbank Quarterly, 62,* 237–250.

McCarthy, I. M., & Tchernis, R. (2010). Search costs and Medicare plan choice. *Health Economics, 19*(10), 1142–1165.

McClellan, M. (2000). Medicare reform: Fundamental problems, incremental steps. *Journal of Economic Perspectives, 14,* 21–44.

McGuire, T. G., Newhouse, J. P., & Sinaiko, A. D. (2011). An economic history of Medicare Part C. *Milbank Quarterly, 89,* 289–332.

Moon, M., Gage, B., & Evans, A. (1997). *An examination of key Medicare provisions in the Balanced Budget Act of 1997.* Washington, DC: Urban Institute.

Morrison, L. (2008). Medicare from A to D: What every nephrologist needs to know. *Clinical Journal of the American Society of Nephrology: CJASN, 3*(3), 899–904.

Petrie, J. T. (1992). Overview of the Medicare program. *Health Care Financing Review Annual Supplement,* 1–22.

Potetz, L., Cubanski, J., & Neuman, T. (2011). *Medicare spending and financing: A primer.* Menlo Park CA: The Henry J. Kaiser Family Foundation.

Pope, G. C., Adamache, K. W., Walsh, E. C., & Khandker, R. K. . (1998). Evaluating alternative risk adjusters for Medicare. *Health Care Financing Review, 20,* 109–129.

Rice, T., & Bernstein, J. (1999). *Supplemental health insurance for Medicare beneficiaries.* Medicare Brief. no. 6. Washington, DC: National Academy of Social Insurance.

Rice, T., & McCall, N. (1985). The extent of ownership and the characteristics of Medicare supplemental policies. *Inquiry, 22,* 188–200.

Rice, T., Graham, M. L., & Fox, P. D. (1997). The impact of policy standardization on the Medigap market. *Inquiry, 34,* 106–116.

Saving, T. R. (2000). Making the transition to prepaid Medicare. *Journal of Economic Perspectives, 14,* 85–98.

Schaum, K. D. (2008). Copayment collection is not an option! *Advances in Skin & Wound Care, 21*(1), 23–28.

Shih, Y. T. (1999). Effect of insurance on prescription drug use by ESRD beneficiaries. *Health Care Financing Review, 20*(3), 39–54.

Smits, H. L., Feder, J., & Scanlon, W. (1982). Medicare's nursing home benefit: Variations in interpretation. *New England Journal of Medicine, 307,* 855–862.

Soumerai, S., & Ross-Degnan, D. (1999). Inadequate prescription drug coverage for Medicare enrollees. *New England Journal of Medicine, 340,* 722–728.

U.S. Department of Health and Human Services. (1983). *The Medicare and Medicaid data book.* HCFA publication no. 03156. Baltimore, MD: Health Care Financing Administration.

U.S. Department of Health and Human Services. (1993). *Medicare and Medicaid statistical supplement.* Baltimore, MD: U.S. Department of Health and Human Services.

U.S. General Accounting Office. (1999). *Medicare and budget surpluses.* Publication no. GAO/TAIMD/HEHS-99–113. Washington, DC: Government Accounting Office.

U.S. Government Accounting Office. (1995). *Medicare managed care.* Document no. GAO/HEHS96–21. Washington, DC: Government Accounting Office.

Wolkstein, I. (1984). Medicare's financial status: How did we get here? *Milbank Quarterly, 62,* 183–206.

Wood, S., Hanoch, Y., Barnes, A., Liu, P. J., Cummings, J., Bhattacharya, C., & Rice, T. (2011). Numeracy and Medicare Part D: The importance of choice and literacy for numbers in optimizing decision making for Medicare's prescription drug program. *Psychology & Aging, 26*(2), 295–307.

Medicaid

Baicker, K., & Finkelstein, A. (2011). The effects of Medicaid coverage—Learning from the Oregon experiment. *New England Journal of Medicine, 365*(8), 683–685.

Battistella, R. M. (1989). National health insurance: Dilemmas and opportunities. *Hospital and Health Services Administration, 34,* 139–156.

Bisgaier, J., & Rhodes, K. V. (2011). Auditing access to specialty care for children with public insurance. *New England Journal of Medicine, 364*(24), 2324–2333.

Blumberg, L. J., Dubay, L., & Norton, S. A. (2000). Did the Medicaid expansions for children displace private insurance? An analysis using the SIPP. *Journal of Health Economics, 19,* 33–60.

Bradford, W. D. (1995). The effects of a relative value reimbursement scheme on the medical market: Lessons from Medicaid. *Review of Industrial Organization, 10,* 511–532.

Brecher, C., & Knickman, J. (1985). A reconsideration of long-term-care policy. *Journal of Health Politics, Policy, and Law, 10,* 245–272.

Bruen, B., & Holahan, J. (1999). *Slow growth in Medicaid spending continues in 1997.* Issue paper. Washington, DC: Kaiser Commission on Medicaid and the Uninsured.

Buchanan, R. J. (1983). Medicaid cost containment: Prospective reimbursement for long-term care. *Inquiry, 20,* 334–342.

Congressional Budget Office. (1981). *Medicaid: Choices for 1982 and beyond.* Washington, DC: Congressional Budget Office.

Cook, P. J., Parnell, A. M., Moore, M. J., & Pagnini, D. (1999). The effects of short-term variation in abortion funding on pregnancy outcomes. *Journal of Health Economics, 18,* 241–257.

Currie, J., & Gruber, J. (1996a). Saving babies: The efficacy and cost of recent changes in the Medicaid eligibility of pregnant women. *Journal of Political Economy, 104,* 1263–1293.

Currie, J., & Gruber, J. (1996b). Health insurance eligibility, utilization of medical care and child health. *Quarterly Journal of Economics, 110,* 431–464.

Cutler, D. M., & Gruber, J. (1996a). The effect of Medicaid expansions on public insurance, private insurance, and redistribution. *American Economic Review, 86,* 378–383.

Cutler, D. M., & Gruber, J. (1996b). Does public insurance crowd out private insurance? *Quarterly Journal of Economics, 110,* 391–426.

Cutler, D. M., & Gruber, J. (1996c). The effect of Medicaid expansions on public insurance, private insurance, and redistribution. *American Economic Review, 86*(2), 378–383.

Davidoff, A., Blumberg, L., & Nichols, L. (2005). State health insurance market reforms and access to insurance for high-risk employees. *Journal of Health Economics, 24*(4), 725–750.

Davis, K. (1989). National health insurance: A proposal. *American Economic Review, 79,* 349–352.

Davis, K., & Schoen, C. (1978). *Health and the war on poverty.* Washington, DC: Brookings Institution.

Ettner, S. L. (1997). Medicaid participation among the eligible elderly. *Journal of Policy Analysis and Management, 16*(2), 237–255.

Fairbrother, G., Madhavan, G., Goudie, A., Watring, J., Sebastian, R. A., Ranbom, L., & Simpson, L. A. (2011). Reporting on continuity of coverage for children in Medicaid and CHIP: What states can learn from monitoring continuity and duration of coverage. *Academic pediatrics, 11*(4), 318–325.

Fossett, J. W., & Peterson, J. A. (1989). Physician supply and Medicaid participation. *Medical Care, 27*, 386–396.

Fox, H. G., Wicks, L. B., & Newacheck, P. W. (1993). State Medicaid health maintenance organization policies and special-needs children. *Health Care Financing Review, 15*(1), 25–37.

Friedman, B., Berdahl, T., Simpson, L. A., McCormick, M. C., Owens, P. L., Andrews, R., & Romano, P. S. (2011). Annual report on health care for children and youth in the United States: Focus on trends in hospital use and quality. *Academic Pediatrics, 11*(4), 263–279.

Gilmer, T. P., & Kronick, R. G. (2011). Differences in the volume of services and in prices drive big variations in Medicaid spending among US states and regions. *Health Affairs, 30*(7), 1316–1324.

Gold, M., Sparer, M., & Chu, K. (1996). Medicaid managed care: Lessons from five states. *Health Affairs, 15*(3), 153–166.

Gruber, J. (1997). Medicaid and uninsured women and children. *Journal of Economic Perspectives, 11*, 199–208.

Gruber, J., Adams, K., & Newhouse, J. P. (1997). Physician fee policy and Medicaid program costs. *Journal of Human Resources, 32*, 611–634.

Gurny, P., Baugh, D. K., & Reilly, T. W. (1992). Payment, administration, and financing of the Medicaid program. *Health Care Financing Review Annual Supplement*, 285–301.

Harrington, C., & Swan, J. H. (1984). Medicaid nursing home reimbursement policies, rates and expenditures. *Health Care Financing Review, 6*(1), 39–49.

Health Care Financing Administration. (2000). *A profile of Medicaid.* Retrieved from http://www.hcfa.gov/ stats/2Tchartbk.pdf

Hemmeter, J. (2011). Health-related unmet needs of supplemental security income youth after the age-18 redetermination. *Health Services Research, 46*, 1224–1242.

Holahan, J. (1975). *Financing health care for the poor.* Lexington, MA: Lexington.

Holahan, J. (1999). *Medicaid managed care payment methods and capitation rates.* Washington, DC: Urban Institute.

Holahan J. & Chen V. (2011). Changes in health insurance coverage in the great recession, 2007-2010. *Issue Paper.* Kaiser Commission on Medicaid and the Uninsured, Kaiser Family Foundation.

Huesch, M. D. (2011). Association between type of health insurance and elective cesarean deliveries: New Jersey, 2004–2007. *American Journal of Public Health, 101*(11), e1–e7.

Iglehart, J. K. (1999). The American health care system—Medicaid. *New England Journal of Medicine, 340*, 403–408.

Joyce, T. (1999). Impact of augmented prenatal care on birth outcomes of Medicaid recipients in New York City. *Journal of Health Economics, 18*, 31–67.

Ku, L., & Coughlin, T. A. (1995). Medicaid disproportionate share and other special financing programs. *Health Care Financing Review, 16*(3), 27–54.

Lee, J. (2011). Restraining Medicaid. More states to cut provider payments: Kaiser study. *Modern Healthcare, 41*(44), 14.

Levincon, A., & Ullman, F. (1998). Medicaid managed care and infant health. *Journal of Health Economics, 17*, 351–368.

Levy, D. E., Rigotti, N. A., & Winickoff, J. P. (2011). Medicaid expenditures for children living with smokers. *BMC Health Services Research, 11*, 125.

Margolis, L. H., Mayer, M., Clark, K. A., & Farel, A. M. (2011). Associations between state economic and health systems capacities and service use by children with special health care needs. *Maternal & Child Health Journal, 15*(6), 713–721.

Maxwell, A. (2011). Access to specialty care for children with public insurance. *New England Journal of Medicine, 365*(11), 1060; author reply, 1060.

McCue, M. J., & Bailit, M. H. (2011). Assessing the financial health of Medicaid managed care plans and the quality of patient care they provide. *Issue Brief (Commonwealth Fund), 11*, 1–16.

Medicare Payment Advisory Commission. (2000). *Report to Congress.* Washington, DC: Medicare Payment Advisory Commission.

Meiners, M. R. (1983). The case for long-term care insurance. *Health Affairs, 2*(2), 55–79.

Miller, M. E., & Gengler, D. J. (1993). Medicaid case management: Kentucky's patient access and care program. *Health Care Financing Review, 15*(1), 55–69.

Oberlander, J. (2011). Health care policy in an age of austerity. *New England Journal of Medicine, 365*(12), 1075–1077.

Ortego, L. S. (2011). Is it unethical to have a policy for Medicaid-enrolled patients that allows termination of the relationship when the patient does not show up or call? *Journal of the American Dental Association, 142*(7), 858–859.

Rask, K. N., & Rask, K. J. (2000). Public insurance substituting for private insurance: New evidence regarding public hospitals, uncompensated care funds, and Medicaid. *Journal of Health Economics, 19*, 1–31.

Rhodes, K. V., & Bisgaier, J. (2011). Limitations in access to dental and medical specialty care for publicly insured children. *LDI Issue Brief, 16*(7), 1–4.

Ricketts, T.C., III, (2011). New models of health care payment and delivery. *North Carolina Medical Journal, 72*(3), 197–200.

Rieselbach, R. E., & Kellermann, A. L. (2011). A model health care delivery system for Medicaid. *New England Journal of Medicine, 364*(26), 2476–2478.

Rosenbaum, S. (2011a). Equal access for Medicaid beneficiaries—The Supreme Court and the Douglas cases. *New England Journal of Medicine, 365*(24), 2245–2247.

Rosenbaum, S. (2011b). Medicaid and access to health care—A proposal for continued inaction? *New England Journal of Medicine, 365*(2), 102–104.

Rowland, D. (1995). Medicaid at 30: New challenges for the nation's safety net. *JAMA, 274*, 271–273.

Saunders, J. (2011). Child health screenings under Medicaid. *NCSL Legisbrief, 19*(43), 1–2.

Schneiderman, L. J. (2011). Rationing just medical care. *American Journal of Bioethics, 11*(7), 7–14.

Shore-Sheppard, L., Buchmueller, T. C., & Jensen, G. A. (2000). Medicaid and crowding out of private insurance: A reexamination using firm level data. *Journal of Health Economics, 19*, 61–91.

Showalter, M. H. (1997). Physicians' cost shifting behavior: Medicaid versus other patients. *Contemporary Economic Policy, 15*, 74–84.

Smith, S. (2011). Transforming the Medicaid transformation . . . or just new packaging? *Journal of the Arkansas Medical Society, 108*(2), 28.

Sommers, B. D., & Epstein, A. M. (2011). Why states are so miffed about Medicaid—Economics, politics, and the "woodwork effect." *New England Journal of Medicine, 365*(2), 100–102.

Sonnenfeld, N., Decker, S. L., & Schappert, S. M. (2011). Trends in emergency department visits among Medicaid patients. *JAMA, 306*(11), 1202–1203; author reply, 1203.

Strumpf, E. (2011). Medicaid's effect on single women's labor supply: Evidence from the introduction of Medicaid. *Journal of Health Economics, 30*(3), 531–548.

Stuart, B. (1972). Equity and Medicaid. *Journal of Human Resources, 7*, 152–178.

Stuart, B., & Zacker, C. (1999). Who bears the burden of Medicaid drug copayment policies? *Health Affairs, 18*(2), 201–212.

Stuart, B., Briesacher, B. A., Ahern, F., Kidder, D., Zacker, C., Erwin, G., ..., & Fahlman, C. (1999). Drug use and prescribing problems in four state Medicaid programs. *Health Care Financing Review, 20*(2), 63–75.

Subramanian, S. (2011). Impact of Medicaid copayments on patients with cancer: Lessons for Medicaid expansion under health reform. *Medical Care, 49*(9), 842–847.

Tallon, J. R., & Rowland, D. (1995). Federal dollars and state flexibility. *Inquiry, 32*, 235–240.

Thompson, F. J. (2011). The Medicaid platform: Can the termites be kept at bay? *Journal of Health Politics, Policy & Law, 36*(3), 549–554.

Tudor, C. G. (1995). Medicaid expenditures and state responses. *Health Care Financing Review, 16*(3), 1–10.

Wade, M., & Berg, S. (1995). Causes of Medicaid expenditure growth. *Health Care Financing Review, 16*(3), 11–25.

Wilensky, G. R. (2011). Improving value in Medicaid. *Healthcare Financial Management, 65*(11), 34, 36.

Wycoff, P. G. (1985). Medicaid: Federalism and the Reagan budget proposals. *Economic Commentary of the Reserve Bank of Cleveland,* (August 15).

Yelowitz, A. S. (1998). Why did the SSI-disabled program grow so much? Disentangling the effect of Medicaid. *Journal of Health Economics, 17,* 321–349.

Yu, H., Dick, A. W., & Szilagyi, P. G. (2008). Does public insurance provide better financial protection against rising health care costs for families of children with special health care needs? *Medical Care, 46*(10), 1064–1070.

Dual Eligible

Atherly, A., & Dowd, B. E. (2005). Effect of Medicare advantage payments on dually eligible Medicare beneficiaries. *Health Care Financing Review, 26*(3), 93–104.

Clemans-Cope, L., & Waidmann, T. (2011). Improving care for dual eligibles through innovations in financing. *New England Journal of Medicine, 365*(11), e21.

Deshpande, M. (2005). The implications of the Medicare Modernization Act for dual eligibles. *American Journal of Geriatric Cardiology, 14*(6), 298–300.

Koroukian, S. M., Dahman, B., Copeland, G., & Bradley, C. J. (2010). The utility of the state buy-in variable in the Medicare denominator file to identify dually eligible Medicare-Medicaid beneficiaries: A validation study. *Health Services Research, 45*(1), 265–282.

Kuttner, R. (1999). The American health care system. Health insurance coverage. *New England Journal of Medicine, 340*(2), 163–168.

Lied, T. R., & Haffer, S. C. (2004). Health status of dually eligible beneficiaries in managed care plans. *Health Care Financing Review, 25*(4), 59–74.

Milligan, C. J., Jr., & Woodcock, C. H. (2008a). Coordinating care for dual eligibles: Options for linking state Medicaid programs with Medicare Advantage Special Needs Plans. *Issue Brief (Commonwealth Fund), 32,* 1–12.

Milligan, C. J., Jr., & Woodcock, C. H. (2008b). Medicare Advantage Special Needs Plans for dual eligibles: A primer. *Issue Brief (Commonwealth Fund), 31,* 1–12.

Nemore, P. (2004). Dual eligibles. *Issue Brief (Center for Medicare Education), 5*(2), 1–6.

Ryan, J., & Super, N. (2003). Dually eligible for Medicare and Medicaid: Two for one or double jeopardy? *Issue Brief/National Health Policy Forum,* (794), 1–24.

Thorpe, K. E., & Philyaw, M. (2010). Impact of health care reform on Medicare and dual Medicare-Medicaid beneficiaries. *Cancer Journal, 16*(6), 584–587.

Uninsured Care

Babu, M. A., Nahed, B. V., Demoya, M. A., & Curry, W. T. (2011). Is trauma transfer influenced by factors other than medical need? An examination of insurance status and transfer in patients with mild head injury. *Neurosurgery, 69*(3), 659–67; discussion, 667.

Barnato, A. E. (2011). The effect of insurance status on mortality and procedure use in critically ill patients: An object lesson in financial incentives. *American Journal of Respiratory & Critical Care Medicine, 184*(7), 750–751.

Birnbaum, H., Naierman, N., Schwartz, M., & Wilson, D. (1979). Focusing the catastrophic illness debate. *Quarterly Review of Economics and Business, 19,* 17–33.

Boukus, E. R., & Cunningham, P. J. (2011). Mixed signals: Trends in Americans' access to medical care, 2007–2010. *Tracking Report,* (25), 1–6.

Cafferata, G. L. (1984). *Private health insurance coverage of the Medicare population.* National Health Care Expenditures Study data preview 18. Rockville, MD: National Center for Health Services Research.

Cleeton, D. (1989). The medical uninsured: A case for market failure. *Public Finance Quarterly 17,* 55–83.

Collins, S. R., Garber, T., & Robertson, R. (2011). Realizing health reform's potential: How the Affordable Care Act is helping young adults stay covered. *Issue Brief (Commonwealth Fund), 5,* 1–26.

De Lew, N., Greenberg, G., & Kinchen, K. (1992). A layman's guide to the U.S. health care system. *Health Care Financing Review, 14*(2), 151–170.

DeLia, D. (2008). A primer on the uninsured and the healthcare safety net in New Jersey. *MD Advisor, 1*(1), 18–23.

DeNavas-Walt, C., Proctor, B. D., & Smith, J. C. (2011). *US Census Bureau, Current Population Reports, P60–239, Income, Poverty, and Health Insurance Coverage in the United States: 2010.* Washington, DC: US Government Printing Office.

DeNavas-Walt, C., Proctor, B. D., & Smith, J. C. (2010). *US Census Bureau, Current Population Reports, P60–238, Income, Poverty, and Health Insurance Coverage in the United States: 2010.* Washington, DC: US Government Printing Office.

Doty, M. M., Collins, S. R., Robertson, R., & Garber, T. (2011). Realizing health reform's potential: When unemployed means uninsured: The toll of job loss on health coverage, and how the Affordable Care Act will help. *Issue Brief (Commonwealth Fund), 18,* 1–18.

Ferayorni, A., Sinha, M., & McDonald, F. W. (2011). Health issues among foreign born uninsured children visiting an inner city pediatric emergency department. *Journal of Immigrant & Minority Health, 13*(3), 434–444.

Fronstin, P. (2011). Sources of health insurance and characteristics of the uninsured: Analysis of the March 2011 current population survey. *EBRI Issue Brief,* (362), 1–35.

Granruth, L. B., & Shields, J. J. (2011). Impact of the level of state tax code progressivity on children's health outcomes. *Health & Social Work, 36*(3), 207–215.

Hadley, J., & Feder, J. (1985). Hospital cost shifting and care for the uninsured. *Health Affairs, 4*(3), 67–81.

Hall, M. A. (2011). Access to care provided by better safety net systems for the uninsured: Measuring and conceptualizing adequacy. *Medical Care Research & Review, 68,* 441–461.

Hellander, I. (2011). The deepening crisis in U.S. health care: A review of data. *International Journal of Health Services, 41*(3), 575–586.

Herman, P. M., Rissi, J. J., & Walsh, M. E. (2011). Health insurance status, medical debt, and their impact on access to care in Arizona. *American Journal of Public Health, 101*(8), 1437–1443.

Kapoor, J. R., Kapoor, R., Hellkamp, A. S., Hernandez, A. F., Heidenreich, P. A., & Fonarow, G. C. (2011). Payment source, quality of care, and outcomes in patients hospitalized with heart failure. *Journal of the American College of Cardiology, 58*(14), 1465–1471.

Levit, K. R., Olin, G. L., & Letsch, S. W. (1992). America's health insurance coverage, 1980–91. *Health Care Financing Review, 14*(1), 31–57.

Lyon, S. M., Benson, N. M., Cooke, C. R., Iwashyna, T. J., Ratcliffe, S. J., & Kahn, J. M. (2011). The effect of insurance status on mortality and procedural use in critically ill patients. *American Journal of Respiratory & Critical Care Medicine, 184*(7), 809–815.

Monheit, A. C., & Short, P. F. (1989). Mandating health coverage for working Americans. *Health Affairs, 8*(4), 22–38.

Mulstein, S. (1984). The uninsured and financing of uncompensated care. *Inquiry, 21,* 214–229.

Schlomann, P., Virgin, S., Schmitke, J., & Patros, S. (2011). Hypertension among the uninsured: Tensions and challenges. *Journal of the American Academy of Nurse Practitioners, 23,* 305–313.

Short, P. F., Monheit, A. C., & Beeauregard, K. (1988). *Uninsured Americans: A 1987 profile.* Rockville, MD: National Center for Health Services Research and Health Care Technology Assessment.

Short, P. F., Swartz, K., Uberoi, N., & Graefe, D. (2011). Realizing health reform's potential: Maintaining coverage, affordability, and shared responsibility when income and employment change. *Issue Brief (Commonwealth Fund), 4,* 1–18.

Wilensky, G. (1987). Viable strategies for dealing with the uninsured. *Health Affairs, 6*(1), 33– 46.

Wilensky, G. (1988). Filling the gaps in health insurance. *Health Affairs, 7*(3), 133–149.

Wolinsky, P., Kim, S., & Quackenbush, M. (2011). Does insurance status affect continuity of care for ambulatory patients with operative fractures? *Journal of Bone & Joint Surgery—American Volume, 93*(7), 680–685.

Pay for Performance

Atta, M. G. (2011). Health care reform and pay for performance: Prognosis uncertain. *Nephrology Times, 4*(1), 2–5.

Christianson, J. B., Leatherman, S., & Sutherland, K. (2007). *Paying for quality: Understanding and assessing physician pay-for-performance initiatives.* Princeton, NJ: Robert Wood Johnson Foundation, The Synthesis Project, Issue 13.

Cromwell, J., Trisolini, M. G., Pope, G. C., Mitchell, J. B., & Greenwald, L. M. (2011). *Pay for performance in health care: Methods and approaches.* Research Triangle Park, NC: RTI Press Publications. Retrieved January 26, 2012, from https://www.rti.org/pubs/bk-0002-1103-mitchell.pdf

Hussey, P. S., Ridgely, M. S., & Rosenthal, M. B. (2011). The PROMETHEUS Bundled Payment experiment: Slow start shows problems in implementing new payment models. *Health Affairs, 30*(11), 2116–2124.

Lindenauer, P. K., Remus, D., Roman, S., Rothberg, M. B., Benjamin, E. M., Ma, A., & Bratzler, D. W. (2007). Public reporting and pay for performance in hospital quality improvement. *New England Journal of Medicine, 356*(5), 486–496.

Mullen, K. J., Frank, R. G., & Rosenthal, M. B. (2010). Can you get what you pay for? Pay-for-performance and the quality of healthcare providers. *RAND Journal of Economics, 41*(1), 64–91.

Rosenthal, M. B. (2008). Beyond pay for performance—Emerging models of provider-payment reform. *New England Journal of Medicine, 359*(12), 1197–1200.

Streit, K., & Kelly, W. (2010). Hospital readmissions. *Patient Safety & Quality Healthcare, 7*(2), 38–41.

Van Herck, P., De Smedt, D., Annemans, L., Remmen, R., Rosenthal, M. B., & Sermeus, W. (2010). Systematic review: Effects, design choices, and context of pay-for-performance in health care. *BMC Health Services Research, 10,* 247

Werner, R. M., Kolstad, J. T., Stuart, E. A., & Polsky, D. (2011). The effect of pay-for-performance in hospitals: Lessons for quality improvement. *Health Affairs, 30*(4), 690–698.

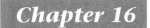

Reform of the Healthcare Market

OBJECTIVES

1. Define the concept of healthcare market reform and explain the need for reform in the context of health care and health insurance markets.

2. Explain the operation of an insurance market that is efficient but not "equitable," in the sense that insurance coverage is not universal.

3. Define each of the following policies and describe their effects in terms of equity and efficiency: premium subsidies, cooperative pools, community rating, mandates, and limits on selection.

4. Define managed care.

5. Describe the key characteristics of a health maintenance organization and explain why it is the prototypical managed care organization.

6. Explain how consumer and provider incentives work to achieve cost reduction in a managed care environment.

7. Define *selection bias* and explain how it might cause an HMO to misleadingly appear more efficient than fee-for-service healthcare provision.

8. Compare the effects of HMOs with the effects of fee-for-service on resource use and quality of care.

9. Explain the conceptual role of consumer sovereignty in hospital markets and identify several reasons why early attempts to achieve it were controversial.

10. Distinguish between employer and individual use of information on health plan performance.

16.1 INTRODUCTION

Health reform is a term that has been applied to insurance and healthcare markets, as well as to the total constellation of health services. In the case of insurance markets, the term refers to specific ways to make the markets perform more like a competitive market, such as by setting rules to prevent insurers from engaging in "biased risk selection," a key factor in market failure, and trying to ensure that insurance is available at a "reasonable" price to those who want it.

In the case of the healthcare market, the main goal of reform has been to increase consumer choice (i.e., to make the healthcare markets more sensitive to consumer rather than provider demands). One of the key efforts has been to increase the degree of competition so that the markets work more like the textbook model of a competitive market.

A competitive market has a number of specific characteristics that impact its performance and efficiency. For one, a competitive market contains a large number of buyers and sellers, with each acting independently. This characteristic means that no one buyer or seller can individually impact the market for the product or service. The interaction of buyers and sellers in the market determine the price and quantity that will result in market equilibrium. A supplier can sell all desired quantity of his/her product or service at the established market price. All suppliers are providing homogenous products. Both buyers and sellers possess complete information about the market. Consumer sovereignty prevails in a competitive market, with consumer preferences determining the services offered in the market.

The goals that market reforms seek to achieve include equity and efficiency. The insurance market reforms have focused largely on equity (i.e., making insurance affordable to those who want it). Possible strategies include subsidies for high-risk consumers. The reforms are only secondarily concerned with increasing provider efficiency or consumer choice. Healthcare market reforms have focused on efficiency—on making the markets more like the competitive ideal.

This chapter examines reforms in healthcare markets and insurance markets and considers the integration of the insurance and healthcare delivery functions into managed care. Section 16.2 reviews insurance market reforms, focusing on alternative mechanisms that have been proposed to make the insurance markets more sensitive to consumer wants. Section 16.3 looks at the role of managed care in changing provider and buyer incentives to promote greater efficiency and limit cost increases. Finally, Section 16.4 describes some of the developments in information and consumer orientation that have affected healthcare markets.

16.2 INSURANCE MARKET REFORM

16.2.1 The Need for Reform

The performance of insurance markets can be judged from the vantage point of efficiency or equity. In looking at economic efficiency performance criteria, the essential question being asked is whether an optimal degree of risk is being shifted by consumers to insurers. This degree is related to the value of risk shifting to the consumers and the cost of risk shifting to insurers. If individuals are willing to pay for greater amounts of coverage (e.g., coverage for more expensive services), and there are insurers who are willing to provide this coverage at the desired price, but there are some impediments to the shifting of the risks so that it does not take place, then the degree of insurance coverage is not optimal. By the same token, if the value to consumers of shifting additional risks is low (below the cost to insurers of accepting these risks), but consumers purchase insurance anyway because of subsidized out-of-pocket prices or lack of good information, then an excess of coverage will result.

Under these conditions, an efficient degree of coverage may mean no coverage at all for healthcare expenditures. If individuals value risk shifting less than they do the cost of insurance, then they will simply not insure. However, these individuals may be very high risk and/or low-income individuals, or may work for small companies, and other society members may think it is inequitable for these individuals to go without insurance coverage. On the grounds of equity, it could be decided that something should be done to remedy the situation. This section will examine the causes of market failure in insurance markets and the remedies that have been proposed. The analysis using a simple economic model to bring out the essential features of insurance market failure and market reform is presented.

16.2.2 The Basic Model

A basic model of a health insurance market is presented, in which there are seven individuals, each with a given degree of risk of being ill. The expected loss for each of these individuals is shown in Table 16-1. Individual 1, the least healthy of the lot, has an expected loss of $120; individual 2 has an expected loss of $80; and so on.

The assumptions about the demand for insurance are now introduced. Each individual has a certain willingness to pay for health insurance coverage. Individual 1 is willing to pay $120, which would indicate that he or she is risk neutral (i.e., puts no additional value on the size of the loss). Individual 2 is willing to pay $100 for coverage, individual 3 is willing to pay $90, and so on. Note that individual 1 might be a high-risk person with limited means to pay for health insurance.

In addition to the individuals' demands, the personal characteristics or circumstances that will affect the insurance market in a systematic way are specified. One such characteristic is age. In this example, two separate age groups are specified—individuals older than 50 and individuals 50 or younger. In general, the expectation is that an individual whose age is above 50 will have greater expected healthcare costs because of poorer health status. Age is a piece of information that might be used by insurers to set premium rates.

Also specified in this example is the individuals' work circumstances, as these are a prime determinant of the cost of providing health insurance and thus of the loading charge. It costs less to provide insurance coverage to individuals in a large group than to individuals who are employed by small companies or who are not employed at all. In this example, it is assumed that it costs $10 to supply insurance coverage to individuals in a large group and $30 to individuals in smaller employment groups or to those who must purchase insurance individually. With regard to the supply side of the market, it is assumed that there is a single supplier. This supplier knows the risk for each

Table 16-1　The Value and Price of Insurance for Individuals

	Individual						
	1	2	3	4	5	6	7
Willingness to pay for insurance coverage (dollars)	$120.00	$100.00	$90.00	$80.00	$70.00	$60.00	$50.00
Expected loss due to illness	$120.00	$80.00	$70.00	$60.00	$50.00	$40.00	$30.00
Age	>50	>50	>50	<50	<50	<50	<50
Employment group type (N = no group, L = large group, S = small group)	N	L	L	L	L	L	S
Cost of administering insurance in absence of pool membership	$30.00	$10.00	$10.00	$10.00	$10.00	$10.00	$30.00
Model 1 prices (experience rating in absence of pool membership)	$150.00	$90.00	$80.00	$70.00	$60.00	$50.00	$60.00
Model 2 prices (complete information asymmetry, first round)	$80.00	$80.00	$80.00	$80.00	$80.00	$80.00	$80.00
Model 3 prices (25 percent subsidy provided to all individuals, experience rating, and information symmetry)	$112.50	$67.50	$60.00	$52.50	$45.00	$37.50	$45.00

person (a situation referred to as *information symmetry*). The supplier sets a price for each person based strictly on his or her expected loss plus the cost of administration (i.e., the supplier engages in experience rating). Thus, for individual 1, the price will be $150 (the expected loss plus the $30 administrative cost). It is also assumed that the insurer has sufficient capacity to insure all consumers who are willing to shift their risks.

The conclusions of this model regarding the availability of insurance can now be drawn. Each individual will purchase insurance as long as the premium rate is less than or equal to what the individual is willing to pay. In our model, individuals 1 and 7 are not willing to pay up to the premium rates that would be charged by the insurer. Individuals 2 through 6 will obtain insurance at the given premium rates. For all individuals, the outcome is the result of rational decisions. Further, this outcome is economically efficient, in that the net benefits from insurance coverage are maximized. If any additional insurance coverage was secured, the result (given the assumptions in this example) would be a net social loss.

However, just because the outcome is economically efficient does not mean that it is "fair" or even "socially acceptable." All individuals in society (1 through 7) may agree that this outcome is unacceptable and that some solution must be found to ensure that all individuals have some degree of coverage. The focus now is on a number of these solutions in subsequent sections of this chapter. However, first, the focus is on one of the critical assumptions of this analysis—the assumption of information symmetry. There is considerable literature on what happens when this assumption does not hold. This simple model will be changed to take the assumption of information asymmetry into account.

16.2.3 Information Asymmetry and Adverse Selection

In a state of information asymmetry, one group of individuals (potentially) engaged in a transaction have better information than another group (potentially) engaged in the transaction. Such a situation can lead to market failure, such that a transaction benefiting both parties never actually takes place. To see how market failure might occur, focus on the previous model, except that it is now assumed that information asymmetry exists. In this case, the information is about the expected loss of the potential purchasers of health insurance. The assumption made is that the consumers have full information about their risks, but the insurer knows nothing about the health status and risks of individual consumers; it only knows about the risks of the entire population.

Given this assumption, the insurer cannot distinguish among insureds in terms of their health status, and it will therefore have to charge each insured the same premium. In total, expected costs are $450, and administrative costs are still the same, $110 for all individuals. Therefore, the insurer must collect $560, or $80 per person. Remember, it is assumed that the insurer has no way of distinguishing among individuals with regard to their risk.

At a price of $80 per person, only four individuals will insure, as the price exceeds the willingness to pay for the other potential insureds. If this situation occurs, then the expected loss per person will be determined by the loss experience of the members of the group who remain in the market. The market will not even insure individuals 1 through 4 because with the other members dropping out the price will have to increase to $97.50 to cover the cost of insuring these individuals. Indeed, the entire market can eventually disappear as people successively drop out. It should be noted that, except for individual 1, each individual would be willing to pay for the cost of his or her insurance. However, the insurer has no way of finding out each person's risk, and so it must charge a group rate.

16.2.4 Underwriting and Group Rating

The phenomenon of adverse selection occurs in extreme cases of information asymmetry. In fact, insurers or underwriters have numerous ways of distinguishing between high- and low-risk insureds. They know, or can obtain information on, many characteristics associated with the risk of loss, such as age, gender, and employment (Giacomini, Luft, & Robinson, 1995). Insurers can also resort to physical exams and tests to determine if individuals have certain conditions that might lead to costly health care. In addition, they have access to the past health records of their potential insureds, and these are often good predictors of future usage. Based on such risk-related information, rates can be set that reflect individual expected costs. Insurers do not have to know exactly how much each person will spend on health care; they must only be able to form separate risk pools and estimate average costs in each pool.

In cases in which there are large groups, insurers need only predict the experience of the entire group. For very large groups, healthcare costs are quite predictable, and therefore information asymmetry does not pose a problem. Indeed, many large employers have realized this and so they self-insure. Of course, this does not solve the problem of those who are not members of large groups.

Nevertheless, these phenomena raise the issue of how relevant adverse selection is. Certainly, if information on projected utilization was not available to insurers, this would be a main problem in the market. But the main problem does not seem to be an absence of information; rather it appears to be what happens when insurers *do* have accurate information about the projected utilization of potential insureds, that is, when they can set very high rates that consumers cannot afford (i.e., are not willing to pay). This leads to a situation in which some individuals are selectively excluded from the insurance market. This situation, called "preferred risk selection," will be discussed in subsequent sections.

16.2.5 Subsidies

The absence of insurance coverage can come about in markets with information symmetry and information asymmetry. Attention is now focused on the former, that is, when there is complete information on the part of both groups, the insurers and the insureds. In Section 16.2.2, it was concluded (under assumed conditions in the example) that two individuals—1 and 7—would not insure. It was noted that this situation, while efficient, might not be considered equitable. If this is the case, some solution would need to be devised that would increase the amount of insurance purchased by the individuals who do not have insurance.

For the moment, retain faith in the market as a mechanism for ensuring that individuals have access to health care when they get sick. At the same time, the policy goal of total population insurance coverage is to be achieved. However, because the "unfettered" market excludes some individuals, a technique must be devised to allow all individuals to obtain insurance coverage. One such technique, widely used in the United States, is an insurance premium subsidy provided by government to individuals who purchase insurance. An example of such a subsidy is the income tax deduction for employer-paid health insurance premiums. Such a deduction reduces the cost of the premium by the individual's personal income tax rate. Some states provide subsidies directly to smaller employers in order to induce them to purchase health insurance for their employees.

In this example, a subsidy of 25% of the premium paid by the individual is now introduced. In this case, each person pays 25% less than before. The postsubsidy premium rates for each individual are shown in Table 16-1. Under initial assumption of experience rating, individual 1 now pays $112.50

(three-quarters of what was paid before), individual 2 pays $67.50, and so on. In this case, all individuals will purchase insurance. The subsidy is successful in achieving full coverage.

However, the postsubsidy situation may not be efficient from a social point of view. In those cases in which the cost of insuring exceeds the individual's willingness to pay in the absence of the subsidy, the social cost of insurance will exceed the social value. Only now, the cost has been shifted on to the taxpayer, and so the true cost of insurance coverage is hidden. A second problem with subsidies is that they may not be successful. Studies of subsidies provided to small firms that focused on small employers in New York State have indicated that even quite large subsidies may not be sufficient to induce the desired increases in the health insurance coverage that firms provide (Thorpe, Hendricks, Garnick, Donelan, & Newhouse, 1992). Because of the design of the subsidy, there may have been a reluctance on the part of the employers to commit to providing health insurance coverage for their employees. The subsidy was only to last for two years, after which time the employers would have to pay the entire amount. Because of the greater eventual financial burden, such a design might well deter employers from providing health insurance coverage.

16.2.6 Cooperative Pools

The provision of insurance is less expensive when it is done in the context of a large group, such as employers or professional associations. Individual and small-group policies are much more expensive to administer. As a result, the loading charge for individual and small-group policies is greater than it is for large-group policies.

There has been a recent trend toward the formation of cooperatives or insurance purchasing groups that individuals or smaller employers could join. These are called health insurance purchasing cooperatives (HIPCs). By forming a cooperative, smaller groups can be rated together as a unit and therefore receive the same rate that a larger group with the same risk profile would receive. Purchasing cooperatives have become commonplace, and a number of market reform proposals focus on this trend (Hall, 1994; Reinhardt, 1993a).

In this analysis, assume that individuals 1 and 7 can join the main group. If they do so, the cost of providing them with health insurance falls to $10. If the assumption of experience rating by individual risk is retained, then individual 1, at least, would not be insured. Individual 1 would still not be willing to pay $130, the premium he or she would have to pay. However, the cooperative would have increased insurance coverage (by extending coverage to individual 7) through lowering the cost of provision. This would be an efficient solution and would increase equity.

16.2.7 Community Rating and Biased Selection

One feature that has been included in some health insurance reform proposals is a requirement for community rating. To determine the effects of community rating, return to the original model presented (see Section 16.2.2).

It is initially assumed that everyone pays the same premium to a single insurer. If the insurer has only to meet its full costs, including administration costs, and if all individuals are to be served, then the single community rate would be $80. At this single rate, individuals 5, 6, and 7 will not insure. This may start a spiral that leads to the eventual drying up of the entire market.

There is another consideration in community rating. Assume that there are two insurers, A and B, and they are competing for business at the community rate. Another assumption is also changed, assuming that the insurers want to maximize their profits. The implications of these changes are as follows. In order to maximize profits, each of the two insurers will seek out insureds with a low risk of loss and low administrative expenses. They will avoid providing insurance to other individuals. There are numerous ways that the insurers could do this. They could screen applicants and if provision is not mandatory, refuse to sell insurance to high-cost individuals. Alternatively, they could make it difficult for potentially high-cost insureds to reach them by locating in areas where younger, healthier individuals live (Light, 1992).

The incentive for insurers to select low-risk individuals is indeed a powerful one, and its relevance needs to be emphasized. A key way for insurers to contain their costs is to make certain that their clients are initially low risk. Numerous health insurance reform proposals have been put forward, and most of them at least try to address this issue. However, under community rating, this issue is especially difficult to address because it relates directly to the profits that the insurers can earn.

Another issue relating to community rating is that if each individual's premium is fixed, there will be no incentive for individuals to reduce their risk through health promotion and disease prevention activities. Under experience rating, individuals can be offered incentives (lower premiums) to engage in behaviors that lead to better health (e.g., no smoking). Such incentives do not exist when everyone pays the same premium.

Community rating can now be evaluated on two grounds: equity and efficiency. From one point of view, community rating can appear to be the most equitable rating method. After all, everyone pays the same rate. However, if everyone is not in the same risk category, then community rating involves the subsidization of the unhealthy by the healthy. If a notion of equity is assumed based on the premise that equals should pay equally and unequals should pay unequally, then community rating might not seem an equitable method. On the other hand, if all individuals are viewed as "equals" (in the sense that, no matter how healthy or unhealthy, they are all human beings), then community rating will indeed appear fair.

On efficiency grounds, there can be little said in favor of community rating. Community rating discourages individuals from engaging in health promotion activities when the social costs would warrant them to do it. Cost savings from such activities are not passed on to the individuals who engage in them. In addition, community rating encourages insurers to seek out the lowest risk individuals, and this can cause individuals who would otherwise buy insurance not to purchase it, which eventually could lead to a drying up of the health insurance market. In response to these problems, two additional innovations have been introduced. One is a mandate requiring individuals or employers to obtain insurance. The second is risk rating—the assignment of individuals to groups according to their risks, and the requirement that they pay different premiums based on these risks.

16.2.8 Mandates

A mandate is a legal requirement that some action be taken, such as the purchasing of health insurance coverage by an individual or an employer. The purpose of a mandate to purchase insurance is to block individuals from leaving the health insurance market. It is maintained that some individuals (primarily low-risk individuals) will not insure until they get older or sick, and the risk of their using services increases. Only then do they insure and "take advantage" of their coverage. When low-risk individuals do not participate in the market, this causes higher group premiums and could even result in the eventual disappearance of the market. Under a mandate, everyone must purchase insurance. Many health insurance reform proposals involve introducing a mandate.

The Patient Protection and Affordable Care Act (PPACA), passed in 2010, contained mandatory coverage provisions. To provide coverage for most Americans meant the population must participate to avoid substantial increases in premiums. The PPACA contained a number of provisions designed to transform the health insurance market in the United States, expanding insurance coverage to about 95% of the population.

Under the health reform plan, discriminatory practices that exclude individuals from coverage because of preexisting conditions will be eliminated. Also, lifetime and unreasonable annual limits of benefits will be eliminated, and policies will be prohibited from being rescinded because of health status. In addition, policies will be required to develop uniform coverage documents, so comparisons can be easily made. Insurance companies would be prohibited from setting rates or denying coverage based on health status, medical condition, claims experience, genetic information, or other health-related factors.

Under PPACA, most individuals would be required to maintain insurance for minimum essential coverage or pay a penalty, with individuals under 18 paying half the established premium. Certain limited exceptions to the mandate would be allowed. Employers with more than 200 employees are required to automatically enroll new full-time employees, and any employer with more than 50 employees not offering coverage must pay a penalty for each employee, if at least one full-time employee receives the premium assistance tax credit. If the employer of more than 50 employees offers a plan deemed unaffordable or does not meet the standard for minimum essential coverage and has at least one employee receiving the premium tax credit, then the employer will pay a penalty per employee.

Starting with our original example, a community rating is assumed and a mandate that all individuals purchase insurance. The premium rate will be $80, and all individuals are mandated to pay this rate.

Such a premium rate might impose a considerable burden on low-income individuals, and so few proposals would stop at a mandate. One way to reduce the burden would be to provide a subsidy for individuals who are designated as low income. The combined reforms would ensure that all individuals were insured and could afford insurance because those who could not otherwise afford it would be subsidized.

The Patient Protection and Affordable Care Act stipulates that insurance premiums will vary only because of family structure, geography, actuarial value, tobacco use, participation in health promotion programs, and age. To ensure the mandatory insurance coverage is affordable, out-of-pocket costs are limited. Coverage is offered at four levels, with actuarial values defining how much the insurer pays, ranging from 90 to 60%. A low benefit catastrophic plan is available to individuals under 30. States must establish a Health Benefits Exchange (also called Health Insurance Exchange) to assist individuals and small employers obtain coverage. The PPACA establishes new, refundable, sliding scale tax credits for Americans with incomes between 100 and 400% of the federal poverty level. In addition, a new tax credit is available for employers with fewer than 25 workers for up to 50% of the total premium cost. The PPACA expands Medicaid and the Children's Health Insurance Plan (CHIP) eligibility to low-income individuals and families.

The main objection to a mandate is that it imposes a welfare loss on some individuals. For example, individuals 5, 6, and 7 are not willing to pay $80 for health insurance coverage. Under a mandate, they would have to pay that amount anyway, and so they would suffer an added burden in order that higher risk and/or lower income individuals be able to obtain insurance (Hall, 1994). In addition, the mandate does not eliminate the powerful incentive insurance companies have to "cherry pick," or engage in other competitive practices that enable them to select low-risk insureds. Other elements of health insurance reform must be introduced if these practices are to be curbed. The most prominent of these is risk adjustment.

16.2.9 Risk Selection Limitation and Risk Adjustment

Some government policies directly limit insurers' ability to select individual risks. Because past or current health may be a good predictor of future health, a decision to accept a person for coverage, or renew a policy, may involve examination of the applicant's current health or past claim experience. The existence of a chronic health condition, or large past expenses, could be the basis for denying coverage. In such cases, decisions to deny coverage have generated significant media and political attention because they can be seen as refusing coverage to people who need it most. In 1996, federal legislation directly addressed this issue by requiring companies to sell insurance policies to groups willing to purchase them and guaranteeing individuals or groups the right to renew policies. This legislation did not however address the premiums that could be charged for such policies.

Risk adjustment is a technique that can be used to modify payments made to prepaid plans on the basis of characteristics of the entire group. The rationale behind this technique is that certain subgroups are more costly to treat (because they use more services) and that health plans should be appropriately compensated for accepting these subgroups as members. Among the variables that have been used in risk-adjustment formulas are age, gender, self-reported health status, and prior period healthcare use.

A problem with risk adjustment, in the present context, is that if a health plan discovers a variable related to healthcare use, it might be able to profit by selecting low-risk individuals. For example, if body weight was associated with healthcare utilization, then a health plan might try to select members, at least partly, on the basis of their weight. Assuming it was successful in attracting lower weight members, it would benefit from having lower costs. Currently, there seem to be a number of risk factors that are not included in the risk-adjustment techniques commonly used. This leaves the door open for health plans to invest in techniques that will identify potentially heavy healthcare users and avoid them. Such actions would reduce the effectiveness of market reforms.

16.3 MANAGED CARE

16.3.1 Introduction

Managed care is a system of healthcare insurance and delivery by which the payer attempts to exert direct influence over the economic behavior of the suppliers. Managed care focuses on efforts to coordinate, rationalize, and channel utilization to achieve desired outcomes and costs. Growth of managed care has been a central aspect of healthcare reform in the United States. In the 1970s, federal legislation endorsed and encouraged the growth of health maintenance organizations (HMOs). Rapid growth of HMO membership occurred during the 1980s, along with the development of other types of managed care organizations and the adoption by traditional insurers of some of the techniques of cost control that had been introduced by HMOs. By the 1990s, managed care was a major part of the healthcare delivery system, as well as an important segment of financial markets. A "backlash" developed as state and federal governments became aware of growing concerns about quality of care and the restriction of consumer choice in the managed care context.

Integration of the insurance function with the healthcare delivery function in one organization changes incentives for use of resources. Under traditional insurance and fee-for-service medical practice, the providers have little reason to be concerned with the cost consequences of their treatment decisions, because the payers bear all the risks of the providers' actions. On the other hand, a managed care organization receives prepayment for members' health care, and because its surplus is the difference between the prepaid amount and the amount spent on health care, it has a clear incentive to provide care as inexpensively as possible. The acceptance of a predefined financial payment for a set of defined benefits for its members places the HMO at financial risk. HMOs were initially seen as a possible means of enhancing two types of economic efficiency. Improvements in productive efficiency could result from using different combinations of inputs to produce a given output level (e.g., the substitution of nonphysician providers of care for physicians and the substitution of outpatient treatment for hospitalization).

Greater allocative efficiency could result from more careful weighing of the marginal health benefits against the marginal costs of particular treatments. Further, competition among HMOs, and between HMOs and traditional insurers, had the potential of reducing healthcare costs through price competition. In addition, it was anticipated that HMOs would shift the emphasis from short-term acute care for sickness to prevention and long-term health maintenance. This section reviews some of the economic issues associated with the development of managed care.

16.3.2 Types of Managed Care Organization

All managed care organizations (MCOs) employ some form of prepayment and some degree of integration of financial risk bearing with healthcare delivery. All MCOs contract to provide fairly comprehensive health services to members in exchange for an annual premium and often small copayments. However, they differ importantly in their relationships with the healthcare providers and in the arrangements for dispensing care. In terms of ability to control provider decision making, the "tightest" type of plan is the staff-model HMO, in which physicians are employees of the HMO. A group-model HMO is similar, except that the health plan and the physician group are separate legal entities. Usually, HMO members make up all or a great majority of the physician group's practice, and the plan and the physician group are in fact managed jointly in many respects. Members of a staff-model or group-model HMO receive care at one of the HMO's medical office locations, which typically have a number of primary care providers and often some specialty care providers under one roof.

An independent practice association (IPA) type of HMO provides a contrast in several respects. In an IPA, the physicians practice in their own offices as solo practitioners or small groups. The health plan contracts with the physicians to provide care for HMO members. Members of the HMO typically would account for only a small proportion of any physician's practice. Indeed, the physician might well be a provider for several different HMOs. Compared with a staff- or group-model HMO, an IPA usually offers members a larger number of providers and a larger number of office locations among which to choose.

A preferred provider organization (PPO) is an arrangement whereby the insurer designates a selected list of providers, including physicians and hospitals. If a patient seeks care from a provider on the list, the insurance coverage will be extensive, with a small or zero copayment. However, a patient may choose to seek treatment from providers not on the list. In that case, there will still be some insurance coverage, but the patient will bear a larger share of the cost.

As the industry evolves, there have emerged various mixed models. The term *network model* is often applied to these. For example, an HMO might offer care through its own health centers and also from a list of physicians in the community. Increasingly popular in HMO contracts is a point-of-service (POS) provision. This provision enables the HMO member to seek care from providers other than the HMO providers but at greater cost.

16.3.3 Control of Resource Use

While it is clear that the overall incentive for a managed care organization is to minimize costs, the specific ways it is done make a large difference in terms of the public and political acceptance of this type of organization. Proponents of managed care point to the elimination of unnecessary or low marginal benefit care, the selection of more cost-effective treatment approaches, the encouragement of wellness, and increased access to care through elimination of financial barriers. Critics note the lack of choice of provider and fear that the cost incentives can lead to lower quality care through the elimination or restriction of necessary treatments. A position in this controversy is not presented here, but rather some of the factors influencing costs and how they might operate in a managed care environment are described.

Incentives provided to both physicians and patients are relevant. The initial decision to seek care is a patient decision. Specific treatment choices require both physician recommendation and patient consent. Decisions with major resource-use implications, such as hospitalization or surgery, are complex, and the physician is still a major decision maker, although patients are becoming more informed and more involved in the decisions made.

The method of physician compensation plays an important role and is best viewed in an agency context. Under fee-for-service compensation, the physician earns more by using more resources. This type of compensation can lead to supplier-induced demand and treatments of low marginal benefit. While some managed care organizations (typically IPAs or PPOs) do use it, alternative forms of compensation are common. One is to provide a straight salary. Under salary compensation, a physician's income is not affected by treatment choices made. Capitation is another alternative. Under this scheme, a physician receives a certain sum per assigned patient, irrespective of what services are provided to the patient. An extreme form of capitation would pay a primary care physician a certain sum per patient and make him or her financially responsible for all care the patient receives during the time period, including specialty or hospital care. This provides a very strong incentive to limit the care provided and puts the physician at great financial risk if a patient should need treatment for catastrophic illness. The risk is somewhat mitigated if the capitation payment goes to a physician group rather than individual providers, and capitation of this type is often used to pay the physician group in a group-model HMO. Individual providers in the group could then be compensated by salary, fees for service, or some other method. Different combinations of compensation schemes are also in use. For example, physicians in an HMO might be paid fees in return for services but have a certain portion of the fees held back by the HMO until the end of the financial year, at which time an amount would be returned to the physician based on the HMO's surplus; or salary payment could be supplemented by a year-end bonus related to the HMO's financial results.

Under a typical traditional insurance plan, copayments and deductibles, to some extent, deter utilization of services. For some types of services (e.g., preventive services), coverage may not be included at all, and patients would have to pay the full cost. Managed care tends to rely less on financial incentives to limit utilization and more on administrative arrangements. Such arrangements are particularly important for influencing the use of specialized referral services. In contrast to traditional insurance, in which a patient can self-refer to a specialist, many managed care plans will have the primary care provider play a "gatekeeper" role. That is, a referral to a specialist must be authorized by the member's primary care provider in order for the expense to be covered by the HMO. The referral may be limited to a small number of visits to the specialist, after which time the patient care responsibility would return to the primary care provider. Concurrent utilization review for hospitalized patients is another example of a managed care strategy that has the potential to influence utilization more than the relatively laissez-faire role of the traditional insurer.

16.3.4 Empirical Evidence: Resource Use, Quality of Care, and Satisfaction

There has been considerable empirical research comparing managed care to traditional insurance. The subject of study has been something of a "moving target," however. New types of managed care organization have emerged that mix features of the "pure" HMO model with elements of a fee-for-service system, and traditional insurers have adopted methods to influence the delivery of care, methods that have undoubtedly had an effect on economic performance. So it must be kept in mind that the evidence reflects a rapidly evolving industry and that research findings can easily become outdated. Nevertheless, with that caveat, a selective review of some of the findings is provided.

The comparison of care under HMOs to that under traditional insurance has faced substantial methodological challenges. Much early research involved statistical comparisons of hospital admission rates, hospital lengths of stay, or the use of particular expensive procedures between members of an HMO and those of a comparison group with traditional insurance (For a detailed review, see Doebbeling & Flanagan, 2011; Elliott, Haviland, Orr, Hambarsoomian, & Cleary, 2011; Luft, 1978, 1980). It was clear in a preponderance of these studies that HMO members seemed to use fewer resources than the comparison group. What was less clear was whether the comparisons were valid in the face of possible selection bias. There was reason to believe that people joining HMOs were different from, and healthier than, the population of people with traditional insurance. If that was the case, it would not be possible to conclude that the observed differences in resource utilization represented greater efficiency.

One way to deal with selection bias in research is to eliminate it through random selection (i.e., to use an experimental study design in which people are assigned at random to different types of insurance coverage). This was in fact done in the RAND Health Insurance Study undertaken in the years 1976–1981 in Seattle. The researchers assigned some people to an HMO and others to a variety of fee-for-service insurance plans with different coinsurance rates. They then observed use of healthcare resources. In the comparison that would best show the HMO effect (i.e., between the HMO group and the traditional insurance with no copayment), there was a clear difference in resource use. Annual hospital admissions (per 100 people) were 8.4 in the HMO group, compared with 13.8 in the traditional insurance group.

Annual hospital days (per 100 people) totaled 49 in the HMO group and 83 in the traditional insurance group (Manning, Leibowitz, Goldberg, Rogers, & Newhouse, 1984).

In a comprehensive literature review covering 37 studies published between 1993 and 1997, comparing managed care and non–managed care groups, Miller and Luft (1997) found a mixed picture of differences in resource use. HMO hospital use was less than non–managed care groups in some studies, but about an equal number of studies showed the opposite result. The four studies that looked at specific costly procedures all found somewhat lower use of such procedures in HMOs. Three of the five studies that examined total spending showed that HMOs spent significantly less, with the other two studies finding no such difference.

Quality of care is another dimension along which managed care and non–managed care may differ. One could hypothesize, *a priori*, that a difference in quality might occur in either direction. Economic incentives to limit resource use could lead HMOs to cut corners, which would lead to deterioration in quality. On the other hand, lack of financial barriers to early treatment and emphasis on wellness could lead to higher quality in the managed care setting. Studies that have investigated the issue empirically have usually focused on one or two specific diseases or patient groups and used clinical measures of outcome (e.g., risk of dying for ICU patients or blood pressure for hypertensive patients). In the Miller and Luft (1997) review, 15 studies examined the quality issue, and the results varied widely: many studies found no significant difference, and about as many found higher quality in HMOs as found lower quality. According to Miller and Luft, "The results show something that is simple, obvious and yet sometimes underemphasized: HMOs produce better, the same, and worse quality of care, depending on the particular organization and particular disease" (p. 15).

A 2004 study by Landon, Zaslavsky, Bernard, Cioffi, & Cleary compared Medicare beneficiaries enrolled in the Medicare managed care program, Medicare Advantage, with those enrolled in the traditional insurance plan. These authors found that the traditional program enrollees scored higher, in the aggregate, on all measures except immunizations, than did Medicare Advantage (MA) enrollees. A recent study by Elliott, Haviland, Orr, Hambarsoomian, & Cleary. (2011) that employed a risk-adjustment factor, found more mixed results. In their study, MA outperformed traditional on five measures, while traditional outperformed MA on three measures. The authors did note that the five instances in which MA outperformed traditional involved prescription drug measures, which didn't exist at the time of the 2004 study. Increased payments to MA plans compared to traditional have also increased their abilities to offer enhanced benefits to their members.

Enrollee satisfaction, as measured by survey responses, has also been a subject of research. The preponderance of the evidence on this issue in the studies reviewed by Miller and Luft (1997) showed a somewhat lower level of overall satisfaction among HMO members than those in fee-for-service plans. When the survey questions were broken down into satisfaction with financial aspects and nonfinancial aspects, however, people in HMOs were more satisfied with financial aspects, while the reverse was true for nonfinancial aspects.

In a large statistical study, Reschovsky & Kemper (1999) provided new evidence regarding differences between HMOs and traditional care. Unlike most of the studies reviewed by Miller and Luft (1997), which used data from a relatively small number of people in a few plans in one location, the data from this later study came from a large national sample ($N = 60,446$) of people who were interviewed by telephone during 1996 and 1997. The study is also noteworthy in that it examined differences for particularly vulnerable population subgroups (e.g., low-income people, children, racial subgroups, and chronically ill people). The major findings of that study were summarized by the authors as follows (Kemper, Reschovsky, & Tu. 1999, pp. 419–420):

- Enrollees in HMOs differ from those not in HMOs, but not with respect to health status.

- HMOs provide more primary and preventive care.

- HMOs use less specialist care, but the study did not find evidence of less use of other types of costly care.

- HMOs reduce financial barriers to care but increase provider access problems and organizational barriers.

- Patients assess HMO care as worse than care under non-HMO insurance.

- The study found no consistent evidence that HMO effects differ for vulnerable subgroups.

As is evident, it is hard to generalize about the effects of managed care. Some of the early findings on resource savings attributable to managed care have not held up in the later work. It is also apparent that the worst fears of HMO critics about quality effects are not borne out by research findings. Not all of the possible economic effects of managed care can be captured by the type of study that compares individual managed care organizations to traditional insurance plans, however. HMOs in a market may affect the economic behavior of other market participants and change the nature of competition, as discussed in the next section.

16.3.5 Managed Care in the Market

The entry of new participants into a market can change the structure of the market and the nature of buyer-seller interactions in it. The specific nature of the change will depend of course on what the market structure and conduct was like before the entry of the new participants. Managed care represents vertical integration of insurance with service delivery and thus has possible effects on two types of market, the market for health insurance and the market for medical care.

In the early years of HMO growth (the 1970s and 1980s), the major issue and subject of research was the effect of HMO market entry on traditional insurers. In a simple theoretical model, entry of new sellers to the insurance market would be expected to shift the supply curve outward and result in lower prices. Particularly, if preentry market power was held by the established firms, one would expect price competition to drive prices down. If the entrants had lower costs than established firms, this would have further downward effects on price, as established firms imitated the lower cost technology and competition forced prices to reflect marginal costs.

This scenario does not accurately reflect the effects of initial HMO entry into insurance markets in several respects, however. In markets with the possibility of nonprice competition, the rivalry among firms may not take the form of price competition, in which case lower costs and prices would not result. Much of the rivalry between HMOs and traditional insurers was not based on price but rather on product differentiation (McLaughlin, 1988). HMOs priced their products somewhat below the traditional insurers and did not fully exploit their cost advantage to lower prices further; instead, they offered a more comprehensive benefits package and lower cost sharing. As a consequence, there was considerable pressure on established health insurers to adopt organizational and product innovations, such as expanded benefits packages and utilization review techniques to control costs. (For a review of the early literature, see Frank & Welch, 1985.)

As HMOs grew into significant market participants, the focus of research shifted to the effects of managed care on medical care markets. An HMO enters medical care markets as a buyer of services, including hospital and physician services. If the buyer side of these markets was initially competitive (i.e., there were many small buyers), the entry of an HMO as a big buyer would introduce monopsony power. Here, theory predicts a downward pressure on price as well as a lower quantity of output. The effects of managed care on hospital costs might come from two directions. First, managed care organizations might simply decrease the use of hospital care, substituting outpatient for inpatient care or reducing lengths of stay through administrative techniques, such as utilization review. Second, they might engage in selective contracting (i.e., directing patients to less expensive and more efficient hospitals).

A number of studies using different research methodologies have explored the relationship between managed care and hospital use and found significant effects. One approach is to examine the relationship between HMO penetration in a market and the rate of hospital cost inflation. One such study, based on California data, examined cost per admission for 298 hospitals during the years 1982–1988. It found that growth in costs per admission was 9.4% lower in markets with high HMO penetration than in markets with low HMO penetration (Robinson, 1991). Another study (Feldman, Chan, Kralewski, Dowd, & Shapiro, 1990) estimated demand for hospital admissions by six HMOs in four metropolitan areas. The researchers found that the HMO demand was sensitive to hospital price, with the elasticity for staff-network-model HMOs being much greater than that for IPAs. A third study took advantage of a "natural experiment" to examine the effect of a change in benefits for Wisconsin state employees. The change made HMO membership a very attractive choice, and as a result the percentage of state employees enrolled in HMOs grew sharply during the years 1983–1993. Hill and Wolfe (1997) examined the changes in hospital resources that took place over that time period in Madison, Wisconsin, where the state is a very large employer, and they found large decreases in resource use. Finally, two studies by Wholey and coworkers (1995, 1997) examined both HMO penetration and the number of HMOs in a market and found that hospital use and premiums were lower when the market was more competitive. This effect was more evident for group-model HMOs than for IPAs.

Another type of medical care market in which changes might result from the increased presence of HMOs is the market for specialized, expensive, high-technology services. Some empirical studies have found evidence that managed care has decreased the demand for such services, while others have failed to find this effect. The Wisconsin study noted earlier (Hill & Wolfe, 1997) examined two services that required expensive capital equipment—magnetic resonance imaging (MRI) and lithotripsy, a method of treating kidney stones. They noted that after the increase in HMO enrollment, area hospitals were much more likely to obtain the necessary equipment jointly, whereas prior to 1983, the pattern was for individual hospitals to acquire them independently. However, Madison was not much different than comparison cities in the proportion of hospitals with selected high-technology facilities. A study of the growth of an innovative surgical procedure, laparoscopic cholecystectomy, found no difference between HMO enrollees and the general fee-for-service population in the use of this technology (Chernew, Fendrick, & Hirth, 1997). One possible effect on market structure results from the pressures of selective contracting by managed care organizations. If HMOs search for the low-cost providers and channel business to them, there is a powerful incentive for providers to seek out and realize economies of scale. A study of mammography found just such a result. HMO market share was associated with consolidation among mammography providers and reductions in cost for mammography services (Baker & Brown, 1999).

16.4 INFORMATION AND CONSUMER CHOICE

In a well-functioning competitive market, the principle of "consumer sovereignty" prevails (i.e., the products to be produced are determined by consumer preferences, and appropriate incentives are in place for economic efficiency to be achieved). This market result, however, depends on consumers having adequate information about prices and product characteristics to be able to choose wisely among alternatives. If market-oriented reforms in health care, particularly managed care, are to be effective, potential buyers must be able to assess the characteristics of managed care products. During the period when managed care was experiencing rapid growth, the technology used for developing and disseminating statistical information also advanced greatly. The combination of these changes resulted in a number of initiatives designed to make information about healthcare organizations more available to consumers, with the goal of improving their decision making and at the same time improving market outcomes. This section reviews some of those developments and the issues they raise.

The characteristic of healthcare organization performance that is perhaps most difficult for consumers to understand is quality, so not surprisingly, that characteristic has received the most attention. A number of reporting or rating systems have been introduced that attempt to define quality in a measurable way, develop statistical information about the quality of specific healthcare organizations, and disseminate that information widely to consumers and employers, often in the form of "report cards." Some of these efforts have been by government agencies, while others have taken place in the private sector. Ratings or reports have been developed for such healthcare providers as hospitals or individual physicians, as well as for managed care organizations.

One of the earliest attempts to report widely on hospital performance was the dissemination by the Health Care Financing Administration (HCFA), beginning in 1986, of hospital mortality rates for all hospitals in the United States. These annual reports provided for each hospital the actual mortality rate of Medicare patients, as well as that predicted statistically based on characteristics of the admitted patients. Frequently, the performance of a particular hospital was the subject of local media attention if it appeared to have an unusually low or high mortality rate compared with other hospitals. The reporting program gave rise to a great deal of controversy and was ended in 1992. Several aspects of the controversy are of continuing interest because they apply to other similar programs.

First, critics questioned whether the statistical methodology used was adequate to adjust for severity of illness. Certainly, hospitals with sicker patients would be expected to have more deaths, so a higher mortality rate in such hospitals would not be indicative of a quality difference but rather a case-mix difference. Indeed, it may be that higher quality hospitals attract the sickest and most difficult to treat patients and have higher mortality rates for that reason. Second, there is a question as to whether it makes sense to consider the hospital's patient population as a whole or whether the analysis should be conducted for individual patient groups. For example, a hospital may be very successful at treating cardiac surgery patients but have less than average success treating cancer patients. An overall assessment would miss these important details. Third, administrative data may not capture clinical information accurately. There may be data errors that occur in the transition from a patient chart to a hospital information system. Moreover, administrative datasets, developed mostly for financial or operational purposes, may not reflect fully the clinical complexity of a patient's illness and treatment. Finally, of course, there is the question of whether the information provided actually influences the choices of consumers and healthcare providers. One careful statistical study of the HCFA experience found only very slight evidence of a relationship between the ratings of hospitals and changes in the numbers of patients who used them (Mennemeyer, Morrisey, & Howard, 1997).

Performance measurement and reporting on managed care organizations has been largely a private sector activity. Several different organizations are involved in this field, but the major one is the National Committee for Quality Assurance (NCQA), a private not-for-profit organization that has been reporting on and accrediting managed care organizations since 1991. NCQA was formed initially with the participation of a group of large employers who were concerned about the cost and quality of health care and who believed that a standardized system for evaluating HMOs would help them make better purchasing decisions when administering their employee health benefits. Although NCQA accreditation is voluntary for HMOs, as of 2000, about half of all HMOs in the United States (with enrollments totaling about three-quarters of all HMO members) were accredited by NCQA or seeking accreditation.

Accreditation is different from, although closely related to, performance measurement. NCQA is also the organization that manages the evolution of a major dataset for assessing health plan performance. The Health Plan Employer Data and Information Set (HEDIS) includes more than 50 statistical measures of a managed care organization's performance, including survey information on member satisfaction, as well as measures based on clinical data on the treatment of specific diseases, such as heart disease, cancer, and diabetes. The goal is to provide a common measure that can be used by purchasers to compare health plans. HEDIS data are often used as the basis for health plan "report cards" made available to consumers by employers and publicized in the media.

Although much effort has gone into developing systems for analyzing health plan performance, creating statistical reports on performance, and disseminating these reports, the actual effect of these activities is, as yet, unclear. From an economic standpoint, the important question is whether actual market decisions are made using such information. It is important to recall here that the health plan enrollment decision is really a two-stage process: first, the employer decides to offer particular plans to its workers as choices, and second, each employee chooses a particular plan from among those in the benefits package. It is reasonable to think that an employer's decision to include a plan in the benefits package would be influenced by performance data, at least in the case of a large employer with sophisticated benefits administrators who have the time and expertise to evaluate the data. Whether smaller employers and individual consumers have the ability and incentive to use such information is less evident. Furthermore, it is hard to know whether the variables chosen by "experts" as measures of plan performance are really about what individual consumers care. One study that examined the influence of HEDIS data on the choices of workers of one large firm found a very weak response to the data in terms of actual plan choice. The researchers suggested that personal experience and word-of-mouth may be more important determinants of individual choices (Scanlon & Chernew, 1999). However, the use of performance data is too new for there to be enough evidence for a clear conclusion. This area is an important one for future research.

16.5 CONSUMER-FOCUSED HEALTH CARE

16.5.1. Patient-Centered Medical Homes

The United States continues to explore and experiment with strategies and designs to transform the functioning of the healthcare system to improve outcomes and control costs. One of these strategies is the patient-centered medical home (PCMH) model. The term *medical home* was coined by the Academy of Pediatrics in 1967 and has evolved into the concept of patient-centered medial home since. PCMH is a supply-side method to enable clinicians to provide care of a higher quality in a more efficient manner. Conceptually, it promotes better relationships between patients and providers, resulting in better access, increased quality, and improved consistency in care. PCMH focuses on and rewards ongoing patient-physician relationships and coordinated care that is of high quality. PCMHs require healthcare providers to reorganize practices into more effective systems in order to deliver high-quality efficient care.

Patient-centered medical homes are designed to offer care that is consistent with the needs and expectations of patients. The provision of needed care is enabled by technology and delivery systems that coordinate care safely. A key component of PCMHs is a payment system aligned to compensate providers for the infrastructure and time costs necessary for the coordination and delivery of patient-centered care. In addition to the reorganization of care delivered, PCMH also focus on self-management strategies for the patient. These last strategies are designed to decrease reliance on the healthcare system and increase patient responsibility for their health outcomes.

The Centers for Medicare and Medicaid Services (CMS) sponsored demonstration projects to create and implement medical homes to provide continuous and coordinated family-centered medical care; the focus on family-centered rather than just patient-centered recognized the important role families have in improved health outcomes. The focus is on coordinated and integrated health care managed by primary care physicians. The integrated care is expected to enhance patient adherence to a treatment plan and avoid unnecessary hospitalizations, office visits, tests, and procedures. PCMHs are also expected to increase use of less expensive technologies and biologicals when appropriate and reduce the risks to patients that are inherent in a fragmented system that results in inconsistent treatment decisions. PCMHs are expected to increase preventive care and improve patient adherence to treatment plans.

CMS has identified six domains of medical services that must be present in a medical home. These are continuity of care; clinical information systems; delivery system design to promote access and communication; decision support; patient/family engagement; and coordination. Criteria are established for each of these domains, and the performance of the practice is measured against these criteria. Providers receive additional funding per member per month to participate; and for aggregate savings to Medicare that are greater than 2%, the providers will receive 80% and Medicare will receive 20%.

As PCMHs evolve and expand, the focus on comprehensive care provided by a team of providers increases. The team approach relies heavily on the easy flow of information, reducing redundancy of tests and information, and improving coordinated decision making. As the concept evolves, increased recognition of the role of the patient and family as team members has occurred. The information exchanged among *all* team members is critical to the success of the PCMH.

For PCMHs to achieve their potential, the payment system will need to be restructured to incorporate appropriate incentives and rewards. The current fee-for-service system rewards providers for delivering more curative services and pays little or nothing for preventive care. In general, physicians receive payment for services delivered, even if the services provided omit some or many of the clinical practice guidelines. Fragmentation is rewarded in the current system because multiple providers are paid for multiple tests on the same patient. Providers are not rewarded for efforts to manage the health of the patient between visits, only for services delivered during the visit. In addition, in the current system, patients do not have financial incentives to adhere to preventive or disease-management recommendations, and insurers lack mechanisms for directing patients to higher value providers. The payment system developed for PCMHs must incorporate features to address the shortcomings of the current payment system if they are to achieve their goals of increased efficiency, better outcomes, and controlled costs.

16.5.2 Accountable Care Organizations

Another concept that has been proposed to improve quality and slow the growth in healthcare costs is Accountable Care Organizations (ACOs). The ACO concept involves considerable flexibility in how ACOs can be organized, which will enable them to develop more quickly and require fewer resources. Also, ACOs are paid on a shared-savings basis, which reflects a percentage of the difference between a benchmark established by the Secretary of Health and Human Services and the costs to Medicare for services provided to ACO-assigned beneficiaries. The ACO faces less financial risk than under a fixed amount capitation system, which pays the same amount per member regardless of amount of services actually used. Under the ACO model, the standard Medicare payment level for beneficiaries using services is generally guaranteed, although the ACO can suffer a loss if expenditures for beneficiaries are too high.

In general, an ACO is defined as a local organization with a related set of providers (at least primary care physicians, specialists, and hospitals) that can be held accountable for costs and quality of care delivered to a defined population. The defined population can be either a subset of Medicare beneficiaries or subscribers in health insurance plans. The organization must be able to provide services and manage patients across a continuum of care, have sufficient financial resources to assume risk, and have sufficient volume to support comprehensive, valid, and reliable performance measurement. Diverse types of organizations can serve as an ACO, as long as they can meet the required criteria of accountability for health, quality, and costs of care over the full continuum of patient care.

The ACO model builds upon earlier models, especially those of the patient-centered medical home and bundled payment for a discrete episode of care. The ACO model goes further than the previous models by aligning payments, benefits, and other healthcare policies with measurable, meaningful progress in improving care while controlling cost increases. As highlighted by the Accountable Care Organization Learning Network (www.acolearningnetwork. org), the foundation of an ACO is clear, patient-focused aims of better overall health through higher quality and lower costs for patients; provider accountability through performance measures that are transparent; and payment reform that uses the measures to align and provide organizations that are focused on these aims directly and meaningfully. As health information technology, performance measurement, and effective medical practices continue to advance, the ability of organizations to meet the aims of ACOs will improve.

A basic feature of the ACO model is the establishment of a spending benchmark that is based on expected spending on the defined population. The benchmark established takes into consideration the health status and characteristics of the defined population. If the ACO can achieve the quality targets while slowing the growth in healthcare costs, then the ACO receives a portion (a share) of the savings from the payer. Medicare initially set the organization's share of the savings at 80%; that percentage varies by payer. If preventive care, coordinated services, patient-centered care, and other quality-improvement strategies achieve better outcomes and lower resource use, then providers will receive bonuses to replace some of the upfront losses they may experience with the ACO model. Such payment reform should increase the sustainability of such services, as the financial incentives are aligned with the desired aims of the system. Another feature of the ACO model is that it reduces or eliminates incentives to expand service capacity that will be underutilized by its members.

ACOs have a number of key design features, regardless of their organizational structure. These features are (1) local accountability, (2) a legal structure with a governing board, (3) a focus on primary care, (4) adequate patient population size, (5) appropriate investments in improvements in the delivery system, (6) realistic and achievable opportunities for providers to achieve shared savings, and (7) transparent and accessible performance measurements. These features are key to the success of the ACO model and will grow and become more sophisticated as experience and technical progress occurs.

A major difference in the ACO model and previous efforts is that it combines care delivery and payment reform. However, change and results cannot be expected to occur overnight. It will take time and experimentation to identify and develop best practices, to redesign work flows in practice settings in order to assemble high-functioning teams, to improve performance measures, and to establish appropriate spending benchmarks. The initial expectations and values established should not be viewed as absolutes or permanent but as temporary benchmarks as the system evolves and more and better information becomes available.

Another key feature of the ACO model is the recognition of the need for local accountability in the system. Instead of establishing a national standard, it recognizes differences in populations in various locations and the diversity of practice types and organizational settings in the healthcare system. To be successful, the model must allow for variation in strategies undertaken to improve care and control costs but must establish boundaries to avoid claims of "uniqueness," which are designed to allow providers to continue to function and perform under current conditions. The focus must be on promoting value, not just on volume and intensity of services. The care must be coordinated across providers and settings to minimize duplication and excessive use.

Finally, the healthcare system must include greater transparency for consumers. For consumers to make truly informed choices in their demand for healthcare services, they must have clear, reliable, valid, and understandable information on the overall quality, cost, and other performance aspects of providers within the system, and the system in general. Consumers need to have confidence in their providers and in the system that the most appropriate care is being provided and that they have the ability to determine the value of care available.

EXERCISES

1. Explain the relationship between information asymmetry and health insurance market failure.
2. Give an example of a health insurance market outcome that is efficient but not acceptable for reasons of equity. Describe a policy to address it.
3. Explain why individual or small-group insurance tends to be more expensive than large-group insurance.
4. Explain the relationship between community rating and economic efficiency.
5. Give two reasons why a person may lack health insurance: one in which an economic efficiency issue is involved and one in which no such issue arises.
6. Distinguish between a staff- or group-model HMO, an IPA, and a PPO with regard to the provider choices and out-of-pocket costs for members.
7. Contrast the incentives for resource use faced by a physician under a salary, under fee-for-service compensation, and under capitation.
8. Explain the problem presented by selection bias for research on the effects of HMOs.
9. Describe the types of effects that the entry of managed care organizations into a market can have on other types of insurance providers.
10. Describe the types of effects that the entry of managed care organizations into a market can have on other types of medical care providers.
11. Describe the potential effects that may be achieved by Accountable Care Organizations (ACOs) and Patient Centered Medical Homes (PCMHs).

BIBLIOGRAPHY

Insurance Market Reform

Abraham, K. S. (1985). Efficiency and fairness in insurance risk selection. *Virginia Law Review, 71*, 403–451.

Antos, J., Bertko, J., Chernew, M., Cutler, D., de Brantes, F., Goldman, D, ..., & Shortell, S. (2010). Bending the curve through health reform implementation. *American Journal of Managed Care, 16*(11), 804–812.

Berkowitz, S. A., & Miller, E. D. (2011). The individual mandate and patient-centered care. *JAMA, 306*(6), 648–649.

Blendon, R. J., Edwards, J. N., & Hymans, A. L., (1992). Making the critical choices. *JAMA, 267*, 2509–2520.

Borger, C., Smith, S., Truffer, C., Keehan, S., Sisko, A., Poisal, J., & Clemens, M. K. (2006). Health spending projections through 2015: Changes on the horizon. *Health Affairs, 25*(2), w61–w73.

Browne, M. J., & Doerpinghaus, H. (1994/1995). Asymmetric information and the demand for Medigap insurance. *Inquiry, 31,* 445–450.

Buchmueller, T. C. (2009). Consumer-oriented health care reform strategies: A review of the evidence on managed competition and consumer-directed health insurance. *Milbank Quarterly, 87*(4), 820–841.

Butler, S. M. (1991). A tax reform strategy to deal with the uninsured. *JAMA, 265,* 2541–2544.

Cogan, J. A., Jr. (2011). The Affordable Care Act's preventive services mandate: Breaking down the barriers to nationwide access to preventive services. *Journal of Law, Medicine & Ethics, 39,* 355–365.

Davis, K. (1991). Expanding Medicare and employer plans to achieve universal health insurance. *JAMA, 265,* 2525–2528.

deShazo, R. D. (2011). Who will care for the newly insured under health reform? *Journal of the Mississippi State Medical Association, 52*(8), 263–269.

Doebbeling, B. N., & Flanagan, M. E. (2011). Emerging perspectives on transforming the health-care system: Key conceptual issues. *Medical Care, 49*(Suppl.), S3–S5.

Dranove, D., Shanley, M., & White, W. D. (1993). Price and concentration in hospital markets: The switch from patient-driven to payer-driven competition. *Journal of Law and Economics, 36,* 179–204.

Dranove, D., Simon, C. J., & White, W. D. (1998). Determinants of managed care penetration. *Journal of Health Economics, 17,* 729–745.

Enthoven, A. C. (1993). The history and principles of managed competition. *Health Affairs, 12*(Suppl.), 24–48.

Enthoven, A. C ., & Kronick, R. (1989). A consumer choice health plan for the 1990s. Parts 1, 2. *New England Journal of Medicine, 320,* 29–37, 94–101.

Enthoven, A. C., & Kronick, R. (1991). Universal health insurance through incentives reform. *JAMA, 265,* 2532–2536.

Flynn, P., Wade, M., & Holahan, J. (1997). State health reform: Effects on labor markets and economic activity. *Journal of Policy Analysis and Management, 16,* 219–236.

Giacomini, M., Luft, H. S., & Robinson, J. C. (1995). Risk adjusting community rated health plan premiums. *Annual Review of Public Health, 16,* 401–430.

Gilmer, T., & Kronick, R. (2005). It's the premiums, stupid: Projections of the uninsured through 2013. *Health Affairs,* (Suppl. Web Exclusives), W5-143–W5-151.

Gonser, G. (2011). Mandated benefits and health insurance costs. *Journal of the Massachusetts Dental Society, 60*(2), 9.

Gostin, L. O., & Garcia, K. K. (2012). Affordable Care Act litigation: The Supreme Court and the future of health care reform. *JAMA, 307*(4), 369–370.

Graves, J. A., Curtis, R., & Gruber, J. (2011). Balancing coverage affordability and continuity under a basic health program option. *New England Journal of Medicine, 365*(24), e44.

Gruber, J., & Perry, I. (2011). Realizing health reform's potential: Will the Affordable Care Act make health insurance affordable? *Issue Brief (Commonwealth Fund), 2,* 1–15.

Grumbach, K., Bodenheimer, T., Himmelstein, D. U., & Woolhandler, S. (1991). Liberal benefits, conservative spending. *JAMA, 265,* 2549–2554.

Gupta, A., & Sao, D. (2011). The constitutionality of current legal barriers to telemedicine in the United States: Analysis and future directions of its relationship to national and international health care reform. *Health Matrix, 21*(2), 385–442.

Hall, M. A. (1994). *Reforming private health insurance.* Washington, DC: American Enterprise Institute.

Hardcastle, L. E., Record, K. L., Jacobson, P. D., & Gostin, L. O. (2011). Improving the population's health: The Affordable Care Act and the importance of integration. *Journal of Law, Medicine & Ethics, 39,* 317–327.

Holahan, J., Moon, M., Welch, W. P., & Zuckerman, S. (1991). An American approach to health system reform. *JAMA, 265,* 2537–2540.

Iglehart, J. K. (2011). Medicare payment reform—Proposals for paying for an SGR repeal. *New England Journal of Medicine, 365*(20), 1859–1861.

Karaca-Mandic, P., Abraham, J. M., & Phelps, C. E. (2011). How do health insurance loading fees vary by group size?: Implications for healthcare reform. *International Journal of Health Care Finance & Economics, 11*(3), 181–207.

Lahey, J. N. (2012). The efficiency of a group-specific mandated benefit revisited: The effect of infertility mandates. *Journal of Policy Analysis & Management, 31*(1), 63–92.

Light, D. W. (1992). The practice and ethics of risk-rated health insurance. *JAMA, 267*, 2503–2508.

Luft, H. S. (1978). How do health maintenance organizations achieve their savings? *New England Journal of Medicine, 298*, 1336–1343.

Luft, H. S. (1980). Assessing the evidence on HMO performance. *Milbank Memorial Fund Quarterly, 58*, 501–536.

Marton, J., Ketsche, P. G., & Zhou, M. (2010). SCHIP premiums, enrollment, and expenditures: A two state, competing risk analysis. *Health Economics, 19*(7), 772–791.

Marton, J., & Talbert, J. C. (2010). CHIP premiums, health status, and the insurance coverage of children. *Inquiry, 47*(3), 199–214.

Morrisey, M. A., Kilgore, M. L., & Nelson, L. J. (2008). Medical malpractice reform and employer-sponsored health insurance premiums. *Health Services Research, 43*(6), 2124–2142.

Pauly, M. V. (1990). The rational nonpurchase of long-term-care insurance. *Journal of Political Economy, 98*, 153–168.

Pauly, M. V., Damon, P., Feldstein, P. & Hoff, J. (1991). A plan for "responsible national health insurance." *Health Affairs, 10*(1), 5–25.

Reinhardt, U. E. (1993a). An "all-American" health reform proposal. *Journal of American Health Policy, 3*(3), 11–17.

Reinhardt, U. E. (1993b). Reorganizing the financial flows in American health care. *Health Affairs, 12*(Suppl.), 173–193.

Rice, T., Brown, E. R., & Wyn, R. (1993). Holes in the Jackson Hole approach to health care reform. *JAMA, 270*, 1357–1362.

Selden, T. M. (1999). Premium subsidies for health insurance: Excess coverage vs. adverse selection. *Journal of Health Economics, 18*, 709–725.

Shortridge, E. F., Moore, J. R., Whitmore, H., O'Grady, M. J., & Shen, A. K. (2011). Policy implications of first-dollar coverage: A qualitative examination from the payer perspective. *Public Health Reports, 126*(3), 394–399.

Summers, L. H. (1989). Some simple economics of mandated benefits. *American Economic Review, 79*(Suppl.), 177–183.

Tanne, J. H. (2011). Cost must be considered in setting essential health benefits under US health reform act. *BMJ, 343*, d6524.

Thomas, K. (1994/1995). Are subsidies enough to encourage the uninsured to purchase health insurance? *Inquiry, 31*, 415–424.

Thorpe, K. E. (1992). Expanding employment-based health insurance: Is small group reform the answer? *Inquiry, 29*, 128–136.

Thorpe, K. E., Hendricks, A., Garnick, D., Donelan, K., & Newhouse, J. P. (1992). Reducing the number of uninsured by subsidizing employment-based health insurance. *JAMA, 267*, 945–948.

Whitmore, H., Gabel, J. R., Pickreign, J., & McDevitt, R. (2011). The individual insurance market before reform: Low premiums and low benefits. *Medical Care Research & Review, 68*(5), 594–606.

Wilper, A. P., Woolhandler, S., Lasser, K. E., McCormick, D., Bor, D. H., & Himmelstein, D. U. (2008). A national study of chronic disease prevalence and access to care in uninsured U.S. adults. *Annals of Internal Medicine, 149*(3), 170–176.

Wilper, A. P., Woolhandler, S., Lasser, K. E., McCormick, D., Bor, D. H., & Himmelstein, D. U. (2009). Health insurance and mortality in US adults. *American Journal of Public Health, 99*(12), 2289–2295.

Zabinski, D., Selden, T. M., Moeller, J. F., & Banthin, J. S. (1999). Medical savings accounts: Microsimulation results from a model with adverse selection. *Journal of Health Economics, 18*, 195–218.

Zweifel, P., & Breuer, M. (2006). The case for risk-based premiums in public health insurance. *Health Economics, Policy, & Law, 1*(Pt. 2), 171–188.

Managed Care

Baker, L. C. & Brown, M. L. (1999). Managed care, consolidation among health care providers and health care: Evidence from mammography. *RAND Journal of Economics, 30,* 351–374.

Berchtold, P., Kunzi, B., & Busato, A. (2011). Differences of the quality of care experience: The perception of patients with either network or conventional health plans. *Family Practice, 28*(4), 406–413.

Brennan, N., & Shepard, M. (2010). Comparing quality of care in the Medicare program. *American Journal of Managed Care, 16*(11), 841–848.

Chapman, R. H., Liu, L. Z., Girase, P. G., & Straka, R. J. (2011). Determining initial and follow-up costs of cardiovascular events in a US-managed care population. *BMC Cardiovascular Disorders, 11,* 11.

Chernew, M., Fendrick, A. M., & Hirth, R. A. (1997). Managed care and medical technology: Implications for cost growth. *Health Affairs, 16*(2), 196–209.

Dalal, A. A., Shah, M., Lunacsek, O., & Hanania, N. A. (2011). Clinical and economic burden of depression/anxiety in chronic obstructive pulmonary disease patients within a managed care population. *Journal of Chronic Obstructive Pulmonary Disease, 8,* 293–299.

Deom, M., Agoritsas, T., Bovier, P. A., & Perneger, T. V. (2010). What doctors think about the impact of managed care tools on quality of care, costs, autonomy, and relations with patients. *BMC Health Services Research, 10,* 331.

Elliott, M. N., Haviland, A. M., Orr, N., Hambarsoomian, K., & Cleary, P. D. (2011). How do the experiences of Medicare beneficiary subgroups differ between managed care and original Medicare? *Health Services Research, 46,* 1039–1058.

Feldman, R., Chan, H. C., Kralewski, J., Dowd, B., & Shapiro, J. (1990). Effects of HMOs on the creation of competitive markets for hospital services. *Journal of Health Economics, 9,* 207–222.

Frakt, A. B. (2011). How much do hospitals cost shift? A review of the evidence. *Milbank Quarterly, 89,* 90–130.

Frank, R. G., & Welch, W. P. (1985). The competitive effects of HMOs: A review of the evidence. *Inquiry, 22,* 148–161.

Grandchamp, C., & Gardiol, L. (2011). Does a mandatory telemedicine call prior to visiting a physician reduce costs or simply attract good risks? *Health Economics, 20,* 1257–1267.

Gruber, J., & Simon, K. (2008). Crowd-out 10 years later: Have recent public insurance expansions crowded out private health insurance? *Journal of Health Economics, 27*(2), 201–217.

Health Policy Tracking Service. (2011). Managed care. Issue brief. *Issue Brief—Health Policy Tracking Service,* 1–32.

Hellerstein, J. K. (1998). Public funds, private funds, and medical innovation: How managed care affects public funds for clinical research. *American Economic Review, 88*(2), 112–116.

Hill, S. C., & Wolfe, B. L. (1997). Testing the HMO competitive strategy: An analysis of its impact on medical care resources. *Journal of Health Economics, 16,* 261–286.

Iglehart, J. K. (2011). Desperately seeking savings: States shift more Medicaid enrollees to managed care. *Health Affairs, 30*(9), 1627–1629.

Iglehart, J. K. (2012). Expanding eligibility, cutting costs—A Medicaid update. *New England Journal of Medicine, 366*(2), 105–107.

Jones, M., Hsu, C., Pearson, D., Wolford, D., & Labby, D. (2011). An alternative to pay-for-performance: One health plan's approach to quality improvement. *Journal for Healthcare Quality, 33,* 22–29.

Kemper, P., Reschovsky, J. D., & Tu, H. T. (1999). Do HMOs make a difference? Summary and implications. *Inquiry, 36,* 419–425.

Kolbasovsky, A. (2011). Strategies for measuring outcomes and ROI for managed care programs. Determining return on investment and improvement of outcomes is essential when new programs are being tried, but the research method must be chosen carefully. *Managed Care, 20*(11), 54–57.

Lake, T. (1999). Do HMOs make a difference? Consumer assessments of health care. *Inquiry, 36,* 411–418.

Landon, B. E., Zaslavsky, A. M., Bernard, S. L., Cioffi, M. J., & Cleary, P. D. (2004). Comparison of performance of traditional Medicare vs Medicare managed care. *JAMA*, *291*(14), 1744–1752.

Manning, W. G., Leibowitz, A., Goldberg, G. A., Rogers, W. H., & Newhouse, J. P. (1984). A controlled trial of the effect of a prepaid group practice on use of services. *New England Journal of Medicine, 310,* 1505–1510.

McLaughlin, C. G. (1988). Market responses to HMOs: Price competition or rivalry? *Inquiry, 25,* 207–218.

Mason, M. V., Poole-Yaeger, A., Lucas, B., Krueger, C. R., Ahmed, T., & Duncan, I. (2011). Effects of a pregnancy management program on birth outcomes in managed Medicaid. *Managed Care, 20*(4), 39–46.

McCue, M. J., & Bailit, M. H. (2011). Assessing the financial health of Medicaid managed care plans and the quality of patient care they provide. *Issue Brief (Commonwealth Fund), 11,* 1–16.

Miller, R. H., & Luft, H. S. (1997). Does managed care lead to better or worse quality of care? *Health Affairs, 16*(5), 7–25.

Mobley, L. R., Subramanian, S., Koschinsky, J., Frech, H. E., Trantham, L. C., & Anselin, L. (2011). Managed care and the diffusion of endoscopy in fee-for-service Medicare. *Health Services Research, 46,* 1905–1927.

Newhouse, J. P. (1996). Health reform in the United States. *Economic Journal, 106,* 1713–1724.

Nugent, M. E. (2011a). Aligning managed care contracts, compensation plans, and incentive models. *Healthcare Financial Management, 65*(11), 88–92, 94, 96.

Nugent, M. E. (2011b). Budget planning under payment reform. *Healthcare Financial Management, 65*(7), 38–42.

Pracht, E. E., Orban, B. L., Comins, M. M., Large, J. T., & Asin-Oostburg, V. (2011). The relative effectiveness of managed care penetration and the healthcare safety net in reducing avoidable hospitalizations. *Journal for Healthcare Quality, 33,* 42–51; quiz, 51–53.

Reschovsky, J. D. (1999a). Do HMOs make a difference? Access to health care. *Inquiry, 36,* 390– 399.

Reschovsky, J. D. (1999b). Do HMOs make a difference? Data and methods. *Inquiry, 36,* 378–389.

Reschovsky, J. D., & Kemper, P. (1999). Do HMOs make a difference? Introduction. *Inquiry, 36,* 374–377.

Robinson, J. C. (1991). HMO market penetration and hospital cost inflation in California. *JAMA, 266,* 2719–2725.

Saunier, B. (2011). The devil is in the details: Managed care and the unforeseen costs of utilization review as a cost containment mechanism. *Issues in Law & Medicine, 27*(1), 21–48.

Shipman, D., Hooten, J., & Roa, M. (2011). Is managed care an oxymoron? *Nursing Ethics, 18*(1), 126–128; discussion, 129–130.

Stern, J. M. (2011). The role of managed care in improving outcomes in epilepsy. *American Journal of Managed Care, 17*(Suppl. 10), S263–S270.

Tu, H. T., Kemper, P., & Wong, H. J. (1999). Do HMOs make a difference? Use of health services. *Inquiry, 36,* 400–410.

Wholey, D., Feldman, R., & Christianson, J. B. (1995). The effect of market structure on HMO premiums. *Journal of Health Economics, 14,* 81–105.

Wholey, D., Christianson, J. B., Engberg, J., & Bryce, C. (1997). HMO market structure and performance, 1985–1995. *Health Affairs, 16*(6), 75–84.

Consumer Information

Alexander, J. A., Hearld, L. R., Hasnain-Wynia, R., Christianson, J. B., & Martsolf, G. R. (2011). Consumer trust in sources of physician quality information. *Medical Care Research & Review, 68,* 421–440.

Baldwin, M., Spong, A., Doward, L., & Gnanasakthy, A. (2011). Patient-reported outcomes, patient-reported information: From randomized controlled trials to the social web and beyond. *The Patient: Patient-Centered Outcomes Research, 4,* 11–17.

Beales, J.H., III (2011). Health related claims, the market for information, and the first amendment. *Health Matrix, 21*(1), 7–30.

Buckley, N. A., & Rossi, S. (2011). Bringing greater transparency to "black box" warnings. Clinical toxicology: *The Official Journal of the American Academy of Clinical Toxicology & European Association of Poisons Centres & Clinical Toxicologists, 49*(6), 448–451.

Cho, J., Noh, H. I. Ha, M. H. Kang, S. N. Choi, J. Y.and Chang. Y. J. (2011). What kind of cancer information do Internet users need? *Supportive Care in Cancer, 19*(9), 1465–1469.

Crutzen, R., Cyr, D., & de Vries, N. K. (2011). Bringing loyalty to e-health: Theory validation using three Internet-delivered interventions. *Journal of Medical Internet Research, 13*(3), e73.

Epstein, A. M. (1998). Rolling down the runway: The challenges ahead for quality report cards. *JAMA, 279,* 1691–1696.

Grabowski, D. C., & Town, R. J. (2011). Does information matter? Competition, quality, and the impact of nursing home report cards. *Health Services Research, 46,* 1698–1719.

Haggstrom, D. A., & Doebbeling, B. N. (2011). Quality measurement and system change of cancer care delivery. *Medical Care, 49*(Suppl.), S21–S27.

Hannan, E. L., Kilburn, H., Jr., Lindsey, M. L., & Lewis, R. (1992). Clinical versus administrative data bases for CABG surgery: Does it matter? *Medical Care, 30,* 892–907.

Harris, P. R., Sillence, E., & Briggs, P. (2011). Perceived threat and corroboration: Key factors that improve a predictive model of trust in Internet-based health information and advice. *Journal of Medical Internet Research, 13*(3), e51.

Hirth, R. A. (1999). Consumer information and competition between nonprofit and for-profit nursing homes. *Journal of Health Economics, 18,* 219–240.

Horden, A., Georgiou, A., Whetton, S., & Prgomet, M. (2011). Consumer e-health: An overview of research evidence and implications for future policy. *Health Information Management Journal, 40*(2), 6–14.

Iezzoni, L. I., Ash, A. S., Shwartz, M., Daley, J., Hughes, J. S., & Mackieman, Y. D. (1996). Judging hospitals by severity-adjusted mortality rates: The influence of the severity-adjustment method. *American Journal of Public Health, 86,* 1379–1387.

Knutson, D. J., Kind, E. A., Fowles, J. B., & Adlis, S. (1998). Impact of report cards on employees: A natural experiment. *Health Care Financing Review, 20*(1), 5–27.

Lober, W. B., & Flowers, J. L. (2011). Consumer empowerment in health care amid the Internet and social media. *Seminars in Oncology Nursing, 27,* 169–182.

Luft, H. S., Garnick, D. W., Mark, D. H., Peltzman, D. J., Phibbs, C. S., Lichtenberg, E., & McPhee, S. J. (1990. Does quality influence choice of hospital? *JAMA, 263,* 2899–2906.

Mackert, M., & Love, B. (2011). Educational content and health literacy issues in direct-to-consumer advertising of pharmaceuticals. *Health Marketing Quarterly, 28*(3), 205–218.

Mennemeyer, S. T., Morrisey, M. A., & Howard, L. Z. (1997). Death and reputation: How consumers acted upon HCFA mortality information. *Inquiry, 34,* 117–128.

Nili, T., Moti, M., & Avner, C. (2011). Dentists' attitudes toward discussing Internet health information with their patients—Does professional self-efficacy matter? *Journal of Public Health Dentistry, 71*(2), 102–105.

Noah, L. (2011). Truth or consequences?: Commercial free speech vs. public health promotion (at the FDA). *Health Matrix, 21*(1), 31–95.

Patel, P. P., Hoppe I. C., Ahuja, N. K., & Ciminello, F. S. (2011). Analysis of comprehensibility of patient information regarding complex craniofacial conditions. *Journal of Craniofacial Surgery, 22*(4), 1179–1182.

Radina, M. E., Ginter, A. C., Brandt, J., Swaney, J., & Longo, D. R. (2011). Breast cancer patients' use of health information in decision making and coping. *Cancer Nursing, 34*(5), E1–E12.

Rickard, L. N. (2011). In backyards, on front lawns: Examining informal risk communication and communicators. *Public Understanding of Science, 20*(5), 642–657.

Scanlon, D. P., & Chernew, M. (1999). HEDIS measures and managed care enrollment. *Medical Care Research and Review, 56*(Suppl. 2), 60–84.

Spoeri R. K., & Ullman, R. (1997). Measuring and reporting managed care performance: Lessons learned and new initiatives. *Annals of Internal Medicine, 127,* 726–732.

Tu, H. T. (2011). Surprising decline in consumers seeking health information. *Tracking Report,* (26), 1–6.

Vranceanu, A. M., & Ring, D. (2011). Factors associated with patient satisfaction. *Journal of Hand Surgery—American Volume, 36*(9), 1504–1508.

Patient Centered Medical Home

Adubato, S. (2008). Don't say "managed care"; Say "patient-centered care." *MD Advisor, 1*(1), 11–13.

Bertakis, K. D., & Azari, R. (2011). Determinants and outcomes of patient-centered care. *Patient Education & Counseling, 85,* 46–52.

Bras, M., Dordevic, V., Milunovic, V., Brajkovic, L., Milicic, D., & Konopka, L. (2011). Person-centered medicine versus personalized medicine: Is it just a sophism? A view from chronic pain management. *Psychiatria Danubina, 23*(3), 246–250.

Burston, S., Chaboyer, W., Wallis, M., & Stanfield, J. (2011). A discussion of approaches to transforming care: Contemporary strategies to improve patient safety. *Journal of Advanced Nursing, 67,* 2488–2495.

Butcher, L. (2011). Medical homes prepare the way for accountable care organizations. *Managed Care, 20*(10), 67–69.

Crabtree, B. F., Nutting, P. A., Miller, W. L., McDaniel, R. R., Stange, K. C., Jaen, C. R., & Stewart, E. (2011). Primary care practice transformation is hard work: Insights from a 15-year developmental program of research. *Medical Care, 49*(Suppl.), S28–S35.

Farmer, J. E., Clark, M. J. Drewel, E. H., Swenson, T. M., & Ge, B. (2011). Consultative care coordination through the medical home for CSHCN: A randomized controlled trial. *Maternal & Child Health Journal, 15,* 1110–1118.

Groene, O. (2011). Patient centeredness and quality improvement efforts in hospitals: Rationale, measurement, implementation. *International Journal for Quality in Health Care, 23*(5), 531–537.

Hjorngaard, T. (2011). Family-centered care: A critical perspective. *Physical & Occupational Therapy in Pediatrics, 31*(3), 243–244.

Hofdijk, J. (2011). Patient-centered integrated clinical resource management. *Studies in Health Technology & Informatics, 169,* 996–999.

Hughes, C. L., Marshall, C. R., Murphy, E., & Mun, S. K. (2011). Technologies in the patient-centered medical home: Examining the model from an enterprise perspective. *Telemedicine Journal & E-Health, 17*(6), 495–500.

Kagan, S. H. (2011). Patient- and family-centered care—Is there individualized care here? *Geriatric Nursing, 32*(5), 365–367.

Luxford, K., Safran, D. G., & Delbanco, T. (2011). Promoting patient-centered care: A qualitative study of facilitators and barriers in healthcare organizations with a reputation for improving the patient experience. *International Journal for Quality in Health Care, 23*(5), 510–515.

Lyon, R. K., & Slawson, J. (2011). An organized approach to chronic disease care. *Family Practice Management, 18*(3), 27–31.

Manahan, B. (2011). The whole systems medicine of tomorrow: A half-century perspective. *Explore: The Journal of Science & Healing, 7*(4), 212–214.

Marsh, H. M., & Schenk, M. J. (2011). Primary care in the new millennium: Affordable, sustainable systems of care. *Michigan Medicine, 110*(5), 8.

Marshall, R. C., Doperak, M., Milner, M., Motsinger, C., Newton, T., Padden, M., …, & Mun, S. K. (2011). Patient-centered medical home: An emerging primary care model and the military health system. *Military Medicine, 176*(11), 1253–1259.

Porterfield, S. L., & DeRigne, L. (2011). Medical home and out-of-pocket medical costs for children with special health care needs. *Pediatrics, 128*(5), 892–900.

Rittenhouse, D. R., Casalino, L. P., Shortell, S. M., McClellan, S. R., Gillies, R. R., Alexander, J. A., & Drum, M. L. (2011). Small and medium-size physician practices use few patient-centered medical home processes. *Health Affairs, 30*(8), 1575–1584.

Romeo, S. J. (2011). The promise of the medical home. *Medical Economics, 88*(20), 59–60, 65.

Roumie, C. L., Greevy, R., Wallston, K. A., Elasy, T. A., Kaltenbach, L., Kotter, K., ..., & Speroff, T. (2011). Patient-centered primary care is associated with patient hypertension medication adherence. *Journal of Behavioral Medicine, 34*(4), 244–253.

Sandman, L., & Munthe, C. (2010). Shared decision making, paternalism and patient choice. *Health Care Analysis, 18*(1), 60–84.

Snyder, C. F., Wu, A. W., Miller, R. S., Jensen, R. E., Bantug, E. T., & Wolff, A. C. (2011). The role of informatics in promoting patient-centered care. *Cancer Journal, 17*(4), 211–218.

Stichler, J. F. (2011). Patient-centered healthcare design. *Journal of Nursing Administration, 41,* 503–506.

Takach, M. (2011). Reinventing Medicaid: State innovations to qualify and pay for patient-centered medical homes show promising results. *Health Affairs, 30*(7), 1325–1334.

Washington, A. E., & Lipstein, S. H. (2011). The Patient-Centered Outcomes Research Institute—Promoting better information, decisions, and health. *New England Journal of Medicine, 365*(15), e31.

Zickafoose, J. S., Gebremariam, A., Clark, S. J., & Davis, M. M. (2011). Medical home disparities between children with public and private insurance. *Academic Pediatrics, 11*(4), 305–310.

Accountable Care Organizations

Accountable Care Organization Learning Network. (2011). *ACO toolkit.* Washington, DC: Engelberg Center for Health Care Reform, The Dartmouth Institute.

Aslin, P. (2011). Unveiling the unicorn: A leader's guide to ACO preparation. *Journal of Healthcare Management, 56*(4), 245–253.

Bailit, M., & Hughes, C. (2011). Key design elements of shared-savings payment arrangements. *Issue Brief (Commonwealth Fund), 20,* 1–16.

Berenson, R. A. (2010). Shared savings program for accountable care organizations: A bridge to nowhere? *American Journal of Managed Care, 16*(10), 721–726.

Berwick, D. M. (2011a). Launching accountable care organizations—The proposed rule for the Medicare Shared Savings Program. *New England Journal of Medicine, 364*(16), e32.

Berwick, D. M. (2011b). Making good on ACOs' promise—The final rule for the Medicare shared-savings program. *New England Journal of Medicine, 365*(19), 1753–1756.

Bliss-Holtz, J. (2011). Accountable care organizations: Characteristics, challenges and responses. *Issues in Comprehensive Pediatric Nursing, 34*(2), 59–61.

Boland, P., Polakoff, P., & Schwab, T. (2010). Accountable care organizations hold promise, but will they achieve cost and quality targets? *Managed Care, 19*(10), 12–16, 19.

Breslau, J., & Lexa, F. J. (2011). A radiologist's primer on accountable care organizations. *Journal of the American College of Radiology, 8*(3), 164–168.

Burke, T. (2011). Accountable care organizations. *Public Health Reports, 126*(6), 875–878.

Centers for Medicare & Medicaid Services (CMS), HHS. (201). Medicare program: Medicare shared-savings program: Accountable care organizations. *Final rule. Federal Register, 76*(212), 67802–67990.

Chu, D. Z. (2011). Future of surgery: Accountable care organizations and the end of private practice? *Journal of the American College of Surgeons, 213*(6), 810–811.

Correia, E. W. (2011). Accountable care organizations: The proposed regulations and the prospects for success. *American Journal of Managed Care, 17*(8), 560–568.

Devore, S., & Champion, R. W. (2011). Driving population health through accountable care organizations. *Health Affairs, 30*(1), 41–50.

Diamond, F. (2009). Accountable care organizations give capitation surprise encore. *Managed Care, 18*(9), 14–15, 21–24.

Dove, J. T., Weaver, W. D., & Lewin, J. (2009). Health care delivery system reform: Accountable care organizations. *Journal of the American College of Cardiology, 54*(11), 985–988.

Eldridge, G. N., & Korda, H. (2011). Value-based purchasing: The evidence. *American Journal of Managed Care, 17*(8), e310–e313.

Filson, C. P., Hollingsworth, J. M., Skolarus, T. A., Clemens, J. Q., & Hollenbeck, B. K. (2011). Health care reform in 2010: Transforming the delivery system to improve quality of care. *World Journal of Urology, 29*(1), 85–90.

Fine, A., & Frazier, B. (2011). Can a hospital benefit from partnering with physicians? *Healthcare Financial Management, 65*(5), 70–76.

Fisher, E. S., & Shortell, S. M. (2010). Accountable care organizations: Accountable for what, to whom, and how. *JAMA, 304*(15), 1715–1716.

Fisher, E. S., Staiger, D. O., Bynum, J. P., & Gottlieb, D. J. (2007). Creating accountable care organizations: The extended hospital medical staff. *Health Affairs, 26*(1), w44–w57.

Ginsburg, P. B., & White, C. (2011). Health care's role in deficit reduction—Guiding principles. *New England Journal of Medicine, 365*(17), 1559–1561.

Goldsmith, J. (2011. Accountable care organizations: The case for flexible partnerships between health plans and providers. *Health Affairs, 30*(1), 32–40.

Gosfield, A. G. (2011). Accountable care organizations versus accountable care: Is there a difference? *Journal of the National Comprehensive Cancer Network, 9*(6), 587–589.

Haywood, T. (2010). The cost of confusion: Healthcare reform and value-based purchasing. *Healthcare Financial Management, 64*(10), 44–48.

Kocher, R., & Sahni, N. R. (2010). Physicians versus hospitals as leaders of accountable care organizations. *New England Journal of Medicine, 363*(27), 2579–2582.

Lieberman, S. M., & Bertko, J. M. (2011). Building regulatory and operational flexibility into accountable care organizations and "shared savings." *Health Affairs, 30*(1), 23–31.

Mackinney, A. C., Mueller, K. J., & McBride, T. D. (2011). The march to accountable care organizations—How will rural fare? *Journal of Rural Health, 27*, 131–137.

Maeng, D. D., Scanlon, D. P., Chernew, M. E., Gronniger, T., Wodchis, W. P., & McLaughlin, C. G. (2010). The relationship between health plan performance measures and physician network overlap: Implications for measuring plan quality. *Health Services Research, 45*(4), 1005–1023.

Marsh, H. M., & Schenk, M. J. (2011). Primary care in the new millennium: Affordable, sustainable systems of care. *Michigan Medicine, 110*(5), 8.

Mulvany, C. (2011). Medicare ACOs no longer mythical creatures. *Healthcare Financial Management, 65*(6), 96–104.

Reynolds, J., & Roble, D. (2011). The financial implications of ACOs for providers. *Healthcare Financial Management, 65*(10), 76–82.

Richman, B. D., & Schulman, K. A. (2011). A cautious path forward on accountable care organizations. *JAMA, 305*(6), 602–603.

Schiller, R. E., & Silverman, D. A. (2011). Accountable care organizations: Before you jump in. *Journal of the American College of Radiology, 8*(9), 661–662.

Schoenbaum, S. C. (2011). Accountable care organizations: Roles and opportunities for hospitals. *Hospital Practice, 39*(3), 140–148.

Shields, M. C., Patel, P. H., Manning, M., & Sacks, L. (2011). A model for integrating independent physicians into accountable care organizations. *Health Affairs, 30*(1), 161–172.

Shortell, S. M., & Casalino, L. P. (2010). Implementing qualifications criteria and technical assistance for accountable care organizations. *JAMA, 303*(17), 1747–1748.

Silversmith, J. (2011). Accountable care organizations: A primer. *Minnesota Medicine, 94*(2), 38–40.

Sinaiko, A. D., & Rosenthal, M. B. (2010). Patients' role in accountable care organizations. *New England Journal of Medicine, 363*(27), 2583–2585.

Singer, S., & Shortell, S. M. (2011). Implementing accountable care organizations: Ten potential mistakes and how to learn from them. *JAMA, 306*(7), 758–759.

Smith, C. (2011). Between the Scylla and Charybdis: Physicians and the clash of liability standards and cost cutting goals within accountable care organizations. *Annals of Health Law, 20*(2), 165–203, 6p preceding i.

Springgate, B. F., & Brook, R. H. (2011). Accountable care organizations and community empowerment. *JAMA, 305*(17), 1800–1801.

Terry, K. (2011). Health IT: The glue for accountable care organizations. Four big systems show how they're using EHRs, connectivity, and data warehouses to drive ACOs. *Healthcare Informatics, 28*(5), 16, 18, 20, passim.

Walker, J., & McKethan, A. (2012). Achieving accountable care—"It's not about the bike." *New England Journal of Medicine, 366*(2), e4.

Weinberg, S. L. (2010). Accountable care organizations—Ready for prime time or not? *American Heart Hospital Journal, 8*(2), E78–E79.

Wood, D. (2011). The move to accountable care organizations includes telemedicine. *Telemedicine & e-Health, 17*(4), 237–240.

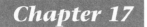

Chapter 17

Regulation and Antitrust Policy in Health Care

OBJECTIVES

1. Define regulation.

2. Describe two different views on why governments regulate markets.

3. Describe the variables that regulators focus on when regulating health care.

4. Identify the regulatory means that are used by regulators of hospitals, physicians, drugs, healthcare insurance, and managed care.

5. Explain the rationale for antitrust policy.

6. Describe market changes that have taken place in health care, and explain how these might affect antitrust enforcement.

7. Describe the key provisions of antitrust legislation in the United States.

8. Explain how antitrust legislation regulates price fixing.

9. Explain how antitrust legislation regulates mergers.

10. Explain how quality issues in health care affect antitrust policy.

17.1 INTRODUCTION

The regulation of markets takes three general forms. *Direct regulation* refers to intervention in markets by regulatory agencies to control price, quantity, or quality by direct action, such as instituting price controls, establishing professional licensure requirements, or assessing and regulating the quality of services. *Indirect regulation* refers to regulatory activities that affect price, quantity, or quality by enforcing the competitive behavior of firms in the market or by changing the structure of the market. Antitrust policy is the leading example of indirect regulation. Governments also intervene in markets through *public ownership* and operation of healthcare facilities and services (Santerre & Neun, 1996). In this chapter, the use of the term *regulation* will generally refer to direct regulation. The chapter will focus on regulation of private sector healthcare providers in the United States and thus will not address public ownership, which is more common in other nations.

Original chapter contributed by Ronald P. Wilder. Revision by Lanis Hicks.

17.1.1 The Concept of Economic Regulation

Economic systems based on competitive markets and private enterprise are characteristic of most of the nations of the world, including the United States. In private enterprise systems, scarce resources are allocated and income is distributed primarily on the basis of supply and demand in markets and the resulting price, income, and profitability signals. In these systems, largely unrestricted free markets are the principal determinants of economic outcomes. Under conditions of perfect competition and complete information, the economic outcome meets the social welfare standards of Pareto optimality. In other words, changes in the allocation of resources could not improve the welfare of some members of society without reducing the welfare of other members of society.

In some instances, including health care, the market outcomes may be viewed as suboptimal by society at-large. Situations in which a market's price, quantity, or product quality does not meet social welfare norms are said, by economists, to be cases of market failure. One form of market failure occurs when prices in a market are above marginal costs as a result of monopoly power. Another type occurs when the external effects of the production or consumption of a product, such as pollution, are not captured in the product's price, creating a wedge between the price and social costs of the product. A third form, especially important for healthcare markets, results from imperfect information. In a market with a low level of information, consumers find it difficult to evaluate the quality of goods and services, and therefore difficult to make decisions regarding whether or not to purchase the goods and services.

Economic regulation consists of governmental interventions intended to affect market outcomes in some manner. There are two different views of why economic regulation exists. According to the first view, economic regulation is generally motivated by the objective of reducing the extent of market failure. According to the second view, it is the result of producers or consumers working through the political process to further their own interests.

17.1.2 Regulation of Health Care

The regulation of health care in the United States and Canada is extensive. Much of this activity is directed toward information and quality issues. Quality-of-care regulation frequently takes the form of control of entry into the market, such as requiring that healthcare professionals be licensed and that new drugs be approved by a regulatory agency. Entry by hospitals is also commonly regulated through policy instruments, such as certificate of need (CON) legislation, which gives permission to a healthcare firm to develop the infrastructure (buildings and equipment) to provide care to specific populations. The regulation of price in health care is generally carried out indirectly through antitrust policy and through the effects of government reimbursement rules on the prices of healthcare services.

17.1.3 Regulation as a Means of Correcting Market Failure

Healthcare markets are characterized by imperfect information on the price and quality of healthcare services. The problem of inadequate information can take a number of forms. Consumers tend to have incomplete information about the quality of healthcare services available from alternative providers and about the probability of a successful outcome for procedures that involve risk. Consumers may also have incomplete information about price because the out-of-pocket price to consumers may be the result of negotiations between providers and third-party payers.

Information can also be impaired as a result of relationships in which a principal delegates responsibility to an agent. One inherent difficulty with such relationships is that the agent possesses information not available to the principal (the person with ultimate authority), and may have different objectives than the principal. An example of an agency relationship is that between a physician and a patient. In health care, the physician is both a healthcare provider and an agent of the consumer. The physician's incentives in the provider role may not be aligned with the incentives of the consumer. This agency relationship between physician and consumer is complicated further by the relationship between the physician and the third-party payer or managed care organization, which also involves agency. These complex relationships have led at least one writer to use the phrase "the doctor as double agent" (Blomqvist, 1991). When the physician serves as both a provider of services and a demander of services in the role of the patient's agent, then the independent relationship between demand and supply is broken and market failure can occur.

Consumers may be handicapped by the lack of information about quality of healthcare services and about quality of alternative providers. Thus, incomplete information may prevent socially optimal outcomes in healthcare markets. The agency relationships between a consumer and his or her physician and between the consumer and other providers may also lead to over- or underconsumption of healthcare services relative to the social optimum that would be realizable with complete information.

Therefore, the direct regulation of healthcare providers may be a response of governments to the perception that the consumer lacks information about quality and thus that the workings of competitive, private-enterprise healthcare markets may not produce the best outcomes in terms of social welfare. Another possibility, as mentioned earlier, is that regulation is fostered as a means for providers to further their private interests.

17.1.4 Regulation as a Political Good

In his seminal work on the economic theory of regulation, George Stigler (1971), supplemented by work by Peltzman (1976) and others, pointed out that regulatory legislation may redistribute wealth. This effect of regulation is important, given that the behavior of legislators is likely to be motivated by their wish to remain in office. If there is competition among special interest groups in the democratic system, that competition may take the form of exchanges of political support for legislation favorable to the objectives of the interest groups. If the political process works in this manner, well-organized interest groups, with a high per capita stake in the outcomes of legislation, will tend to dominate larger interest groups with a smaller per capita stake.

The economic theory of regulation suggests that providers may be able to dominate the legislative and regulatory process. This suggestion is a hypothesis and not a conclusion of the economic theory of regulation. What are the actual healthcare-related outcomes of real-world legislative and regulatory processes is an empirical question. Very active lobbying activities are pursued by healthcare provider groups, as well as healthcare consumer groups.

17.2 REGULATION OF HEALTH CARE

Regulation of health care takes the form of regulation of price, quantity (or utilization), and quality. Sometimes, the quality objectives are achieved through control of entry, such as the licensure of physicians. In other instances, quality is regulated by the setting of technical standards, as in the regulation of pharmaceuticals. In the following sections, the regulation of hospitals and long-term care facilities, the regulation of physician services, and the regulation of pharmaceuticals are discussed separately. Indirect regulation through antitrust policy is subsequently considered.

17.2.1 Regulation of Hospitals and Long-Term Care Facilities

Community hospitals are the major providers of acute medical and surgical care. Many hospitals are tax-exempt nonprofit institutions, supported by government or by charitable organizations. In the United States, there has been an increase in the importance of investor-owned hospitals. In addition, there has been a large number of hospital mergers, as well as formal and informal vertical combinations among hospitals, insurance and managed care companies, and physicians groups (Gaynor & Haas-Wilson, 1999).

Direct regulation of hospitals includes such supply-side measures as certificate-of-need requirements for the entry of new hospitals or the expansion of additional services. Demand-side regulations include price controls imposed through the payment practices of such government programs as Medicare and Medicaid. Price controls may also affect the supply side by motivating greater efficiency and reducing lengths of stay. Regulation of hospital service quality includes licensure, peer review, utilization review, and pay-for-performance systems.

17.2.2 Regulation of Hospital Quality

Hospitals are licensed by a state licensing agency, typically located in the state department of health. The license requires that a minimum level of facilities, services, and personnel be present; the intent is to ensure the quality of services delivered is safe, cost-effective, and compliant with all state and federal laws. In addition to this direct regulation by state governments, hospitals participate in self-regulation by seeking accreditation from The Joint Commission (TJC), formerly known as the Joint Commission on Accreditation of Healthcare Organizations (JCAHO). By the end of 2011, The Joint Commission accredited or certified over 19,000 healthcare organizations and programs in the United States (Joint Comission, 2012).

Hospital quality is also regulated by quality improvement organizations (QIOs), which were originally established as peer-review organizations (PROs) under the Tax Equity and Fiscal Responsibility Act (TEFRA) of 1982, an act that made numerous changes to Medicare. The Centers for Medicare and Medicaid Services (CMS) administers the QIO program, which is designed "to review medical care and help beneficiaries with complaints about the quality of care received, and to implement improvements in the quality of care available throughout the spectrum of care" (http://cms.gov). The mission of the QIO is to improve effectiveness, efficiency, economy, and quality of services delivered to Medicare beneficiaries.

There are 53 QIOs, one in each state, the District of Columbia, Puerto Rico, and the U.S. Virgin Islands. The QIOs are private, usually tax-exempt, organizations. The care functions of the QIOs have been identified by CMS as

- Improving quality of care to beneficiaries;

- Protecting the integrity of the Medicare Trust Fund by ensuring that Medicare pays only for services and goods that are reasonable and necessary, and that are provided in the most appropriate setting; and

- Protecting beneficiaries by expeditiously addressing individual complaints, such as beneficiary complaints, provider-based notice appeals, violations of the Emergency Medical Treatment and Labor Act (EMTALA), and other related responsibilities as articulated in QIO-related laws. (http://cms.gov/QualityImprovementOrgs/)

Through the history of PROs and QIOs, efforts have been directed to advance national efforts to motivate providers to improve quality. They have also focused on measuring and improving outcomes of quality.

17.2.3 Supply-Side Regulation of Hospitals

The quality review improvement organizations, in addition to regulating quality, may also review utilization of care. Utilization deemed inappropriate would be denied payment by Medicare. Since the advent of the prospective payment system, however, the QIOs have been more focused on quality of service than on excessive utilization.

Certificate-of-need regulation is a form of supply-side regulation. Its stated purpose is to restrain health facility costs and allow coordinated planning of new services and construction in order to prevent duplication of facilities or excessive capital expenditures. Certificate-of-need regulation for hospitals played an extensive role during the 1970s and 1980s, but the federal requirement that states have certificate-of-need regulation ended in 1986. Since then, several states have ended certificate-of-need regulation for hospitals. As of December 2009, however, 36 states retained some type of CON law. A retrospective study of the consequences of ending certificate-of-need regulation found that such regulation had only a modest containing effect on hospital costs (Conover & Sloan, 1998). A 2009 study by Hellinger found that CON laws reduced the number of hospital beds by about 10% and healthcare expenditures by almost 2%.

17.2.4 Demand-Side Regulation of Hospitals

Hospital prices and charges are subject to extensive regulation. Rate regulation at the state level was widely practiced during the 1970s and 1980s but has since largely disappeared. Medicare's prospective payment system (PPS), established in the early 1980s, controls hospital charges nationwide, but for Medicare patients only. In addition to their direct effect on hospital charges, Medicare payment rules may influence the charges paid by other payers, such as health insurance companies and HMOs.

Studies of the effectiveness of price regulation of hospitals have generally found that hospitals entered a new competitive era in the early 1980s, as Medicare's PPS, which paid providers prospectively based on diagnosis rather than retrospectively, tended to reduce days of stay and hospital occupancy rates and increase price competition among hospitals (Dranove, Shanley, & White l, 1993). The increase in price competition was reinforced by the rapid development of managed care and the greater purchasing power of large payer groups.

17.2.5 Regulation of Long-Term Care Facilities

Long-term care in the United States is provided in tax-exempt and investor-owned nursing homes, which are regulated by state and federal agencies. Licensing is by state health departments. Nursing homes may also pursue self-regulation by seeking accreditation through The Joint Commission.

Nursing homes are regulated on the supply side by state CON regulation, or moratoriums which restricts construction and capacity increases. Certificate-of-need regulation was most important in the years directly after Medicare and Medicaid began to cover nursing home costs for some patients. It limited the expansion of nursing home providers and hence the financial burden on states, which finance Medicaid jointly with the federal government (Getzen, 1997).

Whatever price regulation of nursing homes exists is primarily a result of the reimbursement systems used by Medicare and Medicaid. Medicaid, which covers the medically needy, generally pays a flat rate per day, although some states have moved to adopt a system in which payment is based on the health status of the patient. Medicare covers skilled nursing services for a limited period of time after certain hospitalizations. Since the changes introduced by the 1997 Balanced Budget Amendments, Medicare uses a prospective payment system in which the daily rate depends on the health status of the patient (Folland, Goodman, & Stano, 2001).

17.2.6 Regulation of Physician Services

Physicians play a central role in health care. They have total or partial control of hospital admissions, specialist referrals, and drug prescriptions. They also advise patients on the necessity or potential benefit of medical services. Traditionally, physicians were paid on a fee-for-service basis. Currently, 80–90% of physician fees are paid by third-party payers, who possess some control over price and utilization. Physicians are also subject to regulations intended to ensure high quality of care.

17.2.7 Regulation of Physician Quality and Utilization

The primary regulation of physician quality is through state licensure—the granting of licenses to practice medicine to those who meet specific criteria. Because state legislatures appoint state licensing boards with input from the state medical associations, licensing is a form of self-regulation.

Quality Improvement Organizations monitor the utilization patterns and the professional quality of hospitals and physicians. In 1986, Congress enacted the Health Care Quality Improvement Act, which provides legal protections to those participating in peer reviews by granting immunity from testifying in malpractice lawsuits. In addition, the act established the National Practitioner Data Base, which is an information clearinghouse that gathers information on malpractice judgments, disciplinary actions, and license suspensions and revocations. Scheutzow (1999) reviewed the practice of peer-review organizations and concluded that because of the failure to report incidents and other problems, the present peer-review process is ineffective. In the early 1990s, the earlier PROs were converted to QIOs, with more emphasis placed on improving quality of care and outcomes. Increased emphasis is being placed on improving measures of quality and assisting providers to achieve these measures.

17.2.8 Regulation of Physician Pricing

Medicare and Medicaid reimburse physicians on a modified fee-for-service basis. In the early years of Medicare and Medicaid, fees were screened on the basis of usual, customary, and reasonable (UCR) payments. The UCR system included the range of fees charged by other physicians in the same geographic area. In 1992, Medicare began using a new method of physician payment. This method, which utilizes the Resource Based Relative Value Scale (RBRVS), includes components for physician time and skill, practice expenses, and professional liability insurance (Medicare Payment Advisory Commission, 2000). The reimbursement rules amount to price controls on the services provided to patients covered by Medicare, and in fact they have an effect on the prices charged by managed care plans and private insurance plans that insure large numbers of private patients.

17.2.9 Regulation of the Pharmaceutical Industry

The production of pharmaceuticals is regulated by the Food and Drug Administration (FDA). The distribution and dispensing of pharmaceuticals is regulated at the state level by the licensing of pharmacists and by requirements that apply to pharmacy operations. At the present time, the prices of pharmaceuticals are not directly controlled, but government agencies, such as Medicaid, and other large purchasers, use their purchasing power to obtain lower prices than those paid by noninsured consumers. In some instances, lower prices are negotiated through the design of drug formularies, which are lists of drugs eligible for prescription under a managed care plan or other insurer. In order to have a drug included on the formulary, the pharmaceutical manufacturer must agree to charge a discounted price (Abbott, 1997).

17.2.10 Food and Drug Administration Regulation of Drugs

The FDA, founded in 1906, is one of the oldest federal regulatory agencies. Prior to 1962, the FDA regulated drugs for safety, although there existed a strong element of self-regulation. The 1962 Drug Amendments strengthened the FDA's regulation of drugs for safety and extended its focus to include effectiveness. The approval of a new drug requires extensive testing by the manufacturer and submission of drug studies to the FDA, so that the agency can evaluate the drug and reach a judgment as to whether its benefits outweigh its risks. Most new drugs are initially approved as prescription medicines, which means their purchase requires a provider's authorization. The FDA also regulates generic drugs (which compete with brand-name products at the end of the life of drug patents) and over-the-counter drugs (those available without a prescription) (U.S. Food and Drug Administration, 2000).

The competition from generic drugs was promoted by a 1984 law that greatly reduced the testing required of generics. Prior to 1984, generic producers were often required to perform tests for safety and effectiveness as part of the approval process. After 1984, they were required only to show the generics were bioequivalent to the name brands. This change promoted the entry of generics and led to lower prices within a relatively short period after patent expiration (Grabowski & Vernon, 1992).

Patents on new drugs provide a monopoly position for a period of time that may extend beyond the 20-year standard for American patents (the possibility of extension is to allow for the considerable time required by the regulatory process). The patent right provides an incentive for manufacturers to develop and test new drugs. This incentive must be balanced against the length of time it takes to develop drugs and the risk of failure. The total time lag from the beginning of research and development of a new drug to bringing it to market may be 10 to 15 years, and the total development cost may run over a billion dollars (Pharmaceutical Research and Manufacturers of America, 2011).

17.2.11 State Regulation of Pharmacists

In addition to their commercial role as sellers of drugs, pharmacists perform a professional role in monitoring prescriptions. State boards of pharmacy regulate registered pharmacists. In most states, the members of the state board are appointed by the governor, and registered pharmacists generally make up the majority of the members. The state boards regulate pharmacist quality through licensure and through requirements for continuing education. The increasing importance of mail-order pharmacies may restrict the ability of state boards to control the quality of dispensing within state boundaries (Conlan, 1997).

17.2.12 Regulation of Health Insurance and Managed Care

In the United States, regulation of insurance is practiced at the state level. This federalist tradition means that state insurance commissions regulate private health insurance companies, both investor-owned and tax-exempt.

The state insurance commissions have oversight control regarding entry and prices for commercial health insurance. Changes in healthcare markets have increased competition in these markets. The growing tendency of large employers to self-insure and utilize third-party administrators is a significant trend (Frech, 1993). As a result of this trend, a larger portion of the market escapes regulation.

In fact, more and more, state regulators have turned their attention to regulating the behavior of managed care organizations. During the 1990s and early 2000s, many state legislatures enacted bills intended to influence the practices of these organizations. Among the provisions were some that placed restrictions on physician communication with patients, placed restrictions on lengths of hospital stay, and mandated the creation of external grievance processes for dissatisfied patients.

A number of Patient's Bill of Rights exist. In 2010, a new Patient's Bill of Rights was created along with the Affordable Care Act, which extends the federal role in the regulation of private health insurance. Earlier bills focused on the right of patients to sue and the ability of managed care organizations to override the professional judgments of physicians (Pear, 2000). Federal regulation of health insurance traditionally has been restricted mostly to Medicare and Medicaid, which are public health insurance programs. The Employee Retirement Income Security Act of 1974 (ERISA) preempts state law related to benefit plans, including health insurance plans, offered by employers. One effect of ERISA has been to free employer self-insured health plans from most state regulatory restrictions, thereby contributing both to the growth of employer-provided plans and to complaints about the lack of patient rights (Havighurst, 2000). Currently, Patient's Bill of Rights address eight key areas: information for patients, choice of providers and plans, access to emergency services, taking part in treatment decisions, respect and nondiscrimination, confidentiality (privacy) of health information, complaints and appeals, and consumer responsibilities. In addition, some states have their own bill of rights.

17.3 ANTITRUST POLICY

17.3.1 Conceptual Framework

The economist's model of perfect competition is generally used as a benchmark in evaluating market outcomes. The perfectly competitive market, with large numbers of buyers and sellers, free entry and exit, and homogeneous products, yields a long-run competitive equilibrium in which all firms in the market are producing at minimum long-run average cost and in which price is equal to marginal cost. This market equilibrium yields both technical efficiency and economic efficiency. (*Technical efficiency* refers to the tendency of firms in a market to produce goods and services at the minimum long-run average cost, a result of the price competition among firms and of the relatively small scale of each firm in comparison to market demand. *Economic efficiency* refers to the equality of price and marginal cost, which suggests that the allocation of resources could not be improved in a perfectly competitive world by moving resources from their present use to a different one.)

A second benchmark in examining market outcomes is found in the monopoly market model. In this market structure, because there is a single seller with blocked entry, long-run market equilibrium may yield a price greater than marginal cost. If the monopolist is a profit maximizer, productive efficiency is still achieved (in the sense that average cost is at the lowest level possible given the monopolist's choice of output). However, the monopolist may not produce at the lowest average cost possible, independent of the rate of output selected.

Monopoly markets also raise the possibility of shifts in the distribution of income, compared with a perfectly competitive organization of the market. Under restrictive assumptions, a competitive market in long-run equilibrium that is transformed into a monopoly market as a result of cartelization or merger would be changed in the way shown in Figure 17-1. Total market output would decline from Q_c to Q_m as a result of monopolization. The corresponding equilibrium price would increase from P_c to P_m. Monopoly profits would appear in the amount shown by area ABDE, while the consumer surplus would decrease from the amount reflected by area FCD under perfect competition to area FAE under monopoly. The consumer surplus is the difference between the sum of the marginal valuations over all quantities of the service and the prices paid over all quantities. It is a reflection of the welfare gains made by the consumer from purchasing the product. The difference between these two levels of consumer surplus, measured by area ABC, is traditionally called the

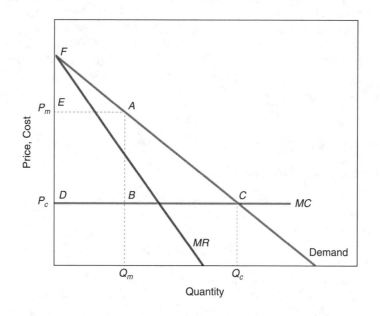

Figure 17-1 Economic Analysis of Monopolization Effects. Under perfect competition, the price is P_c and the quantity is Q_c. Under monopoly, the price is P_m and the quantity is Q_m. Competition yeilds no monopoly profits and a consumer surplus of FCD. Monopoly yields monopoly profits of EABD and a consumer surplus of FAE.

deadweight loss due to monopoly. In sum, the adverse affects of monopoly market structures are related directly to the reduction in market output from Q_c to Q_m. The reduced market output causes redistribution between consumers and producers, as well as allocative effects in the form of deadweight loss.

Many real-world markets, including most healthcare markets, are structured as oligopoly markets. Paucity of sellers and generally large numbers of buyers characterize oligopoly markets. Some healthcare markets are oligopolies on both sides of the market (i.e., both buyers and sellers are few in number). Economic models of markets structured as oligopolies tend not to yield general predictions about market outcome. Depending on whether sellers attempt to engage in price collusion and if not, how they react to one another's price changes, the outcome in oligopoly markets may cover the entire outcome range from monopoly on one extreme to perfect competition on the other.

Antitrust policy economic analysis has traditionally made an attempt to analytically define the boundaries of product markets and geographic markets and to consider whether the structure of markets so defined is close enough to a monopoly structure to suspect that performance in these markets is adversely affected. This approach is reflected, for example, in the merger guidelines that have been developed by the U.S. Department of Justice and the Federal Trade Commission. More recently, antitrust economists have begun to use simulation as a means of predicting the likely outcome of changes in market structure due to horizontal mergers.

It should be noted that, in the previous discussion of competitive and monopoly markets, perfect information on the part of consumers as well as producers is generally assumed. Complete information implies that there is no uncertainty on the part of the consumers regarding product quality. Furthermore, because products are assumed to be homogeneous in a given market, price is the major decision variable for consumers. Clearly, healthcare markets do not meet this information requirement, partly because of the imperfect ability of consumers to link the acquisition of healthcare services with improvements in health status and to compare the quality of alternative providers. Additionally, because third-party payers are dominant in most healthcare markets, the price of a particular healthcare service may be relatively unimportant to the ultimate consumer of that service. The market structure is further complicated by the role of the physician as the agent of the patient in making decisions about whether a particular service should be purchased.

As a result of these differences between healthcare markets and standard consumer goods markets, a discussion of antitrust policy in healthcare markets must take into account their particular economic characteristics. The point of view expressed here favors public policies that oppose monopoly power and promote competitive market structures. In the case of healthcare markets, however, there are even more caveats concerning this generalization than is true of traditional consumer goods markets. It is often asserted that, in traditional goods and services markets, economies of scale and the possibly greater propensity of firms with monopoly power to engage in research and development may justify market concentration. In healthcare markets, in addition to those two factors, high seller concentration may also be justified on the basis of access-to-care or quality-of-care considerations.

17.3.2 The Structure of Healthcare Markets

17.3.2.1 Hospitals

Hospital services in the United States and Canada have historically been provided by private community hospitals, which have traditionally been tax-exempt hospitals sponsored by religious organizations, local governments, and charitable organizations. One major structural trend in the 1980s and 1990s in the United States was the rapid growth of investor-owned hospital corporations.

Another strong trend in the 1980s and 1990s among U.S. hospitals was the increasing rate of mergers. Many of the mergers were related to the rise of investor-owned hospital corporations. Other mergers have occurred among tax-exempt hospitals in response to the rise of investor-owned hospital corporations, or to the increasing market power (on the buyer side) of managed care networks (Schactman & Altman, 1995).

The economic analysis of mergers suggests that mergers may be motivated by the pursuit of increased market power, the pursuit of increased efficiency, or both. The effects of changes in Medicare payment policies after the early 1980s provided a ready source of efficiency gains from mergers. The shift to prospective payment for Medicare resulted in shorter inpatient stays and a shift from inpatient to outpatient treatment. The general effect of these shifts was to create overcapacity in many hospitals, increasing the likelihood that efficiency gains could be realized from mergers, especially mergers within the same geographic market. Such horizontal mergers also increase market power in given geographic markets, raising the issue of whether hospital mergers are in the public interest (Gaynor & Haas-Wilson, 1999).

17.3.2.2 Physician Services

Physician services have traditionally been produced by physicians practicing alone or in small-group practices. Before 1980, when cost containment was less prominent in the healthcare sector, physicians played the dominant role in the management of hospitals, as well as in the management of physician group practices. The cost-containment trend in hospitals has led to the increased power of hospital administrators in hospital management. The development of managed care networks also tended to reduce the discretionary power of physicians in determining the price and quality of service. One response of physicians to these trends is to form larger practices and other physician networks. Regional and even national physician practice corporations have been established. As in the case of hospitals, the combining of physicians into large networks raises issues of efficiency versus market power.

17.3.2.3 Health Insurers and Managed Care Plans

Employers have traditionally provided health insurance in the United States as a tax-exempt fringe benefit. Before about 1980, most Americans were covered by traditional health insurance, which supported fee-for-service transactions with providers. Health insurers competed with one another to obtain insurance contracts with employers, who provided health insurance as a fringe benefit. Until the 1980s, healthcare cost containment had a relatively low priority in the U.S. system.

The early 1980s saw the rise of two important healthcare cost-containment mechanisms. First, Medicare's prospective payment system allowed the program to use its purchasing power to control the pricing and utilization of hospital services and physician services. Second, some states, beginning with California in 1982, began to allow payers to contract selectively with providers. Selective contracting enabled payers to negotiate reduced rates from providers in exchange for volume. Greater coordination of care, utilization review, and other changes caused health maintenance organizations (HMOs) to grow rapidly. As of 2010, HMOs enrolled about 77 million Americans, or about 25% of the population (Sanofi-Aventis, 2012).

The structural change in the payers' markets has important implications for healthcare competition. In effect, increased market power on the buyer side has evolved in response to market power on the provider side, or to rapid price inflation in healthcare markets resulting from the absence of economizing by consumers due to the existence of third-party payers. Mergers and consolidation among payers also raise potential issues of market power versus efficiency.

17.3.2.4 Pharmaceuticals

The pharmaceutical industry is an oligopoly that includes a relatively small number of large multinational firms with broad product lines, along with a large number of small companies with limited product lines. A major competitive dimension is research and development competition—the search for new drugs with broad potential usage. The main incentive for new product development is the patent system, which grants the holder of a patent monopoly rights to manufacture and sell the product for about 20 years. Pharmacy retailers and pharmacy benefits-management companies carry out the distribution of pharmaceuticals, with registered pharmacists licensed by state departments of health.

17.3.3 Antitrust Policy: History and Institutions

The most prominent piece of antitrust legislation in the United States is the Sherman Act of 1890, which was a legislative response to rapid changes occurring in American industry. In the last two decades of the 19th century, innovations in transportation and communication led to the transformation of local and regional markets into national markets. Business consolidation was a major trend, and near-monopoly conditions arose in some markets. The Sherman Act, building on common law traditions against conspiracy and monopolization, had two major sections:

1) Every contract, combination in the form of trust or otherwise, or conspiracy, in restraint of trade or commerce among the several states, or with foreign nations, is declared to be illegal.

2) Every person who shall monopolize, or attempt to monopolize, or combine or conspire with any other person or persons,

to monopolize any part of the trade or commerce among the several states, or with foreign nations, shall be deemed guilty of a felony.

The Clayton Act of 1914, with subsequent amendments, is the other major antitrust legislation in the United States. Two of the more important provisions of the Clayton Act are found in Sections 2 and 7, quoted, in part, as follows:

2a) It shall be unlawful for any person engaged in commerce in the course of such commerce, either directly or indirectly, to discriminate in price between different purchasers of commodities of like grade and quality . . . where the effect of such discrimination may be substantially to lessen competition or tend to create a monopoly.

7) No person engaged in commerce or in activity affecting commerce shall acquire, directly or indirectly, the whole or any part of the stock or other share capital and no person . . . shall acquire the whole or any part of the assets of another person engaged also in commerce . . . where in any line of commerce in any section of the country, the effect of such acquisition may be substantially to lessen competition, or to tend to create a monopoly.

The Federal Trade Commission Act, also passed in 1914, established the Federal Trade Commission (FTC). The FTC shares in the enforcement of the Clayton Act and enforces Section 5A1 of the FTC Act, which holds that "unfair methods of competition in or affecting commerce, and unfair or deceptive acts or practices in or affecting commerce, are declared unlawful."

There are two federal agencies that share the enforcement of antitrust law: the Antitrust Division of the U.S. Department of Justice and the Federal Trade Commission. The Department of Justice has primary responsibility for public enforcement of the Sherman Act; the FTC has primary responsibility for enforcement of the Federal Trade Commission Act and of Section 2 of the Clayton Act. The two agencies combine in enforcing the merger provisions of the Clayton Act. In addition, there are areas of overlap in which the agencies share jurisdiction. In addition to public enforcement of the antitrust laws, private enforcement is also important. The importance of private enforcement is related directly to Section 4 of the Clayton Act, which provides that those injured as a result of "anything forbidden in the antitrust laws" may bring private suit and recover triple damages, including attorney's fees. The triple damages provision provides a strong incentive for injured parties to bring private suits, including class action suits.

Because of the time and expense of fully developing cases and bringing them to trial, the majority of antitrust cases are settled by consent decrees. In a consent decree settlement, a court-supervised agreement is worked out between the parties. In the case of criminal suits, a settlement sometimes involves the use of a no-contest plea in order that the defendant may avoid pleading guilty. In private civil cases, financial settlements, generally involving amounts less than those initially requested by the plaintiffs, are common.

17.3.4 Price Fixing and Conspiracy in Restraint of Trade in Healthcare Markets

Section 1 of the Sherman Act concerns conspiracy in restraint of trade. The legal tradition in the enforcement of this section is that evidence of direct communication among competitors is sufficient to find a violation. This principle is referred to as the "per se rule." The U.S Supreme Court has strongly stated that whether or not the prices established by conspiracy are reasonable is *not* an issue.

Despite the strong *per se* tradition in enforcing price fixing, legal precedent was relatively slow in extending the range of antitrust law to the professions. A landmark case in this regard is *Goldfarb v. Virginia State Bar* (1975), in which the Supreme Court stated that the professions are not exempt from the Sherman Act's prohibition of price fixing. The *Goldfarb* case involved fee schedules set for legal fees by a bar association.

That the *per se* rule also applies to price fixing among physicians was forcefully stated in the U.S. Supreme Court's decision in the case of *Arizona v. Maricopa County Medical Society* (1982). In this case, two physician groups utilized relative value schedules to establish maximum prices for medical services. The Court ruled that this approach to setting maximum physician fees was subject to the *per se* rule against price fixing.

The *Maricopa* case clearly establishes that the healthcare professions fall under the *per se* rule concerning price fixing and conspiracy in restraint of trade. This is not to say that physicians and other health professionals may not form professional associations and discuss issues of mutual concern. Trade association activities, including some exchange of pricing information, generally do not constitute a violation. However, the use of a common fee schedule setting either maximum or minimum fees would likely be a violation of the Sherman Act.

17.3.5 Mergers in Healthcare Markets

A merger is a partial or total combination of two separate business firms. Partial mergers include such combinations as joint ventures and intercorporate stock purchases. Complete mergers are more common. A complete merger involves the purchase of assets or stock in one corporation by a separate corporation and typically results in the blending of identities and the creation of a single succeeding firm.

Mergers are generally described as falling into one of three categories. The first type of merger is the horizontal merger, which is the combination of two firms that compete in the same product market and geographic market. A merger of two community hospitals in the same metropolitan area would be an example of a horizontal merger. The second type of merger is the vertical merger, which involves firms that have a buyer-seller relationship. The acquisition of a physician group practice by an HMO or a hospital would be an example of a vertical merger. The third type of merger is the conglomerate merger, which unites firms that are neither horizontally nor vertically related. The acquisition of a community hospital by a banking corporation would be an example of a conglomerate merger.

Mergers and joint ventures have become very common in healthcare markets. Investor-owned hospital corporations, such as Columbia/HCA, have expanded in size and in geographic scope, primarily through merger. Mergers have also been common in physician group practices, as solo practitioners combine to form local and regional group practices.

The enforcement of Section 7 of the Clayton Act by the Department of Justice and Federal Trade Commission focuses on the seller concentration in the market before and after prospective mergers. The Hart-Scott-Rodino Act of 1976 requires that mergers above a threshold size ($100 million in sales or assets on the part of one premerger firm and $10 million for the other party) must notify the Federal Trade Commission and Department of Justice in advance of the merger. This provision of the law allows the antitrust authorities to intervene before the merger actually occurs rather than wait until asset ownership has changed hands. This provision also allows for modification of the assets to be acquired if seller concentration in certain markets raises objections to parts of the merger.

Hospital markets tend to be local or regional in scope. In addition, because hospitals differ with respect to the array of services offered, the analysis of hospital mergers must consider both product market definition and geographic market definition. The definitions of geographic market and product market for hospitals are based on the interchangeability or cross-price elasticity of the services offered, as viewed by consumers. Two or more hospitals are in the same geographic market if consumers (or their physician agents) consider the hospitals to be reasonably interchangeable when making decisions regarding where to seek care. Two or more hospitals are in the same product market if consumers consider their offerings of a given service to be reasonably interchangeable (Wilder & Jacobs, 1987).

As noted earlier, the Clayton Act prohibits mergers when "the effect of such acquisition may be substantially to lessen competition, or to tend to create a monopoly." In the case of hospital mergers, a potential anticompetitive effect exists if there is overlap in the product and geographic markets of the hospitals prior to the merger. In general, the question of whether two hospitals are in the same geographic and product markets may be more complicated for hospitals than for nonhealthcare service firms. The geographic market definition is likely to vary depending on the medical procedure in question. Because patients are likely to be willing to travel greater distances for more complicated, more expensive procedures, the geographic market definition for hospitals is not independent of the procedure in question. In general, the geographic market is much wider for complicated procedures than for simple procedures, or for tertiary care than for primary care (Wilder & Jacobs, 1987).

Antitrust aspects of hospital mergers must be considered in the light of merger history. During the period 1950–1980, enforcement agencies treated horizontal mergers very strictly, and modest market concentration levels and modest increases in concentration were often sufficient for horizontal mergers to be successfully challenged. After 1980, horizontal merger enforcement became more lenient, as reflected in the Department of Justice and Federal Trade Commission merger guidelines, the most recent version of which was released in 2010.

In evaluating horizontal mergers, the Justice Department guidelines use the Herfindahl-Hirschman Index (HHI) of market concentration. The HHI is defined as the sum of the squares of the individual market shares of all firms in the market, wherein market shares are expressed in percentages. For example, one hospital in a market would result in an HHI of 10,000 (100 × 100). Two hospitals of equal size would result in an HHI of 2,500 (50 × 50). Ten hospitals of equal size would result in an HHI of 1,000. According to the guidelines, in evaluating a proposed merger, the Justice Department and Federal Trade Commission consider both the market concentration and the increase in concentration that would result from the merger. The guidelines establish three categories of horizontal mergers:

1. Post-Merger HHI Below 1,500: The agency regards markets in this region to be unconcentrated. Mergers resulting in unconcentrated markets are unlikely to have adverse competitive effects and ordinarily require no further analysis.

2. Post-Merger HHI Between 1,500 and 2,500: The agency regards markets in this region to be moderately concentrated. Mergers producing an increase in the HHI of less than 100 points in moderately concentrated markets post-merger are unlikely to have adverse competitive consequences and ordinarily require no further analysis. Mergers producing an increase in the HHI of more than 100 points in moderately concentrated markets post-merger potentially raise significant competitive concerns.

3. Post-Merger HHI Above 2,500: The agency regards markets in this region to be highly concentrated. Mergers producing an increase in the HHI of less than 100 points, even in highly concentrated markets post-merger, are unlikely to have adverse competitive consequences and ordinarily require no further analysis. Mergers producing an increase in the HHI of more than 100 points in highly concentrated markets post-merger potentially raise significant competitive concerns, depending on the factors set forth in [other sections] of the guidelines. Where the post-merger HHI exceeds 2,500, it will be presumed that mergers producing an increase in the HHI of more than 200 points are likely to create or enhance market power or facilitate its exercise (U.S. Department of Justice and Federal Trade Commission, 2010).

If hospital mergers were judged entirely on the basis of the 2010 guidelines, it is unlikely that many hospital mergers in a given geographic market would be approved. In research reported elsewhere, it was found that the HHI for hospitals in a medium-sized metropolitan area market was on the order of 2,600 for all diagnoses together. For individual procedures, the HHI ranged from a low of 2,300 for plastic surgery to a high of 4,600 for surgeries of the nervous system (Wilder & Jacobs, 1987).

Hospital mergers have occurred at a rapid rate since 1980. Blackstone and Fuhr (1992) state that 40 to 60 hospital mergers per year occurred in the 1980s, but that the Department of Justice and Federal Trade Commission challenged fewer than 10 hospital mergers during this decade. In some cases, mergers were not challenged because the hospitals were not in the same geographic market. Many of the mergers and acquisitions were part of the hospital consolidation involved in the formation and growth of such firms as Columbia/HCA. Even when hospital mergers were truly horizontal, the Justice Department and Federal Trade Commission applied somewhat different standards to these mergers than to other horizontal mergers. The variation in standards is apparent in the Department of Justice–Federal Trade Commission Antitrust Guidelines for the Business of Health Care, which were released initially in 1993 and updated in August 2010. The purpose of the guidelines is to provide information concerning the types of mergers, joint ventures, and other competition-related actions that might be challenged by the antitrust authorities. In the area of mergers, the guidelines state that the merger of two small hospitals with low occupancy rates, even if they are in the same geographic market, would not be challenged. The guidelines also state that two or more hospitals of any size could engage in joint ventures to buy high-technology equipment, if each hospital by itself could not fully utilize the equipment.

For mergers between larger hospitals, the antitrust agencies state that they will use the "rule of reason" in analyzing mergers. The rule of reason approach considers whether mergers may have a substantial anticompetitive effect and if so, whether the anticompetitive effect is offset by procompetitive efficiencies (Steiger, 1995).

When considering the effect of antitrust policy on hospital mergers, the primary fact to keep in mind is that only a small number of mergers have been challenged by the antitrust authorities out of the hundreds of mergers that have taken place. Another indication of the effects of antitrust policy on hospital mergers may be seen in the outcome of the antitrust review of the Columbia Healthcare Corporation/HCA Healthcare merger. The merger was allowed after the divestiture of three hospitals in Salt Lake City and four hospitals in Louisiana, Florida, and Texas. The resulting Columbia/HCA Corporation included 191 hospitals, with 39,328 acute care beds. Columbia/HCA subsequently merged with HealthTrust, Inc., forming a national hospital corporation with 320 hospitals and more than 100 outpatient surgery centers. The FTC approved this merger after Columbia/HCA agreed to sell seven hospitals and end a joint venture with another hospital. In more recent times, Columbia/HCA has come under attack for Medicare billing irregularities, has negotiated a settlement to pay the federal government $754 million plus interest to resolve the overbilling allegations, has spun off and sold some of its hospitals, and has changed its name to HCA—The Healthcare Co. (Kirchheimer, 2000).

One reason for the relatively lenient antitrust policy toward hospital mergers is the possibility of efficiency gains. Gaynor and Haas-Wilson (1999) point out that some mergers are rational responses to excess capacity and empty hospital beds resulting from the shift to increased use of outpatient treatment. Mergers may also be driven by changes in payment practices that shift more risk to the provider.

State governments have also become players in the merger policy arena. As of 1998, some 20 states had enacted regulatory programs for state approval of hospital actions, including mergers. Under the state action immunity doctrine, state supervision in some circumstances replaces federal antitrust action. This development could, for example, allow some hospital mergers that would otherwise attract federal antitrust action. The effects of state-approved mergers on hospital markets are largely unknown (Hellinger, 1998).

The pharmaceutical industry has experienced a number of mergers. Examples include the Monsanto-Pharmacia Upjohn, Pfizer-Warner Lambert, and Hoechst AG and Rhone-Poulenc Rorer mergers, all of which took place in 1998 and 1999 (Pharmaceutical Researchers and Manufacturers of America, 2000). The industry has relatively high seller concentration in some drug submarkets, but the level of concentration in the broadly defined pharmaceutical preparations industry is relatively low. An example of an FTC merger complaint is that issued by the agency regarding the Hoechst AG and Rhone-Poulenc merger. This complaint argued that Hoechst's acquisition of Rhone-Poulenc would reduce competition in the market for agents used to treat blood-clotting diseases. A consent decree in 2000 allowed the merger subject to the transfer of Rhone-Poulenc's product in this submarket to a separate firm (U.S. Federal Trade Commission, 2000) This case illustrates that the relevant product market in pharmaceutical antitrust cases may be defined quite narrowly.

17.3.6 Antitrust Policy: Monopolization

Section 2 of the Sherman Act makes it illegal to "monopolize, or attempt to monopolize." The use of the verb *monopolize* rather than the noun *monopoly* suggests one of difficulties in enforcing monopoly laws. Conceptually, a monopoly is a single firm with exclusive possession of a market for a good or service. As a practical matter, however, pure monopoly status is highly unusual. Markets with high seller concentration resulting in partial or near-monopoly market structures are the more common objects of monopoly inquiries. As a result, the enforcement of monopoly laws tends to focus on market definition, market share, and specific acts that suggest monopolistic intent.

A good summary of the enforcement tradition in monopoly cases may be found in the U.S. Supreme Court decision in the *Grinnell* case, in which Justice Douglas stated that the offense of monopoly "has two elements: 1) possession of monopoly power in the relevant market and; 2) willful acquisition or maintenance of that power." (*U.S. v. Grinnell Corporation*, 384US 563 [1966]).

Relatively little of the antitrust enforcement activity in health care has involved monopolization issues directly. Instead, most enforcement activity has taken place under the conspiracy statute (Section 1 of the Sherman Act) or the antimerger statute (Section 7 of the Clayton Act). However, as national hospital corporations and healthcare provider networks grow more important in the United States, the likelihood that monopolization issues will become more important will increase.

The major reason that monopolization issues have been less important than other antitrust issues is that the level of seller concentration in most hospital or physician services markets, while relatively high in some instances, does not approach the level that indicates monopoly on the basis of case law. In the most direct statement on the connection between market share and monopoly status, the *Aluminum Company of America* case, Judge Hand stated that a market share over 90% "is enough to constitute a monopoly; it is doubtful whether 60 or 64 percent would be enough; and certainly 33 percent is not" (*U.S. vs. Aluminum Company of America*, 148F. 2nd 416 [1945]).

Since the *Aluminum Company of America* case in the 1940s, the only very large national corporation whose monopoly status was broken up by anti-trust action was AT&T, in a case settled through a consent decree in 1982. A monopolization case against IBM by the Justice Department was dropped at about the same time (in the early 1980s). Because neither of these cases reached the Supreme Court, there is no clear recent judicial statement interpreting monopoly law for today's world.

There are at least three principal market areas within health care in which monopoly issues may come to the fore. First, as national hospital corporations grow and as tax-exempt community hospitals merge and engage in joint ventures, the market structure in some local hospital markets may evolve in such a way that a group of jointly owned hospitals will reach a market share of 60%. Such market evolution could then make monopolization enforcement under Section 2 of the Sherman Act relevant in some hospital markets.

Physician networks may also become subject to monopolization enforcement. Physicians have been rapidly forming networks that operate as unified firms. Such networks may increasingly accumulate market shares in relevant geographic markets in the 60% range or greater. As such market shares arise through continued consolidation, antimonopoly law may become directed toward the larger networks.

HMOs and other managed care organizations may also become the target of monopolization statutes. These organizations tend to increase concentration on the buyer side in markets for hospital and physician services. As the market penetration of HMOs increases, the potential for high market shares on the buyer side of healthcare markets also increases. Some observers believe that the rapid growth of physician networks and the increasing number of hospital mergers and joint ventures are partly responses to the increased purchasing power of HMOs and other managed care organizations.

The 1996 Department of Justice and Federal Trade Commission statement on healthcare and antitrust laws addresses the interaction of physician networks and multiprovider networks. In general, the statement indicates that HMOs and other multiprovider networks might violate antitrust laws if the exclusion of some physicians from a dominant network in a local market makes it impossible for them to practice medicine. A similar argument could be directed at a dominant multiprovider network that excludes hospitals in a local market. Efficiency gains may be an offsetting virtue of provider coordination and combination. Antitrust cases considering monopolization issues would also consider efficiency effects.

17.3.7 Quality Competition and Antitrust Policy

Nonprice competition is particularly important in most sectors of the healthcare market. Quality competition among insurers or managed care organizations is related to such attributes as access to specialists, freedom of choice among providers, and treatment capacity. Quality competition among providers is based on such attributes as credentials, location, and treatment outcomes (Sage & Hammer, 1999). Because of incomplete information in healthcare markets, consumers may be poorly informed about the quality of service. This information problem could mean that antitrust policies that encourage price competition may lead to the provision of lower quality service than is socially optimal (Gaynor & Haas-Wilson, 1999).

There is a developing trend toward greater provision of information about healthcare quality. The Centers for Medicare and Medicaid Services, for example, reports on the characteristics and performance of nursing homes. The Agency for Healthcare Research and Quality (AHRQ) sponsors and conducts research with a focus on providing evidence-based information on healthcare outcomes and quality (Agency for Healthcare Research and Quality, 2005). The National Committee for Quality Assurance (NCQA) issues an annual report on the quality of managed care plans (National Committee for Quality Assurance, 2000). The committee is funded by government and corporate sponsors. The greater availability of information offers the promise of improved quality competition and a reduction in the likelihood that markets will provide service quality that is suboptimal.

17.3.8 Antitrust Issues Related to Managed Care

One of the most important trends in the healthcare sector during the 1980s and 1990s was the rise of managed care plans, selective contracting, and integrated health networks. In a nutshell, what happened is that the market power in the hands of the physicians and hospitals (the suppliers of health care) was met by the growth of market power on the buyer side. The growth of managed care appears to have promoted competitive efficiencies in health care and likely reduced the rate of increase in healthcare costs. At the same time, the rise of managed care could eventually result in increased market power on the part of buyers or sellers of health care and ultimately lead to an increase in the prices paid by consumers (Schactman & Altman, 1995).

The healthcare initiatives put forth by the Clinton Administration in 1993—initiatives that seemed likely to result in greater public sector participation in health care—were not politically popular. However, it is interesting to note that the managed competition approach at the heart of the Clinton plan has been implemented without federal legislation. In other words, the managed care revolution has been a private market response rather than a legislative reaction to increasing healthcare costs.

The managed care industry has followed a path of consolidation through merger. In 1998, the 10 largest HMO providers accounted for almost two-thirds of the total HMO enrollment in the United States (Standard and Poor's, 2000). Since 2005, the share of HMOs that belong to integrated healthcare systems has declined to a low of 18.1% in 2010 (Sanofi-Aventis, 2012). Because competition takes place in geographic markets at the local or regional level, HMO concentration in specific geographic markets may be higher or lower than at the national level. Feldman and colleagues (1999) found that while national HMO concentration increased from 1994 to 1997, most local HMO markets were less concentrated in 1997 than in 1994 because of the entry of new firms.

17.3.9 Federal Antitrust Policy Guidelines

A major landmark in healthcare antitrust policy was the issuing of the *Statements of Enforcement Policy and Analytical Principles Relating to Health Care and Antitrust* by the U.S. Department of Justice and Federal Trade Commission in 1993 (revised in 1994 and 1996). These statements reflect the complexity of markets and provider and purchaser institutions in health care. They also indicate that the antitrust authorities are seeking to adapt antitrust policy, which was developed for broad applicability, to the particular economic characteristics of healthcare markets. The provisions of the statements address the following nine areas:

1. Mergers among hospitals
2. Hospital joint ventures involving high-technology or other expensive healthcare equipment
3. Hospital joint ventures involving specialized clinical or other expensive healthcare services
4. Providers' collective provision of nonfee-related information to purchasers of healthcare services
5. Providers' collective provision of fee-related information to purchasers of healthcare services
6. Provider participation in exchanges of price and cost information
7. Joint purchasing arrangements among healthcare providers
8. Physician network joint ventures
9. Analytical principles relating to multiprovider networks

The purpose of the statements is to reduce uncertainty concerning antitrust policy and to establish "antitrust safety zones" (market conditions under which business conduct will not be challenged). For example, the merger of two small hospitals with low occupancy rates would fall into one of the safety zones. A physician network might attract antitrust scrutiny by collusive agreement on price or by excluding some physicians, making it impossible for them to practice in the market.

Physicians criticized the first version of the statements on the grounds that they favored insurance company and hospital networks over those formed by physicians. Statements 8 and 9 regarding physician networks and multiprovider networks were rewritten in the 1996 revision. The new version stated clearly that physician networks "could act jointly, without sharing financial risk, and not be considered as engaged in per se illegal conduct if they were doing something together that had the potential to create significant efficiencies" (Iglehart, 1998).

The healthcare system in the United States has been transformed by structural change, including the rise of managed care, selective contracting, provider networks, and numerous large mergers. These changes have the potential to increase productive efficiency and to slow the rate of healthcare price inflation. At the same time, the changes may increase market power in some product or geographic markets and may lead to higher consumer prices. In addition, there is increasing concern regarding the quality of healthcare services, leading to such developments as congressional debates on the legal rights of physicians to form unions and on the patient bill of rights. It is likely that as greater consolidation among providers and purchasers occurs and as quality-competition tradeoffs are discussed widely, regulation and antitrust issues will become even more important.

EXERCISES

1. Why are physicians sometimes described as "double agents?"
2. If physicians can gain large per capita wealth effects from state regulation, and consumers can gain relatively small per capita wealth effects from state regulation, which of the two groups does the economic theory of regulation suggest will control the legislative process that enacts regulatory procedures?
3. If physicians can organize at a low cost to influence state regulation, and consumers can organize only at a relatively high cost for this same purpose, which of the two groups does the economic theory of regulation suggest will control the legislative process that enacts regulatory procedures?
4. How can consumers of healthcare services obtain more information about service quality?
5. Explain how the patent right provides a financial incentive for pharmaceutical manufacturers to develop new drugs.
6. Explain the connection between the Employee Retirement Income Security Act (ERISA) and calls for a patient bill of rights.
7. Suppose that you overhear a foursome of physicians on the golf course discussing the prices they charge for an office visit. Suppose further that you hear them reach an agreement to all charge a fee of $100 for an office visit. What is such an agreement called in antitrust policy, and what antitrust law may have been violated?
8. Suppose that emergency room services in the city of Hibiscus are provided by three hospitals. Two of the hospitals each have a market share of 40% and the third hospital has a market share of 20%. The two largest hospitals plan to merge.
   a. Compute the premerger and postmerger HHI for this market.
   b. Based on the 1992 merger guidelines, would this merger likely be challenged by the antitrust authorities?
9. Physician networks have become increasingly popular in the past 25 years. How do the healthcare antitrust guidelines view physician networks, and what benefits of such networks might offset antitrust concerns?

BIBLIOGRAPHY

Regulation

Abbott, T. (1997). The pharmaceutical industry. In T. E. Getzen (Ed.), *Health economics*. New York, NY: John Wiley & Sons.

Aiken, L. H., Sloane, D. M., Cimiotti, J. P., Clarke, S. P., Flynn, L., Seago, J. A., ..., & Smith, H. L. (2010). Implications of the California nurse staffing mandate for other states. *Health Services Research, 45*(4), 904–921.

Anonymous. (2010). Tax exemption and community benefit: Key questions for addressing a critical concern. *Healthcare Financial Management, 64*(8), 52–53.

Arrow, K. J. (1963). Uncertainty and the welfare economics of medical care. *American Economic Review, 53*, 941–947.

Barr, P. (2011). Unwanted clarification. Critical-access hospitals fight CMS over rulemaking on provider taxes. *Modern Healthcare, 41*(9), 32–33, 35.

Blanchard, M. S., Meltzer, D., & Polonsky, K. S. (2009). To nap or not to nap? Residents' work hours revisited. *New England Journal of Medicine, 360*(21), 2242–2244.

Block, A. E., & Norton, D. M. (2008). Nurse labor effects of residency work hour limits. *Nursing Economics, 26*(6), 368–373.

Blomqvist, A. (1991). The doctor as double agent: Information asymmetry, health insurance, and medical care. *Journal of Health Economics, 10*, 411–432.

Conlan, M. (1997). Board games. *Drug Topics, 17*(November), 58–63.

Conover, C., & Sloan, F. (1998). Does removing certificate-of-need regulation lead to a surge in health care spending? *Journal of Health Politics, Policy and Law, 23*, 455–481.

Daly, R. (2011). Oversight overload: Harried hospitals say the growing number of billing audits they face could actually increase costs. *Modern Healthcare, 41*(47), 6–7.

David, G., Helmchen, L. A., & Henderson, R. A. (2009). Does advanced medical technology encourage hospitalist use and their direct employment by hospitals? *Health Economics, 18*(2), 237–247.

Delia, D., Cantor, J. C., Tiedemann, A., & Huang, C. S. (2009). Effects of regulation and competition on health care disparities: The case of cardiac angiography in New Jersey. *Journal of Health Politics, Policy & Law, 34*(1), 63–91.

Department of Veterans Affairs. (2010). Responding to disruptive patients. *Final rule. Federal Register, 75*(220), 69881–69883.

Dranove, D., & White, W. D. (1987). Agency and the organization of health care delivery. *Inquiry, 24*, 405–415.

Dranove, D., Shanley, M., & White, W.D. (1993). Price and concentration in hospital markets: The switch from patient-driven to payer-driven competition. *Journal of Law and Economics, 36*, 179–204.

Evans, M. (2011). Feds widen probe. "Most-favored nation" clauses draw more scrutiny. *Modern Healthcare, 41*(14), 8–9.

Evans, M. (2011). Revamp of IRS rules urged. Not-for-profit hospitals want clear, usable guidance. *Modern Healthcare, 41*(18), 8–9.

Exton, R. (2010). Enterprising health: Creating the conditions for entrepreneurial behaviour as a strategy for effective and sustainable change in health services. *Journal of Health Organization & Management, 24*(5), 459–479.

Fareed, N., & Mick, S. S. (2011). To make or buy patient safety solutions: A resource dependence and transaction cost economics perspective. *Health Care Management Review, 36*(4), 288–298.

Ferrier, G. D., Leleu, H., & Valdmanis, V. G. (2010). The impact of CON regulation on hospital efficiency. *Health Care Management Science, 13*(1), 84–100.

Folland, S., Goodman. A. C., & Stano, M. (2001). *The economics of health and health care* (3rd ed.). Englewood Cliffs, NJ: Prentice Hall.

Fournier, G. M., & McInnes, M. M. (1997). Medical board regulation of physician licensure: Is excessive malpractice sanctioned. *Journal of Regulatory Economics, 12,* 113–126.

Frech, H. E., III (1993). Health insurance: Designing products to reduce costs. In L. Deutsch (Ed.), *Industry studies.* Englewood Cliffs, NJ: Prentice Hall.

Getzen, T. E. (1997). *Health economics.* New York, NY: John Wiley & Sons.

Ginn, G. O., Shen, J. J., & Moseley, C. B. (2009). Community benefit laws, hospital ownership, community orientation activities, and health promotion services. *Health Care Management Review, 34*(2), 109–118.

Ginsburg, P. B. (2010). Wide variation in hospital and physician payment rates evidence of provider market power. *Research Briefs,* (16), 1–11.

Goldsmith, J. (2010). Managing the risks: Healthcare reform's challenge to hospitals. *Healthcare Financial Management, 64*(7), 46–50.

Goodman, K. W., Berner, E. S., Dente, M. A., Kaplan, B., Koppel, R., Rucker, D., ..., & Winkelstein, P. (2011). Challenges in ethics, safety, best practices, and oversight regarding HIT vendors, their customers, and patients: A report of an AMIA special task force. *Journal of the American Medical Informatics Association, 18*(1), 77–81.

Grabowski, H., & Vernon, J. (1992). Brand loyalty, entry, and price competition in pharmaceuticals after the 1984 Drug Act. *Journal of Law and Economics, 35,* 331–350.

Gravelle, H., & Sivey, P. (2010). Imperfect information in a quality-competitive hospital market. *Journal of Health Economics, 29*(4), 524–535.

Gray, B. H., & Schlesinger, M. (2009). Charitable expectations of nonprofit hospitals: Lessons from Maryland. *Health Affairs, 28*(5), w809–w821.

Harrison, J. P., & Ferguson, E. D. (2011). The crisis in United States hospital emergency services. *International Journal of Health Care Quality Assurance, 24*(6), 471–483.

Havighurst, C. (2000). American health care and the law—We need to talk! *Health Affairs, 19*(4), 84–106.

Health Care Financing Administration. (2000). *Peer review organizations (PROs).* Washington DC: U.S. Government Printing Office.

Hellinger, F. J. (2009). The effect of certificate-of-need laws on hospital beds and healthcare expenditures: An empirical analysis. *American Journal of Managed Care, 15*(10), 737–744.

Horwitz, J. R., & Nichols, A. (2011). Rural hospital ownership: Medical service provision, market mix, and spillover effects. *Health Services Research, 46,* 1452–1472.

Joint Commission. (2012). *Facts about the Joint Commission.* Retrieved from http://www.joint commission.org/about_us/fact_sheets.aspx

Joint Commission on Accreditation of Healthcare Organizations. (2000). Retrieved from http://www.jcaho.org

Kamath, A. F., Baldwin, K., Meade, L. K., Powell, A. C., & Mehta, S. (2011). The increased financial burden of further proposed orthopaedic resident work-hour reductions. *Journal of Bone & Joint Surgery—American Volume, 93*(7), e31.

Kelley, P. (2010). Medical device data systems and FDA regulation. Should medical device data systems require FDA clearance? *Journal of Healthcare Information Management, 24*(3), 36–40.

Kronebusch, K. (2009). Quality information and fragmented markets: Patient responses to hospital volume thresholds. *Journal of Health Politics, Policy & Law, 34*(5), 777–827.

Luft, H. S. (2009). Economic incentives to promote innovation in healthcare delivery. *Clinical Orthopaedics & Related Research, 467*(10), 2497–2505.

Marshall, L. W., Jr., Marshall, B. L., & Valladares, G. (2010). Federal and state public health authority and mandatory vaccination: Is Jacobson v Massachusetts still valid? *American Journal of Disaster Medicine, 5*(2), 107–112.

Medicare Payment Advisory Commission. (2000). Report to Congress: Medicare payment policy. Retrieved from http://www.medpac.gov

Mudrick, N. R., & Schwartz, M. A. (2010). Health care under the ADA: A vision or a mirage? *Disability & Health Journal, 3*(4), 233–239.

Mustard, L. W. (2009). Questionable hospital financial relationships with physicians. *Journal of Medical Practice Management, 25*(1), 41–43.

Peltzman, S. (1976). Toward a more general theory of regulation. *Journal of Law and Economics, 19,* 211–240.

Ranawat, A. S., Koenig, J. H., Thomas, A. J., Krna, C. D., & Shapiro, L. A. (2009). Aligning physician and hospital incentives: The approach at hospital for special surgery. *Clinical Orthopaedics & Related Research, 467*(10), 2535–2541.

Raymond, C. (2010). Taking aim at medical identity theft. Document security key element to comply with government regulations. *Journal of Medical Practice Management, 25*(6), 383–385.

Scheutzow, S. O. (1999). State medical peer review: High cost but no benefit—Is it time for a change? *American Journal of Law and Medicine, 25*(1), 7–60.

Sees, D. L. (2009). Impact of the Health Care Financing Administration regulations on restraint and seclusion usage in the acute psychiatric setting. *Archives of Psychiatric Nursing, 23*(4), 277–282.

Sefton, M., Brigell, E., Yingling, C., & Storfjell, J. (2011). A journey to become a federally qualified health center. *Journal of the American Academy of Nurse Practitioners, 23,* 346–350.

Stigler, G. (1971). The theory of economic regulation. *Bell Journal of Economics, 2,* 3–21.

Taylor, M. (2010). Feds refocus on fraud with new tools, fervor. *Hospitals & Health Networks, 84*(10), 2, 46, 48, 50.

Taylor, M. (2011). Feds refocus on fraud. *Trustee, 64*(2), 17–20.

Thompson, C. A. (2010). Government incentivizes hospitals to use EHR technology in meaningful ways. *American Journal of Health-System Pharmacy, 67*(17), 1398, 1401–1402.

Thornton, T., & Saha, S. (2008). The need for tort reform as part of health care reform. *Journal of Long-Term Effects of Medical Implants, 18*(4), 321–327.

Tyrrell, J. E., III (2010). Non-profits under fire: The effects of minimal charity care requirements legislation on not-for-profit hospitals. *Journal of Contemporary Health Law & Policy, 26*(2), 373–402.

U.S. Food and Drug Administration. (2000). *About the Center for Drug Evaluation and Research.* Retrieved from http://www.fda.gov/cder

Umbdenstock, R. (2011). Miles to go. Proposed ACO regs are lacking on clinical integration, increase risks and costs. *Modern Healthcare, 41*(15), 26.

Wartman, S. A., & Steinberg, M. J. (2011). The role of academic health centers in addressing social responsibility. *Medical Teacher, 33*(8), 638–642.

Weir-Hughes, D. (2010). Dickon Weir-Hughes on being good enough. *Health Service Journal, 120*(6226), 12.

Weld, T., & Klein, G. (2011). Future pension accounting changes: Implications for hospitals. *Healthcare Financial Management, 65*(5), 44–46.

Healthcare Antitrust Policy

Adelman, S. A. (2008). Physicians can't unite to stifle competition. *Medical Economics, 85*(23), 36.

Agency for Healthcare Research and Quality. (2005). AHRQ Annual Report on Research and Financial Management, FY 2004. Rockville MD: U.S. Department of Health and Human Services. Retrieved from http://archive.ahrq.gov/about/annrpt04/annrpt04.pdf

Amoresano, G. V. (2007). Branded drug reformulation: The next brand vs. generic antitrust battleground. *Food & Drug Law Journal, 62*(1), 249–256.

Balto, D. (2010). Enforcing reform. It's time for federal authorities to bring antitrust scrutiny to insurers. *Modern Healthcare, 40*(21), 24.

Barr, P. (2011). FTC scores antitrust win. Federal judge puts ProMedica deal on hold in Ohio. *Modern Healthcare, 41*(14), 8–9.

Becker, C. (2006). Police thyself. From GPOs and QIOs to not-for-profit hospitals, leaders hope a voluntary-compliance approach can stave off more regulation. *Modern Healthcare, 36*(41), 28–30.

Bissegger, M. R. (2006). The Evanston initial decision: Is there a future for patient flow analysis? *Journal of Health Law, 39*(1), 143–159.

Blackstone, E., & Fuhr, J. P. (1992). An antitrust analysis of non-profit hospital mergers. *Review of Industrial Organization, 8,* 473–490.

Blesch, G. (2010a). Easing the way for ACOs. Feds aim to create antitrust "safe harbor" for new healthcare delivery model. *Modern Healthcare, 40*(41), 12.

Blesch, G. (2010b). How far can providers go? Regulators grapple with antitrust, fraud-and-abuse issues under reform. *Modern Healthcare, 40*(38), 36–37.

Brewbaker, W. S., III (2006). Learning to love the state action doctrine. *Journal of Health Politics, Policy & Law, 31*(3), 609–621.

Brockmeier, M. S. (2010). The "reverse payment paradox": An overview of the legality of reverse exclusionary payments in the pharmaceutical industry. *Health Care Law Monthly, 2010*(3), 2–10.

Burns, J. (2011). What can be done to counteract growing power of providers? Three health plans outline steps they are taking to deal with the effects of growing consolidation of providers. *Managed Care, 20*(7), 14–16, 19–21.

Carlson, J. (2011a). Dodging an ACO chilling effect. Regulators ease up on provider collusion warnings. *Modern Healthcare, 41*(44), 17.

Carlson, J. (2011b). Leaping hurdles. Antitrust clearance costly, offers no guarantee: AHA. *Modern Healthcare, 41*(23), 7, 16.

Carrier, M. A. (2009). Unsettling drug patent settlements: A framework for presumptive illegality. *Michigan Law Review, 108*(1), 37–80.

Carroll, J. (2011). FTC antitrust rules offer hope of limiting ACO market power. *Managed Care, 20*(5), 5–7.

Casalino, L. P. (2006). The Federal Trade Commission, clinical integration, and the organization of physician practice. *Journal of Health Politics, Policy & Law, 31*(3), 569–585.

Claiborne, A. B., Hesse, J. R., & Roble, D. T. (2009). Legal impediments to implementing value-based purchasing in healthcare. *American Journal of Law & Medicine, 35*(4), 442–504.

Dranove, D., & Ludwick, R. (1999). Competition and pricing by nonprofit hospitals. *Journal of Health Economics, 18,* 87–98.

Dranove, D., & Sfekas, A. (2009). The revolution in health care antitrust: New methods and provocative implications. *Milbank Quarterly, 87*(3), 607–632.

Dranove, D., & White, W. D. (1998). Emerging issues in the antitrust definition of healthcare markets. *Health Economics, 7,* 167–170.

Evans, M. (2011). Feds widen probe. "Most-favored nation" clauses draw more scrutiny. *Modern Healthcare, 41*(14), 8–9.

Feldman, R., & Given, R. S. (1998). HMO mergers and Medicare: The antitrust issues. *Health Economics, 7,* 171–174.

Feldman, R., Wholey, & Christianson, J. B. (1999). HMO consolidations: How national mergers affect local markets. *Health Affairs, 18*(4), 96–104.

Frech, H. E., & Danger, K. L. (1998). Exclusive contracts between hospitals and physicians. *Health Economics, 7,* 175–178.

Freudenheim, M. (1994, June 27). Health industry is changing itself ahead of reform. *New York Times,* p. 1.

Gaynor, M. (2006). Why don't courts treat hospitals like tanks for liquefied gases? Some reflections on health care antitrust enforcement. *Journal of Health Politics, Policy & Law, 31*(3), 497–510.

Gaynor, M., & Haas-Wilson, D. (1999). Change, consolidation and competition in health care markets. *Journal of Economic Perspectives, 13,* 141–164.

Gibofsky, A. (2005). An analysis of recent antitrust issues affecting specialty practice: Is dermatology immune? *Seminars in Cutaneous Medicine & Surgery, 24*(3), 137–143.

Graham, J. (2005). The Federal Trade Commission and physician practice. *Journal of Medical Practice Management, 20*(5), 259–262.

Greaney, T. L. (2006). Antitrust and hospital mergers: Does the nonprofit form affect competitive substance? *Journal of Health Politics, Policy & Law, 31*(3), 511–529.

Guttler, S. D. (2010). The case for integrated delivery systems. *New England Journal of Medicine, 362*(1), 86; author reply, 86.

Haas-Wilson, D., & Gaynor, M. (1998). Physician networks and their implications for competition in health care markets. *Health Economics, 7,* 179–182.

Haskel, M. A. (2008). Should antitrust principles be used to assess insurance residual market mechanisms, such as New York's Medical Malpractice Insurance Plan? *Albany Law Review, 71*(1), 229–298.

Havighurst, C. C. (2006). Contesting anticompetitive actions taken in the name of the state: State action immunity and health care markets. *Journal of Health Politics, Policy & Law, 31*(3), 587–607.

Hellinger, F. J. (1998). Antitrust enforcement in the healthcare industry: The expanding scope of state activity. *Health Services Research, 33*(5, Pt. 2), 1477–1494.

Iglehart, J. K. (1998). The Federal Trade Commission in action: The FTC's Robert F. Leibenluft. Interview. *Health Affairs, 17*(5), 65–74.

Kesselheim, A. S., Murtagh, L., & Mello, M. M. (2011). "Pay for delay" settlements of disputes over pharmaceutical patents. *New England Journal of Medicine, 365*(15), 1439–1445.

Kinney, E. D. (2008). The corporate transformation of medical specialty care: The exemplary case of neonatology. *Journal of Law, Medicine & Ethics, 36*(4), 611, 790–802.

Kirchheimer, B. (2000). Move over Columbia, HCA is back. *Modern Healthcare, 19*(June).

Kuttner, R. (1997). Physician-operated networks and the new antitrust guidelines. *New England Journal of Medicine, 336,* 386–391.

Lee, J. (2011). Robust blood market. FTC attaches strings to merger, but competition concerns remain. *Modern Healthcare, 41*(23), 14.

Leibenluft, R. F. (2011). ACOs and the enforcement of fraud, abuse, and antitrust laws. *New England Journal of Medicine, 364*(2), 99–101.

Lynk, W. J., & Neumann, L. R. (1999). Price and profit. *Journal of Health Economics, 18,* 99–116.

Mantone, J. (2006). Trade wars. While our annual group purchasing survey shows continued growth, organizations face ongoing battles involving government inquiries, vendor disputes. *Modern Healthcare, 36*(35), S1–S5, following 24.

McIntire, T. (2005). OIG opinions on malpractice subsidies and gainsharing: A legal analysis. *Tennessee Medicine, 98*(4), 178–179.

McLaughlin, N. (2010). Cost questions. How antitrust, uniformity and exercise play their roles. *Modern Healthcare, 40*(43), 20.

McLean, T. R. (2005). Antitrust law and a tale of two health care industries. *American Heart Hospital Journal, 3*(1), 24–30.

Meier, M. H. (2010). More on integrated delivery systems. *New England Journal of Medicine, 362*(13), 1247–1248.

National Committee for Quality Assurance. (2000). *State of managed care quality 2000.* Retrieved from http://www.ncqa.org

Pear, R. (1996, April 8). Doctors may get leeway to rival large companies. *New York Times.*

Pear, R. (2000, July 1). Doctor's antitrust hopes face a roadblock from Lott. *New York Times.*

Pharmaceutical Research and Manufacturers of America. (2000). *Pharmaceutical industry profile 2000.* Retrieved from http://www.phrma.org/publications

Pharmaceutical Research and Manufacturers of America. (2011). *Pharmaceutical Industry Profile 2011.* Washington, DC: PhRMA.

Portman, R. M. (2007). Exclusive contracts in the hospital setting: A two-edged sword, part 1: Legal issues. *Journal of the American College of Radiology, 4*(5), 305–312.

Portman, R. M. (2007). Exclusive contracts in the hospital setting: A two-edged sword: part 2: Pros and cons, avoidance strategies, and negotiating tips. *Journal of the American College of Radiology, 4*(6), 401–405.

Rakestraw, E. (2009). A conflict of interest: Why peer review committees need heightened scrutiny under federal antitrust law. *Journal of Legal Medicine, 30*(4), 563–578.

Rawlings, R. B. (2011). At the crossroads: Accountable care organizations and antitrust law. *Health Care Law Monthly, 2011*(5), 2–11.

Sage, W. M., & Hammer, P. J. (1999). Competing on quality of care: The need to develop a competition policy for health care markets. *University of Michigan Journal of Law Reform, 32,* 1069–1118.

Sanofi-Aventis (2012). *Managed Care Digest Series, HMO-PPO Digest, 2011-2012.* Bridgewater NJ: Author.

Santerre, R. E., & Neun, S. (1996). *Health economics: Theories, insights and industry studies.* Chicago, IL: Dryden.

Schactman, D., & Altman, S. H. (1995). *Market consolidation, antitrust, and public policy in the health care industry: Agenda for future research.* Princeton, NJ: Robert Wood Johnson Foundation.

Schiff, A. H. (2009). Physician collective bargaining. *Clinical Orthopaedics & Related Research, 467*(11), 3017–3028.

Schreiber, J. C, Wachsstock, S. E., & Willcox, J. N. (2006). Network contracting and the antitrust laws: Giving "messenger models" a tune-up. *Caring, 25*(4), 54–60.

Schulte, D. (2010). Why antitrust laws are important to understand. *Journal of Michigan Dental Association, 92*(4), 18–19.

Sfikas, P. M. (2005). Are covenants not to compete becoming unenforceable? A growing trend explored. *Journal of the American Dental Association, 136*(9), 1309–1311.

Silvia, L., & Leibenluft, R. F. (1998). Health economics research and antitrust enforcement. *Health Economics, 7,* 163–166.

Standard and Poor's. (2000). Healthcare: Managed care. *Industry Surveys, 31*(August).

Steiger, J. D. (1995, November 9). *Health care enforcement issues.* Prepared remarks of Commissioner Janet D. Steiger, Federal Trade Commission, before the Health Trustee Institute, Cleveland, OH.

Steinhauer, E. H. (2006). Is Noerr-Pennington immunity still a viable defense against antitrust claims arising from Hatch-Waxman litigation? *Food & Drug Law Journal, 61*(4), 679–700.

Taylor, M. (2008). Working through the frustrations of clinical integration. *Hospitals & Health Networks, 82*(1), 2, 34–40.

U.S. Department of Justice and Federal Trade Commission. (1992). *Horizontal merger guidelines,* Washington, DC.

U.S. Department of Justice and Federal Trade Commission. (1996). *Statements of antitrust enforcement policy in health care.* Washington, DC.

U.S. Federal Trade Commission. (2000). *FTC antitrust actions in pharmaceutical services and products.* Retrieved from http://www.ftc.gov

Welch, S. (2008). OIG considers pay-for-call arrangements. *Journal of the Medical Association of Georgia, 97*(1), 47–49.

White, C. L., & Good, H. (2009). All together now? Evolving antitrust approaches to bundled discounting. *Journal of Health & Life Sciences Law, 2*(3), 47–71.

Wilder, R. P., & Jacobs, P. (1987). Antitrust considerations for hospital mergers: Market definition and market concentration. In R. M. Scheffler & L. F. Rossiter (Eds.), *Advances in health economics and health services research.* Stamford, CT: JAI Press.

Wolfram, R. (2009). Clinical practice guideline development and antitrust law. *JAMA, 301*(24), 2548–2549; author reply, 2549–2550.

Wooley, J. M. (1993). Hospitals: Price-increasing competition. In L. Deutsch (Ed.), *Industry studies.* Englewood Cliffs, NJ: Prentice Hall.

Zain, S. (2007). Sword or shield? An overview and competitive analysis of the marketing of "authorized generics." *Food & Drug Law Journal, 62*(4), 739–777.

Chapter 18

Evolving Issues in Health Care

OBJECTIVES

1. Identify several of the current and future issues confronting and changing the healthcare system.

2. Describe the implications of current and future issues for market efficiency of the healthcare system.

3. Discuss the rationale for and implications of a value-added focus for the healthcare system.

4. Explore the implications and potential consequences of consumer engagement in the healthcare system.

5. Assess the implications of alternative financing mechanism for the healthcare industry.

18.1 INTRODUCTION

The healthcare industry is a major sector in the economy of the United States, accounting for over 17% of the gross domestic product (GDP). Because the healthcare industry represents such a substantial portion of economic activities, it both impacts and is impacted by the general economy. As the healthcare industry continues to grow and evolve, a number of transformational changes are occurring in its organizational structure and in the arrangements of healthcare providers, in its financial systems, in new technologies and advances in medical science, and in the introduction and implementation of new and modifications of existing healthcare policies. Consequently, the healthcare industry continues to present a dynamic environment for the application of economic evaluation and analysis.

18.2 ISSUES FACING THE HEALTHCARE SYSTEM

The passage of the Patient Protection and Affordable Care Act (P.L. 111–148) in 2010 stimulated significant activity in the healthcare system, as each sector of the healthcare industry reacted to and prepared for the implementation of the various features of the act. A major contributor to the passage of the act was the continued rapid rise in healthcare expenditures and the projections regarding the growth in those expenditures. As the data in Figure 18-1 illustrate, health-care costs were projected to continue consuming an ever-increasing percentage of the GDP in the United States.

Every sector of the healthcare industry is facing tremendous pressure to cut costs, improve quality, and prepare for fundamental change in how health care is provided, financed, and consumed. An initial reaction in the hospi-tal industry has been to acquire and merge organizations, and to purchase or develop extensive physician networks. As hospital organizations grow, they have also begun to undertake direct approaches with employers with insurance-like options, eliminating the health insurance plan in the middle. Vertical collaborative arrangements have also been undertaken to integrate better control over the coordination of care across providers and institutions. In addition, insurance plans have increased direct involvement with provid-ers, and employers are seeking different ways to reduce benefit costs for their employees. Government programs are seeking alternative payment methods and reducing payment schedules to providers. Pressures continue to mount to control costs, increase access, and improve the quality of care delivered in the healthcare system.

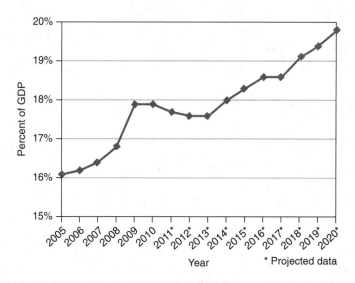

Figure 18-1 Historical and Projected Health Expenditures as Percent of GDP, 2005–2020

Source: Data from historical data obtained from NHE Summary Including Share of GDP, CY 1960–2010, https://www.cms.gov/Research-Statistics-Data-and-Systems/Statistics-Trends-and-Reports/NationalHealthExpendData/NationalHealthAccountsHistorical.html and from projected data obtained from Table 1: Economic Indicators, Levels and Annual Percent Change: Calendar Years 2005 – 2020. Retrieved on February 12, 2012 from: https://www.cms.gov/Research-Statistics-Data-and-Systems/Statistics-Trends-and-Reports/NationalHealthExpendData/NationalHealthAccountsProjected.html.

18.2.1 Contributions of Technology

A major contributor to the growth of healthcare expenditures has been the rapid development and widespread diffusion of new medical technologies and services; this is expected to continue or even grow in the future. These procedure, equipment, and process innovations enable the diagnosis and treatment of previously untreatable terminal conditions and acute healthcare problems, and change the diagnosis and treatment of existing healthcare problems by identifying secondary conditions and expanding the indications for treatment. Many of these new innovations require costly new pharmaceuticals, expensive equipment, and a more highly skilled healthcare workforce. These innovations also enable the expansion of the scope of medical interventions into areas outside previous boundaries of the healthcare system. (Kaiser Family Foundation, 2007). Unlike other industries in which the adoption of new innovations typically reduce the per-unit cost of output, many of these innovations in health care usually increase the costs of the output. Economics has an important role in assisting in the evaluation of the value-added of existing and new technologies.

In addition to determining the impact of existing and new innovations on the per-unit cost of output, determining the impact of the innovation on the total healthcare expenditures is another crucial role for economics. In examining the impact, it is important to determine if the innovation supplements an existing treatment, or if it is a partial or total substitute for an existing treatment, and then if the use of the innovation results in higher or lower expenditures for each patient treated.

It is also important to examine the number of patients treated by the new innovation. For example, does the new innovation enable the provision of services to a broader population, either because access is increased or because previously unidentified or untreatable individuals now receive services? Does the innovation allow new populations to be diagnosed for existing treatments, or does it extend existing treatments for new conditions in the population? Or does the new innovation reduce utilization by improving screening and diagnosis capacity, allowing more targeted treatments to be provided to the population?

While it is often possible to identify new innovations and determine when they were first introduced into the healthcare system, it is usually very difficult to measure the impact that the technology has on the costs of health care. One reason for this difficulty is that the introduction and adoption of innovations do not occur in a linear fashion or in similar ways in organizations or systems. Oftentimes, multiple innovations are introduced into the healthcare system in a short time span, and the impacts of the different innovations are often interrelated, making measurement of the impact of a single innovation difficult, if not impossible. In addition, the wide diversity of the innovations and of the structure and organization of the healthcare delivery system makes direct measurement of the impact of a single innovation on the entire system difficult, although assessing the impact of the adoption and implementation on a single organization or practice is more manageable. Economic tools are certainly appropriate and applicable on the micro level, and also make valuable contributions at the macro level.

One of the technologies changing the healthcare industry is health information technology. The introduction of health information technologies was established as a national priority in efforts to assist in the improvement of quality, safety, and efficiency in health care. As electronic health records (EHRs) are adopted, implemented, and used by practices and organizations, they will increase the complexity of changes occurring in the healthcare system. The focus and incentives provided for the adoption and use of EHRs create particular problems for individual and small practices because they often have very limited resources, small staff numbers, and lack the expertise to deploy and integrate these EHRs into their practices. As health information exchanges continue to expand and create the need for interoperability of automated data systems, the expectation is that the sharing of information across organizations will reduce the number of laboratory and imaging procedures, emergency department visits, and the number of provider visits, especially referrals to specialists, significantly impacting the processes of healthcare delivery and outcomes.

If EHRs are to be deployed successfully so that providers achieve meaningful use, then a good understanding of the current processes of delivering care is needed. These processes must be mapped so that they can be changed to adapt to the new requirements of the EHR system. To be successful, support for the technical aspects of the EHR is needed, as well as support for change management within the practices or organizations. Much of this support will need to come from outside sources because the necessary human capital is often not available internally, especially in the small practices or small organizations.

In addition to the EHR, health information technology is also expected to reduce the current lengthy process of translating scientific findings into general clinical practice. Part of these translations into generalizable results involves performing comparative effectiveness research. The tools of health economics are especially relevant in this environment, as the processes, tools, and resources needed for the successful transformation of the healthcare industry must be employed in the translation.

18.2.2 Hospital Contributions

The hospital industry is certainly a major sector of the healthcare industry. In 2010, expenditures on hospital services were $814 billion, accounting for 31.1% of total expenditures in the healthcare system. This amount translated into $2,637 per capita. The relative size of the industry makes it a focal point of many policies and regulations in the healthcare market. It also means that hospitals undertake a number of different strategies in efforts to reduce their risks and uncertainties. In decisions to implement changes in the hospital sector, systematic economic analysis is crucial.

There has been a flurry of mergers and acquisitions in recent years as the hospital industry reacted to the many changes occurring in health care. In many ways, these activities reflect typical supply and demand theories, as institutions that had investment capital available acquired or merged with other institutions that were short of capital reserves. The increase in such activities following the passage of the Accountable Care Act also reflected more vertical integrations as larger tertiary hospitals purchased smaller referring hospitals and also purchased physician practices to build a more diverse enterprise and ensure a larger market.

The vertical integration movement was also supported by the growth in information technology, which enabled the larger systems to share medical information and develop a unified medical record. These shared records also enabled better communications among physicians and between the hospitals and physicians, leading to opportunities for better coordinated care. The sharing of information allowed economies of scale and economies of scope to occur, adding further value to the consolidation of resources. It was also expected that the improved communications and coordination of care would result in improved health outcomes in the system and lower costs.

As a hospital system grows, it typically expands the geographical boundaries of its market and its share of services provided in the market. This increased market share enables the system to identify and develop high-volume, high-impact programs and to funnel resources into them. This activity involves a systematic assessment of the organization and the environment to ensure success. For mergers and acquisitions to be successful, an understanding of the cultural similarities and differences among the organizations is essential, as is the development of a common set of goals to add value for moving forward.

As the healthcare industry turns its focus to patient-centered care, increased sharing of information and communication is critical. This patient-centered focus reflects a new framework for organizing and evaluating health care. For a patient-centered system to function in a truly efficient and effective way, the organizational structure of the former healthcare system must change. The new organizational structure is reflected in the increase in mergers and acquisitions and in the merging of the previous boundaries separating physicians and hospitals in the market for healthcare services.

In this time of mergers and acquisitions, the historical boundaries between investor-owned and tax-exempt organizations are also becoming blurred. This is partly the result of the mergers and acquisitions of the two types of organizations into a new entity, and partly because the changes in the structure, operations, and financing of tax-exempt organizations is forcing them to function more and more like their investor-owned counterparts. As the number of individuals without health insurance declines with the expanded coverage under health reform, it becomes harder for tax-exempt organizations to be able to demonstrate a sufficient volume of community benefits to maintain their tax-exempt status.

As hospitals acquire more physician practices, the boundaries between the markets for physician and hospital services continue to be blurred. The absorption of physicians into the hospital sector changes referral patterns and utilization of services. The coordination of patient information across previously separate boundaries should decrease duplication of services and the need to perform repeated tests and procedures to obtain needed information. As the medical records of patients with multiple providers are centralized and shared, patient outcomes should improve and costs should decrease.

18.3 FINANCING MECHANISMS

The healthcare industry has also been facing a number of changes in payment systems recently, and indications are that even more changes are looming in the future. A difficulty emerging is that there is a disconnect between the external payment systems being implemented and the internal methods that have been used to distribute resources within the organization. Historically, the healthcare system has been a production-based system, receiving compensation for services produced. The incentive in any production-based system is simply to produce more units, as long as the cost of production is less than the market price received for the unit. Complicating the production decisions in health care is the existence of insurance programs that isolate production decisions from the cost of services utilized and the ability of insurance companies to simply pass the increased costs on to employers and governments, the purchasers of the majority of insurance plans. As healthcare costs began to impinge significantly on the other sectors of the economy, efforts emerged to change the payment incentives in the healthcare industry, especially as the increasing costs did not result in a concomitant improvement in the health status of the population. As attention has focused on controlling the rate of increase in healthcare expenditures, such alternative payment methods as pay for performance, shared savings, bundled payments, and global capitation have been introduced.

18.3.1 Pay for Performance

Pay for performance was introduced to provide incentives to providers to improve the quality of care delivered as evidence mounted regarding the underuse, overuse, and misuse of treatments within the healthcare system. The Committee on Redesigning Health Insurance Performance Measures, Payment, and Performance Improvement Programs (2007) defined pay for performance (P4P) as "the systematic and deliberate use of payment incentives that recognize and reward high levels of quality and quality improvement" (p. 5). Pay for performance is designed to offer incentives to encourage the healthcare system to move from its current structure toward different organizational and individual behaviors, which will result in better quality and improved outcomes.

In most markets, incentives induce producers and/or consumers to behave or respond in predictable ways, and desired attributes are identified and rewarded in order to stimulate additional production of those attributes. The goal of the P4P model in health care is to motivate constructive change in the system by explicitly linking incentives to the quality and performance. The difficulty in implementing P4P is in developing a framework that incorporates the complexity of the clinical situations to be included, the diversity of the environments in which care is provided, and the resources necessary to comply with the requirements of the system. A critical and difficult issue in any P4P system is the selection of the priority quality dimensions and the establishment of the measures to be used to assess performance and quality, especially because focusing on one domain of quality may lead to reductions in other domains of quality. Another aspect to be considered is whether the focus should be on improvement or on achieving a recognized threshold of desired quality, or both. The system must also be capable of incorporating new measures as the healthcare system evolves; innovations and discoveries should be encouraged. The incentive created should have a sufficient impact upon the revenues of the provider to influence their decisions.

18.3.2 Bundled Payments

The bundled payments model is known by a variety of names, such as case rate, global payment, package pricing, episode-based payment, comprehensive care payment, and evidence-based case rate. Regardless of the term used, it is a payment method based on the costs expected to be incurred in the provision of a clinically defined episode of care, adjusted for severity and complexity of a patient's condition. Bundled payments are viewed as a blend of fee-for-service and capitation payments, discouraging the provision of unnecessary care and encouraging the coordination of care across providers, but not penalizing providers who care for sicker patients in their practice. The goal of bundled payment is to reduce fragmentation of care thereby improving quality and reducing costs. The use of bundled payments should encourage providers within the system to reorganize how care is delivered so that it is coordinated and responsive to the needs of patients.

Under a bundled payment system, the services that are required by patients during a single illness or a course of treatment for a chronic disease are defined across providers and settings—the services are bundled into a single package of services. Once the required services are defined, a target price is established for the bundle. This target price reflects the total amount that will be paid for the episode of care, and all providers involved in the provision of services are covered under that price. This comprehensive price provides an incentive for the coordination of care in order to keep the costs of producing the services below the price established. Within the provider network, decisions have to be made on how to allocate the global revenue among the participating providers rendering services to the patient.

A number of barriers are encountered in the development of a bundled payment system. A major problem encountered is deciding just when an episode of care begins and ends. For an acute illness of limited duration, this is manageable. For chronic conditions lasting for extended periods of time, this is difficult to determine because, by definition, a chronic condition is a disease or illness that is persistent and long-lasting. Currently, an episode is typically defined for a specified period of time, such as 30 to 90 days after discharge from an acute care facility or after the first visit to a provider for the condition. The bundled payment is applied only to that particular illness or disease, which differs from capitation, which covers all illnesses experienced by an enrolled member for a specified period of time.

Because the target payment to be made is fixed, providers have an incentive to coordinate care and minimize the provision of any marginal or unnecessary care. A concern raised is that the incentive may encourage providers to underutilize services, negatively impacting the patient's outcome. Careful monitoring is needed to ensure that quality is not negatively impacted and that patients receive necessary care.

18.3.3 Value-Based Purchasing

Value-based purchasing (VBP) programs are also sometimes known as shared-savings programs, the goals of which are similar to those of the bundled payment programs: to improve care coordination and redesign the processes of care to produce high quality and efficient care delivery. Incentives are created within these programs to provide care that has higher value to the patient and to the system; they move away from paying providers based only on the volume of services provided to patients. Under these programs, if the provider is able to achieve savings and meet the quality performance standards, then the amount of the savings is shared between the providers and the payer. These programs focus on better care for individuals, better health for the population, and reducing the rate of growth in healthcare expenditures.

Similar to bundled payment systems, VBP programs also require the establishment of clinical measures, measures of effective resource utilization, and incentives within the payment structure to link the two measures to the price paid for services. The focus on these systems is to foster joint clinical and financial accountability within the healthcare system. As with any of the performance-based payment systems, it is critical to communicate among the various providers in order to coordinate care. This communication requires electronic health records with interoperability (the ability to link to each other) capability.

VBP programs are demand-side strategies that impact the utilization of healthcare services by rewarding excellence in the healthcare delivery by enhancing revenue through differential payment and by increasing market share by consumer selection. A key component of VBP is the development of standardized performance measures, including involving consumers in changing their lifestyle and self-managing their chronic diseases. The Institute of Medicine (2001) has established the STEEEP—Safe, Timely, Efficient, Effective, Equitable, and Patient-centered—typology of the dimensions of healthcare performance, which need to be incorporated into the system. To be effective, it is necessary to access and aggregate data on these dimensions from different sources and from different providers. As indicated, a key component of this model is patient-centeredness, which involves engaging the consumer in the process.

18.4 CONSUMER ENGAGEMENT

As efforts continue to improve quality and control the costs of health care, attention is focused on ways of influencing consumers to be more informed decision makers. For consumers to become more engaged in the decision-making process, it is necessary for them to have a better understanding of the availability of alternatives and options, and of the quality of care offered, in order to demand and choose appropriate services. As outlined in Aligning Forces for Quality (AF4Q), sponsored by the Robert Wood Johnson Foundation, to be successful in transforming health care, a communitywide consumer-engagement strategy must help consumers to

- Understand their risks or actual conditions, and take actions to manage them.

- Understand and make informed treatment choices.

- Understand the difference between good care and bad care, and demand good care.

- Advocate for public reporting by hospitals and doctors on nationally recognized indicators of quality care.

- Choose providers based on information about their ability to deliver effective care. (http://www.rwjf.org/qualityequality/af4q/focusareas/consumer.jsp)

For consumers to be informed decision makers in the healthcare system, literacy, and especially health literacy, is critical. A patient's literacy skills are critical in interactions in the healthcare field, impacting the ability of the patient to navigate the services needed and the healthcare delivery system. Literacy skills are also important in enabling the patient to be an advocate for their needs within the system, and the role of consumer self-advocacy is increasingly important. The complexity of the healthcare system and the incentives being created in many of the reform activities increasingly require patients to take a proactive role in the utilization of healthcare services and in the self-management of medical conditions.

As increased emphasis is placed on consumer engagement and access to online information and health information technologies is becoming more widespread, care must be taken that the medically underserved and disadvantaged populations are not further disenfranchised from the system. Health disparities currently exist, and increased reliance on health information technologies for seeking and managing personal health conditions and for communicating between patients and providers may widen the disparity gap rather than solve it. The deployment of health information and health information technology is intended to impact the demand for healthcare services, but care must be taken that this doesn't negatively impact various subgroups of the population.

Patient engagement is also a critical component of the patient-centered medical home model, which involves the provision of quality care that is coordinated, comprehensive, and cost-effective. The patient-centered medical home requires a strong patient-provider relationship through the use of a team approach to care that increases access to care and the continuity of the care provided. In addition to improving quality of care in order to improve health outcomes, the patient-centered medical home is expected to reduce demand for health services through the reduction of duplication of tests, procedures, emergency department visits, hospitalizations, and provider visits as care becomes coordinated across providers.

18.5 SUMMARY AND CONCLUSIONS

The U.S. healthcare industry continues to be faced with pressures to reduce costs and improve access to and quality of healthcare services. As the industry continues to consume an ever-increasing share of the gross domestic product, federal and state governments and private industry continue to look for ways to reduce the rate of increase in healthcare costs while increasing access to necessary and appropriate healthcare services.

The demand for healthcare services is influenced by a number of factors, including population demographics. The elderly population has poorer health status than other subgroups of the population and use a greater share of health services. This has major implications, as the population 65 and older has been projected to grow almost 90% between 2007 and 2030 as the Baby Boomer generation ages. Without increased personal responsibility for lifestyle and self-management of health, the demand for healthcare services will continue to expand with the growing aging population.

Efforts to contain healthcare costs have also been the focus of legislation and regulations, and such efforts are likely to continue in the future as government payments for healthcare services increase. While some interventions are focused on a reduction in the price per unit of service, much more focus is on reducing the volume of services provided. Providers within the system must develop a decision-making system that enables them to respond appropriately and quickly in order to deliver high-quality health care and achieve positive health outcomes. As the healthcare industry struggles to improve efficiency and efficacy, the need for systematic economic evaluations will grow. While health economics is not viewed as "the" answer to the problems in the healthcare system, it can be used to provide substantial assistance to improved decision making.

EXERCISES

1. What are the major contributors to rising healthcare expenditures, and how can the Patient Protection and Accountable Care Act affect these areas?
2. What is the responsibility of individuals in the healthcare system?
3. What are the incentives created by the various payment methods?
4. How can technology innovations impact healthcare costs?
5. What are the driving forces behind the mergers and acquisitions occurring in the healthcare system?

BIBLIOGRAPHY

Health Information Technology

Bergh, B. (2009). "In the same boat": Considerations on the partnership between healthcare providers and manufacturers of health IT products and medical devices. *Yearbook of Medical Informatics*, 33–36.

Blakeman, T., Chew-Graham, C., Reeves, D., Rogers, A., & Bower, P. (2011). The Quality and Outcomes Framework and self-management dialogue in primary care consultations: A qualitative study. *British Journal of General Practice*, 61(591), e666–e673.

Buckner, M., & Gregory, D. D. (2011). Point-of-care technology: Preserving the caring environment. *Critical Care Nursing Quarterly*, 34(4), 297–305.

Cegarra-Navarro, J. G., Wensley, A. K., & Sanchez-Polo, M. T. (2011). Improving quality of service of home healthcare units with health information technologies. *Health Information Management Journal*, 40(2), 30–38.

Collins, S. A., Stein, D. M., Vawdrey, D. K., Stetson, P. D., & Bakken, S. (2011). Content overlap in nurse and physician handoff artifacts and the potential role of electronic health records: A systematic review. *Journal of Biomedical Informatics, 44*(4), 704–712.

Dennehy, P., White, M. P., Hamilton, A., Pohl, J. M., Tanner, C., Onifade, T. J., & Zheng, K. (2011). A partnership model for implementing electronic health records in resource-limited primary care settings: Experiences from two nurse-managed health centers. *Journal of the American Medical Informatics Association, 18*(6), 820–826.

Doebbeling, B. N., & Flanagan, M. E. (2011). Emerging perspectives on transforming the healthcare system: Redesign strategies and a call for needed research. *Medical Care, 49*(Suppl.), S59–S64.

Encinosa, W. E., & Bae, J. (2011/2012). Health information technology and its effects on hospital costs, outcomes, and patient safety. *Inquiry, 48*(4), 288–303.

Freeland, M. S., Heffler, S. K., & Smith, S. D. (1998). *The impact of technological change on health care cost increases: A brief synthesis of the literature.* Office of the Actuary, Health Care Financing Administration.

Geissbuhler, A. (2011). How can eHealth help fix broken health systems? *Methods of Information in Medicine, 50*(4), 297–298.

Jaen, C. R. (2011). Successful health information technology implementation requires practice and health care system transformation. *Annals of Family Medicine, 9*(5), 388–389.

Kaiser Family Foundation. (2007, March). How changes in medical technology affect health care costs. *Snapshots: Health Care Costs.* Retrieved from http://www.kff.org/insurance/snapshot/chcm030807oth.cfm#back1

Kern, L. M., Ancker, J. S., Abramson, E., Patel, V., Dhopeshwarkar, R. V., & Kaushal, R. (2011). Evaluating health information technology in community-based settings: Lessons learned. *Journal of the American Medical Informatics Association, 18*(6), 749–753.

Kuperman, G. J. (2011). Health-information exchange: Why are we doing it, and what are we doing? *Journal of the American Medical Informatics Association, 18*(5), 678–682.

Leonard, K. J., & Dalziel, S. (2011). How and when eHealth is a good investment for patients managing chronic disease. *Healthcare Management Forum, 24*(3), 122–136.

Luxford, K., Safran, D. G., & Delbanco, T. (2011). Promoting patient-centered care: A qualitative study of facilitators and barriers in healthcare organizations with a reputation for improving the patient experience. *International Journal for Quality in Health Care, 23*(5), 510–515.

Ord, E. W., Huerta, T. R., Thompson, M. A., & Patry, R. (2011/2012). The impact of accelerating electronic prescribing on hospitals' productivity levels: Can health information technology bend the curve? *Inquiry, 48*(4), 304–312.

Pauly, M. V. (2005). Competition and new technology. *Health Affairs, 24*(6), 1523–1535.

Russ, A. L., Saleem, J. J., Justice, C. F., Woodward-Hagg, H., Woodbridge, P. A., & Doebbeling, B. N. (2010). Electronic health information in use: Characteristics that support employee workflow and patient care. *Health Informatics Journal, 16*(4), 287–305.

Sequist, T. D. (2011). Health information technology and disparities in quality of care. *Journal of General Internal Medicine, 26*(10), 1084–1085.

Sittig, D. F., & Ash, J. S. (2011). On the importance of using a multidimensional sociotechnical model to study health information technology. *Annals of Family Medicine, 9*(5), 390–391.

Walker, J., & McKethan, A. (2012). Achieving accountable care—"It's not about the bike." *New England Journal of Medicine, 366*(2), e4.

Zheng, K., Guo, M. H., & Hanauer, D. A. (2011). Using the time and motion method to study clinical work processes and workflow: Methodological inconsistencies and a call for standardized research. *Journal of the American Medical Informatics Association, 18*(5), 704–710.

Mergers and Acquisitions

Afendulis, C. C., & Kessler, D. P. (2011). Vertical integration and optimal reimbursement policy. *International Journal of Health Care Finance & Economics, 11*(3), 165–179.

Carlson, J. (2011). All eyes on Ascension. New for-profit system is called workable model. *Modern Healthcare, 41*(9), 14.

Centers for Medicare and Medicaid. (2011). *National health expenditure projections 2010–2020: Table 1: Economic indicators, levels and annual percent change: Calendar years 2005–2020.* Retrieved February 12, 2012, from https://www.cms.gov/NationalHealthExpendData/downloads/proj2010.pdf

Costello, M. M., West, D. J., & Ramirez, B. (2011). Hospitals for sale. *Hospital Topics, 89*(3), 69–73.

Cutler, D. M. (2009). The next wave of corporate medicine—How we all might benefit. *New England Journal of Medicine, 361*(6), 549–551.

Dranove, D., & Sfekas, A. (2009). The revolution in health care antitrust: New methods and provocative implications. *Milbank Quarterly, 87*(3), 607–632.

Evans, M. (2011). Another cost of capital. Cash infusion can mean survival for a hospital, but also loss of independence. *Modern Healthcare, 41*(31), 32

Franey, H. J. (2011). Henry J. Franey: Mergers should create economic value. *Healthcare Financial Management, 65*(4), 30–31.

Galloro, V. (2011). Losing their distinctions. Attributes of deals by not-for-profits, investor-owned chains begin to blur. *Modern Healthcare, 41*(27), 31.

Healthcare Financial Management Association Principles and Practices Board. (2011). Mergers and acquisitions: What has changed. *Healthcare Financial Management, 65*(1), 105–108.

Humphreys, L. R. (2011). Stronger together: Merging to serve the community. *Frontiers of Health Services Management, 27*(4), 33–37; discussion, 39–41.

Kaufman, K., & Grube, M. E. (2009). Making the right decisions in a consolidating market. *Healthcare Financial Management, 63*(7), 44–52.

Manas, J. S. (2011). Lessons learned in mergers and acquisitions. *Frontiers of Health Services Management, 27*(4), 19–23; discussion, 39–41.

Mathis, D. R., & Lewis, M. S. (2011). Is bigger better? The urge to merge. *Journal of Medical Practice Management, 26*(4), 236–238.

Myers, C., & Lineen, J. (2009). Hospital consolidation outlook: Surviving in a tough economy. *Healthcare Financial Management, 63*(11), 56–60, 62.

Nakamura, S. (2010). Hospital mergers and referrals in the United States: Patient steering or integrated delivery of care? *Inquiry, 47*(3), 226–241.

Neumann, M. E. (2011). Is the bundle leading to a tighter provider market? Key acquisition, merger mark activity in 2010–2011. *Nephrology News & Issues, 25*(8), 32–33.

Pozniak, A. S., Hirth, R. A., Banaszak-Holl, J., & Wheeler, J. R. (2010). Predictors of chain acquisition among independent dialysis facilities. *Health Services Research, 45*(2), 476–496.

Riley, J. B., Jr., & Soldato, D. C. (2011). Consolidating physician practices: A guide. *Nephrology News & Issues, 25*(3), 32–33.

Schlossberg, S. (2009). Supergroups and economies of scale. *Urologic Clinics of North America, 36*(1), 95–100, vii.

Zuckerman, A. M. (2011). Healthcare mergers and acquisitions: Strategies for consolidation. *Frontiers of Health Services Management, 27*(4), 3–12; discussion, 39–41.

Payment Systems

Bhargavan, M., Sunshine, J. H., & Hughes, D. R. (2011). Clarifying the relationship between nonradiologists' financial interest in imaging and their utilization of imaging. *AJR. American Journal of Roentgenology, 197*(5), W891–W899.

Bobinac, A., Van Exel, N. J., Rutten, F. F., & Brouwer, W. B. (2010). Willingness to pay for a quality-adjusted life-year: The individual perspective. *Value in Health, 13,* 1046–1055.

Carlson, J. J., Sullivan, S. D., Garrison, L. P., Neumann, P. J., & Veenstra, D. L. (2010). Linking payment to health outcomes: A taxonomy and examination of performance-based reimbursement schemes between healthcare payers and manufacturers. *Health Policy, 96*(3), 179–190.

Chang, G. M., Cheng, S. H., & Tung, Y. C. (2011). Impact of cuts in reimbursement on outcome of acute myocardial infarction and use of percutaneous coronary intervention:

A nationwide population-based study over the period 1997 to 2008. *Medical Care, 49*(12), 1054–1061.

Chen, H. F., Bazzoli, G. J., Harless, D. W., & Clement, J. P. (2010). Is quality of cardiac hospital care a public or private good? *Medical Care, 48*(11), 999–1006.

Colla, C. H., Escarce, J. J., Buntin, M. B., & Sood, N. (2010). Effects of competition on the cost and quality of inpatient rehabilitation care under prospective payment. *Health Services Research, 45*, 1981–2006.

Committee on Redesigning Health Insurance Performance Measures, Payment, and Performance Improvement Programs (2007). *Rewarding provider performance: Aligning incentives in Medicare.* Washington DC: The National Academies Press.

Conrad, D. A., Lee, R. S., Milgrom, P., & Huebner, C. E. (2010). Estimating determinants of dentist productivity: New evidence. *Journal of Public Health Dentistry, 70*(4), 262–268.

Cooke, V., Arling, G., Lewis, T., Abrahamson, K. A., Mueller, C., & Edstrom, L. (2010). Minnesota's Nursing Facility Performance-Based Incentive Payment Program: An innovative model for promoting care quality. *Gerontologist, 50*(4), 556–563.

Coulam, R. F., Feldman, R. D., & Dowd, B. E. (2011). Competitive pricing and the challenge of cost control in Medicare. *Journal of Health Politics, Policy & Law, 36*, 649–689.

Dummit, L. A. (2010). Medicare physician fees: The data behind the numbers. *Issue Brief/National Health Policy Forum*, (838), 1–16.

Duszak, R., Jr., & Saunders, W. M. (2010). Medicare's physician quality reporting initiative: Incentives, physician work, and perceived impact on patient care. *Journal of the American College of Radiology, 7*(6), 419–424.

Eapen, Z. J., Reed, S. D., Curtis, L. H., Hernandez, A. F., & Peterson, E. D. (2011). Do heart failure disease management programs make financial sense under a bundled payment system? *American Heart Journal, 161*(5), 916–922.

Ferrante, J. M., Cohen, D. J., & Crosson, J. C. (2010). Translating the patient navigator approach to meet the needs of primary care. *Journal of the American Board of Family Medicine: JABFM, 23*(6), 736–744.

Filson, C. P., Hollingsworth, J. M., Skolarus, T. A., Clemens, J. Q., & Hollenbeck, B. K. (2011). Health care reform in 2010: Transforming the delivery system to improve quality of care. *World Journal of Urology, 29*(1), 85–90.

Flodgren, G., Eccles, M. P., Shepperd, S., Scott, A., Parmelli, E., & Beyer, F. R. (2011). An overview of reviews evaluating the effectiveness of financial incentives in changing healthcare professional behaviours and patient outcomes. *Cochrane Database of Systematic Reviews*, (7), CD009255.

Fry, D. E., Pine, M., Jones, B. L., & Meimban, R. J. (2010). Surgical warranties to improve quality and efficiency in elective colon surgery. *Archives of Surgery, 145*(7), 647–652.

Fry, D. E., Pine, M., & Pine, G. (2010). Virtual partnerships: Aligning hospital and surgeon incentives. *American Journal of Surgery, 200*(1), 105–110.

Gabbay, R. A., Bailit, M. H., Mauger, D. T., Wagner, E. H., & Siminerio, L. (2011). Multipayer patient-centered medical home implementation guided by the chronic care model. *Joint Commission Journal on Quality & Patient Safety, 37*(6), 265–273.

Herring, B., & Lentz, L. K. (2011/2012). What can we expect from the "Cadillac Tax" in 2018 and beyond? *Inquiry, 48*(4), 322–337.

Hull-Grommesh, L., Ellis, E. F., & Mackey, T. A. (2010). Implications for cardiology nurse practitioner billing: A comparison of hospital versus office practice. *Journal of the American Academy of Nurse Practitioners, 22*(6), 288–291.

Kapoor, J. R., Kapoor, R., Hellkamp, A. S., Hernandez, A. F., Heidenreich, P. A., & Fonarow, G. C. (2011). Payment source, quality of care, and outcomes in patients hospitalized with heart failure. *Journal of the American College of Cardiology, 58*(14), 1465–1471.

Kim, M. O., Lee, K. S., Kim, J. H., & Joo, J. S. (2011). Willingness to pay for hospice care using the contingent valuation method. *Yonsei Medical Journal, 52*(3), 510–521.

Korda, H., & Eldridge, G. N. (2011/2012). Payment incentives and integrated care delivery: Levers for health system reform and cost containment. *Inquiry, 48*(4), 277–287.

Landon, B. E., Reschovsky, J. D., O'Malley, A. J., Pham, H. H., & Hadley, J. (2011). The relationship between physician compensation strategies and the intensity of care delivered to Medicare beneficiaries. *Health Services Research, 46,* 1863–1882.

Lee, D. W., Neumann, P. J., & Rizzo, J. A. (2010). Understanding the medical and nonmedical value of diagnostic testing. *Value in Health, 13*(2), 310–314

Leigh, J. P., Tancredi, D., Jerant, A., & Kravitz, R. L. (2010). Physician wages across specialties: Informing the physician reimbursement debate. *Archives of Internal Medicine, 170*(19), 1728–1734.

McCullough, J., Casey, M., Moscovice, I., & Burlew, M. (2011). Meaningful use of health information technology by rural hospitals. *Journal of Rural Health, 27,* 329–337.

Messori, A., Fadda, V., & Trippoli, S. (2011). A uniform procedure for reimbursing the off-label use of antineoplastic drugs according to the value-for-money approach. *Journal of Chemotherapy, 23*(2), 67–70.

National Research Council. (2007). *Rewarding provider performance: Aligning incentives in Medicare* (Pathways to Quality Health Care Series). Washington DC: The National Academies Press.

Newhouse, J. P., Huang, J., Brand, R. J., Fung, V., & Hsu, J. T. (2011). The structure of risk adjustment for private plans in Medicare. *American Journal of Managed Care, 17*(6 Spec. no.), e231–e240.

Nugent, M. E. (2011). Aligning managed care contracts, compensation plans, and incentive models. *Healthcare Financial Management, 65*(11), 88–92, 94, 96

O'Malley, A. S., Bond, A. M., & Berenson, R. A. (2011). Rising hospital employment of physicians: Better quality, higher costs? *Issue Brief/Center for Studying Health System Change,* (136), 1–4.

Pine, M., Fry, D. E., Jones, B. L., Meimban, R. J., & Pine, G. J. (2010). Controlling costs without compromising quality: Paying hospitals for total knee replacement. *Medical Care, 48*(10), 862–868.

Pirson, M., Delo, C., Martins, D., & Leclercq, P. (2011). Comparison of cost-weights scales methodologies in the perspective of a financing system based on pathologies. *European Journal of Health Economics, 12*(6), 503–508.

Rana, A. J., Iorio, R., & Healy, W. L. (2011). Hospital economics of primary THA decreasing reimbursement and increasing cost, 1990 to 2008. *Clinical Orthopaedics & Related Research, 469*(2), 355–361.

Rittenhouse, D. R., Casalino, L. P., Shortell, S. M., McClellan, S. R., Gillies, R. R., Alexander, J. A., & Drum, M. L. (2011). Small and medium-size physician practices use few patient-centered medical home processes. *Health Affairs, 30*(8), 1575–1584.

Russell, G., Dahrouge, S., Tuna, M., Hogg, W., Geneau, R., & Gebremichael, G. (2010). Getting it all done. Organizational factors linked with comprehensive primary care. *Family Practice, 27*(5), 535–541.

Severson, M. A., Wood, D. L., Chastain, C. N., Lee, L. G., Rees, A. C., Agerter, D.C., ..., & Larusso, N. F. (2011). Health reform: A community experience using design research as a guide. *Mayo Clinic Proceedings, 86*(10), 973–980.

Shortell, S. M., & McCurdy, R. K. (2010). Integrated health systems. *Studies in Health Technology & Informatics, 153,* 369–382.

Song, Z., Safran, D. G., Landon, B. E., He, Y., Ellis, R. P., Mechanic, R. E., ..., & Chernew, M. E. (2011). Health care spending and quality in year 1 of the alternative quality contract. *New England Journal of Medicine, 365*(10), 909–918.

Toussaint, J. S., Queram, C., & Musser, J. W. (2011). Connecting statewide health information technology strategy to payment reform. *American Journal of Managed Care, 17*(3), e80–e88.

Trentman, T. L., Mueller, J. T., Ruskin, K. J., Noble, B. N., & Doyle, C. A. (2011). Adoption of anesthesia information management systems by US anesthesiologists. *Journal of Clinical Monitoring & Computing, 25*(2), 129–135.

Van Kleef, R. C., van de Ven, W. P. M. M., & van Vliet, R. C. J. A. (2011/2012). Risk-adjusting the doughnut hole to improve efficiency and equity. *Inquiry, 48*(4), 313–321.

Wranik, D., & Durier-Copp, M. (2011). Framework for the design of physician remuneration methods in primary health care. *Social Work in Public Health, 26*(3), 231–259.

Yau, G. L., Williams, A. S., & Brown, J. B. (2011). Family physicians' perspectives on personal health records: Qualitative study. *Canadian Family Physician, 57*(5), e178–e184.

Patient-Centered Medical Home

Allen, T., Brailovsky, C., Rainsberry, P., Lawrence, K., Crichton, T., Carpentier, M. P., & Visser, S. (2011). Defining competency-based evaluation objectives in family medicine: Dimensions of competence and priority topics for assessment. *Canadian Family Physician, 57*(9), e331–e340.

Amiel, J. M., & Pincus, H. A. (2011). The medical home model: New opportunities for psychiatric services in the United States. *Current Opinion in Psychiatry, 24*(6), 562–568.

Baxley, L., Borkan, J., Campbell, T., Davis, A,. Kuzel, T., & Wender, R. (2011). In pursuit of a transformed health care system: From patient-centered medical homes to accountable care organizations and beyond. *Annals of Family Medicine, 9*(5), 466–467.

Bertakis, K. D., & Azari, R. (2011). Determinants and outcomes of patient-centered care. *Patient Education & Counseling, 85*, 46–52.

Bras, M., Dordevic, V., Milunovic, V., Brajkovic, L., Milicic, D., & Konopka, L. (2011). Person-centered medicine versus personalized medicine: Is it just a sophism? A view from chronic pain management. *Psychiatria Danubina, 23*(3), 246–250.

Clayton, M. F., Latimer, S., Dunn, T. W., & Haas, L. (2011). Assessing patient-centered communication in a family practice setting: How do we measure it, and whose opinion matters? *Patient Education & Counseling, 84*(3), 294–302.

Cooper, L. A., Roter, D. L., Carson, K. A., Bone, L. R., Larson, S. M., Miller, E. R., III., ..., & Levine, D. M. (2011). A randomized trial to improve patient-centered care and hypertension control in underserved primary care patients. *Journal of General Internal Medicine, 26*(11), 1297–1304.

Davis, K., Abrams, M., & Stremikis, K. (2011). How the Affordable Care Act will strengthen the nation's primary care foundation. *Journal of General Internal Medicine, 26*(10), 1201–1203.

Golden, B. R., Hannam, R., Fraser, H., Leung, M., Downey, S., Stewart, J., & Grichko, E. (2011). Improving the patient experience through design. *Healthcare Quarterly, 14*(3), 32–41.

Groene, O. (2011). Patient centredness and quality improvement efforts in hospitals: Rationale, measurement, implementation. *International Journal for Quality in Health Care, 23*(5), 531–537.

Hofdijk, J. (2011). Patient-centered integrated clinical resource management. *Studies in Health Technology & Informatics, 169*, 996–999.

Hughes, C. L., Marshall, C. R., Murphy, E., & Mun, S. K. (2011). Technologies in the patient-centered medical home: Examining the model from an enterprise perspective. *Telemedicine Journal & E-Health, 17*(6), 495–500.

Ijas-Kallio, T., Ruusuvuori, J., & Perakyla, A. (2010). Patient involvement in problem presentation and diagnosis delivery in primary care. *Communication & Medicine, 7*(2), 131–141.

Janosky, J. E., Joyce, N., & Kingsbury, D. (2011). Turning smaller practices into patient-centered medical homes. *Health Affairs, 30*(9), 1807.

Kuehn, B. M. (2012). Patient-centered care model demands better physician-patient communication. *JAMA, 307*(5), 441–442.

Lawn, S., McMillan, J., & Pulvirenti, M. (2011). Chronic condition self-management: Expectations of responsibility. *Patient Education & Counseling, 84*(2), e5–e8

Lyon, R. K., & Slawson, J. (2011). An organized approach to chronic disease care. *Family Practice Management, 18*(3), 27–31.

Marshall, R. C., Doperak, M., Milner, M., Motsinger, C., Newton, T., Padden, M., ..., & Mun, S. K. (2011). Patient-centered medical home: An emerging primary care model and the military health system. *Military Medicine, 176*(11), 1253–1259.

Moran, W. P., Davis, K. S., Moran, T. J., Newman, R., & Mauldin, P. D. (2012). Where are my patients? It is time to automate notification of hospital use to primary care practices. *Southern Medical Journal, 105*(1), 18–23.

Porterfield, S. L., & DeRigne, L. (2011). Medical home and out-of-pocket medical costs for children with special health care needs. *Pediatrics, 128*(5), 892–900.

Romeo, S. J. (2011). The promise of the medical home. *Medical Economics, 88*(20), 59–60, 65.

Roumie, C. L., Greevy, R., Wallston, K. A., Elasy, T. A., Kaltenbach, L., Kotter, K, ..., & Speroff, T. (2011). Patient-centered primary care is associated with patient hypertension medication adherence. *Journal of Behavioral Medicine, 34*(4), 244–253.

Sandman, L., & Munthe, C. (2010). Shared decision making, paternalism and patient choice. *Health Care Analysis, 18*(1), 60–84.

Snyder, C. F., Wu, A. W., Miller, R. S., Jensen, R. E., Bantug, E. T., & Wolff, A. C. (2011). The role of informatics in promoting patient-centered care. *Cancer Journal, 17*(4), 211–218.

Stephan, B. (2011). Population health management: The next frontier. *Nebraska Nurse, 44*(3), 12.

Stichler, J. F. (2011). Patient-centered healthcare design. *Journal of Nursing Administration, 41*, 503–506.

Stange, K. C., Miller, W. L., Nutting, P. A., Crabtree, B. F., Stewart, E. E., & Jaen, C. R. (2010). Context for understanding the National Demonstration Project and the patient-centered medical home. *Annals of Family Medicine, 8*(Suppl. 1), S2–S8, S92.

Takach, M. (2011). Reinventing Medicaid: State innovations to qualify and pay for patient-centered medical homes show promising results. *Health Affairs, 30*(7), 1325–1334.

Zickafoose, J. S., Gebremariam, A., Clark, S. J., & Davis, M. M. (2011). Medical home disparities between children with public and private insurance. *Academic Pediatrics, 11*(4), 305–310.

Accountable Care Organizations

Anderson, G. F. (2011). Leadership in creating accountable care organizations. *Journal of General Internal Medicine, 26*(11), 1368–1370

Bailit, M., & Hughes, C. (2011). Key design elements of shared-savings payment arrangements. *Issue Brief (Commonwealth Fund), 20*, 1–16

Baxley, L., Borkan, J., Campbell, T., Davis, A., Kuzel, T., & Wender, R. (2011). In pursuit of a transformed health care system: From patient-centered medical homes to accountable care organizations and beyond. *Annals of Family Medicine, 9*(5), 466–467.

Boland, P., Polakoff, P., & Schwab, T. (2010). Accountable care organizations hold promise, but will they achieve cost and quality targets? *Managed Care, 19*(10), 12–16, 19

Burke, T. (2011). Accountable care organizations. *Public Health Reports, 126*(6), 875–878.

Correia, E. W. (2011). Accountable care organizations: The proposed regulations and the prospects for success. *American Journal of Managed Care, 17*(8), 560–568.

Crosson, F. J. (2011). Analysis & commentary: The accountable care organization: Whatever its growing pains, the concept is too vitally important to fail. *Health Affairs, 30*(7), 1250–1255.

Davis, M. A., Whedon, J. M., & Weeks, W. B. (2011). Complementary and alternative medicine practitioners and accountable care organizations: The train is leaving the station. *Journal of Alternative & Complementary Medicine, 17*(8), 669–674.

Devore, S., & Champion, R. W. (2011). Driving population health through accountable care organizations. *Health Affairs, 30*(1), 41–50.

Dorn, S. D. (2009). United States health care reform in 2009: A primer for gastroenterologists. *Clinical Gastroenterology & Hepatology, 7*(11), 1168–1173.

Emanuel, E. J., & Pearson, S. D. (2012). Physician autonomy and health care reform. *JAMA, 307*(4), 367–368.

Filson, C. P., Hollingsworth, J. M., Skolarus, T. A., Clemens, J. Q., & Hollenbeck, B. K. (2011). Health care reform in 2010: Transforming the delivery system to improve quality of care. *World Journal of Urology, 29*(1), 85–90.

Fisher, E. S., McClellan, M. B., & Safran, D. G. (2011). Building the path to accountable care. *New England Journal of Medicine, 365*(26), 2445–2447.

Hagland, M. (2011). Ready to catch the next wave? The new accountability agenda in healthcare. *Healthcare Informatics, 28*(12), 8–16.

Harolds, J. A. (2010). Will accountable care organizations deliver greater quality and lower cost health care? *Clinical Nuclear Medicine, 35*(12), 935–936.

Higgins, A., Stewart, K., Dawson, K., & Bocchino, C. (2011). Early lessons from accountable care models in the private sector: Partnerships between health plans and providers. *Health Affairs, 30*(9), 1718–1727.

Kocher, R., & Sahni, N. R. (2010). Physicians versus hospitals as leaders of accountable care organizations. *New England Journal of Medicine, 363*(27), 2579–2582.

Lund, I. V., & Hartman, J. (2011). Roadmap for reform: Outlook for imaging under accountable care. *Radiology Management, 33*(6), 22–26; quiz, 27–28.

Norman, G., & Schulte, D. (2011). How collaborative care platforms can make ACOs a reality for all physicians. *Physician Executive, 37*(6), 24–28.

Reynolds, J., & Roble, D. (2011). The financial implications of ACOs for providers. *Healthcare Financial Management, 65*(10), 76–82.

Schoenbaum, S. C. (2011). Accountable care organizations: Roles and opportunities for hospitals. Hospital practice (1995) *Hospital Practice, 39*(3), 140–148.

Shields, M. C., Patel, P. H., Manning, M., & Sacks, L. (2011). A model for integrating independent physicians into accountable care organizations. *Health Affairs, 30*(1), 161–172.

Shulkin, D. J. (2011). PRIDE in accountable care. *Population Health Management, 14*(5), 211–214.

Silversmith, J. (2011). Accountable care organizations: A primer. *Minnesota Medicine, 94*(2), 38–40

Sinaiko, A. D., & Rosenthal, M. B. (2010). Patients' role in accountable care organizations. *New England Journal of Medicine, 363*(27), 2583–2585.

Singer, S., & Shortell, S. M. (2011). Implementing accountable care organizations: Ten potential mistakes and how to learn from them. *JAMA, 306*(7), 758–759.

Smith, C. (2011). Between the Scylla and Charybdis: Physicians and the clash of liability standards and cost cutting goals within accountable care organizations. *Annals of Health Law, 20*(2), 165–203, 6p preceding i.

Stremikis, K., Schoen, C., & Fryer, A. K. (2011). A call for change: The 2011 Commonwealth Fund survey of public views of the U.S. health system. *Issue Brief (Commonwealth Fund), 6*, 1–23

Tollen, L., Enthoven, A., Crosson, F. J., Taylor, N., Audet, A. M., Schoen, C., & Ross, M. (2011). Delivery system reform tracking: A framework for understanding change. *Issue Brief (Commonwealth Fund), 10*, 1–18

Walker, J., & McKethan, A. (2012). Achieving accountable care—"It's not about the bike." *New England Journal of Medicine, 366*(2), e4.

Weinberg, S. L. (2010). Accountable care organizations—Ready for prime time or not? *American Heart Hospital Journal, 8*(2), E78–E79.

Value-Based Health Care

Chodroff, C. H., & Krivenko, C. (1994). The role of the coordinator of care. *Physician Executive, 20*(11), 11–14.

Eldridge, G. N., & Korda, H. (2011). Value-based purchasing: The evidence. *American Journal of Managed Care, 17*(8), e310–e313.

Institute of Medicine. (2001). Crossing the quality chasm: A new health system for the 21st century. Washington DC: National Academy Press.

Kenagy, J. W., McCarthy, S. M., Young, D. W., Barrett, D., & Pinakiewicz, D. C. (2001). Toward a value-based health care system. *American Journal of Medicine, 110*(2), 158–163.

Kim, L. S. (2011). How will accreditation of your ambulatory endoscopy center be an essential component of showing value-based health care? *Clinical Gastroenterology & Hepatology, 9*(1), 21–23.

Lee, D. W., Neumann, P. J., & Rizzo, J. A. (2010). Understanding the medical and nonmedical value of diagnostic testing. *Value in Health, 13*(2), 310–314.

Mohlenbrock, W. C. (1998a). Value-based health care, Part 2. The physician imperative: Define, measure, and improve health care quality. *Physician Executive, 24*(3), 47–54.

Mohlenbrock, W. C. (1998b). Value-based health care. Part I: Physicians reestablishing clinical autonomy. *Physician Executive, 24*(1), 26–29.

O'Kane, M. E. (2007). Performance-based measures: The early results are in. *Journal of Managed Care Pharmacy, 13*(2 Suppl. B), S3–S6.

Pollock, R. E. (2008). Value-based health care: The MD Anderson experience. *Annals of Surgery, 248*(4), 510–516; discussion, 517–518.

Porter, M. E. (2008). Value-based health care delivery. *Annals of Surgery, 248*(4), 503–509.

Robinson, J. C. (2008). Slouching toward value-based health care. *Health Affairs, 27*(1), 11–12.

Shannon, D. (2011). Managing the critical transition from volume to value. *Physician Executive, 37*(3), 4–9.

Strite, S., & Stuart, M. E. (2005). What is an evidence-based, value-based health care system? (Part 1). *Physician Executive, 31*(1), 50–54.

Glossary of Health Economics Terms

ABSOLUTE ADVANTAGE

The ability of a given amount of resources to produce more of some goods or services in one industry or organization than in another one.

ABUSE (HEALTH CARE)

Excessive, unnecessary, or improper treatment, including failure to provide medically necessary care.

ACCESS

Potential and actual entry of a population into the healthcare delivery system (U.S. Congress, 1988).

ACCOUNTABILITY

Duty to provide evidence necessary to establish confidence that the activity for which one is responsible is performed and described in a way that reflects transparently the activity that has been performed to all concerned.

ACCOUNTABLE CARE ORGANIZATION (ACO)

A group of doctors, hospitals, and other healthcare providers who come together voluntarily to give coordinated high-quality care to their Medicare patients (https://www.cms.gov/Medicare/Medicare-Fee-for-Service-Payment/ACO/index.html?redirect=/ACO/).

ACCOUNTABLE CARE PLAN

Form of health plan proposed in the 1990s as part of the managed competition approach to health care, accountable for meeting federal requirements for providing a defined set of standardized services.

ACCREDITATION

Process performed by a nongovernmental agency to evaluate an institution or education program to determine if a set of standards has been met.

ACTIVITIES OF DAILY LIVING (ADL)

Activities that are typically done for oneself, such as eating, dressing, brushing teeth, etc.

ACUITY

Level or severity of an illness.

ACUTE CARE

Inpatient diagnostic and short-term treatment of patients.

ADJUSTED COMMUNITY RATE

Term used in Medicare risk contracts to indicate the premium to be charged for providing exactly the same Medicare-covered benefits to a community-rated group, adjusted to allow for greater intensity and frequency of utilization by Medicare recipients.

ADMINISTERED PRICE

Price set by the seller or payer instead of by impersonal market forces.

ADMISSION

Formal acceptance of a patient by a hospital or other healthcare institution in order to provide care to that patient.

ADVERSE DRUG EVENT

Harm (illness or injury) resulting from the use or administration of a drug or medication.

ADVERSE SELECTION

The systematic selection by high-risk consumers of insurance plans with greater degrees of coverage. The insurers who offer these plans end up with insureds who incur greater than normal costs.

ADVOCACY

Attempt to persuade regarding the rightness of a cause or point of view regarding an issue.

AFFILIATION

Number of arrangements among providers outlining relationships and individual responsibilities.

AGENCY (AGENT)

A group or individual who has been delegated authority to make decisions and perform activities on behalf of those doing the delegating. Physicians are often said to act as agents for their patients, indicating that the physicians make decisions about treatments based on their knowledge.

AGGREGATE DEMAND

Total desired purchases by all buyers of goods or services produced.

AGGREGATE SUPPLY

Total desired sales by all producers of goods or services.

ALGORITHM

Set of rules for carrying out a process or the calculation of a statistic.

ALLOCATIVE EFFICIENCY

No reorganization of production or consumption could make one person better off without making someone else worse off.

ALL-PAYER SYSTEM

A system of reimbursing providers in which all separate insurers coordinate to set uniform payment policies. Individual providers will then receive the same reimbursement from different insurers for cases with similar characteristics.

ALTERNATE LEVEL OF CARE (ALC)

A level of care other than the appropriate one, such as that given to a non-acute-treatment patient occupying an acute-care bed.

AMBULATORY CARE

Care rendered to individuals under their own cognizance any time when they are not resident in an institution.

AMBULATORY CARE GROUPS (ACGs)

A case-mix classification system incorporating related ambulatory care visits, based on ICD-9-CM diagnostic codes and patient age and gender (Starfield, Weiner, Mumbord, & Steinwachs, 1991).

AMBULATORY VISIT GROUPS (AVGs)

A classification system by which ambulatory care visits with associated procedures are classified into similar resource-using groups based on diagnosis, procedure, age, and gender.

ANCILLARY SERVICES

Hospital services other than room and board (nursing services are included as part of room and board).

ANTIKICKBACK STATUTE

Federal legislation making it a felony for an individual to receive or offer a bribe, or kickback, in exchange for a referral from another person in any federally financed healthcare program.

ANTITRUST

Laws seeking to prevent monopolies or unfair competition in a market, or other activities that unreasonably restrain trade.

ANY WILLING PROVIDER

State laws requiring a managed care organization to grant participation to any provider who is legally qualified as a practitioner and who is willing to become a member of the organization.

APACHE III

System designed to predict risk of dying in a hospital, generally used to measure the severity of illness of intensive care unit (ICU) patients.

APPROPRIATENESS OF CARE

Degree to which tests, medications, procedures, education, and other healthcare services is clearly indicated, adequate, not excessive, and provided in the setting most appropriate to meet the needs of the patient.

AREA WAGE ADJUSTMENT

Part of the prospective payment formula allowing for differences in wage scales in different parts of the country.

ASSIGNMENT OF BENEFITS

Voluntary action by an insured beneficiary to have insurance benefits paid directly to the provider of services.

ASYMMETRIC INFORMATION

An imbalance of information between buyers and sellers of a service, by which one group is better informed than the other.

ATYPICAL PATIENTS

Patients who exhibit patterns of care different from typical cases, either because they do not complete a full and successful course of treatment in a single institution or because their length of stay exceeds the statistical trim point.

AUTONOMY

Right of an individual to make decisions for his/her health or life.

AVAILABILITY

The supply of services, generally in relation to the demand for the services.

AVERAGE ADJUSTED PER CAPITA COST (AAPCC)

An estimate of the average cost incurred by Medicare per beneficiary in the fee-for-service system, adjusted by county for geographic cost differences related to age, gender, disability status, Medicaid eligibility, and institutional status.

AVERAGE COST (AC)

The unit cost for a selected volume of output; total cost divided by total quantity of output. The average cost is equal to the average variable cost plus the average fixed cost.

AVERAGE FIXED COST (AFC)

The unit fixed cost for a specific volume of output. The average fixed cost is equal to the total fixed cost divided by the volume of output.

AVERAGE LENGTH OF STAY

See **length of stay**.

AVERAGE PRODUCT (AP)

Total product divided by number of units used in its production.

AVERAGE REVENUE (AR)

Total revenue divided by number of units (quantity) sold.

AVERAGE VARIABLE COST (AVC)

The unit variable cost for a specific volume of output; total variable cost divided by quantity of output.

BABY BOOMERS

Individuals born in the United States from 1946 to 1964.

BALANCE BILLING

Practice of physicians to charge patients the difference between their charges and the amount paid by the insurance company for the service.

BALANCED BUDGET ACT OF 1997 (BBA)

Federal law enacting many changes in health care, including the creation of the State Children's Health Insurance Program (S-CHIP), as well as changed design to extend the Medicare Trust Fund's financial life and created the Medicare + Choice program.

BASIS OF PAYMENT

The unit of output in terms for which the provider is paid. This can be on any of a per day of care, per service provided, per case, or per person (capitation).

BED CAPACITY

The number of patients a hospital can house.

BED DAYS

The number of days in a period that beds are available. In a year, bed days are the number of regularly maintained available beds multiplied by 365.

BEHAVIORAL HEALTH

Umbrella term including mental health, substance abuse, and used to distinguish services provided for physical health.

BENCHMARK

Reference point for each element being monitored; used to compare performance or outcomes of an institution or a provider against the defined measure or best practice.

BENEFIT

(1) Money, care, or other services that an individual is entitled to receive because of insurance coverage. (2) The compensation of labor that is additional to wages (e.g., health insurance, life insurance, pension rights, etc.).

BENEFIT COST

The relationship between the dollar impact of an intervention and its opportunity cost. It can be expressed as a ratio (benefits divided by costs) or as a net value (benefits minus costs).

BIASED SELECTION

The deliberate choice, by a provider or insurer, of a group of patients (insureds) with preselected characteristics associated with low utilization of health care.

BREAK-EVEN POINT

Volume of activity where revenues and expenses are equal.

BUDGET NEUTRALITY

Requirement that payment under a new system cannot be larger or smaller than under the previous system.

BUNDLING

Grouping goods and services together into a package for delivery or payment.

BURDEN

With reference to a tax, the reduction in real income resulting from the tax (Due, 1957, p. 6).

CAFETERIA PLAN

Allows employees to choose from a menu of different healthcare coverage and provider options.

CAPACITY

A measure of the output that can be reached when existing resources are fully and efficiently used; output corresponds to the firm's minimum short-run average total cost.

CAPITAL

Human, physical, and financial means of production, usually long-term assets that are primarily fixed and not bought and sold in the course of operations.

CAPITALIST ECONOMY

When capital is predominately owned privately rather than by the state.

CAPITATION

A payment system in which the entity financially responsible for the patients' healthcare services receives a fixed periodic sum for each patient (per capita) that covers the costs of utilization by the patient. The sum can be adjusted for specific patient characteristics, such as age and gender.

CARTEL

Organization of producers who agree to act as a single seller in order to maximize joint profits.

CASE MANAGEMENT

A collection of organized activities to identify high-cost patients as early as possible, locate and assess alternative treatment methods, and manage healthcare benefits for these patients in a cost-effective manner (Scheffler R. M., Sullivan, S. D., Ko. T. H., 1991). Sometimes used interchangeably with care management and disease management.

CASE MIX

Grouping of patients according to characteristics (age, gender, diagnoses, treatments, severity of illness, etc.) and then determining the proportion of total falling into each group.

CASE-MIX GROUPS (CMGs)

A Canadian system for classifying hospital inpatients into groups using similar quantities of resources according to selected patient characteristics such as diagnosis, procedure, age, and comorbidity. CMGs are maintained by the Canadian Institute for Health Information.

CASE-MIX INDEX

An index or measure of the average level of resource requirements for a group of cases sorted and weighted according to type of case. The weights represent the estimated resource use for each type of case.

CENSUS

Number of patients in a hospital at a given point in time.

CHANGE AGENT

Individual whose efforts facilitate change in an organization.

CHANGE IN DEMAND

Increase or decrease in the quantity demanded at each possible price of the good or service represented by a shift in the entire demand curve.

CHANGE IN QUANTITY DEMANDED

Increase or decrease in the specific quantity bought at a specified price, represented by a movement along a given demand curve.

CHANGE IN QUANTITY SUPPLIED

Increase or decrease in the specific quantity sold at a specified price, represented by a movement along a given supply curve.

CHANGE IN SUPPLY

Increase or decrease in the quantity supplied at each possible price of the goods or services, represented by a shift in the entire supply curve.

CHARGES

A price set for a product by the supplier. Charges may not equal cash received, because some payers may receive a discount or fail to pay.

CHARITY CARE

Healthcare services provided free of charge to those who do not have the ability to pay for care.

CHERRY PICKING (ALSO CALLED CREAM SKIMMING)

Practice by insurers of selling policies only to low-risk individuals.

CHRONIC

Illness that lasts a long time and usually without prospect of immediate change for either improvement or deterioration.

CHURNING

Practice of discharging a patient from the hospital and readmitting the patient for what is really a single episode of care in order to increase payment.

COGNITIVE SERVICES

Activities of a health professional other than the performance of a procedure.

COINSURANCE

A system of provider payment in which the patient is responsible for a portion/percentage of the payment, and the insurer or third party is responsible for the rest.

COLLUSION

Overt or covert, explicit or tacit, agreement among suppliers to act jointly in their common interests.

COMMUNITY CARE

Care provided in a noninstitutional setting, including in the home or in the patient's "neighborhood."

COMMUNITY RATING

A method of setting insurance premiums for healthcare coverage. In this method, all insureds in the group pay the same premium, regardless of their risk-related characteristics, such as age or health problems.

COMORBIDITY

A disease or condition that is present at the same time as the principal disease or condition of the patient.

COMPARATIVE ADVANTAGE

Ability of one supplier to produce goods or services at a lower cost than other suppliers.

COMPETITION

A state of competition exists in a market if no single firm or consumer is large enough to influence the market price. This state usually occurs if there are many buyers and sellers in the market.

COMPETITIVE PRICE

The price at which demand and supply are in equilibrium in a competitive market.

COMPLEMENTS

Two goods or services that are consumed together, such as surgeons' services and operating room services. The economic relevance of complementarity is that a change in the direct price of a complement will cause a shift in the demand curve of the other service.

COMPLEX ADAPTIVE SYSTEM

Collection of individual components possessing the freedom to act in ways that are not always predictable and whose actions are interconnected.

COMPLICATIONS

Adverse patient conditions that arise during the process of medical care.

CONCENTRATION (MARKET)

The extent to which market activity is confined to a limited number of firms.

CONCIERGE PHYSICIAN PRACTICE (ALSO CALLED BOUTIQUE MEDICINE)

Arrangement between healthcare provider and a patient in which the patient pays a retainer fee to the provider and, in return, is provided a special class of care and services.

CONCURRENT REVIEW

A process of ongoing review while the patient is undergoing treatment in the hospital and of certifying the length of stay that is appropriate for the approved admission (Scheffler, Sullivan, & Ko, 1991).

CONSPIRACY OF SILENCE

Alleged tacit agreement among health professionals not to testify against one another in malpractice lawsuits.

CONSUMER-DRIVEN HEALTH PLAN

Option designed to influence consumer behavior, typically offering a cost-sharing health plan in conjunction with discretionary healthcare dollars (high-deductible health plan combined with a health savings account).

CONSUMERISM

A view that health care should be directly driven by the interests of consumers.

CONSUMER'S SURPLUS

The difference between what an individual is willing to pay for a given quantity of goods or services and what is actually paid. This is equal to the area under the demand curve between no consumption and that specified quantity minus the amount paid for all the units (price times quantity).

CONSUMPTION

The use of goods or services to satisfy current wants.

CONTINGENT VALUATION

The valuation that a person would place on a service if he/she had the option of having it available.

CONTINUUM OF CARE

The entire spectrum of specialized health, rehabilitative, and residential services available to the frail and chronically ill. The services focus on the social, residential, rehabilitative, and supportive needs of individuals, as well as needs that are essentially medical in nature (U.S. Department of Health and Human Services, 1994).

CONVERSION FACTOR

Dollar amount for one base unit in the relative value scale or the diagnosis-related group.

COPAYMENTS

Out-of-pocket payments for health services made by users at the time a service is rendered.

CORE SERVICES

In Canada, health services that must be available to every resident of a province (Saskatchewan Health, 1993). See also **insured services**. Also, the set of services that must be provided by U.S. hospitals if they are to be eligible for registration with the American Hospital Association.

COST

The expense incurred in producing goods and services. See **opportunity cost** and **money cost**.

COST CURVE

The relationship between cost and volume of output. It can be specified in terms of total costs, average or unit costs, and marginal costs. See **long-run cost curve** and **short-run cost curve**.

COST EFFECTIVENESS

The relationship between the additional cost and the additional health outcome (expressed in physical terms) of one intervention compared with another.

COST FUNCTION

A behavioral relationship between cost (viewed from either a marginal, average, or total perspective) and the variables that influence cost, including volume of output, quality of output, input prices, and variables affecting organizational efficiency. See **cost curve**, **long-run cost curve**, and **short-run cost curve**.

COST SHARING

The joint payment or sharing of a price by the consumer and the payer (insurer).

COST SHIFTING

The charging of different prices for differentially insured patients, usually including the subsidization of care for another group of patients for which the costs are not covered and for nonpaying patients.

COST UTILITY

The relationship between the additional cost and the additional health outcome (expressed in terms of a utility index) of one intervention compared with another.

CRITICAL ACCESS HOSPITAL (CAH) PROGRAM

Medicare's Rural Hospital Flexibility Program, designed to assist rural communities preserve access to primary care and emergency services by paying rural hospitals on a cost-plus basis and having different operating requirements for these hospitals, providing the hospitals meet certain conditions.

CRITICAL CARE

See **intensive care**.

CURRENT PROCEDURAL TERMINOLOGY (CPT)

A classification of procedures and services, primarily for physicians, widely used for coding in billing and payment for physician services.

CUSTOMARY, PREVAILING, REASONABLE CHARGE (CPR)

The charge that is the lowest of the following: actual charge made for the service, the provider's customary (usual) charge for the service, or the fee prevailing in the community for the service.

DAY PROCEDURE GROUPS (DPGs)

A classification system for ambulatory patients in which patients are assigned to classes according to principle procedures that use similar resources. The DPG system was developed from New York's PAS system and is used by the Canadian Institute for Health Information.

DEDUCTIBLE

A fixed amount that a consumer must spend out of pocket before insurance coverage begins. For example, if the deductible is $200, the individual must pay for the first $200 of medical expenditures out of pocket before the insurance company begins to pay its share of the remaining costs.

DEFENSIVE MEDICINE

Provision of services, mainly diagnostic services, in anticipation of defending against a possible lawsuit alleging malpractice.

DEFINED BENEFIT

Type of health insurance in which specific benefits are promised to the purchaser (employee).

DEFINED CONTRIBUTION

Type of health insurance in which the purchaser (employee) of the insurance is provided a specific amount for the insurance premium.

DEMAND

Consumer willingness to purchase alternative quantities of services at various specified prices, represented by the position of the demand curve.

DEMAND CURVE (SCHEDULE)

A schedule indicating the quantities of a service that an individual or group is willing to purchase at different prices of that service, all other factors (income, tastes, other prices) held constant.

DERIVED DEMAND

A good or service that is desired or wanted, not for its own sake, but for its contribution to another good or service. For example, the demand for a physician visit is derived from our demand for better health, not for the direct utility of a physician visit.

DIAGNOSIS

A determination of the specific physical ailment of an individual.

DIAGNOSIS-RELATED GROUPS (DRGs)

A system of classifying hospital inpatients into groups using similar quantities of resources according to selected characteristics, such as diagnoses, procedure, age, and any complications or comorbidities. DRGs were used for hospital reimbursement in the U.S. Medicare system (Fetter, 1992) (see MS-DRGs for current classification system.).

DIMINISHING MARGINAL RATE OF SUBSTITUTION

The marginal rate of substitution changes systematically as the amount of two goods or services being consumed vary.

DIRECT COST

(1) In social cost accounting, the cost of all resources incurred by providers of health care; usually refers to paid resources. (2) In hospital cost accounting, the cost of resources (doctors, nurses, lab techs) that are directly involved in the provision of care; overhead costs are excluded.

DIRECT PRICE

See **out-of-pocket price.**

DIRECT TEACHING COSTS

As regards hospital care, the costs in a teaching hospital that can be directly traced to educational rather than patient care functions. These include resident and intern salaries.

DISCHARGE

The formal release of patient from a hospital or physician's care.

DISCHARGE PLANNING

The process of assessing needs and making sure arrangements are made outside the hospital to receive the patient upon discharge and ensuring appropriate continuity of care is provided.

DISCOUNT (TIME DISCOUNT)

A constant applied to future costs and benefits in order to value them as equivalent to costs and benefits occurring in the present period.

DISEASE PREVENTION

See **prevention.**

DISEQUILIBRIUM

A state in which a market is not in equilibrium (demand and supply are not equal). As a result of a shift in demand or supply, a market will be in disequilibrium until the price and quantity adjust to the new equilibrium levels. A state of disequilibrium can be permanent if there is some barrier (e.g., government price control) that permanently maintains the price at a level above or below that of equilibrium.

DISRUPTIVE INNOVATION

New technology or processes that upset current conditions, but in such a way that progress, in terms of better results or lower costs, is the final result.

DISTRIBUTIVE JUSTICE

Principles of ethics used to allocate resources that are limited in supply; many different approaches are available, such as egalitarianism, desert-based principle, libertarianism, difference principle, resource-based principle, welfare-based principle.

DOCTOR-PATIENT RELATIONSHIP

Legal term for relationship between a patient and a healthcare provider that gives rise to legal obligations.

DOUGHNUT HOLE

Gap in Medicare Part D prescription drug coverage.

DRG

See **diagnosis-related groups**.

DRG COST WEIGHT

Weight assigned to each DRG to reflect the DRG's use of resources relative to the cost of the average Medicare patient. The average Medicare patient's cost, when multiplied by the DRG cost weight, gives the price for the DRG.

DRG CREEP

Change in the distribution of patients among DRGs without a real change in the distribution of patients treated in the hospital.

DUAL ELIGIBLE

Individual qualified for both Medicare and Medicaid coverage.

ECONOMIC COST

See **opportunity cost**.

ECONOMIC EFFICIENCY

Least costly method of producing an output.

ECONOMIC RENT

Surplus of total earnings over amount required to prevent a factor from transferring to another use.

ECONOMIC SYSTEM

Way in which goods and services are produced, distributed, and consumed.

ECONOMIES OF SCALE

Reductions in operating costs associated with larger-scale operations.

ECONOMIES OF SCOPE

Reductions in the operating costs of two or more related services (e.g., home care and hospital care) associated with joint production (e.g., production of both services by the same organization).

EFFECTIVENESS

The relationship between an intervention and its health outcome, usually measured in physical units (e.g., life years saved). Some definitions specify that effectiveness is a measure of the ability of an intervention to bring about an outcome under actual practice conditions.

EFFICACY

The relationship between an intervention and its health outcome under ideal (usually experimental) clinical conditions.

EFFICIENCY

Relationship between amount of output and the amount of effort. (1) Technical efficiency is a measure of how close a given combination of resources is to producing a maximum amount of output. (2) Allocative or economic efficiency is a measure of how close a given combination of resources is to yielding maximum consumer satisfaction.

ELASTICITY OF DEMAND

The quantity of a service demanded in response to the out-of-pocket price of a service or product. Elasticity is calculated by dividing the percentage change in the product demanded by the percentage change in the direct price. The price and quantity in terms of which change is measured can be the original price and quantity (point elasticity) or an average of the original and the new prices and quantities (arc elasticity).

ELASTICITY OF SUPPLY

Measure of the responsiveness of quantity of goods or services supplied to a change in the market price, and is calculated by dividing percentage change in quantity supplied by the percentage change in market price.

EMERGENCY CARE

Involves immediate decision making and action to prevent death or any further disability for patients in a health crisis.

ENCOUNTER

A single visit to a provider (sometimes used as an output measure).

ENDOGENOUS VARIABLE

Variable that is explained within a theory (e.g., price is the endogenous variable in the theory of demand and theory of supply).

ENROLLEE

Person covered (receives benefits) under a contract for care.

ENTRY BARRIER

Natural or created impediment to entry into an industry.

EPISODE OF CARE

A series of temporally contiguous healthcare services related to treatment of a given spell of illness, or provided in response to a specific request by the patient or other relevant entity (Hornbrook, Hurtado, & Johnson, 1985, p. 171).

EPISODE OF ILLNESS

A single unbroken interval of time during which the patient suffers from a continuous spell of signs and/or symptoms that are perceived as sickness or ill-health (Hornbrook, Hurtado, & Johnson, 1985, p. 170).

EQUILIBRIUM

A situation in which all forces are in balance so there is no tendency to change. (1) *Consumer equilibrium* occurs where the individual consuming unit has acquired a composition of goods that gives the unit its maximum attainable satisfaction (utility) given the constraints (prices, incomes) it faces. (2) *Producer or provider equilibrium* occurs when the firm is producing the level of output that achieves its objectives (e.g., maximum profits, maximum output). (3) *Market or competitive equilibrium* occurs when all buyers and sellers simultaneously achieve their maximized positions; demand and supply are therefore in balance at these determined levels of price and quantity.

EQUITY

Fairness (e.g., in the provision of health care). See **horizontal equity** and **vertical equity**.

EVIDENCE-BASED MEDICINE

Using current best information in making decisions regarding care of individual patients.

EXOGENOUS VARIABLE

Variable that influences endogenous variables in a theory but is itself determined by factors outside the theory.

EXPERIENCE RATING

A method of setting health premiums for healthcare coverage. In this method, each insured in the group pays a premium that is based on his or her risk-related characteristics.

EXPLICIT

Specifically stated conditions.

EXTRA BILLING

Billing for an insured health service rendered to an insured person by a medical practitioner in an amount in addition to any amount paid for that service by the provincial or territorial health insurance plan (Canada Health Act, 1984).

EXTERNALITIES

Effects, good or bad, that occur to parties not directly involved in the production or consumption of goods or services.

FACTORS OF PRODUCTION

See **resources**.

FEE

Charge for a service provided.

FEE-FOR-SERVICE PAYMENT

Payment for each item or service provided.

FEE SCHEDULE

List of prices for specific procedures and services. The schedule may be negotiated between provider and payer or set externally.

FINAL GOODS

Goods that are not used as inputs by other firms.

FIRM

A self-contained organization that engages in the production or provision of a service or product. The production can occur in more than one facility. See **plant**.

FIXED COSTS

Costs that remain the same despite changes in the volume of output.

FIXED INPUTS

Inputs that, within a selected range, do not vary with output. Examples include office space and equipment.

FLAT-OF-THE-CURVE MEDICINE

Medical care that has no impact on health status. The allusion is to the curve relating medical care inputs to health status output. Eventually, if medical care is provided in large enough quantities, its additional effectiveness is hypothesized to be zero (i.e., the output will be constant and the curve will be flat).

FLEXIBLE SPENDING ACCOUNT (FSA)

Account managed by employer allowing employees to set aside pretax funds for medical, dental, legal, and daycare services.

FORMULARY

List of pharmaceutical products covered by a health plan.

FRAUD

Obtaining goods or services or payment by intentional false statements.

FREEDOM OF CHOICE

Policy permitting individuals to select their own physician or hospital.

FULL COST

The cost that a provider incurs in producing services. The total cost covers *all* inputs, direct and indirect, used in the production of the services.

FUNDING

A payment made to a provider to cover expenses for services rendered. The funding is not necessarily related to the costs incurred for specific patients or services.

GAG RULE

Practice employed by health plans to forbid physicians to tell patients about alternative, more expensive forms of treatment that are not covered or authorized by the plan.

GAMING

Manipulating the system in an illegal or unethical way.

GAPS

Services not covered by insurance.

GATEKEEPER

Person responsible for determining services to be provided to a person and coordinating the provision of appropriate care.

GLOBAL BUDGET

A fixed annual operating grant paid to a provider that is to cover all services (regardless of location) provided to all patients who are treated; it encompasses all sources of payment.

GLOBAL FEE

Single fee charged for certain medical services, such as pregnancy and delivery, instead of a fee charged for each service or procedure.

GROSS DOMESTIC PRODUCT (GDP)

The money amount of all final goods and services (consumer, investment, and government) produced within defined geographical boundaries during a defined period of time. A standard measure of relative health expenditures for a given state, province, or country is total health spending divided by GDP.

GROSS NATIONAL PRODUCT (GNP)

The money amount of all final goods and services produced by residents of a country during a defined period of time, regardless of where the actual production took place.

GROUP MODEL HMO

A health maintenance organization in which the HMO contracts with an independent group practice to provide care for its members. The contractual arrangements are usually on a per capita basis.

GROUP PRACTICE

A medical practice in which several practitioners share some inputs, such as office staff and space.

HEALTH

(1) A complete state of physical, mental, and social well-being, and not merely the absence of disease or illness (Preamble to the Constitution of the World Health Organization, 1948). (2) A state characterized by anatomic integrity; ability to perform personally valued family, work, and community roles; ability to deal with physical, biologic, and social stress; a feeling of well-being; and freedom from the risk of untimely disease (Stokes, Noren, & Shindell, 1982).

HEALTH CARE

A range of services and products whose end purpose is the preservation or enhancement of health.

HEALTH ECONOMICS

Branch of economics dealing with the provision, delivery, and use of healthcare goods and services.

HEALTH INSURANCE

The payment for the expected costs of a group resulting from medical utilization based on the expected expenses incurred by the group. The payment can be based on community or experience rating.

HEALTH INSURANCE PORTABILITY AND ACCOUNTABILITY ACT OF 1996 (HIPAA)

Federal legislation whose primary function is to provide continuity of healthcare coverage; it also imposed protection of patient privacy.

HEALTH INSURANCE PURCHASING COOPERATIVE (HIPC)

An insurance organization that acts as a broker between payers of health insurance (households, businesses, governments) and healthcare providers. The HIPC sets standards for healthcare services and seeks competitive bids for these services; consumers can then select from among the competing providers.

HEALTH MAINTENANCE ORGANIZATION (HMO)

An organization in which a provider or management group takes on the responsibility for providing health services to a specific group of enrollees in exchange for a set annual fee for each enrollee. The HMO can be the provider or it can contract for services with outside providers.

HEALTH PLAN

An organization that acts as an insurer for an enrolled group of members (Prospective Payment Assessment Commission, 1993).

HEALTH PROMOTION

Education and/or other supportive services that will assist individuals or groups to adopt healthy behaviors and/or reduce health risks, increase self-care skills, improve management of common minor ailments, use healthcare services effectively, and/or improve understanding of medical procedures and therapeutic regimens (American Hospital Association, 1991).

HEALTH-RELATED QUALITY OF LIFE (HRQOL)

A measure of health status that can incorporate physical, emotional, social, and role functioning; pain; and many other factors. It is usually based on the responses of patients to questions in professionally devised instruments.

HEALTH SAVINGS ACCOUNT (HSA)

Replaced the medical savings account and is available to anyone who has a qualified high-deductible health plan and is not covered by other health insurance. Contributions up to a defined amount are tax deductible, and cash in the account is available to pay for qualified health expenditures.

HEALTH STATUS

State of health of an individual or population.

HEALTH TECHNOLOGY

All procedures, devices, equipment, and drugs used in the maintenance, restoration, and promotion of health.

HEALTH TECHNOLOGY ASSESSMENT

A comprehensive form of policy research that looks at the technical, clinical, economic, and social consequences of the introduction and use of health technology.

HERFINDAHL INDEX (ALSO CALLED HERFINDAHL-HIRSCHMAN INDEX, OR HHI)

A measure of market concentration, computed as the sum of the square of firms' market shares.

HIGH-DEDUCTIBLE HEALTH PLAN

Health insurance with a very high deductible for which the insured individual is responsible.

HOME CARE

Care provided in the home for a wide variety of purposes, including health maintenance, preventive care, and substitution for acute care (Hollander and Pallan, 1995). See also **home support.**

HOME SUPPORT

Home- and community-based long-term care services provided by persons other than such professionals as nurses or rehabilitation therapists (Hollander and Pallan, 1995).

HORIZONTAL EQUITY

Fairness in the treatment of individuals who are at the same level with regard to some scale (e.g., people who are equally wealthy or have the same degree of health).

HORIZONTAL INTEGRATION

The combining under one management or ownership of two or more previously independent producers of the same type of service.

HOSPICE

A combination of services for terminally ill patients and their caregivers that is based on a humanistic philosophy of care.

HUMAN CAPITAL

Capitalized value of productive investments in individuals.

HUMAN CAPITAL APPROACH

A method of valuing outcomes that is based on lost productivity.

IMPLICIT

A part of, but not specifically stated.

INAPPROPRIATE CARE

See **appropriateness of care**.

INCENTIVE

Reward for desired behavior.

INCIDENCE

Number of new events occurring in a defined period of time.

INCOME EFFECT

Effect of a change in real income on quantity demanded.

INCOME ELASTICITY OF DEMAND

Measure of the responsiveness (sensitivity) of quantity demanded to a change in income, calculated by percentage change in quantity demanded divided by percentage change in income.

INCREASING RETURNS

When output increases more in proportion to input as the scale of a firm's production increases.

INCREMENTAL COST

The additional cost resulting from a change in output by one or more than one unit.

INDEMNITY

A type of insurance contract in which the insurer pays for care received up to a fixed amount per episode of illness.

INDEPENDENT PRACTICE ASSOCIATION (IPA)

A type of HMO that contracts with independent physician practices to provide health care for the enrollees. Payment to providers is usually on a fee-for-service basis.

INDIFFERENCE CURVE

Curve showing all combinations of two goods or services that provide an equal amount of satisfaction and between which the consumer is indifferent.

INDIGENT

An individual who cannot pay for his or her own care.

INDIRECT COST

(1) In social cost accounting, the cost of time lost due to illness (i.e., resources that are not directly paid for). (2) In hospital cost accounting, the cost of resources not directly related to patient care.

INDIRECT TEACHING COSTS

The additional costs that a teaching hospital incurs in the process of training interns and residents. These costs cannot be measured directly because they are inseparably joined with treatment costs.

INELASTIC DEMAND

For a given percentage change in price, there is a smaller percentage change in quantity demanded.

INFERIOR GOOD

Goods or services for which income elasticity is negative; as income increases, quantity demanded of the goods or services decreases.

INFORMED CONSENT

Legal permission to provide a treatment or to release information.

INPATIENT CARE

Care provided to individuals lodged within a healthcare facility.

INPUTS

See **resources**.

INSURANCE

Method of paying for specific types of losses that may occur; a contract between one party, the insurer, and another party, the insured.

INTENSITY OF CARE

The amount of resources and services embodied in a unit of care (e.g., a day of hospitalization, a hospital stay, or a physician visit).

INTENSIVE CARE

Care provided to patients with life-threatening conditions who require intensive treatment and continuous monitoring.

INTERMEDIATE CARE FACILITY (ICF)

A facility providing a lower level of nursing care than a skilled nursing facility. Medicare no longer pays for ICF-level care.

INTERMEDIATE PRODUCT

Outputs that are used as inputs by other producers in another stage of production.

INTERNATIONAL CLASSIFICATION OF DISEASES, INJURIES, AND CAUSES OF DEATH, TENTH REVISION (ICD-10)

A comprehensive disease coding system developed by the World Health Organization.

INTERNATIONAL CLASSIFICATION OF DISEASES, INJURIES, AND CAUSES OF DEATH, TENTH REVISION, CLINICAL MODIFICATION (ICD-10-CM)

A two-part medical information coding system used in abstracting systems and for classifying patients for DRGs. The first part consists of a comprehensive list of diseases with corresponding codes compatible with the World Health Organization list of disease codes. The second part contains procedure codes that are independent of the disease codes. ICD-10-CM was developed in the

United States based on the World Health Organization system, and is the U.S. coding standard. Some Canadian provinces also use ICD-10-CM diagnosis and procedure codes.

INTERVENTION

A task or set of tasks performed by a health professional with the object of influencing health status by interrupting or changing the course of events in progress.

INVENTORY

Stock of raw materials, goods in process, and finished goods held by firms to mitigate effects of short-term fluctuations in production or sales.

INVESTMENT

The employment of physical or human capital to create the conditions for further production.

JOINT VENTURE

Business arrangement to share profits, losses, and control in health care, often between a hospital and physicians.

LAW OF DIMINISHING RETURNS

If increasing quantities of a variable factor are applied to a given quantity of fixed factors, the marginal product and average product of the variable factor will eventually decrease.

LEADING HEALTH INDICATORS

Set of 10 key determinants that influence health and are used to measure the health of the nation. (US Department of Health and Human Services, 2000).

LENGTH OF STAY

Number of days an individual remains in an institution.

LIFE EXPECTANCY

Estimate of how much longer an individual with a given characteristic may be expected to live; a common measure is life expectancy at birth.

LOADING CHARGE

The portion of an insurance premium that is over and above the amount expected to cover payment for insured services.

LONG RUN

A period over which all inputs can be increased, including capital stock and specialized labor.

LONG-RUN COST CURVE

The relation between the cost of production and volume of output or scale of plant for a period during which all inputs, including capital equipment, have sufficient time to vary.

LONG-TERM CARE

Services that address the health, social, and personal care needs of individuals who, for one reason or another, have never developed or have lost the capacity for self-care. These services may be continuous or intermittent, but it is generally presumed that they will be delivered indefinitely.

MALPRACTICE

Loss or injury to a patient resulting from failure of care or skill by a professional, leading to legal liability.

MANAGED CARE

Any system of health service payment or delivery arrangements in which the health plan attempts to control or coordinate the use of health services by its enrolled members in order to contain health expenditures, improve quality, or both. Arrangements often involve a defined delivery system of providers who have some form of contractual arrangements with the plan (Physician Payment Review Commission, 1994).

MANAGED CARE PLAN

Organization providing managed care.

MANAGED COMPETITION

A manner of funneling payments for health services from a collective insurance fund to competing providers (Enthoven, 1993; Reinhardt, 1993).

MANDATE

A legal requirement that certain actions be carried out. For example, the requirement that businesses provide health insurance coverage to their employees.

MANDATORY ASSIGNMENT

Requirement for physicians to accept Medicare payment as payment in full for their services.

MARGINAL COST (MC)

The change in cost resulting from a change in output by one unit. Because fixed costs do not change with output, marginal cost is related only to variable cost.

MARGINAL PRODUCTIVITY

The additional output due to the application of one or more units of an input or resource, holding all other inputs constant. Marginal productivity can be increasing, constant, or diminishing.

MARGINAL RATE OF SUBSTITUTION

In consumption, how much more of one product or service must be provided to compensate for giving up one unit of another product or service, if the level of satisfaction is to remain constant. In production, how much more of one factor of production must be used to compensate for the use of one less unit of another factor of production, if production is to remain constant.

MARGINAL REVENUE (MR)

The additional revenue that a firm obtains from selling one more unit of a service.

MARGINAL VALUE PRODUCT

The money value of additional output that is produced by one extra unit of an input (e.g., labor).

MARKET

A network of buyers and sellers whose interaction determines the price and quantity traded of goods and services.

MARKET CLEARING PRICE

Price at which quantity demanded equals quantity supplied: the equilibrium price.

MARKET STRUCTURE

Those organizational characteristics of a market that determine the relationship of sellers to sellers, buyers to buyers, and sellers to buyers.

MEDICAID

A federally aided, state-administered program that provides medical assistance to certain low-income people.

MEDICAL CARE

A component of health care. A process or activity, guided by medical practitioners, in which certain inputs or factors of production (e.g., physician services, medical instruments, and pharmaceuticals) are combined in varying quantities to yield an output (medical care services) or outcome (health status). The totality of diagnostic efforts and treatment involved in the care of patients.

MEDICAL DEVICES

Apparatus, instrument, or machine used for diagnosis, treatment, or prevention that does not depend upon chemical action on or within the body (distinguished from a drug).

MEDICAL HARM

Physical injury resulting from, or contributed to by, medical care (or the absence of medical care) and requiring additional monitoring, treatment, hospitalization, or results in death (Conway, Federico, Stewart, & Campbell, 2011).

MEDICAL LOSS RATIO (MLR)

Percentage of insurance premium that must be paid out to care for patients.

MEDICALLY NECESSARY

A medical service that a health professional has determined to be medically required, or indicated, for the diagnosis or treatment of a patient in a particular instance, and not mainly for the convenience of patient or provider.

MEDICARE

(1) In the United States, a nationwide, federally administered program that covers hospital, physician care, some related services, and prescription drugs for eligible persons age 65 and older, persons receiving Social Security disability insurance payments, and persons with end-stage renal disease or Lou Gehrig's disease. (2) In Canada, the health insurance system that is jointly financed by the federal and provincial governments and administered by the provincial governments.

MEDICARE ADVANTAGE (FORMERLY MEDICARE + CHOICE)

A program of benefits for Medicare beneficiaries that provides choice among different types of health plans, including capitation coverage.

MEDICATION ERROR

A failure in the process of drug administration that violates one of the following: right medication, right dosage, right patient, right time, or right route of administration.

MEDIGAP

A class of insurance policies designed to cover gaps in coverage left by Medicare, such as deductibles, coinsurance, copayments, and gaps in coverage.

MONEY COST

Expenditures incurred (paid out) for a given volume of output.

MONOPOLISTIC COMPETITION

A state of monopolistic competition exists in a market if there are many sellers, but each is able to achieve a certain degree of customer loyalty and thus, has some influence over price.

MONOPOLY

A state of monopoly exists in a market if there is a single supplier. The supplier will then have control over prices in the market.

MONOPSONY

A single buyer in a market. The monopsonist generally uses market power to achieve a satisfactory price.

MORAL HAZARD

The risk to an insurer that its insureds will increase their consumption of insured services because of the reduction in the out-of-pocket price resulting from the insurance coverage.

MORBIDITY

Illness, injury, or other than normal health. The morbidity rate is the rate of illness or injury in a population.

MORTALITY

Death. The mortality rate is the number of individuals who died divided by those at risk.

MOST RESPONSIBLE DIAGNOSIS

The ICD-10 code identifying the disease or condition considered by the physician to be most responsible for the patient's stay in the institution. In a case in which multiple diseases or conditions may be classified as most responsible, it is the one responsible for the greatest length of stay (Juurlink, Preyra, Croxford, Chong, Austin, Tu, & Laupacis, 2006). This is the Canadian coding convention. For the U.S. convention, see **principal diagnosis**.

MULTIPRODUCT FIRM

A firm that produces a variety of products with different specifications (e.g., types of medical services).

NATURAL MONOPOLY

Industry characterized by sufficiently large economies of scale to supply the entire market demand.

NEED

A quantity of services that an expert (doctor, planner, etc.) judges that a patient or group of patients should have in order to achieve a desired level of health status (Boulding, 1966).

NETWORK

An entity providing comprehensive, integrated health services to a defined population of individuals. Historically, a network was associated with a health maintenance organization composed of several different medical groups under contract to provide care to enrollees; currently, it refers to a broader set of arrangements than just HMOs.

NONCOMPLIANCE

Failure or refusal of a patient to take medications as instructed or follow through on recommended or prescribed therapy.

NORMAL GOOD

Good for which income elasticity is positive; the higher the income, the greater the quantity of the goods or services demanded.

NORMAL PROFITS

Opportunity cost of capital and risk-taking needed to keep the owners in the industry.

NOT FOR PROFIT

A not-for-profit organization has as its prime purpose the provision of services to a specified population rather than the earning of profits for shareholders. The term "not-for-profit" organization is being replaced with "tax-exempt organization" to decrease confusion regarding the role of normal profits in the organization and its mislabeling as nonprofit. Every organization must make some profit if it is to survive and grow in the long run.

NURSING HOME

An institution providing supervised, personal care for people who are not ill enough to require hospitalization in an acute care or auxiliary hospital, but who require assistance with the activities of daily living.

OLIGOPOLY

Industry that contains two or more firms, at least one of which produces a significant portion of the industry's total output.

OPEN ACCESS PLAN

The beneficiary or member of a health plan can go directly to a healthcare specialist without going through a gatekeeper.

OPEN ENROLLMENT PERIOD

A limited time period during which individuals are given the opportunity to enroll in a health insurance plan without medical screening and without regard to health status.

OPPORTUNITY COST

The value of the alternative use of resources that was highest valued but not selected. With some exceptions (e.g., when resources are overpaid), this equals the market value of all resources used to produce a given volume of output.

OUTLIER

A patient who has a long length of stay (or a long length of treatment) or generates unusually high costs, compared with other patients with the same diagnosis.

OUT OF AREA

Beyond the geographical service area of a managed care plan, and those providers that are not participating in the plan. Services of these providers are usually covered only for emergency or urgent care.

OUT OF PLAN

Either providers or services that are not part of the enrollee's health plan.

OUT-OF-POCKET PRICE

The price that is directly paid for healthcare services by the consumer and is not subsequently recovered from an insurer or government. The out-of-pocket price is the burden that falls directly on the consumer as a result of his or her use of medical care.

OUTPATIENT CARE

Hospital-provided care that does not involve an overnight stay.

OUTPUT

The goods and services that result from the process of production; an activity or process during which a patient is treated or "cared for" by healthcare resources with the object of improving the patient's health.

PARETO-OPTIMALITY

Situation in which it is not possible to reallocate production or consumption activities to make someone better off without simultaneously making someone else worse off.

PATIENT

Person who is receiving services from a healthcare provider.

PATIENT CARE

Totality of diagnostic, treatment, and preventive services provided to an individual to meet their physical, mental, social, and spiritual needs.

PATIENT-CENTERED CARE

Care that takes into consideration the patient's preferences, values, lifestyle, family, and friends; care approached from the patient's point of view.

PATIENT-CENTERED MEDICAL HOME

A team-based model of care led by a personal physician who provides continuous and coordinated care throughout a patient's lifetime to maximize health outcomes.

PATIENT DAYS

The number of days that patients are under inpatient hospital or nursing-home care during a year.

PATIENT EMPOWERMENT

Enabling individuals to control their own health and healthcare decisions.

PATIENT PROTECTION AND AFFORDABLE CARE ACT

On March 23, 2010, President Obama signed the Patient Protection and Affordable Care Act. The law puts in place comprehensive health insurance reforms that will roll out over four years and beyond, with most changes taking place by 2014. Challenges have been lodged against the bill, including hearings by the Supreme Court, which has upheld the constitutionality of the law.

PATIENT SAFETY

Protection of patients from injury and illness during the provision of healthcare services.

PAY FOR PERFORMANCE (P4P)

Model of payment for healthcare services designed to provide incentives to providers to improve quality and reduce costs, either through payment of bonuses for meeting a target or through withholding payments for failure to meet a target.

PEER REVIEW

Review of performance by individuals from the same discipline and with essentially equal qualifications (peers).

PER CAPITA PAYMENT

A fixed annual payment per person made to a provider or health maintenance organization. The totality of payments is intended to cover the cost of care for all enrollees during the year.

PER DIEM PAYMENT

A flat-rate payment to a hospital or other institution for each day the patient is an inpatient in the institution.

PERFECT COMPETITION

Market structure in which all firms are price takers and in which there is freedom of entry into and exit from the industry.

PERSPECTIVE

The viewpoint (of the person or group) with respect to which economic assessment is taken.

PLANT

A single facility engaged in production. See **firm**.

POINT ELASTICITY

Measure of the responsiveness of quantity to price at a particular point on the demand curve.

POINT OF DIMINISHING AVERAGE PRODUCTIVITY

Level of output at which average product reaches a maximum.

POINT OF DIMINISHING MARGINAL PRODUCTIVITY

Level of output at which marginal product reaches a maximum.

POINT-OF-SERVICE PLAN (POS)

A health maintenance organization plan that allows members to use providers not on the organization's panel at the time (and each time) service is needed. To gain access to such providers, the members must pay an added premium or additional out-of-pocket payment.

POPULATION

Group of individuals occupying a specified area at the same time.

PORTABILITY

Ability of a beneficiary to move from one employer to another without loss of benefits or having to go through a waiting period for coverage.

POTENTIAL YEARS OF LIFE LOST (PYLL)

Sum of years that a group of individuals would have lived had they not died prematurely.

PREADMISSION CERTIFICATION

The prospective review and evaluation of proposed elective hospital admissions using acceptable medical criteria as the standard for determining the appropriateness of the site or level of care and certifying the length of stay required (Scheffler, Sullivan, & Ko, 1991).

PREDATORY PRICING

Practice by insurers of giving low premiums to a low-risk small group or individual and then raising premiums when the insured file claims; also called churning the books.

PREEXISTING CONDITION

Physical or mental condition discovered before an individual applies for health insurance, often leading to insurance company denying coverage for the individual or condition, or requiring a waiting period before the condition is covered.

PREFERRED PROVIDER ORGANIZATION (PPO)

An arrangement in which a group of health providers agrees to provide services to a defined group of patients at an agreed-upon rate for each service (Ermann, de Lissovoy, Gabel, & Rice, 1986).

PREMIUM

The payment made to an insurance company in return for insurance coverage.

PREPAID GROUP PRACTICE (PGP)

A group practice that charges patients on an annual per capita basis and bears the risk for providing the insured services.

PRESENT ON ADMISSION (POA)

A diagnosis, condition, disease, or cause of injury that an individual had at time of admission to the hospital.

PREVALENCE

Number of events or cases present in a given population at a given time.

PREVENTION

Any intervention that reduces the likelihood that a disease or disorder will affect an individual or that interrupts or slows the progress of the disorder. *Primary prevention* reduces the likelihood that a particular disease or disorder will develop in a person. *Secondary prevention* interrupts or minimizes the progress of a disease or irreversible damage from a disease by early detection and treatment. *Tertiary prevention* slows the progress of the disease and reduces the resultant disability through treatment of established diseases (Spitzer, 1990).

PREVENTIVE MEDICINE

That aspect of the physician's practice in which he applies, to individual patients, the knowledge and techniques from medical, social, and behavioral science to promote and maintain health and well-being and prevent disease or its progression (Hilleboe, 1971; Last, 1988).

PRICE

An amount of money paid or received per unit of a service or commodity.

PRICE CEILING

A government-imposed maximum permitted price at which a good or service may be sold.

PRICE DISCRIMINATION

The charging of different prices for the same product to different customers, made possible by the inability of consumers to resell the product to each other. The charging of different prices is usually due to the existence of different demand conditions for different groups of customers.

PRICE FIXING

Two or more competitors agree on prices.

PRICE FLOOR

A government-imposed minimum permitted price at which goods or services may be sold.

PRICE TAKER

A supplier that has no influence over the price of the goods or services it sells; the supplier can alter its rate of production and sales without significantly impacting the market price of its product.

PRIMARY CARE

A type of medical care that emphasizes first-contact care and assumes ongoing responsibility for the patient in health maintenance and therapy for illness. Primary care is comprehensive in scope and includes overall coordination of treatment of the patient's health problems.

PRINCIPAL

The person in whose interests an agent is contracted to act.

PRINCIPAL DIAGNOSIS

The diagnosis that, after investigation, is found to have been responsible for the patient's admission to the hospital. This is the U.S. coding convention.

For example, if a patient is admitted to the hospital for a minor TURP (trans ure-theral resection of the prostate) procedure, and it is discovered he has carcinoma of the lung, the prostate diagnosis would be the one coded under this convention. For the Canadian convention, see **most responsible diagnosis.**

PRINCIPLE OF SUBSTITUTION

Method of production will change if the relative prices of inputs change, with rel-atively more of the less expensive input and relatively less of the more expensive input being used.

PROCEDURE

An operative or nonoperative intervention or course of action designed to improve the health of an individual.

PRODUCER SURPLUS

The difference between the total amount that producers receive for all units sold and the total variable cost of producing the goods or services.

PRODUCT DIFFERENTIATION

Existence of similar, but not identical, products sold by a single industry.

PRODUCTION

The act of combining resources to yield output.

PRODUCTION FUNCTION

A quantitative relationship expressing how outputs vary when the quantity of inputs changes. Also called **production relation.**

PRODUCTION POSSIBILITY BOUNDARY

Curve that shows alternative combinations of goods and services that can be attained if all available resources are used; the boundary between attainable and unattainable output combinations.

PRODUCTIVITY

The ratio of physical inputs to physical outputs. The inputs can be one single input (e.g., labor), with others held constant, or all inputs combined.

PRODUCTIVITY EFFICIENCY

Production of any output at the lowest attainable cost for that level of output.

PRODUCTS OF AMBULATORY CARE (PACs)

An ambulatory care classification system developed in New York State primarily for the funding of nonsurgical, nonemergency ambulatory care visits, based on body parts and purpose of visit (Tenan, Fillmore, Caress, Kelly, Nelson, Grazono, & Johnson, 1988).

PRODUCTS OF AMBULATORY SURGERY (PASs)

An ambulatory surgery classification system developed in New York State for funding ambulatory surgery procedures, based on similar resource-using procedures (Kelly, Fillmore, Tenan, & Miller, 1990).

PROFIT

Total revenue minus total cost. Accounting profit is defined as total revenue for a period's sales minus costs matched to those sales. Economic profit is total revenue minus economic costs.

PROGRESSIVE TAX

Tax that takes a higher percentage of income the higher the level of income.

PROSPECTIVE PAYMENT

Payment to providers based on predetermined rates unrelated to current or past costs of the individual provider.

PROVIDER

A supplier of healthcare services.

PUBLIC HEALTH

The combination of science, practical skills, and beliefs that is directed to the maintenance and improvement of the health of all the population. It is one of the efforts organized by society to protect, promote, and restore the people's health through collective or social actions (Last, 1988).

QUALITY-ADJUSTED LIFE YEAR (QALY)

A numerical assessment of the proportion of an individual's state of full health experienced over a year. QALY values generally range from 0 (assigned to death) to 1 (full health), although certain states of health can be valued at less than 0. QALY values can be directly derived from individuals' utility measurements or can be based on existing values of health states.

QUALITY OF CARE

The degree to which the process of medical care increases the probability of outcomes desired by patients and reduces the probability of undesired outcomes, given the state of medical knowledge (U.S. Congress, Office of Technology Assessment 1988).

QUALITY OF LIFE (QOL)

The degree to which an individual enjoys everything. It has been defined, by a philosopher, as the possession and enjoyment of all the real goods in the right order and proportion. Nonphilosophers, see **health-related quality of life (HRQOL)** or **health status** for terms only slightly less stratospheric.

QUANTITY DEMANDED

The quantity of goods or services that an individual or group is willing to buy at one specific rate during a specified time; a change in quantity demanded refers to a movement along a given demand curve in response to a change in price.

QUANTITY EXCHANGED

The identical amount of goods or services that individuals actually purchase and producers actually sell in some time period.

QUANTITY SUPPLIED

The amount of goods or services a supplier or market is willing to supply at any one price during a specified time; a change in quantity supplied refers to a movement along a given supply curve in response to a change in price.

RATE

The price per unit charged by an institution for its services.

RATE OF RETURN

The ratio of net profits earned by a firm to total invested capital.

RATE REVIEW

Review by a regulatory agency of a budget and financial picture in order to determine the reasonableness of the proposed rate change.

RATE SETTING

The setting of institutional prices by a paying or regulatory agency.

RATIONING

Process of making choices regarding who will receive scarce resources.

REAL INCOME

Income expressed in terms of the purchasing power of money income; the quantity of goods and services that can be purchased with money income.

REFERRAL

Sending of a patient by one physician (the referring physician) to another physician (or some other service), either for consultation or for care.

REFINED DIAGNOSIS-RELATED GROUPS (RDRGs)

Also called **refined group numbers (RGNs)**. A classification system in which resource-use patterns and secondary diagnoses are used to refine the assignment of patients to severity classes (RDRGs).

REGRESSION ANALYSIS

Quantitative measure of the systematic relationship among two or more variables.

REGRESSIVE TAX

Tax that takes a lower percentage of income the higher the level of income.

REGULATION

(1) A law or rule imposing government or government-mandated standards and significant economic responsibilities on individuals or organizations outside the government establishment. (2) The process carried out by government or mandated agencies through such means as setting or approving prices, rates, fares, profits, interest rates, and wages; awarding licenses, certificates, and permits; devising safety rules; setting quality levels; enacting public disclosure of financial information regulations; and enacting prohibitions against price, racial, religious, or sexual discrimination (Khemani & Shapiro, 1993).

REIMBURSEMENT

The payment made by an insurer to a provider for specific services provided to an insured patient. Reimbursement is usually associated with payments based on a service-by-service, or patient-by-patient basis.

RELATIVE PRICE

Ratio of the money price of one product or service to the money price of another product or service; a ratio of two absolute prices.

RELATIVE VALUE

A value placed on a specific unit of service (e.g., a follow-up office visit, a blood test, or an inpatient cholecystectomy) expressed in relation to some standard (e.g., a minute of lab test time or physician care).

RESOURCE ALLOCATION

Distribution of an economy's (or firm's, industry's) scarce resources of land, labor, and capital among alternative uses.

RESOURCE-BASED RELATIVE VALUE SCALE (RBRVS)

A resource-weighted service-classification system that aims at setting resource weights according to the total relative cost of each service, including "psychological" costs of the provider, time costs, and training costs.

RESOURCE INTENSIVE WEIGHTS (RIW)

Canadian relative weightings for inpatient groups. RIWs combine Canadian length-of-stay and U.S. cost-per-day data to form hybrid cost-per-case weights. Separate weights are calculated for "typical" and "atypical" cases.

RESOURCES

The means used in producing services, which can include physical capital (beds and equipment) and human capital (physicians, nurses, etc.). Also called *inputs* and *factors of production*.

RESOURCE UTILIZATION GROUPS (RUGs)

Clusters of nursing home residents, defined by residents' characteristics, that explain resource use (Fries, Schneider, Foley, Gavazzi, Burke, & Cornelius, 1994, p. 668).

RETROSPECTIVE PAYMENT

Payment to a provider for services provided based on actual costs incurred by the provider. Since the payment is based on costs incurred, the amount to be paid must be determined after the service has been provided (i.e., retrospectively).

RETROSPECTIVE REVIEW

A review of claims after the episode of care is concluded and the claim is submitted to the insurer (Scheffler, Sullivan, & Ko, 1991).

RETURNS TO SCALE

The relationship between total output and scale of operations, which are measured as proportional increases in all resources. Because all resources are allowed to increase in proportion, this is a long-run relationship.

REVENUE

Income earned from the provision of services. Gross revenues equal income earned overall, while net revenues equal income earned minus costs or expenses.

RISK

Uncertainty as to loss; in the case of health care, the loss can be due to the cost of medical treatment or other losses arising from illness. Risk can be objective (relative variations between the difference between actual and probable losses) and subjective (psychological uncertainty relating to the occurrence of an event) (Howarth, 1988). See also **risk averse, risk neutral,** and **risk taker.**

RISK AVERSE

A person is said to be risk averse if losses of a given amount create more disutility than the utility that comes from gains of the same amount (and so losses will tend to be avoided).

RISK FACTOR

Behavior or condition that, based on evidence or theory, is thought to directly influence the level of a specific health problem.

RISK NEUTRAL

A person is said to be risk neutral if he or she values losses and gains of the same amount equally.

RISK POOLING

The sharing of the costs incurred by members of a population. The payment method can vary but will not be based on the risk of individuals.

RISK TAKER

A person is said to be a risk taker if, for that person, the utility of gains is greater than the disutility of losses of equal value. A risk taker is therefore predisposed to gamble.

SAFE HARBOR

Assurance that a certain specified behavior or action will not result in civil or criminal penalties when done in a specified way.

SAFE HARBOR REGULATION

Describes certain acts or behaviors that will not be illegal under a specific law, even though they might otherwise be illegal.

SAFETY NET PROVIDER

Provider obligated to provide health care to patients whether or not they are able to pay for the services.

SCARCE GOOD

Good or service for which the quantity demanded is greater than the quantity supplied.

SECONDARY CARE

Specialist-referred care for conditions of a relatively low level of complication and risk. Secondary care can be provided in an office or hospital and can be diagnostic or therapeutic.

SECOND SURGICAL OPINION

Patients are sometimes required to get a second or even a third consulting opinion for specified nonemergency surgical procedures (Scheffler, Sullivan, & Ko, 1991).

SELECTIVE CONTRACTING

A procedure whereby an insurer can legally exclude providers from its list of participating providers (Melnick & Zwanzinger, 1988, p. 2669).

SELF-INSURANCE

Assumption of risk by an individual or entity by setting aside own resources instead of purchasing an insurance policy.

SENSITIVITY ANALYSIS

Determining the extent to which the conclusions or results of a model depend on the model's assumptions.

SEVERITY OF ILLNESS

Gravity of a patient's illness.

SEVERITY SCORE

Mathematical score that expresses the severity of illness of a patient according to a predefined method.

SHORTAGE

An excess of supply over demand at a given price.

SHORT RUN

A period in which all of the inputs cannot be adjusted (increased or reduced). Those inputs that cannot be adjusted are called "fixed" and include capital stock. *Short run* also refers to lengths of time insufficient for new firms to enter a market or industry.

SHORT-RUN COST CURVE

The relation between cost and volume of production of a plant during a short adjustment period in which only some inputs are variable (and the rest are fixed).

SIDE EFFECT

Effect of a drug or treatment that is other than the intended, desired effect.

SIGN-OUT CASE

A patient who leaves the hospital against medical advice.

SINGLE-PAYER SYSTEM

A reimbursement system in which there is a single payer or one dominant payer.

SINGLE-PRODUCT FIRM

A production unit that produces a single, homogeneous product.

SIN TAX

Tax on goods, services, or activities that are allegedly harmful, such as taxes on alcohol and tobacco products.

SKILLED NURSING FACILITY (SNF)

A facility that provides skilled nursing care to residents who do not need acute hospital care but who do need inpatient professional nursing care and other social and health needs.

SOCIAL BENEFIT

Contribution that an activity makes to society's welfare.

SOCIAL COST

The cost to all members of society of any activity or service. It can be the sum of private and external costs or of direct and indirect costs. It is also viewed as the value of the best alternative use of the resources available to society as valued by society.

SOLO PRACTICE

A single physician medical practice.

SPECIALIZATION OF LABOR

Organization of production in which individual workers specialize in the production of particular goods or services (and satisfy their wants and needs by trading) rather than producing everything they consume.

STAFF MODEL HMO

A health maintenance organization whose practitioner staff are employees of the health plan. Usually the practitioners are paid on a salary rather than fee-for-service basis.

STANDARDIZED MORTALITY RATE (SMR)

A single mortality rate for a large group of individuals who are in different age and gender categories. The total rate for the entire group is made up of the rates in different age and gender subgroups, which are weighted or averaged according to a given structure of a standard population (e.g., the population of an entire country or the population in a base year).

STOP-LOSS INSURANCE

Insurance purchased to pay a health plan or a group of providers for costs of care for individual patients or a panel of patients over a ceiling amount; designed to protect against catastrophic claims.

SUBSTITUTES

Goods or services that compete with each other, such as aspirin and Tylenol. The direct price of one of the substitutes will cause a shift in the demand curve for the other.

SUBSTITUTION EFFECT

The shift from one product to another as a result of a price change, after compensating for any increase or reduction in real income that accrues from the price change.

SUPPLIER-INDUCED DEMAND

The amount of shift in the demand for services resulting from the suppliers' influence on consumers' tastes (intensity of desire for the services).

SUPPLY

A supply curve. The quantity supplied at each price.

SUPPLY CURVE

(1) For a single firm, the quantity the firm is willing to supply of a service at alternative prices of the commodity. (2) For the market, the relationship between the quantity that all firms are willing to supply and alternative prices of the service.

SUPPLY FUNCTION

(1) For a single provider, a quantitative relationship between the quantity the supplier is willing to supply and a series of variables that influence the supplier's behavior, such as price, technology, case mix, quality, and input prices. (2) For a market, the quantitative relationship between the quantity that all suppliers in the market are willing to supply and a series of variables that influence all of the suppliers' behavior, including price, technology, case mix, quality, input prices, and the number of suppliers in the market.

SURPLUS

(1) For a tax-exempt firm, total revenue minus total expense (the counterpart of profit for a investor-owned firm). (2) For a market, the excess of quantity supplied over quantity demanded at a given price.

TASTES

Consumer preferences for goods and services expressed in terms of an index of satisfaction or utility. Taste is a catchall concept for everything other than prices and incomes that affect demand, including health status, age, gender, level of education, and so on.

TECHNOLOGY

See **health technology.**

TECHNOLOGY ASSESSMENT

See **health technology assessment.**

TERTIARY CARE

Highly specialized care administered to patients who have complicated conditions or require high-risk pharmaceutical treatments or surgery. Tertiary care is provided in a setting that houses high-technology services, specialists and subspecialists, and intensive care and other highly specialized services.

THIRD-PARTY PAYMENT

Payment by a private insurer or government to a medical provider for care given to a patient.

TIME COST

The value of time required to conduct an activity. This variable has two components: value per unit of time and time actually spent in the activity. Value per unit of time is taken as equivalent to lost earnings or the value placed on forgone leisure activities.

TOTAL COSTS (TC)

The sum of fixed and variable costs. All of the costs required to produce a specified level of output.

TOTAL FIXED COSTS (TFC)

All of the fixed costs required to produce a specified level of output.

TOTAL PRODUCT

The total amount of output produced.

TOTAL VARIABLE COSTS (TVC)

All of the variable costs required to produce a specified level of output.

TRANSACTION COSTS

The costs of reaching an agreement and coordinating activity among participants in a market. These include the costs of searching for potential buyers or sellers and for product quality and cost; negotiating an agreement; monitoring that the agreement conditions are met; and enforcing the terms of the agreement.

TRANSFER CASE

A hospital inpatient who is admitted from or discharged to another institution.

TRANSFER PAYMENT

A payment made to an individual or institution that does not arise out of current productive activity.

TRIM POINT

A point, calculated using a statistical formula, applied to all lengths of stays (or cost per case) within a single DRG (or CMG) in order to separate outlier cases from the rest.

TYPICAL PATIENT

A patient who receives a full, successful course of treatment in a single institution and is discharged when he or she no longer requires acute-care services.

UNIT COSTS

Costs per unit of output, equal to total costs divided by total output.

UTILITY

(1) An index comparing various levels of an individual's satisfaction with alternative quantities of specified goods, services, or situations under certainty. The index that allows the quantification of differences between the levels is called *cardinal utility* (Pigou, 1932). (2) A ranking of alternative bundles of goods and services under certainty, on the basis of better, equal, or worse, with no indication as to *degrees* of satisfaction (ordinal utility). (3) A ranking of alternative risky situations on the basis of an individual's own preferences regarding probabilities (von Neumann-Morgenstern utility) (Torrance, Feeny, Furlong, Barr, Zhang, & Wang, 1996).

UTILIZATION

The actual use of services by consumers (the services must be demanded and supplied).

UTILIZATION MANAGEMENT

A set of techniques used by or on behalf of purchasers of healthcare benefits to manage healthcare costs by influencing patient care decision making through case-by-case assessments of the appropriateness of care prior to provision (Institute of Medicine, 1989).

UTILIZATION REVIEW (UR)

Examination and evaluation of the efficiency and appropriateness of any health-care service that has already been provided.

VALUE-ADDED

Reflects the position that an activity performed on a given product or service has increased its value.

VALUE-ADDED TAX (VAT)

Tax imposed on goods and services at each stage of production.

VALUE-BASED PURCHASING

Obtaining the highest quality health care at the most reasonable price; links payment for care to the quality of care and rewards cost-effective practices.

VALUE-DRIVEN HEALTH CARE

Healthcare system in which price and quality are made visible (transparent) so purchasers of care can make choices based on value.

VALUE JUDGMENT

A pronouncement that states or implies that something is desirable (or undesirable) and is not derived from any technical or objective data but instead from considerations of ultimate value, that is, ethical considerations (Nath, 1969).

VARIABLE COSTS

Costs that change in response to changes in output. Variable costs can be expressed as total, average, or marginal.

VARIABLE INPUTS

Inputs that can vary in quantity during a specified time period.

VERTICAL EQUITY

Fairness in the treatment of individuals who are at different levels with regard to some scale (e.g., people who fall into different income classes).

VERTICAL INTEGRATION

The combining under one management of activities at different stages of the production process.

VIRTUAL MERGER

Loosely defined concept in which healthcare organizations agree to cooperate in some areas in which they had previously competed.

VOLUME

The number of cases (or other service units) provided.

WANTS

Consumer tastes or desires.

WEALTH

Sum of all the valuable assets owned minus liabilities.

WILLINGNESS-TO-PAY APPROACH

A method of valuing an outcome that is based on the consumer's own preferences.

WINDFALL PROFITS

Change in profits that arises out of an unanticipated change in market conditions.

X-INEFFICIENCY

Use of resources at a lower level of productivity than is possible, even if they are allocated efficiently, so that the economy is at a point inside its production possibility curve.

BIBLIOGRAPHY

Accountable Care Organizations (ACO). Retrieved on June 3, 2012, from https://www.cms.gov/Medicare/Medicare-Fee-for-Service-Payment/ACO/index.html?redirect=/ACO/.

American Hospital Association (1991). *AHA Guide*. Chicago IL: Author.

Boulding, K. E. (1966). The concept of need for health services. *Milbank Memorial Fund Quarterly, 44(4)*, 202–223.

Canada Health Act, R.S.C. 1984, C-6 (1984). Published by the Minister of Justice.

Conway, J., Federico, F., Stewart, K., & Campbell, M. (2011). *Respectful Management of Serious Clinical Adverse Events (2nd edition). IHI Innovation Series white paper*. Cambridge MA: Institute for Healthcare Improvement.

Due, J. F. (1957). *Government Finance: Economics of the Public Sector*. Homewood IL: Richard D. Irwin, Inc.

Enthoven, A. C. (1993). Achieving effective cost control in comprehensive health care reform. The Jackson Hole "managed care managed competition" approach. *Health Pac Bulletin, 23(1)*, 13–15.

_____ (1993). The history and principles of managed competition. *Health Affairs, 12 Suppl*, 24–28.

Ermann, D., deLissovoy, G., Gabel, J., & Rice, T. (1986). Preferred provider organizations: issues for employers. *Health Care Management Review, 11(4)*, 26–36.

Fetter, R.B. (1992). Hospital payment based on diagnosis-related groups. *Journal of the Society for Health Systems*, 3(4), 4–15.

Fries, B. E., Schneider, D. P., Foley, W. J., Gavazzi, M., Burke, R., & Cornelius, E. (1994). Refining a case-mix measure for nursing homes: resource utilization groups (RUG-III). *Medical Care, 32(7)*, 668–685.

Hilleboe, H. E. (1971). Modern concepts of prevention in community health. *American Journal of Public Health, 61(5)*, 1000–1006.

Hollander, M. J. and Pallan, P. (1995). The British Columbia Continuing Care system: service delivery and resource planning. *Aging-Clinical & Experimental Research, 7(2),* 94–109.

Hornbrook, M. C., Hurtado, A. V., & Johnson, R. E. (1985). Health care episodes: definition, measurement and use. *Medical Care Review, 42(2),* 163–218.

Howarth, C. I. (1988). The relationship between objective risk, subjective risk and behaviour. *Ergonomics, 31(4),* 527–535.

Institute of Medicine (1989). *Controlling Costs and Changing Patient Care? The Role of Utilization Management.* Washington DC: National Academy Press.

Juurlink, D., Preyra, C., Croxford, R., Chong, A., Austin, P., Tu, J., Laupacis, A. (2006). *A Canadian Institute for health Information Discharge Abstract Database: A Validation Study.* Toronto: Institute for Clinical Evaluative Sciences.

Kelly, W. P., Fillmore, H., Tenan, P. M., & Miller, H. C. (1990). The classification of resource use in ambulatory surgery: The products of ambulatory surgery. *Journal of Ambulatory Care Management.* 13(1), 55–63.

Khemani, R. S. and Shapiro, D.M. (1993). *Glossary of Industrial Organisation Economics and Competition Law.* Geneva: Directorate for Financial, Fiscal and Enterprise Affairs, OECD.

Last, J. M. (1988). The future of health in Canada. *Canadian Journal of Public Health. Revue Canadienne de Sante Publique, 79(3),* 147–149.

Melnick, G. A. and Zwanziger, J. (1988). Hospital behaviour under competition and cost-containment policies. The California experience, 1980 to 1985. *JAMA, 260(18),* 2669–2675.

Nath, S. K. (1969). *A Reappraisal of Welfare Economics.* London: Routledge and Kegan Paul.

Physician Payment Review Commission (1994). *Annual Report to Congress.* Washington DC: Author. Pigou, A. C. (1932). *The Economics of Welfare.* London: Macmillan and Co.

Preamble to the Constitution of the World Health Organization as adopted by the International Health Conference, New York, 19–22 June, 1946; signed on 22 July 1946 by the representatives of 61 States (Official Records of the World Health Organization, no. 2, p. 100) and entered into force on 7 April 1948.

Prospective Payment Assessment Commission (1993). *Report and Recommendations to the Congress.* Washington DC: Author.

Reinhardt, U. E. (1993). Comment on the Jackson Hole initiatives for a twenty-first century American health care system. *Health Economics, 2(1),* 7–14.

Saskatchewan Statutes (1993). The Occupational Health and Safety Act, 1993. Chapter 0–1.1 of the Statutes of Saskatchewan, Canada.

Scheffler, R. M., Sullivan, S. D., Ko. T. H. (1991). The impact of Blue Cross and Blue Shield Plan utilization management programs, 1980–1988. *Inquiry, 28(3),* 263–275.

Spitzer, P. G. (1990). Building a model for the development of better healthcare systems. *Health Informatics, 7(12),* 42, 44.

Starfield, B., Weiner, J., Mumford, L., & Steinwachs, D. (1991). Ambulatory care groups: A categorization of diagnoses for research and management. *Health Services Research, 26(1),* 53–74.

Stokes, J. III, Noren, J., & Shindell, S. (1982). Definition of terms and concepts applicable to clinical preventive medicine. *Journal of Community Health, 8(1),* 33–41.

Tenan, P. M., Fillmore, H. H., Caress, B., Kelly, W. P., Nelson, H., Grazino, D., & Johnson, S. C. (1988). PACs: Classifying ambulatory care patients and services for clinical and financial management. *Journal of Ambulatory Care Management.* 11(5), 36–53.

Torrance, G. W., Feeny, D. H., Furlong, W. J., Barr, R. D., Zhang, Y. & Wang, Q. (1996). Multiattribute utility function for a comprehensive health status classification system: health utilities index mark 2. *Medical Care, 34(7),* 702–722.

US Congress, Office of Technology Assessment (1988). *The Quality of Medical Care: Information for Consumers,* OTA-I-I-386. Washington DC: US Government Printing Office.

US Department of Health and Human Services (1994). *Public Financing of Long-Term Care: Federal and State Roles.* Washington DC: Office of the Assistant Secretary for Planning and Evaluation.

US Department of Health and Human Services (2000). *Healthy People 2010: Understanding and Improving Health.* 2nd ed. Washington DC: US Government Printing Office.

Answers to Odd-Numbered Questions

CHAPTER 1

1. Quality can be judged from a structure, process, or outcome perspective. Structure measures reflect the characteristics of the care providers, the tools they use, and the resources available, such as the physical or organizational setting. The training of physicians is an example of a structure-related quality issue. Process encompasses both the interpersonal and technical aspects of the process of treating patients; the types of procedures done are a process-related quality issue. Outcomes reflect changes that occur in the patient's functioning or symptoms; the health status of patients after the treatment is an outcome-related quality issue.

3. Morbidity is the amount or rate of illness (the number or proportion of people in a given population who are ill); utilization concerns the services provided to treat the illness experienced by the population. Hospitalization is often used to measure both, although hospitalization is influenced by such factors as availability of care and practice patterns, as well as illness. If only hospitalization is used as the measure of illness within a population, it fails to count the individuals who did not use hospital services for the illness; these individuals may have been treated at home or in another institution and so didn't use hospital services, although they were also ill.

5. A health-related quality-of-life index is a multidimensional composite measure of different components (physical, mental, emotional, and social functioning) of health on the quality of life experienced by an individual. Level values measure the amount or quantity of each component. Social importance weights measure the relative importance (value) persons place on each component.

7. If the study group has relatively many old or ill persons in it, the mortality rate is liable to be high merely because of the underlying poor health status of the group; in which case, it would be wrong to interpret the rate as indicating poor performance on the part of the healthcare providers.

9. Health status is hypothesized to be positively influenced by medical care; however, as more medical care is provided to a given population, eventually additional units of medical care will improve their health at an increasingly lower rate. The "flat of the curve" describes the situation in which additional units of medical care provided do not continue to contribute to improved outcomes for the patient.

CHAPTER 2

1. A premium is a payment to an insurer in return for the insurer's acceptance of the financial risk associated with health care (if and when it is consumed). A deductible is a payment by the consumer for care that has been provided before the insurance company begins to pay its share of the costs of services provided.

3. Medicare primarily serves the elderly (individuals 65 and older), those with permanent disabilities, and those with end-stage renal disease or Lou Gehrig's Disease. Part A covers hospitalization and posthospitalization care (home care and nursing home care for rehabilitative purposes; Medicare does not cover the long-term custodial nursing home care). There is no premium, but there are deductibles and copayments.

5. Medicare Part C (also known as Medicare Advantage) is a health plan choice available to Medicare participants that provides both Part A and Part B coverage. These plans may offer extra coverage for the premiums paid, and most will also include the Part D prescription drug program. These plans can charge additional premiums and can have deductibles and copayments as well.

7. Medicaid covers certain categories of low-income populations, including the aged (for services not covered by Medicare). There are no deductibles, but occasionally there are small copayments. There are no premiums because the low-income persons could not afford them. While low-income is a necessary condition for coverage by Medicaid, it is not a sufficient condition; other categorical conditions must also be met.

9. In a preferred provider organization, consumers can obtain services from providers who are not PPO members, although they must pay a differential price. In a traditional HMO, members must use providers designated by the HMO to receive insurance coverage for the service.

11. An opportunity cost is the value of services that are given up by choosing alternative courses of action. Opportunity cost is a broader concept than paid expenses or money costs and becomes important to consider when you need to determine what you have to give up (the next-best use of resources) to undertake an activity.

13. A cost-of-illness study measures the direct and indirect costs of illness for a population. Using the prevalence approach, costs are related to the health care provided in a certain year to all individuals suffering from that illness, regardless of the time of the onset of the illness.

If death occurs during that year, future costs are attached to that death. Using the incidence approach, costs (including related future costs) are assigned to the reporting or occurrence of the illness during that period of time. Using the incidence approach, only new cases of the illness are considered in the measurement of the cost; using the prevalence approach, all individuals who suffer from the illness during the period are considered, regardless of when the illness started.

CHAPTER 3

1. Demand is the relationship between price and quantity demanded along the entire demand curve, and changes in demand reflect movement of the entire demand curve. Quantity demanded is the amount demanded at a certain price, and a change in quantity demanded is reflected by a movement along a given demand curve.

3. (a) It will shift the demand curve to the right. (b) It will shift the demand curve to the right. (c) It will shift the demand curve to the left. (d) It will shift the demand curve to the right. (e) It will shift the demand curve to the right. Each of these factors will change the position of the demand curve, changing the quantity demanded at each of the prices on the curve.

5. It will shift the demand curve to the right because of an increase in total demand; each individual in the market will base quantity-demanded decisions on the price of the aspirin, but because there are more people, the total demand curve will shift to the right.

7. The elasticity is
$$[(Q_2 - Q_1)/(Q_2 + Q_1)]/[(P_2 - P_1)/(P_2 + P_1)] = [(50 - 60)/(50 + 60)]/$$
$$[(\$0.60 - \$0.50)/(\$0.60 - \$0.50)] = [-10/110]/[0.10/1.10]$$
$$= [-0.0909]/[0.0909] = -1.$$

9. (a) No effect on demand would occur because the consumer's out-of-pocket cost has not changed. (b) There would be a movement along the curve, not a shift, because this is a change in price. (c) The demand curve would shift to the right because the total population in the market has increased. (d) No effect on demand would occur because this is a supply cost change (unless the increased productivity enabled the nursing home to reduce the price charged for care). (e) The demand curve would shift to the left because the total population in the market has increased.

11. The current quantity of visits is 3 million population times 2.4 visits per person, or 7.2 million visits. Q_2 is the unknown quantity, and using the elasticity formula $[(Q_2 - Q_1)/(Q_2 + Q_1)] / [(P_2 - P_1/(P_2 + P_1)]$ (with an elasticity value of -0.2), we can solve for Q_2 as follows:

$$-0.2 = [Q_2 - (3,000,000 \times 2.4)]/[Q_2 + (3,000,000 \times 2.4)]/$$
$$[(\$0.50 - 0)/(\$0.50 + 0)]$$

$$-0.2 = [Q_2 - 7,200,000]/(Q_2 + 7,200,000)/[0.50/0.50] = Q_2$$
$$= 4,800,000$$

CHAPTER 4

1. The reduction in health status will eventually cause an increase in demand for health care.

3. Her travel time costs equal $100 (travel time equals 2.5 hours times 2 times $20 per hour equals $100); 150 miles time $0.50 per mile equals $75 for direct travel expenses. Her waiting costs equal $20 (1 hour times $20). The travel and waiting time cost is $195 ($100 + $75 + $20). Her total costs would be $215, because she also loses one hour for the consultation at $20 per hour.

5. Information asymmetry occurs when one party of the transaction has better information than the other party. This asymmetry of information precludes effective monitoring of the decisions involved in the transaction. The information asymmetry can be either in the form of the one party (the principal) having more information than the other party (the agent) or the other way around. Either way, such asymmetry usually results in less than optimal decisions and transactions occurring in the market.

7. Supplier-induced demand occurs when physicians directly cause a shift in the demand curve by influencing their patients' belief in the efficacy of health care or in the need for recommended services. The problem arises from the fact that physicians act as agents for their patients in addition to being suppliers of health care thus violating the independence assumed in market transactions between the buyer and the seller.

9. The present value of exercise equals $1,900 + ($1,900/1.1) + $2,000/ $(1.1)^2$ = $5,280. The present value of medicine equals $2,000 + $1,900/1.1 + $1,900/(1.1)^2$ = $5,297.

CHAPTER 5

1. The total product for May equals 100 patients treated. The total product for June equals 120 patients treated. The marginal product is the change in total output divided by the change in inputs (nursing hours) equals (120 − 100)/(22 − 20) = 20/2 = 10 patients per nursing hour.

3. (a) A change in nurse remuneration from salary to fee for service will shift the production function curve upward. (b) A change in the case mix of patients, with more having leukemia and fewer having common colds, will shift the production function curve downward. (c) A change in policy to provide more thorough examinations will shift the production function curve downward. (d) Higher nurse wages will have no effect on the production function curve. (e) A requirement that each patient now be told all his or her legal rights before an examination will shift the production function curve downward. (f) An increase in the total number of nurses who are

hired will have no effect on the production function curve. (g) An increase in the clinic's budget will have no effect on the production function curve.

5. The average and marginal costs are as follows:

Total Cost	Marginal Cost	Average Cost	Quantity
$100	$100	$100	1
160	60	80	2
200	40	60	3
260	60	65	4
360	100	72	5

7. The fixed costs per month total $4,200 (office = $2,000; phones = $200; secretary = $2,000). The variable costs are shown in the following table:

	Variables Costs at 1,200 Visits	Variable Costs at 1,300 Visits
Nurses	30 × $4,000 = $120,000	32.5 × $4,000 = $130,000
Supplies	20 × 400 = $8,000	20 × $433 = $8,660
Total Variable Costs	$120,000 + $8,000 = $128,000	$130,000 + $8,660 = $138,660

9. The fixed costs total $200 (difference between total costs and total variable costs).

11. The fixed costs total $17,000 (physician: $50 × 200 hours = $10,000; nurse: $15 × 200 hours = $3,000; secretary: $10 × 200 hours = $2,000; rent: $2,000). The variable costs equal $10,000 (supplies: $10 × 1,000).

13. The costs are shown in the following table:

Patient Visits	Nurse Hours	Nurse Cost	TFC	TVC	Total Cost	AC	MC
1	2	$40.00	$150.00	$41.00	$191.00	$191.00	$ —
2	4	80.00	150.00	82.00	232.00	116.00	41.00
3	8	160.00	150.00	163.00	313.00	104.33	81.00
4	14	280.00	150.00	284.00	434.00	108.50	121.00
5	22	440.00	150.00	445.00	595.00	119.00	161.00
6	32	640.00	150.00	646.00	796.00	132.67	201.00

15. The costs are shown in the following table:

Quantity	TC	TFC	TVC	MC
0	$100.00	$100.00	$ —	$ —
1	120.00	100.00	20.00	20.00
2	150.00	100.00	50.00	30.00
3	200.00	100.00	100.00	50.00
4	300.00	100.00	200.00	100.00

CHAPTER 6

1. Dr. Kalikorn supplies two thousand operations.
3. Marginal revenue is the additional unit price received per day, or $180.
5. (a) Four units. (b) Four units.
7. (a) At $10, the quantity supplied is zero. (b) At $20, the quantity supplied is zero. (c) At $30, the quantity supplied is four.
9. (a) The quantity of visits supplied will decrease with an increase in the wage rates for clinic nursing staff. (b) An increase in fixed overhead costs will have no impact on quantity of visits supplied. (c) An increase in the intensity of illness of patients will increase costs, causing a decrease in quantity supplied. (d) An increase in productivity will reduce costs, causing an increase in quantity supplied. (e) An increase in quality (under conditions stated) will increase costs, resulting in a decrease in quantity supplied.

CHAPTER 7

1. Insurers must incur contract costs. These are the costs of negotiating contracts, monitoring performance, and enforcing the terms of the contracts.
3. A salary basis of payment may encourage a reduction in services because the income received by the physician is not directly linked to the number of services provided, the productivity of the physician. Per-service payment may encourage an increase in services, visits, and patients, because the physicians' income is directly tied to the quantity provided. Per-visit payment may encourage a reduction in services per visit and an increase in visits and patients, because the physician receives a total payment based on number of visits and not on the services provided during the visit; the fewer services provided per visit, the higher the difference between revenue and costs. Per-patient payment may encourage a reduction in services and visits and an increase in patients, because the physician receives the same amount regardless of the number of visits or the amount of service per visit provided.

5. RBRVS is a fee-for-service system based on a detailed analysis of time costs, mental effort and judgment, physical effort, technical skill, and stress associated with each service or procedure. Also included were practice costs and professional liability insurance costs. Implementation of the system led to a reduction in surgical fees relative to fees for nonsurgical services.

7. In prospective reimbursement, payment is based on predetermined rates. Payment can be made on the basis of services, days, and cases.

9. The answers are contained in the following table:

Payment System	Degree of Risk Incurred by Insurer	Degree of Risk Incurred by Hospital
Retrospective payment	High	None
Prospective fee-for service payment	High	Low
Per diem fees	High	Low
Per case payment	Low to Moderate	Moderate to High
Per case payment plus outlier adjustments	Moderate	Moderate

11. Information on the national Medicare conversion rate for urban hospitals would need to be provided to answer the question, because total amount received is the weight times the conversion rate. Taking the fee per weighted case as $3,951 (the national Medicare conversion rate for urban hospitals), the hospital would receive $12,236 per craniotomy ($3,951 × 3.0970).

13. Nursing homes can be funded on a per diem basis, which can be adjusted to reflect the characteristics of the residents in the nursing homes.

15. Members can be recruited on the basis of age, type of employment, gender, and other characteristics that can be used to predict potential utilization rates.

17. (a) They have an incentive to increase membership, especially among populations expected to be low users (healthier populations). (b) They have an incentive to reduce services per member as long as that reduction doesn't result in greater use later if the member remains with the HMO.

CHAPTER 8

1. (a) An increase in the degree of insurance coverage (lower copayments) would allow consumers to purchase more at the original market price because their out-of-pocket price decreases, so price and quantity will increase (the demand curve will shift to right).

(b) An increase in the number of ophthalmologists will result in a decrease in price and an increase in quantity (demand curve shifts to right in response to a change in the supply curve). (c) An increase in the average age of the population will result in greater demand, causing the price to increase and quantity to increase (demand curve shifts to right). (d) A reduction in the price of optometry services (a substitute) will cause price and quantity increases (demand curve of ophthalmologists shifts to left). (e) An increase in price of eyeglasses (a complement) will result in price and quantity decreases (demand curve shifts to left).

3. (a) An increase in the wages of nurses will result in price increases and quantity decreases (supply curve shifts to left). (b) An increase in the number of clinics will result in price decreases and quantity increases (supply curve shifts to right). (c) An increase in clinic productivity will result in price decreases and quantity increases (supply curve shifts to right). (d) A reduction in supply costs for clinics will result in price decreases and quantity increases (supply curve shifts to right).

5. The FPL made $2.8 million in profits with an $8 million investment. Its return on capital (35%) is greater than in other industries. Capital will be attracted to this industry. Supply will increase and price and profits will fall.

7. Quantity demanded will increase to 250. Quantity supplied will fall to 50. There will be a shortage of 200. Quantity utilized will be 50.

9. A total of 300 days are demanded at all rates. At a rate of $450, 200 days are supplied. At a rate of $600, some 300 days are supplied. At a rate of $450, funding is $90,000, and 200 days are utilized. At a rate of $600, funding is $180,000, and total utilization is 300.

CHAPTER 9

1. The answers are contained in the following tables:

Price	Quantity of Visits Demanded
$100	0
90	1
80	2
70	3
60	4
50	5
40	6

Price	Quantity of Visits Demanded	Total Revenue	Marginal Revenue
$100	0	$0	$ —
90	1	90	90
80	2	160	70
70	3	210	50
60	4	240	30
50	5	250	10
40	6	240	−10

At a marginal cost of $35, the monopolist will supply up to the point at which *MC* is above *MR*. This is at a volume of 3 and a price of $70.

3. The statistics for Groups A and B are as follows:

Demand Schedule A				Demand Schedule B			
Price	No. of Visits	Total Revenue	Marginal Revenue	Price	No. of Visits	Total Revenue	Marginal Revenue
$100	1	$100	$100	$100	5	$500	$500
90	2	180	80	90	6	540	40
80	3	240	60	80	7	560	20
70	4	280	40	70	8	560	0
60	5	300	20	60	9	540	−20

The price in each market should be set where *MR* = *MC*. This is $90 for group A and $100 for group B.

5. The marginal cost to the hospital is given in the following table:

Price	Units Supplied	Total Cost	Marginal Cost	Price	Units Demanded (nurse)	Total Cost	Marginal Cost
$10	1	$10	$10	$100	1	$100	$100
20	2	40	30	90	2	180	80
30	3	90	50	80	3	240	60
40	4	160	70	70	4	280	40
50	5	250	90	60	5	300	20
60	6	360	110	50	6	300	0
				40	7	280	−20
				30	8	240	−40

The monopsonist will hire up to four nurses, at which point the marginal value of a nurse equals the marginal cost.

7. The consumers in the market may be influenced by the physicians to purchase more health care (supplier-induced demand). In other words, the physicians could increase the elasticity of the demand curve.

CHAPTER 10

1. (a) With no insurance, the expected utility equals $(0.2 \times 84.4) + (0.8 \times 100) = 96.88$. With insurance, the expected utility is 98.8. The individual should purchase insurance. (b) At a price of $60, expected utility is 95.8, which is the utility of $940, or $1,000 − 60. This is less than a utility of 96.88, which is the expected utility if no insurance were bought. She would not buy insurance. (c) If she got sick, and had no insurance, her wealth level would be $800 and utility would be 57.0. The expected utility with no insurance would be 91.4 ($-0.2 \times 57 + 0.8 \times 100$). This is less than the utility of 95.8, which is the utility if she buys insurance. She would therefore buy insurance. (d) Mrs. Smith is risk averse.

3. The price is $500 \times (1 − 0.3)$, or $350.

5. The elasticity is $(\Delta Q/Q)/(\Delta P/P) = (400/1800)/(−40/100) = −5/9$.

7. (a) For healthy persons, the expected utility with no insurance is $0.2(87) + 0.8(100) = 97.8$. The expected utility with insurance is $U(\$975)$, which is greater than 98.8 (the utility of $970). A healthy person should buy insurance. For unhealthy persons, the expected utility with no insurance is $0.2(76) + 0.8(100) = 95.2$. An unhealthy person should buy insurance. (b) For healthy persons, the utility with no insurance equals $0.2(89) + 0.8(100) = 97.8$. The utility with insurance equals $U(\$980) = 99.4$. A healthy person should buy insurance. For unhealthy persons, the utility with no insurance equals $0.2(76) + 0.8(100) = 95.2$. The utility with insurance equals 0.8 (utility at $950) + 0.2(utility at $980) = 98.4. An unhealthy person should buy insurance. In group A, the total cost is $20 per person. In group B, the total cost is $70 each, the $20 premium plus the $50 out-of-pocket costs not paid by the insurance plan.

9. Administrative costs increase and payouts fall. Indeed, despite the improvement in utilization management, the added administrative costs could be enough to push the total costs higher than they were.

11. Information asymmetry occurs when the insurer and the consumer possess different information about risks. If the insurer had no information that it could use to distinguish risks among persons, it would charge a single premium rate.

CHAPTER 11

1. The relevant data for this exercise are contained in the following table:

Number of Nursing Hours	Number of Clinic Visits	Total Revenue	Marginal Revenue	Total Cost	Marginal Cost
1	12	$120	$120	$50	$50
2	22	220	100	100	50
3	30	300	80	150	50
4	36	360	60	200	50
5	40	400	40	250	50

Midwest will hire additional nurses up to the point at which the wage equals the value of the marginal product. In this case, the quantity hired will be four. If $15 is added to the wage of each worker to pay for health insurance, marginal cost increases to $65, and the number of nurses hired would be three.

3. (a) There is no effect on the curve, but there is a movement down the curve. (b) The demand curve shifts outward. (c) The demand curve shifts outward. (d) There is no effect on the curve. (e) The demand curve shifts outward. (f) The demand curve shifts inward.

5. The supply curve (relating wage rates and labor supplied) will shift downward; if insurance is valued equally with wages, the curve will shift by the amount of the premium paid because this is viewed as an increase in the cost of production.

7. The supply of labor is lower for persons with poor health. At any given wage rate, persons with poor health will offer less labor and their incomes will be lower.

CHAPTER 12

1. He should use the concept of cost-utility, because survival and quality of life are both relevant outcomes. Also, two competing interventions are being compared.

3. She should use the concept of benefit-cost, as the question is whether the intervention should be used.

5. A total of 960 people lived the entire year. The 40 who died lived, on average, half a year, making a total of 20 extra life years. Therefore, the grand total is 980 life years.

7. Efficacy is the difference in outcomes under ideal conditions. Because 60 deaths per 100 would occur without the drug, and 40 deaths per 100 would occur if everyone used the drug, the difference (efficacy) is 20 deaths fewer per 100 persons. Effectiveness equals 60 − [(60/100)

$\times 25 + (40/100) \times 75] = 60 - 45 = 15$; that is, the effectiveness equals 15 deaths fewer per 100 persons.

9. The result for the case in which she doesn't take the medicine is 1/2 year $\times 0.8 = 0.4$ QALYs. The result if she does take the medicine is 7/12 years $\times 0.9 = 0.525$ QALYs. The difference is 0.125 QALYs.

CHAPTER 13

1. In the Paretean system, everyone's preferences count, and in the delegatory system, a person or group chooses for the society.
3. Under the socially optimal level of medical care, no further reallocation of resources can increase the net value of resources (i.e., $MV - MC$).
5. No, because if the MC is positive, persons will eventually receive so much care that the MV of this additional care will be low or zero and below the marginal cost of the care.
7. No, because the private market ensures only that each person obtains health care in relation to his or her own valuations and associated costs. If there are consumption externalities, there may be room for increases in social valuations through the philanthropic transfer of funds.
9. No, because the marginal cost of insurance may exceed gains (marginal value of insurance coverage) when the degree of coverage is already high.
11. With the extra-welfarist approach, judgments about social benefits are delegated to an authority. In health care, the delegated authority makes judgments on the valuations of the health states of the population. In the Paretean system, each person evaluates his or her own use of care.

CHAPTER 14

1. Out-of-pocket expenditures account for 11.6%, government for 52.1%, private insurance for 32.7% of total healthcare expenses, and other private sources for 3.6%.
3. The subsidy will increase the demand for insurance because the price paid by the individual decreases. The amount of insurance purchased will increase because of the lower price to the individual.
5. A payroll tax is a tax on employment income. Payroll taxes lead to a reduction in employment and wages because, under the U.S. system, employers are responsible for paying part of the payroll tax of their employees.
7. The income tax burden increases with income. The sales tax burden falls with income. The payroll tax burden falls with income. The insurance premium burden falls with income.

CHAPTER 15

1. Older persons (65 and older), persons with permanent and total disabilities, persons with renal disease, and persons with amyotrophic lateral sclerosis (ALS, or Lou Gehrig's disease).

3. Part A is funded by dedicated taxes levied by the federal government on salary and wages. Part B is funded by general government revenues and by premiums paid by beneficiaries voluntarily enrolled in the program. Part C is not separately funded, but is funded the same way as Parts A, B, and D. Part D receives funding from general revenues, premiums from beneficiaries, and state payments for dual eligibles.

5. Hospital care, physician services, long-term care, and pharmaceuticals.

7. Medigap is private insurance that can be purchased to cover gaps in coverage due to Medicare premiums, deductibles, and copayments. The coverage serves to limit the financial responsibilities of additional costs not covered by Medicare.

9. A substantial number of the uninsured are young and healthy, but also many who were in fair or poor health. About 7.3 million children were uninsured in 2010, and 28 million uninsured people were employed.

11. The stated goals are affordability, equity of payment, adequacy of care, feasibility of policies, and acceptance by concerned groups (providers, intermediaries, and consumers).

13. Medicaid faces the challenge of ensuring that there is adequate coverage (i.e., that persons who are eligible actually enroll) and acceptance by providers. Ensuring coverage can be achieved by extending the program's scope, and gaining acceptance can be achieved by setting adequate reimbursement rates.

CHAPTER 16

1. If insurers cannot determine consumer risk, then they will set prices at the group average. Low-risk persons may drop out of the market because the marginal benefits are less than the marginal costs to them, leaving higher risk persons enrolled in insurance plans. Rates will spiral upward and the market may disappear, even though persons would be willing to buy insurance, and there are potential suppliers who would provide it at rates acceptable to the consumers (if the risks could be adequately determined).

3. The risk for small groups is higher than for large ones, because there is a large variance in outcomes in small groups, which imposes a higher degree of risk on suppliers of insurance. In addition, the administrative costs of enrolling and managing the plans are higher for small groups than for large groups in which enrollment can be handled through the employer.

5. If there was community rating and the premiums exceeded the risk experience of some (more healthy) consumers, these consumers would not buy insurance, even though they could have it at a rate that would cover their medical risks. In the second case, a person may simply choose not to insure and be willing to retain the risks.

7. Salary provides a weak incentive to increase the volume of services, because the physician receives the same income regardless of volume of services provided. Fee-for-service provides a strong incentive to increase the volume of services, because the income of the provider increases with the increase in volume of services. Capitation provides a weak

incentive to decrease services per person because additional services add cost (but not income) and a strong incentive to enroll more members, because income is tied to number of members, not number of additional services provided.

9. Non–managed care insurers might lower their premiums, increase the monitoring of providers, or try to attract less costly consumers.

CHAPTER 17

1. The physician acts as an agent for two principals: the insurer and the patient.

3. If physicians can organize at a lower cost, they will tend to control the legislative process.

5. Patent rights allow drug companies sufficient time to recover their investment in the development of drugs (the development of a single drug can take many years and millions of dollars in investment).

7. It is called a combination in restraint of trade, and it is prohibited by Section 1 of the Sherman Act.

9. If the networks keep other physicians from practicing in a region (e.g., by denying them the right to admit patients to hospitals), then they would be illegal. However, if the networks result in greater efficiencies and enable physicians to lower costs, then this would be a justification for them to continue.

CHAPTER 18

1. A major contributor to the growth in expenditures has been the development and widespread diffusion of new medical technologies and services; another contributor is the growing size and age of the population, increasing the use of hospital services. The Patient Protection and Accountable Care Act may impact rising costs by reducing the fragmentation of health care and reducing the number of uninsured individuals, enabling them to get more timely and appropriate care.

3. Pay for performance provides incentives to providers to improve the quality of care delivered and to move from its current structure toward different organizational and individual behaviors that will result in better quality and improved outcomes. Bundled payment is viewed as a blend between fee-for-service and capitation payments and so will discourage the provision of unnecessary care and encourage the coordination of care across providers. Value-based purchasing, or shared-savings programs, have incentives similar to bundled payments and are designed to improve care coordination and redesign the processes of care to produce high quality and efficient care delivery.

5. The industry is facing tremendous pressure to cut costs, improve quality, and prepare for fundamental change in how health care is provided, financed, and consumed. As an attempt to prepare for these changes, economies of scale and economies of scope are seen as important elements, enabling better control over coordination of care and providers.

Index